Neuroplasticity: Clinical Frontiers and Functions

Neuroplasticity: Clinical Frontiers and Functions

Edited by Christopher Mosley

hayle medical

New York

Hayle Medical,
750 Third Avenue, 9th Floor,
New York, NY 10017, USA

Visit us on the World Wide Web at:
www.haylemedical.com

ISBN: 978-1-63241-857-9

Cataloging-in-Publication Data

Neuroplasticity : clinical frontiers and functions / edited by Christopher Mosley.
    p. cm.
Includes bibliographical references and index.
ISBN 978-1-63241-857-9
1. Neuroplasticity. 2. Developmental neurobiology. 3. Neurophysiology.
4. Adaptation (Physiology). I. Mosley, Christopher.
QP363.3 .N48 2020
612.8--dc21

Table of Contents

Preface

The ability of the brain to reorganize itself by forming new neural connections throughout a person's life is known as neuroplasticity. This mechanism allows neurons to compensate for disease and injury, and adjust their activities to changes in their environment. The fundamental processes underlying neuroplasticity is that individual synaptic connections are continually removed and recreated depending upon the activity of the neurons. An important consequence of neuroplasticity and one with clinical implications is that the brain activity related to a given function can be transferred to a different location. This can be the basis of the treatment of acquired brain injury and rehabilitation of brain injury. Various rehabilitation techniques such as functional electrical stimulation, virtual reality therapy, constraint-induced movement therapy and treadmill training with body-weight support work due to cortical reorganization. Much research is being undertaken to use neuroplasticity for binocular vision improvement, stereopsis recovery, learning disabilities management, sensory function development, etc. This book provides comprehensive insights into the clinical frontiers and functions of neuroplasticity. It will also provide interesting topics for research, which interested readers can take up. With state-of-the-art inputs by acclaimed experts of this field, this book targets students and professionals.

After months of intensive research and writing, this book is the end result of all who devoted their time and efforts in the initiation and progress of this book. It will surely be a source of reference in enhancing the required knowledge of the new developments in the area. During the course of developing this book, certain measures such as accuracy, authenticity and research focused analytical studies were given preference in order to produce a comprehensive book in the area of study.

This book would not have been possible without the efforts of the authors and the publisher. I extend my sincere thanks to them. Secondly, I express my gratitude to my family and well-wishers. And most importantly, I thank my students for constantly expressing their willingness and curiosity in enhancing their knowledge in the field, which encourages me to take up further research projects for the advancement of the area.

Editor

Persistent Stress-Induced Neuroplastic Changes in the Locus Coeruleus/Norepinephrine System

Olga Borodovitsyna, Neal Joshi, and Daniel Chandler (iD)

Department of Cell Biology and Neuroscience, Rowan University School of Osteopathic Medicine, Stratford, NJ 08084, USA

Correspondence should be addressed to Daniel Chandler; chandlerd@rowan.edu

Academic Editor: Jason H. Huang

Neural plasticity plays a critical role in mediating short- and long-term brain responses to environmental stimuli. A major effector of plasticity throughout many regions of the brain is stress. Activation of the locus coeruleus (LC) is a critical step in mediating the neuroendocrine and behavioral limbs of the stress response. During stressor exposure, activation of the hypothalamic-pituitary-adrenal axis promotes release of corticotropin-releasing factor in LC, where its signaling promotes a number of physiological and cellular changes. While the acute effects of stress on LC physiology have been described, its long-term effects are less clear. This review will describe how stress changes LC neuronal physiology, function, and morphology from a genetic, cellular, and neuronal circuitry/transmission perspective. Specifically, we describe morphological changes of LC neurons in response to stressful stimuli and signal transduction pathways underlying them. Also, we will review changes in excitatory glutamatergic synaptic transmission in LC neurons and possible stress-induced modifications of AMPA receptors. This review will also address stress-related behavioral adaptations and specific noradrenergic receptors responsible for them. Finally, we summarize the results of several human studies which suggest a link between stress, altered LC function, and pathogenesis of posttraumatic stress disorder.

1. Introduction

Stressful stimuli and events engage a number of brain circuits that ultimately activate the hypothalamic-pituitary-adrenal (HPA) axis. During periods of stress, the paraventricular nucleus of the hypothalamus (PVN) releases the stress peptide corticotropin-releasing factor (CRF), which stimulates both direct central and indirect peripheral effects, activating signal transduction pathways that enhance catabolism of energy stores and mobilize physiological and psychological resources of the organism to permit an appropriate behavioral response to the stressor. These pathways become dysregulated following chronic or traumatic stress, which leads to destabilization of homeostasis and impaired immune, cardiovascular, and gastrointestinal functions, and promoting central nervous system (CNS) changes associated with depressive and anxiety-like behaviors that contribute to the diagnosis of stress-associated disorders [1–10]. The ability to mobilize CNS function to respond to stressful stimuli

and ensure survival is explained in part by changes in neuroplastic adaptations. Several CNS structures have been demonstrated to undergo neuroplastic changes following stress [2, 11–24] which may contribute to stress-associated anxiety and mood disorders [12, 14, 19, 25, 26]. Chronically altered noradrenergic transmission is a characteristic of many neuropsychiatric and neurodegenerative disorders [12, 27–34], and therefore, short- and long-term stress-induced adaptations in norepinephrine- (NE-) containing cell bodies may contribute to these conditions. For the purposes of this review, we consider short-term effects to refer to the immediate and primary action CRF signaling during stressor exposure and the stress response on electrophysiological properties such as membrane depolarization and action potential generation that result from the opening of channels already inserted in the membrane. Long-term effects on the other hand include persistent changes that continue long after the stress response and CRF signaling have ceased and resulted from intracellular signaling cascades that promote receptor and channel trafficking, altered gene expression, and neurite outgrowth.

A major node in the stress response that promotes noradrenergic signaling in the CNS is the brain stem nucleus locus coeruleus (LC). The LC and other smaller noradrenergic brainstem nuclei, such as A1/C2 region in the solitary tract, are activated by CRF and reciprocally communicate with the HPA axis. Activation of A1/C2 promotes a positive feedback loop in stress circuitry by releasing NE in the PVN which stimulates CRF production and release by engaging α_1-adrenoreceptors (α_1AR) [35, 36]. The LC is the primary source of NE to the forebrain [37–45], where its actions affect sleep/wake cycles, sensory signal discrimination and detection, and cognition [2, 37, 46, 47]. It is innervated by a number of stress-responsive CRF-containing brain regions which when released, acts on CRF receptor 1 (CRFR1) receptor to produce acute changes in LC physiology and responsiveness to synaptically released transmitters [48–51]. Additionally, activation of CRFR1 stimulates Gs proteins and cAMP production [48, 52], which promotes numerous genetic and cellular effects [28, 50, 53–57]. These observations suggest that LC neurons may undergo many long-lasting stress-induced adaptations (Figure 1). These changes include receptor trafficking [58–60], altered expression of genes necessary for transmitter synthesis and release [28, 54–56, 61], protein kinases that activate transcription factors [57] and growth factors [18], electrophysiological properties [53, 62], and morphological changes [50, 53, 63], all of which would directly impact LC function at both immediate and chronic time point poststress.

While most investigations have focused on the transient effects of stress and CRF on LC function [48, 49, 51, 64–66], some have examined their lasting impact [28, 50, 52–54, 56, 57, 62]. This review will summarize how stress and CRF signaling persistently modify morphological and physiological features of the locus coeruleus/norepinephrine (LC/NE) system and its associated behaviors from a genetic, cellular, and neuronal circuitry/transmission perspective. While the stress-induced plastic changes that occur in LC and other brain regions during disease pathogenesis are not entirely clear, identifying how stress can chronically alter the function of this broadly projecting brainstem nucleus across multiple levels of regulation represents an important step forward in clarifying the mechanisms of conditions characterized by hyperactive noradrenergic transmission.

2. LC/NE Synaptic Plasticity Changes during Stress

2.1. Adaptive Functional and Anatomical Changes of LC after Stress. HPA axis activation is pivotal for mediating the central stress response. Through the release of peripheral and central neurohormones, it mobilizes various body tissues and brain areas to orchestrate an appropriate physiological and behavioral response. Importantly, during stressor exposure, CRF is released onto the LC by the PVN and other CRF-containing stress-responsive structures, such as the bed nucleus of the stria terminalis, Barrington's nucleus, and the central nucleus of the amygdala [67–73] which

increase its tonic discharge [51, 62, 65, 66]. LC activity correlates highly with an animal's behavioral state: during quiet rest, LC discharges slowly in a highly regular fashion. During periods of focused attention, a phasic mode of operation dominates such that LC responds to salient stimuli with high-frequency bursts of action potentials that facilitate orientation and sustained attention towards behaviorally relevant stimuli [74]. During stress, CRF causes increased tonic discharge which compromises the ability of LC to respond to salient sensory stimuli with phasic bursts. This leads to impairments in sensory signal discrimination, several aspects of cognition, and a generally anxious state [2, 37, 74–77]. While this might seem generally maladaptive, a consequence of short-term stress-induced LC activation is to promote behaviors that increase the likelihood of survival in a threatening situation [2, 66]. By increasing LC discharge [51, 62, 65, 66] and therefore forebrain NE release [78–82], prefrontal cortical operations are inhibited [3, 78], promoting a behavioral phenotype characterized by broad scanning attention and vigilance [2, 66, 81, 83], which facilitates escape from a threatening situation.

The role of LC in stress has been the subject of study since 1970, when karyometric studies of sleep-resistant rabbits demonstrated an increase in nuclear size during stress [84]. Subsequently, an extensive body of literature has shown that LC is critical for mediating stress-induced behavioral and neuroendocrine responses. The electrophysiological effects of stress and CRF on LC have been well characterized in a number of *in vivo* and ex vivo studies [48, 49, 51, 53, 62, 65, 85]. *In vivo*, CRF increases tonic/spontaneous LC discharge [65, 86, 87] through a cyclic AMP (cAMP)/protein kinase A-dependent mechanism that depolarizes the membrane by decreasing potassium conductance [48]. Additionally, CRF has been demonstrated to decrease sensory-evoked phasic responses by LC [65, 86]. This effect could partially be explained by recent findings from our laboratory that show that a high concentration of bath-applied CRF [49] and preexposure to acute stress [62] both diminish excitatory glutamatergic synaptic transmission in LC. We found that these electrophysiological effects persist for at least a week poststress in adolescent rats. Moreover, electrophysiological changes which were absent immediately after stressor exposure develop over seven days, including increased intrinsic excitability and a hyperpolarized threshold for action potential generation [62]. These findings suggest that LC cells in adolescent rat brain undergo long-lasting changes following even short-term acute stressor exposure and lead to chronically increased forebrain NE concentration and behavioral changes.

2.2. CRF and Morphological Changes. CRF orchestrates a series of neuroplastic changes in LC neurons and LC-derived cell cultures [50, 52, 53, 58, 63]. Specifically, CRF triggers morphological changes in immortalized catecholaminergic neurons, such as the formation of long neurites with prominent growth cones [52]. Similarly, another study demonstrated the ability of CRF to promote neuronal outgrowth in organotypic slice cultures of rat LC [50]. In this study, it was found that 12 hours of CRF exposure increased

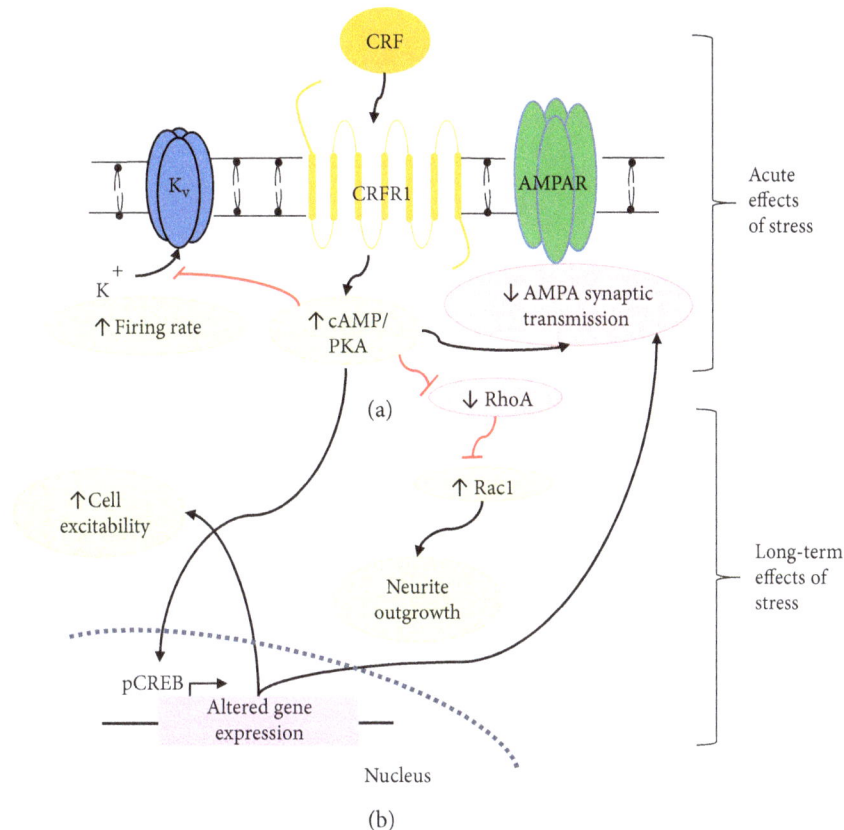

FIGURE 1: Model of signal transduction pathways induced by stress in LC neurons. (a) Pathways which mediate short-term effects of stressor exposure. CRF interacts with CRFR1, which through Gs-coupled receptor mechanisms increases intracellular cAMP levels, reducing potassium conductance resulting in cell depolarization. Through unknown mechanisms, CRF decreases glutamatergic synaptic transmission through AMPARs. (b) Pathways which mediate long-term effects of stressor. Initial CRF activation of Gs-coupled CRFR1 increases PKA activity, which phosphorylates CREB to initiate expression of stress-induced genes. These could potentially include genes regulating AMPAR and voltage-gated ion channel expression. Inactivation of RhoA by PKA phosphorylation disinhibits Rac1 to increase neurite outgrowth via actin remodeling and microtubule stabilization.

the number of primary processes and branching pattern of neurites. Mechanisms of dendritic growth regulation by CRF have been proposed to occur through Rac and RhoA GTPases (Figure 1), which regulate intracellular actin dynamics and spine length [88]. Elsewhere in the brain, inhibition of Rac1 has been shown to promote strong effects on dendritic spines from apical and basal dendrites on pyramidal neurons with relative absence of branching effects [89].

Additional unpublished observations from our laboratory also suggest that in animals subjected to acute intense stressor exposure, LC cells might undergo morphological changes. We have previously shown that fifteen minutes of combined physical restraint and exposure to predator odor induces a number of long-lasting changes in LC function that are accompanied by chronically increased anxiety-like behavior [62]. During whole-cell patch clamp electrophysiological recordings, some neurons were filled with biocytin so their morphology could be recovered. Preliminary findings show that LC cells from stressed animals have larger and more complex dendritic arbors than those from control rats. Additionally, using RNA-Seq, we identified that expression of Ntf3, the gene for neurotrophin 3, which promotes neuronal survival, differentiation, and neurite outgrowth [18, 90],

was approximately twice as high in rats one week after stressor exposure than in their control counterparts (Figure 2). These observations, in combination with earlier reports of stress-induced morphological alterations in LC neurons [50, 52, 53, 75, 91–93], suggest that stress may cause long-lasting changes in noradrenergic transmission throughout the CNS in response to even acute stressor exposure. Such an effect on CNS noradrenergic transmission might be achieved through morphological plasticity because as LC dendrites and axons proliferate, there would be more sites of afferent input to excite LC neurons and a greater density of release points from which NE efflux could occur upon this enhanced excitation, respectively. Such findings could have important implications for posttraumatic stress disorder (PTSD), a condition in which evidence suggests that NE transmission is impaired [12, 31, 79, 94].

It is interesting to note that rodent LC neurons are sexually dimorphic with respect to their morphological characteristics and response to stress/CRF exposure. Female LC dendritic arbors have been reported to extend further into the peri-LC region where synaptic contacts with CRF-positive afferents are made [71, 95, 96] and are larger with more branching points than those of males [68, 97]. This

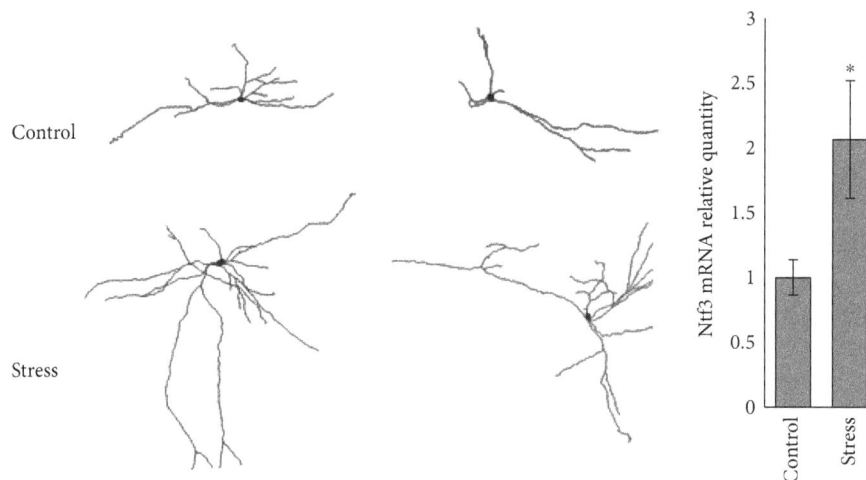

FIGURE 2: LC neurons from stressor-exposed animals show a trend for increased dendritic complexity. Representative traced neurons from control (top) and stressor exposed (bottom) animals filled with biocytin reveal a tendency for LC cells from stressed rats to possess larger and more complex dendritic arbors a week after stressor exposure. Additionally, neurotrophin 3, which promotes neurite outgrowth and dendritic proliferation, is upregulated in LC one week after stressor exposure. $^*p < 0.05$ versus control.

suggests that the female LC might be subjected to greater afferent regulation by CRF and therefore more stress-responsive. This sexual dimorphism might provide a structural basis for differences in emotional arousal between sexes and the greater increased susceptibility of females to anxiety disorders [98]. Interestingly, in mice that genetically overexpress CRF, the complexity of male dendritic morphology increases to resemble the morphology of wild-type and CRF-overexpressing females. This further suggests that enhanced CRF signaling produces neurite proliferation and extension in LC [58]. Such observations provide further evidence for stress and CRF-induced central noradrenergic reorganization.

2.3. CRF and Modified AMPA Receptor-Dependent Synaptic Transmission. Plasticity is highly dependent on the AMPA receptor (AMPAR), an ionotropic glutamate receptor, permeable to Na^+ and Ca^{2+} ions. It is composed of four subunits: GluA1, GluA2, GluA3, and GluA4, which form a heterotetramer. [99–103]. We have previously shown that both stressor exposure *in vivo* [62] and CRF exposure ex vivo [49] alter LC AMPAR signaling. Given that stress and CRF can alter AMPAR-dependent transmission, this receptor might play a critical role in stress-induced neural plasticity. Several mechanisms could account for altered AMPAR functioning in LC following CRF exposure. CRF signaling in LC causes internalization of its own receptor [59, 60, 63], and thus, if CRF and AMPARs are in close apposition to one another on postsynaptic LC membranes, CRF receptor trafficking might inadvertently induce AMPAR internalization as well. This is particularly important with respect to some of the intracellular proteins that AMPARs interact with. AMPARs interact directly and indirectly with kinases and GTPases that regulate actin cytoskeletal dynamics [50, 53, 99–101, 104, 105]. In particular, Rho GTPase activity is modulated by guanine nucleotide exchange factors (GEFs), which are known to interact with *surface-expressed* AMPARs and

promote synaptic plasticity [104]. Thus, if CRF causes shuttling of vesicular AMPARs to the cell membrane, which, based on our prior observations, might occur during high concentrations of CRF exposure [49], their association with GEFs could promote structural plasticity in LC neurons through interaction with Rho GTPases and modulation of cytoskeletal structure. Identifying the mechanisms that link CRF and AMPA receptor function and trafficking could be informative of how LC cells adapt morphologically following stress, thus providing insights to a number of disease states in which LC plasticity is perturbed [29, 50, 53, 106, 107]. In addition to receptor trafficking and altered gene expression, there are other posttranslational modifications that can be made to the AMPAR and its subunits which could promote plastic changes to LC neurons. Using data from both LC and non-LC studies of AMPAR function and modification, we will review possible mechanisms for AMPAR regulation.

There are multiple mechanisms of posttranslational regulation of AMPAR function, which include reversible phosphorylation, ubiquitination, and palmitoylation [108–110]. CRF stimulates cAMP synthesis and PKA activity [48, 50, 52], and therefore, stress could potentially alter AMPAR phosphorylation states. The GluA1 subunit is phosphorylated at different positions at the C-terminal end. For example, phosphorylation at Ser-845 by PKA [101] and Ser-831 by PKC and CaMKII [111, 112] increase single channel conductance. Phosphorylation of Ser-818 and Thr–840 by PKC increases the mean channel conductance [113]. Importantly, mechanisms that increase channel conductance have been shown to promote activity-dependent plasticity [99, 114]. PKCλ was found to phosphorylate Ser-818 on the GluA1 subunit which mediates PI3K-induced AMPAR insertion [115]. GluR2 can also regulate synaptic plasticity through Ser-880 phosphorylation-dependent interactions with PDZ domain-containing proteins, which regulate receptor internalization in the hippocampus [116] and cerebellum [117].

Thus, due to the actions of CRF on cAMP production and PKA activity, stress could potentially impact LC plasticity through modulation of AMPAR function which we have demonstrated in the past [49, 62].

Another modification of AMPARs is ubiquitination, which promotes endocytosis and degradation [108, 109, 118–120] and can occur at multiple places across the subunits. One effect of stress on AMPAR ubiquitination is to decrease glutamatergic synaptic transmission in the prefrontal cortex (PFC), which requires specific ubiquitin ligases Nedd4-1 and Fbx2, an effect which can be blocked by a proteasome inhibitor [121]. Identification of LC-specific ubiquitin ligases would help to find a precise target for stress response control and intervention. In contrast to ubiquitination, AMPAR C-terminal cysteine residue palmitoylation protects from degradation [122] and regulates its internalization [123]. Palmitoylation of the transmembrane domain promotes accumulation of AMPAR in the Golgi, possibly performing a quality control step for proper folding, while depalmitoylation stimulates membrane insertion of AMPAR [123–125]. Identifying any potential mechanisms linking CRF signaling to AMPAR ubiquitination in LC or elsewhere would be informative of means of promoting or inhibiting stress-induced plasticity within the nucleus.

2.4. CRF and Intracellular Signal Transduction. CRF mediates its action through CRFR1, which through Gs-coupled mechanisms increases the concentration of cAMP that phosphorylates PKA [52]. However, there is another mechanism caused by CRFR1 activation which acts through a MAPK cascade, in which a Gq-coupled mechanism increases concentration of phospholipase C (PLC), which activates metabolites which phosphorylate PKC, which in turn phosphorylates ERK1/2 [50, 126]. CRF has been shown to cause an increase in LC neurite length, an effect that is abolished by specific inhibition of PKA or MAPK, but not PKC [50]. PKC appears to also trigger a RhoA-activating cascade through downstream Rho-associated protein kinase (ROCK), which subsequently phosphorylates the collapsin response mediator protein 2 (CRMP-2) and causes growth cone collapse [127] (Figure 2).

Such receptor-mediated acute cellular changes could occur through the aforementioned mechanisms, but long-term changes could also potentially occur through regulation of gene expression. A study of single and repeated restraint stress demonstrated an increase in immunoreactivity of c-Fos, pERK, pCaMKII, and pCREB in the LC two hours following the stressor [128]. The same study also showed that pERK and pCREB had the same expression pattern and were colocalized to the same neurons, suggesting that activation of the MAPK/ERK pathways with CREB phosphorylation promote changes in gene expression. The exact mechanism of transcriptional changes following CRF expression in the LC is not clear. However, another study demonstrated increased c-Fos expression and CREB phosphorylation after acute immobilization stress, while repeated stress increased phosphorylation of p38, cJun N-teminal kinase (JNK 1/2/3), and ERK1/2 [129]. CREB is a transcriptional factor which regulates transcription of multiple downstream genes including c-Fos, brain-derived neurotrophic factor (BDNF), tyrosine hydroxylase (TH), and neuropeptides [130, 131]. These observations corroborate other studies that have shown altered expression of trophic factors and NE synthetic enzymes [18, 28, 54–57, 61].

BDNF stimulates dendritic outgrowth and increased synaptic connectivity. Mice genetically overexpressing the receptor for neurotrophin 3, TrkC, show increased anxiety-like behavior, as well as increased LC neuronal density [132], suggesting that some degree of positive feedback might exist between stress, neurotrophin 3 signaling, and LC plasticity. This is particularly interesting in light of preliminary observations by our laboratory that show that one week after acute stressor exposure, neurotrophin mRNA is increased, an effect accompanied by a trend for increased LC dendritic length and complexity (Figure 2). Others have also reported increased neurotrophin 3 expression in LC following stress, which can be normalized with antidepressant treatment [18]. Interestingly, in addition to sexual dimorphism of LC morphology and stress responsiveness, there are also sex differences in LC intracellular signaling induced by CRF: specifically, CRFR1 is more strongly coupled to β-arrestin in males, promoting receptor internalization and potentially blunted responsiveness to CRF in the future. In females, however, CRFR1 is more strongly coupled to Gs signaling pathways, which promotes increased LC discharge and dendritic proliferation, potentially increasing future sensitivity to stress by providing more space for synaptic contacts with CRF-positive afferents [63, 133]. In this way, the male and female LC may be differentially aligned to respond to stress with specific neuroplastic adaptations that promote disease.

3. CNS Neural Plasticity Changes in Response to NE Volume Transmission Changes

LC contributes to major CNS functions such as waking, arousal, attention, sensory discrimination, and cognition. Because stress promotes both short- and long-term functional and neuroplastic changes in LC, some of these functions might also be impacted by stressor exposure, either directly or indirectly. Through modulation of intrinsic and synaptic features of LC neurons, stress likely modifies noradrenergic volume transmission in target brain areas such as the amygdala, hippocampus, and PFC, where it potently modulates neural plasticity [134–138]. Because stress acutely and chronically alters LC discharge [53, 62, 66, 86] and NE release [78–82], different adrenergic receptors might become engaged during and after stressor exposure. The adrenergic receptors vary in their affinity for NE [3, 78, 139, 140], and different receptors promote different forms of plasticity and learning [134, 135, 137, 141]. Low concentrations of NE engage the high-affinity α_1 receptor, particularly in the prefrontal cortex, which promotes working memory, sustained attention, and other cognitive functions [3, 142, 143].

Conversely, high NE concentration which occurs in response to stress causes engagement of the α_1 and β adrenergic receptors. The α_1 receptor promotes LTD of prefrontal synapses [137] and inhibition of prefrontal-dependent cognitive functions such as working memory and sustained attention [2, 83]. Indeed, enhanced α_1 signaling in PFC is associated with increased behavioral flexibility [144]. Furthermore, stressor exposure has been shown to increase tonic LC discharge and promote scanning attention and behavioral flexibility [65, 66]. It has been proposed that such a change would permit lower-order sensorimotor regions to guide behavior with little modulation by prefrontal circuitry, allowing disengagement from specific stimuli and goal-oriented behaviors to instead promote rapid impulsive responses [2]. Such a stress-induced shift might be beneficial when an animal is faced with a threatening stimulus and a quick escape must be made. Additionally, engagement of the β receptor promotes hippocampal plasticity and encoding and recall of contextual fear memory [141, 145, 146]. Therefore, persistent stress-induced changes in LC function would elevate NE concentration in prefrontal cortex and hippocampus enhancing plasticity in both areas through signaling at α_1 and β receptors to synergistically promote encoding and recall of fear memories, impaired cognition, hypervigilance, and behaviors that allow an appropriate behavioral response to be generated. Therefore, an inverted U relationship between LC firing and arousal/behavioral performance model has been proposed [2, 37, 139], with maximal cognitive function corresponding to "ideal" levels of LC tonic firing [147] and hyperarousal and vigilance corresponding with excessive levels of discharge. During stress, increased tonic LC firing is enhanced, which leads to increased levels of NE in LC projection fields, promoting broad scanning attention, hyperarousal, hypervigilance, and other anxiety-like behavioral symptoms in stressed subjects.

4. Role of Stress-Induced LC/NE Changes in PTSD

Chronic stress-induced alterations in LC structure and function that lead to behavioral impairments might contribute to disease pathogenesis and symptomatology. Many studies show the involvement or potential involvement of the LC in stress-related disease states, particularly PTSD. Both peripheral and central measures of NE activity are increased in PTSD patient populations, including enhanced sympathetic nervous system function [148–151], and increased functional connectivity between LC and the basolateral amygdala during conscious processing of threatening stimuli [152]. This enhanced connectivity is particularly important because of the role that the basolateral amygdala and its noradrenergic inputs in particular [153–157] play in fear conditioning. Furthermore, PTSD patients frequently show disturbances in sleep patterns [158–160], which may be related to chronically elevated LC discharge due to its well-established role in mediating arousal and a forebrain EEG associated with waking [161]. Such an effect could potentially be related to dysregulation of other stress-sensitive systems, such as the HPA axis which releases CRF. LC is potently activated by CRF, and increased levels of the peptide have been found in the cerebrospinal fluid of combat veterans afflicted with PTSD [162, 163], providing a potential means for maintaining LC hyperactivity even in the absence of a stressor. More recently, an fMRI study showed that PTSD patients

showed exaggerated behavioral and autonomic responses to loud sounds, suggesting sensitized phasic responses of LC neurons [34]. Evidence for LC as a central mediator of PTSD-like symptoms comes from observations that yohimbine, an α_{2A} receptor antagonist which disinhibits LC neurons, produces panic attacks in up to 70% of PTSD patients and in 89% of patients with comorbid PTSD and panic disorder, but not in control subjects. Additionally, plasma levels of a NE metabolite postyohimbine administration were twice as high in PTSD patients [163]. These findings suggest that NE release is altered presynaptically at the level of the LC in PTSD patients, which may affect many downstream targets [164].

In contrast to the actions of yohimbine, clonidine, a presynaptic α_{2A} receptor agonist which limits noradrenergic transmission in the forebrain, has been shown to have beneficial effects on hyperarousal, hypervigilance, sleep disruption, exaggerated startle responses, and nightmares in veterans with PTSD [31]. The notion that increased NE release promotes some behaviors associated with PTSD and anxiety is further supported by observations that the β-receptor antagonist propranolol attenuates PTSD symptoms, possibly due to the actions that the β receptor plays in fear memory consolidation and emotion [31, 134, 135, 165–167]. Prazosin, an α_1-adrenergic antagonist, has also been shown to be beneficial for alleviating nightmares and sleep disturbances in both veteran [168] and children PTSD patients [169], as well as for improving symptoms of hyperarousal, avoidance/numbing, and traumatic recall of past events [170]. It is also interesting to note that an *in vivo* PET study that the availability of the NE transporter in the LC is decreased in PTSD patients [171]. This could be indicative of elevated extracellular NE concentration and would be consistent with other reports of LC hyperactivity in this population. Thus, due to the well-documented ability of stress to promote forebrain NE release through short-term physiological activation and enduring molecular and cellular changes in the LC, stress-induced neuroplastic adaptations in the LC likely contribute to disease pathogenesis. This could occur at the level of the LC as a primary site of stress-induced plasticity or in downstream targets of the LC due to the well-established role of NE in mediating neuroplastic changes throughout the brain: fMRI studies have also shown changes in hippocampal volume and altered function in the amygdala, hippocampus, mPFC, orbitofrontal cortex, anterior cingulate, and insular cortex in PTSD patients [172], all of which may be related to maladaptive plastic changes in the LC or the plastic changes promoted by it [134, 135, 137, 165].

Based on these clinical reports, there is clear evidence that LC hyperfunction is at least characteristic of, if not causal to, PTSD symptomatology. However, some clinical observations suggest a more complicated relationship that exists between LC function and PTSD disease progression and treatment. As mentioned above, there is clinical evidence for decreased NE transporter availability in the LC of PTSD patients. This could be explained by elevated extracellular NE concentration; another potential explanation could be LC neuronal loss. Indeed, a postmortem neuromorphometric analysis of veterans with probable or possible war-related PTSD showed a lower LC cell count compared to controls [173], suggesting that the LC plays in the role in the pathophysiology of PTSD, or that a lower LC cell count may predispose individuals to PTSD. While decreased LC cell numbers would suggest reduced forebrain NE levels, in other pathologies in which LC cell counts are decreased such as Alzheimer's disease, the surviving neurons show evidence for hyperactivity [174] and dendritic sprouting and remodeling [107]. Additionally, recent clinical trials using 3,4-methylenedioxymethamphetamine (MDMA) have shown promising results in reduction or remission of PTSD symptoms: specifically, six phase II clinical trials have shown that combined MDMA and psychotherapy are safe and efficacious such that 52.7% of patients receiving active drug no longer meet PTSD criteria [175]. Despite a wealth of evidence showing that enhanced noradrenergic transmission contributes to PTSD etiology, MDMA increases release of catecholamines, including NE. One potential explanation for MDMA's somewhat paradoxical efficacy is that memory reconsolidation is enhanced via plastic changes in the hippocampus due to elevated NE levels [141, 145]. MDMA also facilitates fear extinction learning [176], and thus, enhanced NE efflux following MDMA administration might also promote plastic changes within the amygdala [12]. Additionally, because NE is generally increased in PTSD patients, the benefits of MDMA on symptom improvement are likely due to the drug complex polypharmacological interactions and its effects on brainwide neurotransmission. It is hypothesized that in addition to enhanced plasticity and memory reconsolidation, heightened monoaminergic neurotransmission following MDMA administration promotes a number of subjective psychological effects such as increased introspection and receptiveness for psychotherapy that lead to improved outcomes in PTSD patients [175]. Collectively, however, many clinical observations strongly suggest that hyperactive noradrenergic transmission contributes to PTSD symptomology and anxiety-like behavior.

5. Conclusions

Stressor exposure induces a series of neuroendocrine, physiological, and behavioral adaptations that promote an appropriate response to the stressor. Central to these diverse functions is CRF signaling which in a number of brain regions promotes a number of immediate [48, 49, 51, 177–184] and persistent [50, 52, 60, 121, 185–187] cellular changes. These effects are of particular interest in LC, where the interaction of CRF with its receptor CRFR1 activates cAMP-dependent intracellular signaling cascades, increasing tonic discharge and promoting anxiety-like behavior [64, 77, 188, 189]. Evidence suggests that chronic stressor exposure is able to alter LC gene expression [18, 28, 54–57, 61], promote long-term changes in synaptic transmission and excitability [53, 62] and receptor trafficking [58–60, 185], and, importantly, induce morphological changes and dendritic remodeling (Figure 1) [50, 52, 53, 57, 190]. These actions appear to be dependent on a number of kinases and GTPases and their associated signaling pathways [50, 52, 57] and potentially on AMPAR function

[191, 192] which is modulated by CRF in the short term [49] and stressor exposure in the long term [62]. Through its complex signaling cascades, CRFR1 activation in LC induces a number of long-lasting cellular effects which ultimately impact the function of the nucleus itself as well as other target brain regions which are heavily innervated by LC and modulated by noradrenergic transmission. Critically, the LC promotes plasticity in other structures including the PFC, amygdala, and hippocampus by promoting noradrenergic transmission at α_1 and β receptors [137, 141, 145, 146]. Therefore, stress and CRF can induce neuroplastic changes in LC, which can lead to subsequent neuroplastic changes elsewhere, ultimately promoting causing chronic anxiety-like behavior. Specifically, increased tonic discharge in the short term will drive an animal to display such behavior [62, 64, 77]. Maintenance of increased LC discharge in the long term [62] along with enhanced expression of genes necessary for NE synthesis and release [54–56] will lead to chronically elevated forebrain NE levels. This promotes network adaptations and plasticity in target regions which facilitate fear memory encoding and drive an animal towards a behavioral state characterized by vigilance, impulsivity, and impaired cognition [3, 78, 83, 193]. Meanwhile, morphological plasticity and dendritic outgrowth into the peri-LC area [50, 52, 53, 68, 194] will make LC subject to greater afferent regulation by stress-responsive structures such as PVN and CeA [58, 63, 194]. Through these mechanisms, chronic or traumatic stress could permanently alter forebrain noradrenergic transmission to promote long-lasting changes in behavior, manifesting in humans as mood and anxiety disorders such as depression and posttraumatic stress disorder. Thus, identifying how stress and CRF promote synaptic and morphological plasticity in LC to chronically elevate forebrain NE concentration represents an important step in understanding disease pathogenesis and symptomatology for mood, anxiety, and other neuropsychiatric disorders.

Conflicts of Interest

The authors declare that there is no conflict of interest regarding the publication of this paper.

Acknowledgments

The authors wish to acknowledge Mr. Matthew Flamini for his assistance in reviewing and editing the manuscript.

References

[1] P. E. Greenberg, T. Sisitsky, R. C. Kessler et al., "The economic burden of anxiety disorders in the 1990s," *The Journal of Clinical Psychiatry*, vol. 60, no. 7, pp. 427–435, 1999.

[2] A. F. T. Arnsten, "Through the looking glass: differential noradenergic modulation of prefrontal cortical function," *Neural Plasticity*, vol. 7, no. 1-2, 146 pages, 2000.

[3] A. F. T. Arnsten, "Prefrontal cortical network connections: key site of vulnerability in stress and schizophrenia," *International Journal of Developmental Neuroscience*, vol. 29, no. 3, pp. 215–223, 2011.

[4] R. Crupi, A. Marino, and S. Cuzzocrea, "New therapeutic strategy for mood disorders," *Current Medicinal Chemistry*, vol. 18, no. 28, pp. 4284–4298, 2011.

[5] G. C. Curtis, J. L. Abelson, and P. W. Gold, "Adrenocorticotropic hormone and cortisol responses to corticotropin-releasing hormone: changes in panic disorder and effects of alprazolam treatment," *Biological Psychiatry*, vol. 41, no. 1, pp. 76–85, 1997.

[6] J. F. W. Deakin, "Depression and 5HT," *International Clinical Psychopharmacology*, vol. 6, pp. 23–32, 1991.

[7] J. Ho, S. P. C. Ngai, W. K. K. Wu, and W. K. Hou, "Association between daily life experience and psychological well-being in people living with nonpsychotic mental disorders: protocol for a systematic review and meta-analysis," *Medicine*, vol. 97, no. 4, article e9733, 2018.

[8] T. L. Tay, C. Béchade, I. D'Andrea et al., "Microglia gone rogue: impacts on psychiatric disorders across the lifespan," *Frontiers in Molecular Neuroscience*, vol. 10, p. 421, 2018.

[9] S. K. Wood, H. E. Walker, R. J. Valentino, and S. Bhatnagar, "Individual differences in reactivity to social stress predict susceptibility and resilience to a depressive phenotype: role of corticotropin-releasing factor," *Endocrinology*, vol. 151, no. 4, pp. 1795–1805, 2010.

[10] C. S. Wood, R. J. Valentino, and S. K. Wood, "Individual differences in the locus coeruleus-norepinephrine system: relevance to stress-induced cardiovascular vulnerability," *Physiology & Behavior*, vol. 172, pp. 40–48, 2017.

[11] O. Berton, C. McClung, R. J. Dileone et al., "Essential role of BDNF in the mesolimbic dopamine pathway in social defeat stress," *Science*, vol. 311, no. 5762, pp. 864–868, 2006.

[12] J. D. Bremner, B. Elzinga, C. Schmahl, and E. Vermetten, "Structural and functional plasticity of the human brain in posttraumatic stress disorder," *Progress in Brain Research*, vol. 167, pp. 171–186, 2008.

[13] A. C. Campos, F. R. Ferreira, W. A. da Silva Jr, and F. S. Guimarães, "Predator threat stress promotes long lasting anxiety-like behaviors and modulates synaptophysin and CB1 receptors expression in brain areas associated with PTSD symptoms," *Neuroscience Letters*, vol. 533, pp. 34–38, 2013.

[14] C. Challis, J. Boulden, A. Veerakumar et al., "Raphe GABAergic neurons mediate the acquisition of avoidance after social defeat," *Journal of Neuroscience*, vol. 33, no. 35, pp. 13978–13988, 2013.

[15] A. Chocyk, B. Bobula, D. Dudys et al., "Early-life stress affects the structural and functional plasticity of the medial prefrontal cortex in adolescent rats," *European Journal of Neuroscience*, vol. 38, no. 1, pp. 2089–2107, 2013.

[16] V. Krishnan, M. H. Han, D. L. Graham et al., "Molecular adaptations underlying susceptibility and resistance to social defeat in brain reward regions," *Cell*, vol. 131, no. 2, pp. 391–404, 2007.

[17] S. D. Kuipers, A. Trentani, J. A. den Boer, and G. J. ter Horst, "Molecular correlates of impaired prefrontal plasticity in response to chronic stress," *Journal of Neurochemistry*, vol. 85, no. 5, pp. 1312–1323, 2003.

[18] M. A. Smith, S. Makino, M. Altemus et al., "Stress and antidepressants differentially regulate neurotrophin 3 mRNA expression in the locus coeruleus," *Proceedings of the National Academy of Sciences of the United States of America*, vol. 92, no. 19, pp. 8788–8792, 1995.

[19] A. Veerakumar, C. Challis, P. Gupta et al., "Antidepressant-like effects of cortical deep brain stimulation coincide with pro-neuroplastic adaptations of serotonin systems," *Biological Psychiatry*, vol. 76, no. 3, pp. 203–212, 2014.

[20] P. R. Zoladz, C. R. Park, J. D. Halonen et al., "Differential expression of molecular markers of synaptic plasticity in the hippocampus, prefrontal cortex, and amygdala in response to spatial learning, predator exposure, and stress-induced amnesia," *Hippocampus*, vol. 22, no. 3, pp. 577–589, 2012.

[21] F. Jeanneteau, C. Barrère, M. Vos et al., "The stress-induced transcription factor NR4A1 adjusts mitochondrial function and synapse number in prefrontal cortex," *The Journal of Neuroscience*, vol. 38, no. 6, pp. 1335–1350, 2018.

[22] F. F. Scarante, C. Vila-Verde, V. L. Detoni, N. C. Ferreira-Junior, F. S. Guimarães, and A. C. Campos, "Cannabinoid modulation of the stressed hippocampus," *Frontiers in Molecular Neuroscience*, vol. 10, p. 411, 2017.

[23] K. G. Bath, S. J. Russo, K. E. Pleil, E. S. Wohleb, R. S. Duman, and J. J. Radley, "Circuit and synaptic mechanisms of repeated stress: perspectives from differing contexts, duration, and development," *Neurobiology of Stress*, vol. 7, pp. 137–151, 2017.

[24] Y. S. Nikolova, K. A. Misquitta, B. R. Rocco et al., "Shifting priorities: highly conserved behavioral and brain network adaptations to chronic stress across species," *Translational Psychiatry*, vol. 8, no. 1, p. 26, 2018.

[25] I. A. Paul and P. Skolnick, "Glutamate and depression: clinical and preclinical studies," *Annals of the New York Academy of Sciences*, vol. 1003, no. 1, pp. 250–272, 2003.

[26] P. J. Lucassen, J. Pruessner, N. Sousa et al., "Neuropathology of stress," *Acta Neuropathologica*, vol. 127, no. 1, pp. 109–135, 2014.

[27] B. E. Leonard, "Psychopathology of depression," *Drugs of Today*, vol. 43, no. 10, pp. 705–716, 2007.

[28] E. Mamalaki, R. Kvetnansky, L. S. Brady, P. W. Gold, and M. Herkenham, "Repeated immobilization stress alters tyrosine hydroxylase, corticotropin-releasing hormone and corticosteroid receptor messenger ribonucleic acid levels in rat brain," *Journal of Neuroendocrinology*, vol. 4, no. 6, pp. 689–699, 1992.

[29] D. Weinshenker, "Functional consequences of locus coeruleus degeneration in Alzheimer's disease," *Current Alzheimer Research*, vol. 5, no. 3, pp. 342–345, 2008.

[30] J. D. Bremner, "Traumatic stress: effects on the brain," *Dialogues in Clinical Neuroscience*, vol. 8, no. 4, pp. 445–461, 2006.

[31] J. R. Strawn and T. D. Geracioti, "Noradrenergic dysfunction and the psychopharmacology of posttraumatic stress disorder," *Depression and Anxiety*, vol. 25, no. 3, pp. 260–271, 2008.

[32] O. Borodovitsyna, M. Flamini, and D. Chandler, "Noradrenergic modulation of cognition in health and disease," *Neural Plasticity*, vol. 2017, Article ID 6031478, 14 pages, 2017.

[33] R. A. Eser, A. J. Ehrenberg, C. Petersen et al., "Selective vulnerability of brainstem nuclei in distinct tauopathies: a postmortem study," *Journal of Neuropathology and Experimental Neurology*, vol. 77, no. 2, pp. 149–161, 2018.

[34] C. Naegeli, T. Zeffiro, M. Piccirelli et al., "Locus coeruleus activity mediates hyperresponsiveness in posttraumatic stress disorder," *Biological Psychiatry*, vol. 83, no. 3, pp. 254–262, 2018.

[35] E. T. Cunningham, M. C. Bohn, and P. E. Sawchenko, "Organization of adrenergic inputs to the paraventricular and supraoptic nuclei of the hypothalamus in the rat," *The Journal of Comparative Neurology*, vol. 292, no. 4, pp. 651–667, 1990.

[36] J. P. Herman, H. Figueiredo, N. K. Mueller et al., "Central mechanisms of stress integration: hierarchical circuitry controlling hypothalamo–pituitary–adrenocortical responsiveness," *Frontiers in Neuroendocrinology*, vol. 24, no. 3, pp. 151–180, 2003.

[37] C. W. Berridge and B. D. Waterhouse, "The locus coeruleus–noradrenergic system: modulation of behavioral state and state-dependent cognitive processes," *Brain Research Reviews*, vol. 42, no. 1, pp. 33–84, 2003.

[38] D. J. Chandler, W. J. Gao, and B. D. Waterhouse, "Heterogeneous organization of the locus coeruleus projections to prefrontal and motor cortices," *Proceedings of the National Academy of Sciences of the United States of America*, vol. 111, no. 18, pp. 6816–6821, 2014.

[39] S. L. Foote, F. E. Bloom, and G. Aston-Jones, "Nucleus locus ceruleus: new evidence of anatomical and physiological specificity," *Physiological Reviews*, vol. 63, no. 3, pp. 844–914, 1983.

[40] S. E. Loughlin, S. L. Foote, and F. E. Bloom, "Efferent projections of nucleus locus coeruleus: topographic organization of cells of origin demonstrated by three-dimensional reconstruction," *Neuroscience*, vol. 18, no. 2, pp. 291–306, 1986.

[41] S. D. Robertson, N. W. Plummer, J. de Marchena, and P. Jensen, "Developmental origins of central norepinephrine neuron diversity," *Nature Neuroscience*, vol. 16, no. 8, pp. 1016–1023, 2013.

[42] D. Chandler and B. D. Waterhouse, "Evidence for broad versus segregated projections from cholinergic and noradrenergic nuclei to functionally and anatomically discrete subregions of prefrontal cortex," *Frontiers in Behavioral Neuroscience*, vol. 6, p. 20, 2012.

[43] D. J. Chandler, "Evidence for a specialized role of the locus coeruleus noradrenergic system in cortical circuitries and behavioral operations," *Brain Research*, vol. 1641, Part B, pp. 197–206, 2016.

[44] D. J. Chandler, C. S. Lamperski, and B. D. Waterhouse, "Identification and distribution of projections from monoaminergic and cholinergic nuclei to functionally differentiated subregions of prefrontal cortex," *Brain Research*, vol. 1522, pp. 38–58, 2013.

[45] D. J. Chandler, B. D. Waterhouse, and W. J. Gao, "New perspectives on catecholaminergic regulation of executive circuits: evidence for independent modulation of prefrontal functions by midbrain dopaminergic and noradrenergic neurons," *Frontiers in Neural Circuits*, vol. 8, p. 53, 2014.

[46] D. M. Devilbiss, M. E. Page, and B. D. Waterhouse, "Locus ceruleus regulates sensory encoding by neurons and networks in waking animals," *Journal of Neuroscience*, vol. 26, no. 39, pp. 9860–9872, 2006.

[47] B. D. Waterhouse, H. C. Moises, and D. J. Woodward, "Phasic activation of the locus coeruleus enhances responses of primary sensory cortical neurons to peripheral receptive field stimulation," *Brain Research*, vol. 790, no. 1-2, pp. 33–44, 1998.

[48] H. P. Jedema and A. A. Grace, "Corticotropin-releasing hormone directly activates noradrenergic neurons of the locus

ceruleus recorded *in vitro*," *Journal of Neuroscience*, vol. 24, no. 43, pp. 9703–9713, 2004.

[49] E. W. Prouty, B. D. Waterhouse, and D. J. Chandler, "Corticotropin releasing factor dose-dependently modulates excitatory synaptic transmission in the noradrenergic nucleus locus coeruleus," *European Journal of Neuroscience*, vol. 45, no. 5, pp. 712–722, 2017.

[50] J. D. Swinny and R. J. Valentino, "Corticotropin-releasing factor promotes growth of brain norepinephrine neuronal processes through Rho GTPase regulators of the actin cytoskeleton in rat," *European Journal of Neuroscience*, vol. 24, no. 9, pp. 2481–2490, 2006.

[51] R. J. Valentino, S. L. Foote, and G. Aston-Jones, "Corticotropin-releasing factor activates noradrenergic neurons of the locus coeruleus," *Brain Research*, vol. 270, no. 2, pp. 363–367, 1983.

[52] G. Cibelli, P. Corsi, G. Diana, F. Vitiello, and G. Thiel, "Corticotropin-releasing factor triggers neurite outgrowth of a catecholaminergic immortalized neuron via cAMP and MAP kinase signalling pathways," *European Journal of Neuroscience*, vol. 13, no. 7, pp. 1339–1348, 2001.

[53] J. D. Swinny, E. O'Farrell, B. C. Bingham, D. A. Piel, R. J. Valentino, and S. G. Beck, "Neonatal rearing conditions distinctly shape locus coeruleus neuronal activity, dendritic arborization, and sensitivity to corticotrophin-releasing factor," *The International Journal of Neuropsychopharmacology*, vol. 13, no. 04, pp. 515–525, 2010.

[54] Y. Fan, P. Chen, Y. Li, and M. Y. Zhu, "Effects of chronic social defeat on expression of dopamine β-hydroxylase in rat brains," *Synapse*, vol. 67, no. 6, pp. 300–312, 2013.

[55] M. Rusnák, R. Kvetňanský, J. Jeloková, and M. Palkovits, "Effect of novel stressors on gene expression of tyrosine hydroxylase and monoamine transporters in brainstem noradrenergic neurons of long-term repeatedly immobilized rats," *Brain Research*, vol. 899, no. 1-2, pp. 20–35, 2001.

[56] S. A. George, D. Knox, A. L. Curtis, J. W. Aldridge, R. J. Valentino, and I. Liberzon, "Altered locus coeruleus–norepinephrine function following single prolonged stress," *European Journal of Neuroscience*, vol. 37, no. 6, pp. 901–909, 2013.

[57] S. Salim, B. Hite, and D. C. Eikenburg, "Activation of the CRF_1 receptor causes ERK1/2 mediated increase in GRK3 expression in CATH.a cells," *FEBS Letters*, vol. 581, no. 17, pp. 3204–3210, 2007.

[58] D. A. Bangasser, B. A. S. Reyes, D. Piel et al., "Increased vulnerability of the brain norepinephrine system of females to corticotropin-releasing factor overexpression," *Molecular Psychiatry*, vol. 18, no. 2, pp. 166–173, 2013.

[59] B. A. S. Reyes, D. A. Bangasser, R. J. Valentino, and E. J. Van Bockstaele, "Using high resolution imaging to determine trafficking of corticotropin-releasing factor receptors in noradrenergic neurons of the rat locus coeruleus," *Life Sciences*, vol. 112, no. 1-2, pp. 2–9, 2014.

[60] B. A. S. Reyes, R. J. Valentino, and E. J. Van Bockstaele, "Stress-induced intracellular trafficking of corticotropin-releasing factor receptors in rat locus coeruleus neurons," *Endocrinology*, vol. 149, no. 1, pp. 122–130, 2008.

[61] E. L. Sabban, L. I. Serova, E. Newman, N. Aisenberg, and I. Akirav, "Changes in gene expression in the locus coeruleus-amygdala circuitry in inhibitory avoidance PTSD model," *Cellular and Molecular Neurobiology*, vol. 38, no. 1, pp. 273–280, 2018.

[62] O. Borodovitsyna, M. D. Flamini, and D. J. Chandler, "Acute stress persistently alters locus coeruleus function and anxiety-like behavior in adolescent rats," *Neuroscience*, vol. 373, pp. 7–19, 2018.

[63] R. J. Valentino, D. Bangasser, and E. J. Van Bockstaele, "Sex-biased stress signaling: the corticotropin-releasing factor receptor as a model," *Molecular Pharmacology*, vol. 83, no. 4, pp. 737–745, 2013.

[64] J. G. McCall, R. al-Hasani, E. R. Siuda et al., "CRH engagement of the locus coeruleus noradrenergic system mediates stress-induced anxiety," *Neuron*, vol. 87, no. 3, pp. 605–620, 2015.

[65] A. L. Curtis, S. C. Leiser, K. Snyder, and R. J. Valentino, "Predator stress engages corticotropin-releasing factor and opioid systems to alter the operating mode of locus coeruleus norepinephrine neurons," *Neuropharmacology*, vol. 62, no. 4, pp. 1737–1745, 2012.

[66] K. Snyder, W. W. Wang, R. Han, K. McFadden, and R. J. Valentino, "Corticotropin-releasing factor in the norepinephrine nucleus, locus coeruleus, facilitates behavioral flexibility," *Neuropsychopharmacology*, vol. 37, no. 2, pp. 520–530, 2012.

[67] L. A. Schwarz, K. Miyamichi, X. J. Gao et al., "Viral-genetic tracing of the input–output organization of a central noradrenaline circuit," *Nature*, vol. 524, no. 7563, pp. 88–92, 2015.

[68] D. A. Bangasser, X. Zhang, V. Garachh, E. Hanhauser, and R. J. Valentino, "Sexual dimorphism in locus coeruleus dendritic morphology: a structural basis for sex differences in emotional arousal," *Physiology & Behavior*, vol. 103, no. 3-4, pp. 342–351, 2011.

[69] A. Kreibich, B. A. S. Reyes, A. L. Curtis et al., "Presynaptic inhibition of diverse afferents to the locus ceruleus by κ-opiate receptors: a novel mechanism for regulating the central norepinephrine system," *Journal of Neuroscience*, vol. 28, no. 25, pp. 6516–25, 2008.

[70] B. A. S. Reyes, R. J. Valentino, G. Xu, and E. J. Van Bockstaele, "Hypothalamic projections to locus coeruleus neurons in rat brain," *European Journal of Neuroscience*, vol. 22, no. 1, pp. 93–106, 2005.

[71] B. A. S. Reyes, G. Zitnik, C. Foster, E. J. Van Bockstaele, and R. J. Valentino, "Social stress engages neurochemically-distinct afferents to the rat locus coeruleus depending on coping strategy," *eNeuro*, vol. 2, no. 6, 2015.

[72] R. J. Valentino, C. Rudoy, A. Saunders, X. B. Liu, and E. J. van Bockstaele, "Corticotropin-releasing factor is preferentially colocalized with excitatory rather than inhibitory amino acids in axon terminals in the peri-locus coeruleus region," *Neuroscience*, vol. 106, no. 2, pp. 375–384, 2001.

[73] R. J. Valentino, M. Page, E. van Bockstaele, and G. Aston-Jones, "Corticotropin-releasing factor innervation of the locus coeruleus region: distribution of fibers and sources of input," *Neuroscience*, vol. 48, no. 3, pp. 689–705, 1992.

[74] G. Aston-Jones and J. D. Cohen, "Adaptive gain and the role of the locus coeruleus–norepinephrine system in optimal performance," *The Journal of Comparative Neurology*, vol. 493, no. 1, pp. 99–110, 2005.

[75] D. A. Bangasser and R. J. Valentino, "Sex differences in stress-related psychiatric disorders: neurobiological perspectives," *Frontiers in Neuroendocrinology*, vol. 35, no. 3, pp. 303–319, 2014.

[76] R. J. Valentino, S. L. Foote, and M. E. Page, "The locus coeruleus as a site for integrating corticotropin-releasing factor and noradrenergic mediation of stress responses," *Annals of the New York Academy of Sciences*, vol. 697, no. 1 Corticotropin, pp. 173–188, 1993.

[77] J. G. McCall, E. R. Siuda, D. L. Bhatti et al., "Locus coeruleus to basolateral amygdala noradrenergic projections promote anxiety-like behavior," *eLife*, vol. 6, 2017.

[78] A. F. T. Arnsten, "Catecholamine modulation of prefrontal cortical cognitive function," *Trends in Cognitive Sciences*, vol. 2, no. 11, pp. 436–447, 1998.

[79] A. K. Rajbhandari, B. A. Baldo, and V. P. Bakshi, "Predator stress-induced CRF release causes enduring sensitization of basolateral amygdala norepinephrine systems that promote PTSD-like startle abnormalities," *Journal of Neuroscience*, vol. 35, no. 42, pp. 14270–14285, 2015.

[80] G. Bouchez, M. J. Millan, J. M. Rivet, R. Billiras, R. Boulanger, and A. Gobert, "Quantification of extracellular levels of corticosterone in the basolateral amygdaloid complex of freely-moving rats: a dialysis study of circadian variation and stress-induced modulation," *Brain Research*, vol. 1452, pp. 47–60, 2012.

[81] G. Patki, F. Atrooz, I. Alkadhi, N. Solanki, and S. Salim, "High aggression in rats is associated with elevated stress, anxiety-like behavior, and altered catecholamine content in the brain," *Neuroscience Letters*, vol. 584, pp. 308–313, 2015.

[82] M. J. Mana and A. A. Grace, "Chronic cold stress alters the basal and evoked electrophysiological activity of rat locus coeruleus neurons," *Neuroscience*, vol. 81, no. 4, pp. 1055–1064, 1997.

[83] A. F. T. Arnsten, R. Mathew, R. Ubriani, J. R. Taylor, and B.-M. Li, "α-1 noradrenergic receptor stimulation impairs prefrontal cortical cognitive function," *Biological Psychiatry*, vol. 45, no. 1, pp. 26–31, 1999.

[84] J. Korf, G. K. Aghajanian, and R. H. Roth, "Increased turnover of norepinephrine in the rat cerebral cortex during stress: role of the locus coeruleus," *Neuropharmacology*, vol. 12, no. 10, pp. 933–938, 1973.

[85] B. Bingham, K. McFadden, X. Zhang, S. Bhatnagar, S. Beck, and R. Valentino, "Early adolescence as a critical window during which social stress distinctly alters behavior and brain norepinephrine activity," *Neuropsychopharmacology*, vol. 36, no. 4, pp. 896–909, 2011.

[86] R. J. Valentino and S. L. Foote, "Corticotropin-releasing hormone increases tonic but not sensory-evoked activity of noradrenergic locus coeruleus neurons in unanesthetized rats," *The Journal of Neuroscience*, vol. 8, no. 3, pp. 1016–1025, 1988.

[87] F. Lejeune and M. J. Millan, "The CRF₁ receptor antagonist, DMP695, abolishes activation of locus coeruleus noradrenergic neurones by CRF in anesthetized rats," *European Journal of Pharmacology*, vol. 464, no. 2-3, pp. 127–133, 2003.

[88] A. Tashiro and R. Yuste, "Regulation of dendritic spine motility and stability by Rac1 and Rho kinase: evidence for two forms of spine motility," *Molecular and Cellular Neuroscience*, vol. 26, no. 3, pp. 429–440, 2004.

[89] A. Y. Nakayama, M. B. Harms, and L. Luo, "Small GTPases Rac and Rho in the maintenance of dendritic spines and branches in hippocampal pyramidal neurons," *The Journal of Neuroscience*, vol. 20, no. 14, pp. 5329–5338, 2000.

[90] L. Van Aelst and H. T. Cline, "Rho GTPases and activity-dependent dendrite development," *Current Opinion in Neurobiology*, vol. 14, no. 3, pp. 297–304, 2004.

[91] E. J. Van Bockstaele, B. A. S. Reyes, and R. J. Valentino, "The locus coeruleus: a key nucleus where stress and opioids intersect to mediate vulnerability to opiate abuse," *Brain Research*, vol. 1314, pp. 162–174, 2010.

[92] Y. Liu and S. Nakamura, "Stress-induced plasticity of monoamine axons," *Frontiers in Bioscience*, vol. 11, no. 1, pp. 1794–1801, 2006.

[93] S. Nakamura, T. Sakaguchi, and F. Aoki, "Electrophysiological evidence for terminal sprouting of locus coeruleus neurons following repeated mild stress," *Neuroscience Letters*, vol. 100, no. 1–3, pp. 147–152, 1989.

[94] A. M. Rasmusson, R. L. Hauger, C. A. Morgan III, J. D. Bremner, D. S. Charney, and S. M. Southwick, "Low baseline and yohimbine-stimulated plasma neuropeptide Y (NPY) levels in combat-related PTSD," *Biological Psychiatry*, vol. 47, no. 6, pp. 526–539, 2000.

[95] B. A. S. Reyes, J. D. Glaser, and E. J. Van Bockstaele, "Ultrastructural evidence for co-localization of corticotropin-releasing factor receptor and μ-opioid receptor in the rat nucleus locus coeruleus," *Neuroscience Letters*, vol. 413, no. 3, pp. 216–221, 2007.

[96] E. J. Van Bockstaele, E. E. O. Colago, and R. J. Valentino, "Amygdaloid corticotropin-releasing factor targets locus coeruleus dendrites: substrate for the co-ordination of emotional and cognitive limbs of the stress response," *Journal of Neuroendocrinology*, vol. 10, no. 10, pp. 743–757, 1998.

[97] D. A. Bangasser, S. R. Eck, A. M. Telenson, and M. Salvatore, "Sex differences in stress regulation of arousal and cognition," *Physiology & Behavior*, vol. 187, pp. 42–50, 2018.

[98] R. C. Kessler, P. Berglund, O. Demler, R. Jin, K. R. Merikangas, and E. E. Walters, "Lifetime prevalence and age-of-onset distributions of DSM-IV disorders in the National Comorbidity Survey Replication," *Archives of General Psychiatry*, vol. 62, no. 6, pp. 593–602, 2005.

[99] T. G. Banke, D. Bowie, H. K. Lee, R. L. Huganir, A. Schousboe, and S. F. Traynelis, "Control of GluR1 AMPA receptor function by cAMP-dependent protein kinase," *The Journal of Neuroscience*, vol. 20, no. 1, pp. 89–102, 2000.

[100] J. A. Esteban, S. H. Shi, C. Wilson, M. Nuriya, R. L. Huganir, and R. Malinow, "PKA phosphorylation of AMPA receptor subunits controls synaptic trafficking underlying plasticity," *Nature Neuroscience*, vol. 6, no. 2, pp. 136–143, 2003.

[101] K. W. Roche, R. J. O'Brien, A. L. Mammen, J. Bernhardt, and R. L. Huganir, "Characterization of multiple phosphorylation sites on the AMPA receptor GluR1 subunit," *Neuron*, vol. 16, no. 6, pp. 1179–1188, 1996.

[102] I. H. Greger, J. F. Watson, and S. G. Cull-Candy, "Structural and functional architecture of AMPA-type glutamate receptors and their auxiliary proteins," *Neuron*, vol. 94, no. 4, pp. 713–730, 2017.

[103] A. S. Kato and J. M. Witkin, "Auxiliary subunits of AMPA receptors: the discovery of a forebrain-selective antagonist, LY3130481/CERC-611," *Biochemical Pharmacology*, vol. 147, pp. 191–200, 2018.

[104] M. G. Kang, Y. Guo, and R. L. Huganir, "AMPA receptor and GEF-H1/Lfc complex regulates dendritic spine development through RhoA signaling cascade," *Proceedings of the National*

Academy of Sciences of the United States of America, vol. 106, no. 9, pp. 3549–3554, 2009.

[105] Z. Szíber, H. Liliom, C. O. O. Morales et al., "Ras and Rab interactor 1 controls neuronal plasticity by coordinating dendritic filopodial motility and AMPA receptor turnover," *Molecular Biology of the Cell*, vol. 28, no. 2, pp. 285–295, 2017.

[106] M. Gesi, P. Soldani, F. S. Giorgi, A. Santinami, I. Bonaccorsi, and F. Fornai, "The role of the locus coeruleus in the development of Parkinson's disease," *Neuroscience & Biobehavioral Reviews*, vol. 24, no. 6, pp. 655–668, 2000.

[107] P. J. McMillan, S. S. White, A. Franklin et al., "Differential response of the central noradrenergic nervous system to the loss of locus coeruleus neurons in Parkinson's disease and Alzheimer's disease," *Brain Research*, vol. 1373, pp. 240–252, 2011.

[108] W. Lu and K. W. Roche, "Posttranslational regulation of AMPA receptor trafficking and function," *Current Opinion in Neurobiology*, vol. 22, no. 3, pp. 470–479, 2012.

[109] J. Widagdo, S. Guntupalli, S. E. Jang, and V. Anggono, "Regulation of AMPA receptor trafficking by protein ubiquitination," *Frontiers in Molecular Neuroscience*, vol. 10, p. 347, 2017.

[110] M. P. Lussier, A. Sanz-Clemente, and K. W. Roche, "Dynamic regulation of N-methyl-d-aspartate (NMDA) and α-amino-3-hydroxy-5-methyl-4-isoxazolepropionic acid (AMPA) receptors by posttranslational modifications," *Journal of Biological Chemistry*, vol. 290, no. 48, pp. 28596–28603, 2015.

[111] A. L. Mammen, K. Kameyama, K. W. Roche, and R. L. Huganir, "Phosphorylation of the α-amino-3-hydroxy-5-methylisoxazole4-propionic acid receptor GluR1 subunit by calcium/calmodulin-dependent kinase II," *Journal of Biological Chemistry*, vol. 272, no. 51, pp. 32528–32533, 1997.

[112] M. A. Jenkins and S. F. Traynelis, "PKC phosphorylates GluA1-Ser831 to enhance AMPA receptor conductance," *Channels*, vol. 6, no. 1, pp. 60–64, 2012.

[113] M. A. Jenkins, G. Wells, J. Bachman et al., "Regulation of GluA1 α-amino-3-hydroxy-5-methyl-4-isoxazolepropionic acid receptor function by protein kinase C at serine-818 and threonine-840," *Molecular Pharmacology*, vol. 85, no. 4, pp. 618–629, 2014.

[114] V. Derkach, A. Barria, and T. R. Soderling, "Ca^{2+}/calmodulin-kinase II enhances channel conductance of α-amino-3-hydroxy-5-methyl-4-isoxazolepropionate type glutamate receptors," *Proceedings of the National Academy of Sciences of the United States of America*, vol. 96, no. 6, pp. 3269–3274, 1999.

[115] S. Q. Ren, J. Z. Yan, X. Y. Zhang et al., "PKCλ is critical in AMPA receptor phosphorylation and synaptic incorporation during LTP," *The EMBO Journal*, vol. 32, no. 10, pp. 1365–1380, 2013.

[116] C. H. Kim, H. J. Chung, H. K. Lee, and R. L. Huganir, "Interaction of the AMPA receptor subunit GluR2/3 with PDZ domains regulates hippocampal long-term depression," *Proceedings of the National Academy of Sciences of the United States of America*, vol. 98, no. 20, pp. 11725–11730, 2001.

[117] J. Xia, H. J. Chung, C. Wihler, R. L. Huganir, and D. J. Linden, "Cerebellar long-term depression requires PKC-regulated interactions between GluR2/3 and PDZ domain–containing proteins," *Neuron*, vol. 28, no. 2, pp. 499–510, 2000.

[118] A. N. Hegde, "The ubiquitin-proteasome pathway and synaptic plasticity," *Learning & Memory*, vol. 17, no. 7, pp. 314–327, 2010.

[119] M. S. Goo, S. L. Scudder, and G. N. Patrick, "Ubiquitin-dependent trafficking and turnover of ionotropic glutamate receptors," *Frontiers in Molecular Neuroscience*, vol. 8, p. 60, 2015.

[120] J. Jiang, V. Suppiramaniam, and M. W. Wooten, "Posttranslational modifications and receptor-associated proteins in AMPA receptor trafficking and synaptic plasticity," *Neurosignals*, vol. 15, no. 5, pp. 266–282, 2006.

[121] E. Y. Yuen, J. Wei, W. Liu, P. Zhong, X. Li, and Z. Yan, "Repeated stress causes cognitive impairment by suppressing glutamate receptor expression and function in prefrontal cortex," *Neuron*, vol. 73, no. 5, pp. 962–977, 2012.

[122] G. Yang, W. Xiong, L. Kojic, and M. S. Cynader, "Subunit-selective palmitoylation regulates the intracellular trafficking of AMPA receptor," *European Journal of Neuroscience*, vol. 30, no. 1, pp. 35–46, 2009.

[123] T. Hayashi, G. Rumbaugh, and R. L. Huganir, "Differential regulation of AMPA receptor subunit trafficking by palmitoylation of two distinct sites," *Neuron*, vol. 47, no. 5, pp. 709–723, 2005.

[124] D. T. Lin, Y. Makino, K. Sharma et al., "Regulation of AMPA receptor extrasynaptic insertion by 4.1N, phosphorylation and palmitoylation," *Nature Neuroscience*, vol. 12, no. 7, pp. 879–887, 2009.

[125] G. M. Thomas and R. L. Huganir, "Palmitoylation-dependent regulation of glutamate receptors and their PDZ domain-containing partners," *Biochemical Society Transactions*, vol. 41, no. 1, pp. 72–78, 2013.

[126] B. K. Brar, A. Chen, M. H. Perrin, and W. Vale, "Specificity and regulation of extracellularly regulated kinase1/2 phosphorylation through corticotropin-releasing factor (CRF) receptors 1 and 2β by the CRF/urocortin family of peptides," *Endocrinology*, vol. 145, no. 4, pp. 1718–1729, 2004.

[127] N. Arimura, C. Menager, Y. Kawano et al., "Phosphorylation by Rho kinase regulates CRMP-2 activity in growth cones," *Molecular and Cellular Biology*, vol. 25, no. 22, pp. 9973–9984, 2005.

[128] M. S. Kwon, Y. J. Seo, E. J. Shim, S. S. Choi, J. Y. Lee, and H. W. Suh, "The effect of single or repeated restraint stress on several signal molecules in paraventricular nucleus, arcuate nucleus and locus coeruleus," *Neuroscience*, vol. 142, no. 4, pp. 1281–1292, 2006.

[129] M. A. Hebert, L. I. Serova, and E. L. Sabban, "Single and repeated immobilization stress differentially trigger induction and phosphorylation of several transcription factors and mitogen-activated protein kinases in the rat locus coeruleus," *Journal of Neurochemistry*, vol. 95, no. 2, pp. 484–498, 2005.

[130] E. J. Nestler, "Chapter six—role of the brain's reward circuitry in depression: transcriptional mechanisms," *International Review of Neurobiology*, vol. 124, pp. 151–170, 2015.

[131] L. Aurelian, K. T. Warnock, I. Balan, A. Puche, and H. June, "TLR4 signaling in VTA dopaminergic neurons regulates impulsivity through tyrosine hydroxylase modulation," *Translational Psychiatry*, vol. 6, no. 5, article e815, 2016.

[132] M. Dierssen, M. Gratacòs, I. Sahún et al., "Transgenic mice overexpressing the full-length neurotrophin receptor TrkC exhibit increased catecholaminergic neuron density in specific brain areas and increased anxiety-like behavior and

panic reaction," *Neurobiology of Disease*, vol. 24, no. 2, pp. 403–418, 2006.

[133] G. A. Zitnik, "Control of arousal through neuropeptide afferents of the locus coeruleus," *Brain Research*, vol. 1641, Part B, pp. 338–350, 2016.

[134] N. Hansen and D. Manahan-Vaughan, "Hippocampal long-term potentiation that is elicited by perforant path stimulation or that occurs in conjunction with spatial learning is tightly controlled by beta-adrenoreceptors and the locus coeruleus," *Hippocampus*, vol. 25, no. 11, pp. 1285–1298, 2015.

[135] N. Hansen and D. Manahan-Vaughan, "Locus coeruleus stimulation facilitates long-term depression in the dentate gyrus that requires activation of β-adrenergic receptors," *Cerebral Cortex*, vol. 25, no. 7, pp. 1889–1896, 2015.

[136] N. Lemon, S. Aydin-Abidin, K. Funke, and D. Manahan-Vaughan, "Locus coeruleus activation facilitates memory encoding and induces hippocampal LTD that depends on β-adrenergic receptor activation," *Cerebral Cortex*, vol. 19, no. 12, pp. 2827–2837, 2009.

[137] A. Marzo, J. Bai, J. Caboche, P. Vanhoutte, and S. Otani, "Cellular mechanisms of long-term depression induced by noradrenaline in rat prefrontal neurons," *Neuroscience*, vol. 169, no. 1, pp. 74–86, 2010.

[138] H. Salgado, M. Trevino, and M. Atzori, "Layer- and area-specific actions of norepinephrine on cortical synaptic transmission," *Brain Research*, vol. 1641, Part B, pp. 163–176, 2016.

[139] A. F. T. Arnsten, "Catecholamine and second messenger influences on prefrontal cortical networks of "representational knowledge": a rational bridge between genetics and the symptoms of mental illness," *Cerebral Cortex*, vol. 17, Supplement 1, pp. i6–15, 2007.

[140] M. Atzori, R. Cuevas-Olguin, E. Esquivel-Rendon et al., "Locus ceruleus norepinephrine release: a central regulator of CNS spatio-temporal activation?," *Frontiers in Synaptic Neuroscience*, vol. 8, p. 25, 2016.

[141] K. Schutsky, M. Ouyang, and S. A. Thomas, "Xamoterol impairs hippocampus-dependent emotional memory retrieval via $G_{i/o}$-coupled β_2-adrenergic signaling," *Learning & Memory*, vol. 18, no. 9, pp. 598–604, 2011.

[142] C. W. Berridge and R. C. Spencer, "Differential cognitive actions of norepinephrine a2 and a1 receptor signaling in the prefrontal cortex," *Brain Research*, vol. 1641, Part B, pp. 189–196, 2016.

[143] S. Amemiya, N. Kubota, N. Umeyama, T. Nishijima, and I. Kita, "Noradrenergic signaling in the medial prefrontal cortex and amygdala differentially regulates vicarious trial-and-error in a spatial decision-making task," *Behavioural Brain Research*, vol. 297, pp. 104–111, 2016.

[144] R. E. Nicholls, J. M. Alarcon, G. Malleret et al., "Transgenic mice lacking NMDAR-dependent LTD exhibit deficits in behavioral flexibility," *Neuron*, vol. 58, no. 1, pp. 104–117, 2008.

[145] C. F. Murchison, X. Y. Zhang, W. P. Zhang, M. Ouyang, A. Lee, and S. A. Thomas, "A distinct role for norepinephrine in memory retrieval," *Cell*, vol. 117, no. 1, pp. 131–143, 2004.

[146] M. Ouyang, M. B. Young, M. M. Lestini, K. Schutsky, and S. A. Thomas, "Redundant catecholamine signaling consolidates fear memory via phospholipase C," *Journal of Neuroscience*, vol. 32, no. 6, pp. 1932–1941, 2012.

[147] F. M. Howells, D. J. Stein, and V. A. Russell, "Synergistic tonic and phasic activity of the locus coeruleus norepinephrine

(LC-NE) arousal system is required for optimal attentional performance," *Metabolic Brain Disease*, vol. 27, no. 3, pp. 267–274, 2012.

[148] S. P. Orr, N. B. Lasko, L. J. Metzger, and R. K. Pitman, "Physiologic responses to non-startling tones in Vietnam veterans with post-traumatic stress disorder," *Psychiatry Research*, vol. 73, no. 1-2, pp. 103–107, 1997.

[149] S. P. Orr, N. B. Lasko, A. Y. Shalev, and R. K. Pitman, "Physiologic responses to loud tones in Vietnam veterans with posttraumatic stress disorder," *Journal of Abnormal Psychology*, vol. 104, no. 1, pp. 75–82, 1995.

[150] S. P. Orr, L. J. Metzger, N. B. Lasko et al., "Physiologic responses to sudden, loud tones in monozygotic twins discordant for combat exposure: association with posttraumatic stress disorder," *Archives of General Psychiatry*, vol. 60, no. 3, pp. 283–288, 2003.

[151] R. K. Pitman and S. P. Orr, "Twenty-four hour urinary cortisol and catecholamine excretion in combat-related posttraumatic stress disorder," *Biological Psychiatry*, vol. 27, no. 2, pp. 245–247, 1990.

[152] R. A. Lanius, D. Rabellino, J. E. Boyd, S. Harricharan, P. A. Frewen, and M. C. McKinnon, "The innate alarm system in PTSD: conscious and subconscious processing of threat," *Current Opinion in Psychology*, vol. 14, pp. 109–115, 2017.

[153] S. Soya, H. Shoji, E. Hasegawa et al., "Orexin receptor-1 in the locus coeruleus plays an important role in cue-dependent fear memory consolidation," *Journal of Neuroscience*, vol. 33, no. 36, pp. 14549–14557, 2013.

[154] A. Uematsu, B. Z. Tan, and J. P. Johansen, "Projection specificity in heterogeneous locus coeruleus cell populations: implications for learning and memory," *Learning & Memory*, vol. 22, no. 9, pp. 444–451, 2015.

[155] A. Uematsu, B. Z. Tan, E. A. Ycu et al., "Modular organization of the brainstem noradrenaline system coordinates opposing learning states," *Nature Neuroscience*, vol. 20, no. 11, pp. 1602–1611, 2017.

[156] T. F. Giustino, P. J. Fitzgerald, and S. Maren, "Revisiting propranolol and PTSD: memory erasure or extinction enhancement?," *Neurobiology of Learning and Memory*, vol. 130, pp. 26–33, 2016.

[157] T. F. Giustino and S. Maren, "Noradrenergic modulation of fear conditioning and extinction," *Frontiers in Behavioral Neuroscience*, vol. 12, p. 43, 2018.

[158] R. J. Ross, W. A. Ball, D. F. Dinges et al., "Rapid eye movement sleep disturbance in posttraumatic stress disorder," *Biological Psychiatry*, vol. 35, no. 3, pp. 195–202, 1994.

[159] R. J. Ross, W. A. Ball, L. D. Sanford et al., "Rapid eye movement sleep changes during the adaptation night in combat veterans with posttraumatic stress disorder," *Biological Psychiatry*, vol. 45, no. 7, pp. 938–941, 1999.

[160] T. A. Mellman, R. Kulick-Bell, L. E. Ashlock, and B. Nolan, "Sleep events among veterans with combat-related posttraumatic stress disorder," *The American Journal of Psychiatry*, vol. 152, no. 1, pp. 110–115, 1995.

[161] M. E. Page, C. W. Berridge, S. L. Foote, and R. J. Valentino, "Corticotropin-releasing factor in the locus coeruleus mediates EEG activation associated with hypotensive stress," *Neuroscience Letters*, vol. 164, no. 1-2, pp. 81–84, 1993.

[162] D. G. Baker, S. A. West, W. E. Nicholson et al., "Serial CSF corticotropin-releasing hormone levels and adrenocortical activity in combat veterans with posttraumatic stress disorder," *American Journal of Psychiatry*, vol. 156, no. 4, pp. 585–588, 1999.

[163] J. D. Bremner, R. B. Innis, C. K. Ng et al., "Positron emission tomography measurement of cerebral metabolic correlates of yohimbine administration in combat-related posttraumatic stress disorder," *Archives of General Psychiatry*, vol. 54, no. 3, pp. 246–254, 1997.

[164] C. S. Fullerton, H. B. Herberman Mash, K. N. Benevides, J. C. Morganstein, and R. J. Ursano, "Distress of routine activities and perceived safety associated with post-traumatic stress, depression, and alcohol use: 2002 Washington, DC, sniper attacks," *Disaster Medicine and Public Health Preparedness*, vol. 9, no. 5, pp. 509–515, 2015.

[165] H. Hagena, N. Hansen, and D. Manahan-Vaughan, "β-adrenergic control of hippocampal function: subserving the choreography of synaptic information storage and memory," *Cerebral Cortex*, vol. 26, no. 4, pp. 1349–1364, 2016.

[166] B. Huang, H. Zhu, Y. Zhou, X. Liu, and L. Ma, "Unconditioned- and conditioned- stimuli induce differential memory reconsolidation and β-AR-dependent CREB activation," *Frontiers in Neural Circuits*, vol. 11, p. 53, 2017.

[167] H. Villain, A. Benkahoul, P. Birmes, B. Ferry, and P. Roullet, "Influence of early stress on memory reconsolidation: implications for post-traumatic stress disorder treatment," *PLoS One*, vol. 13, no. 1, article e0191563, 2018.

[168] M. A. Raskind, D. J. Dobie, E. D. Kanter, E. C. Petrie, C. E. Thompson, and E. R. Peskind, "The α_1-adrenergic antagonist prazosin ameliorates combat trauma nightmares in veterans with posttraumatic stress disorder: a report of 4 cases," *The Journal of Clinical Psychiatry*, vol. 61, no. 2, pp. 129–134, 2000.

[169] B. R. Keeshin, Q. Ding, A. P. Presson, S. J. Berkowitz, and J. R. Strawn, "Use of prazosin for pediatric PTSD-associated nightmares and sleep disturbances: a retrospective chart review," *Neurology and Therapy*, vol. 6, no. 2, pp. 247–257, 2017.

[170] M. A. Raskind, E. R. Peskind, E. D. Kanter et al., "Reduction of nightmares and other PTSD symptoms in combat veterans by prazosin: a placebo-controlled study," *American Journal of Psychiatry*, vol. 160, no. 2, pp. 371–373, 2003.

[171] R. H. Pietrzak, J. D. Gallezot, Y. S. Ding et al., "Association of posttraumatic stress disorder with reduced in vivo norepinephrine transporter availability in the locus coeruleus," *JAMA Psychiatry*, vol. 70, no. 11, pp. 1199–1205, 2013.

[172] I. Liberzon and K. L. Phan, "Brain-imaging studies of posttraumatic stress disorder," *CNS Spectrums*, vol. 8, no. 9, pp. 641–650, 2003.

[173] H. S. Bracha, E. Garcia-Rill, R. E. Mrak, and R. Skinner, "Postmortem locus coeruleus neuron count in three American veterans with probable or possible war-related PTSD," *The Journal of Neuropsychiatry and Clinical Neurosciences*, vol. 17, no. 4, pp. 503–509, 2005.

[174] W. J. G. Hoogendijk, M. G. P. Feenstra, M. H. A. Botterblom et al., "Increased activity of surviving locus ceruleus neurons in Alzheimer's disease," *Annals of Neurology*, vol. 45, no. 1, pp. 82–91, 1999.

[175] A. A. Feduccia and M. C. Mithoefer, "MDMA-assisted psychotherapy for PTSD: are memory reconsolidation and fear extinction underlying mechanisms?," *Progress in Neuro-Psychopharmacology & Biological Psychiatry*, vol. 84, Part A, pp. 221–228, 2018.

[176] M. B. Young, R. Andero, K. J. Ressler, and L. L. Howell, "3,4-Methylenedioxymethamphetamine facilitates fear extinction learning," *Translational Psychiatry*, vol. 5, no. 9, article e634, 2015.

[177] A. L. Curtis, S. M. Lechner, L. A. Pavcovich, and R. J. Valentino, "Activation of the locus coeruleus noradrenergic system by intracoerular microinfusion of corticotropin-releasing factor: effects on discharge rate, cortical norepinephrine levels and cortical electroencephalographic activity," *Journal of Pharmacology and Experimental Therapeutics*, vol. 281, no. 1, pp. 163–172, 1997.

[178] A. Asok, J. Schulkin, and J. B. Rosen, "Corticotropin releasing factor type-1 receptor antagonism in the dorsolateral bed nucleus of the stria terminalis disrupts contextually conditioned fear, but not unconditioned fear to a predator odor," *Psychoneuroendocrinology*, vol. 70, pp. 17–24, 2016.

[179] G. Aston-Jones, M. T. Shipley, G. Chouvet et al., "Chapter 4 - afferent regulation of locus coeruleus neurons: anatomy, physiology and pharmacology," *Progress in Brain Research*, vol. 88, pp. 47–75, 1991.

[180] G. F. Koob, S. C. Heinrichs, F. Menzaghi, E. M. Pich, and K. T. Britton, "Corticotropin releasing factor, stress and behavior," *Seminars in Neuroscience*, vol. 6, no. 4, pp. 221–229, 1994.

[181] S. Kratzer, C. Mattusch, M. W. Metzger et al., "Activation of CRH receptor type 1 expressed on glutamatergic neurons increases excitability of CA1 pyramidal neurons by the modulation of voltage-gated ion channels," *Frontiers in Cellular Neuroscience*, vol. 7, p. 91, 2013.

[182] A. R. Howerton, A. V. Roland, J. M. Fluharty et al., "Sex differences in corticotropin-releasing factor receptor-1 action within the dorsal raphe nucleus in stress responsivity," *Biological Psychiatry*, vol. 75, no. 11, pp. 873–883, 2014.

[183] L. G. Kirby, E. Freeman-Daniels, J. C. Lemos et al., "Corticotropin-releasing factor increases GABA synaptic activity and induces inward current in 5-hydroxytryptamine dorsal raphe neurons," *Journal of Neuroscience*, vol. 28, no. 48, pp. 12927–12937, 2008.

[184] C. M. Lamy and S. G. Beck, "Swim stress differentially blocks CRF receptor mediated responses in dorsal raphe nucleus," *Psychoneuroendocrinology*, vol. 35, no. 9, pp. 1321–1332, 2010.

[185] K. D. Holmes, A. V. Babwah, L. B. Dale, M. O. Poulter, and S. S. G. Ferguson, "Differential regulation of corticotropin releasing factor 1α receptor endocytosis and trafficking by β-arrestins and Rab GTPases," *Journal of Neurochemistry*, vol. 96, no. 4, pp. 934–949, 2006.

[186] R. Zhao-Shea, S. R. DeGroot, L. Liu et al., "Increased CRF signalling in a ventral tegmental area-interpeduncular nucleus-medial habenula circuit induces anxiety during nicotine withdrawal," *Nature Communications*, vol. 6, no. 1, p. 6770, 2015.

[187] N. V. Gounko, J. D. Swinny, D. Kalicharan et al., "Corticotropin-releasing factor and urocortin regulate spine and synapse formation: structural basis for stress-induced neuronal remodeling and pathology," *Molecular Psychiatry*, vol. 18, no. 1, pp. 86–92, 2013.

[188] D. A. Bangasser, "Sex differences in stress-related receptors: "micro" differences with "macro" implications for mood and anxiety disorders," *Biology of Sex Differences*, vol. 4, no. 1, p. 2, 2013.

[189] F. G. Graeff, "Neuroanatomy and neurotransmitter regulation of defensive behaviors and related emotions in mammals," *Brazilian Journal of Medical and Biological Research*, vol. 27, no. 4, pp. 811–829, 1994.

[190] K. L. Widnell, J. S. Chen, P. A. Iredale et al., "Transcriptional regulation of CREB (cyclic AMP response element-binding protein) expression in CATH.a cells," *Journal of Neurochemistry*, vol. 66, no. 4, pp. 1770–1773, 1996.

[191] M. P. Lussier, Y. Nasu-Nishimura, and K. W. Roche, "Activity-dependent ubiquitination of the AMPA receptor subunit GluA2," *Journal of Neuroscience*, vol. 31, no. 8, pp. 3077–3081, 2011.

[192] R. Malinow and R. C. Malenka, "AMPA receptor trafficking and synaptic plasticity," *Annual Review of Neuroscience*, vol. 25, no. 1, pp. 103–126, 2002.

[193] B. Aisa, R. Tordera, B. Lasheras, J. del Río, and M. J. Ramírez, "Cognitive impairment associated to HPA axis hyperactivity after maternal separation in rats," *Psychoneuroendocrinology*, vol. 32, no. 3, pp. 256–266, 2007.

[194] R. J. Valentino, B. Reyes, E. van Bockstaele, and D. Bangasser, "Molecular and cellular sex differences at the intersection of stress and arousal," *Neuropharmacology*, vol. 62, no. 1, pp. 13–20, 2012.

2

Functional Connectivity Alterations in Children with Spastic and Dyskinetic Cerebral Palsy

Yun Qin [ID],[1] Yanan Li,[2] Bo Sun,[1] Hui He [ID],[1] Rui Peng,[1] Tao Zhang [ID],[1] Jianfu Li,[1] Cheng Luo [ID],[1] Chengyan Sun [ID],[2] and Dezhong Yao [ID][1]

[1]*The Clinical Hospital of Chengdu Brain Science Institute, MOE Key Lab for Neuroinformation, High-Field Magnetic Resonance Brain Imaging Key Laboratory of Sichuan Province, University of Electronic Science and Technology of China, Chengdu 610054, China*
[2]*Sichuan Rehabilitation Hospital, Chengdu, China*

Correspondence should be addressed to Cheng Luo; chengluo@uestc.edu.cn and Chengyan Sun; 279798774@qq.com

Academic Editor: Carlo Cavaliere

Cerebral palsy (CP) has long been investigated to be associated with a range of motor and cognitive dysfunction. As the two most common CP subtypes, spastic cerebral palsy (SCP) and dyskinetic cerebral palsy (DCP) may share common and distinct elements in their pathophysiology. However, the common and distinct dysfunctional characteristics between SCP and DCP on the brain network level are less known. This study aims to detect the alteration of brain functional connectivity in children with SCP and DCP based on resting-state functional MRI (fMRI). Resting-state networks (RSNs) were established based on the independent component analysis (ICA), and the functional network connectivity (FNC) was performed on the fMRI data from 16 DCP, 18 bilateral SCP, and 18 healthy children. Compared with healthy controls, altered functional connectivity within the cerebellum network, sensorimotor network (SMN), left frontoparietal network (LFPN), and salience network (SN) were found in DCP and SCP groups. Furthermore, the disconnections of the FNC consistently focused on the visual pathway; covariance of the default mode network (DMN) with other networks was observed both in DCP and SCP groups, while the DCP group had a distinct connectivity abnormality in motor pathway and self-referential processing-related connections. Correlations between the functional disconnection and the motor-related clinical measurement in children with CP were also found. These findings indicate functional connectivity impairment and altered integration widely exist in children with CP, suggesting that the abnormal functional connectivity is a pathophysiological mechanism of motor and cognitive dysfunction of CP.

1. Introduction

Cerebral palsy (CP) is the most common cause of physical disability in early childhood, occurring at a rate of around 2 per 1000 live births [1, 2]. CP encompasses a range of motor and postural disorders resulting from nonprogressive injury during the prenatal or infant development, causing serious activity limitation often accompanied by various degrees of sensation and cognition impairments [3, 4]. Spastic cerebral palsy (SCP) is the most common CP subtype, which is usually presented with bilateral spastic or hemiplegic disability with increased muscle tone, hyperreflexia, and persistence of primitive reflexes [5]. Dyskinetic CP (DCP) is the second common subtype, affecting 15%–20% of children with CP

[6]. The new definition of dyskinetic CP includes dystonic and choreoathetoid CP, which is characterized by abnormal movement or posture, with involuntary, recurring, uncontrolled, and occasionally stereotyped movements [7, 8]. Besides motor function impairment, both SCP and DCP subtypes tend to be associated with visual and auditory impairment and cognitive impairments such as intellectual and learning disability [1, 7]. Furthermore, evidence points to abnormal sensorimotor reorganization, attention, and executive function deficits, as well as visual-perceptual impairments in children with DCP and SCP [9–11].

The wide array of dysfunction in CP is due to the heterogeneous nature of the underlying cerebral lesions. Depending on the location, extent, and timing of the insult, clinical symptoms vary largely [12]. Brain maldevelopment, white matter (WM) lesions, basal ganglia lesions, and cortical/subcortical lesions [13, 14] are the most common pathological findings in CP. Bilateral spastic CP (diplegia and tetraplegia) is foremost associated with white matter injury especially periventricular leukomalacia (PVL), in particular in children born preterm or prolonged hypoxic-ischemic events [15, 16]. Some MR studies have showed that brain injury pattern of DCP was associated with basal ganglia and thalamic injury following profound hypoxic insults and commonly seen in term infants [17, 18]. Cortical injury and WM involvement have also been reported in DCP cases [13]. Nevertheless, the heterogeneity among neuroimaging studies makes it ambiguous to systematically understand the relationship between the dysfunction and the brain state in children with CP.

Previous studies have widely applied diffusion tensor imaging to focus on the microstructural damage of white matter fiber tract of CP [19, 20]. Inverse correlation was found between the quantitative indicators of sensory-motor tracts and gross motor clinical grade in CP group [21]. In addition, some voxel-based morphometry studies have investigated that the gray matter abnormality in CP was associated with clinical features [22–24]. However, the common and distinguished brain dysfunctional characteristics associated with clinical features between DCP and SCP are relatively less explored.

Functional magnetic resonance imaging (fMRI) has been effectively used in children with CP to map the regional motor and cognitive processing [25–27]. Applications of fMRI in children with CP have mainly focused on the somatosensory, motor, and language tasks which are directly associated with the sensorimotor dysfunction in CP [28, 29]. Other cognitive impairments widely existing in children with CP, such as visual-perceptual, attention, and executive function [9–11, 30], are less explored because performing relative tasks during fMRI scanning may be difficult for children with CP. In contrast, the resting-state fMRI scanning is simple and easy to execute for these children [31]. Functional connectivity, referring to an analysis for identifying spatial patterns of coherent BOLD activity in distributed brain regions, has been used to detect the abnormal pathways (e.g., somatosensory, motor, and thalamocortical pathway) in children with CP using resting-state fMRI data [22, 32, 33]. For defining distinct modes of long-distance interactions, independent component analysis (ICA) has been a popular method to generate resting-state networks (RSNs) [34, 35], and resting-state functional network connectivity (FNC) [36] can be used to represent the temporal correlation among these RSNs. Therefore, investigations of the RSNs and FNC may provide more information to advance the understanding of the underlying physiopathology mechanisms in children with SCP and DCP. We hypothesized that common and distinct functional connectivity patterns may exist in SCP and DCP.

To test our hypothesis, 16 children with DCP, 18 children with SCP, and 18 healthy controls were included to explore the resting-state functional connectivity within and between RSNs. Group-level independent component analysis [37, 38] was used to extract the RSNs, and FNC analysis was

performed. Group comparisons were then conducted for RSNs and FNC. The relationship between functional disconnection and motor-related clinical measurement in CP was also examined.

2. Material and Methods

2.1. Participants. A total of 43 children with CP were recruited from Sichuan Rehabilitation Hospital: 22 DCP (10 female, mean age: 9 years, age range: 3–18 years) and 21 SCP (10 female, mean age: 9.2 years, age range: 3–16 years) were involved. The diagnosis for the two subtypes of CP was made through standardized assessment by neurologists based on clinical features and MRI scanning [7]. All children with SCP were diplegic, and all children with DCP were dystonic. The inclusion criteria for the study were as follows: (1) a diagnosis of DCP and SCP with predominant spastic diplegic or dyskinetic features, (2) age under 18 years old, and (3) no history of trauma or brain operation. Children with serious brain loss or lesions (lesion size > 1 cm^3, including 4 DCP children and 2 SCP children) were excluded based on MRI brain image. No child was on medication. 20 healthy children without history of neurological disorder or brain injury (7 female, mean age: 9.3, age range: 5–12) were included in the healthy control group (HC). Parents of all participants gave written informed consent in accordance with the Declaration of Helsinki. This study was performed according to the guidelines approved by the Ethics Committee of the University of Electronic Science and Technology of China (UESTC).

2.2. Clinical Measurement. Motor function was assessed for the DCP and SCP groups by the Gross Motor Function Classification System (GMFCS) [39]. GMFCS scores range from level I, which indicates children with no disability for community mobility, to level V, which includes children who are totally dependent on assistance for mobility. Everyday activities of daily living (ADL) [40] were also evaluated by the Assessment of Motor and Process Skills (AMPS) to access the self-care ability during everyday life. Both GMFCS and ADL evaluations were conducted by physical therapists in the Rehabilitation Assessment Department, Sichuan Rehabilitation Hospital.

2.3. Imaging Data Acquisition. Images were acquired on a 3 T MRI scanner (GE Discovery MR750) at the MRI Research Center of UESTC. Children with CP underwent MRI scanning under monitored sedation induced by midazolam (0.1 mg/kg) and propofol (1-2 mg/kg), which is approved by the Department of Anaesthesia of the Sichuan Rehabilitation Hospital, and written informed consent was obtained from participants' parents. The HC children were instructed simply to keep their eyes closed and remain still without sedation. The same scanning protocol was used for both CP and HC children as follows. High-resolution T1-weighted images were acquired using a 3-dimensional fast spoiled gradient-echo (T1-3D FSPGR) sequence (repetition time (TR) = 5.956 ms, echo time (TE) = 1.964 ms, flip angle (FA) = 9°, matrix = 256 × 256, field of view (FOV) = $25.6 \times 25.6 \, \text{cm}^2$, slice thickness = 1 mm, no gap, 152 slices). T2 images were also acquired using OAx T2 fluid-attenuated inversion recovery (OAx T2 FLAIR) (TR = 8400 ms, TE = 150 ms, FA = 111°, matrix = 256 × 256, FOV = $25.6 \times 25.6 \, \text{cm}^2$, slice thickness = 4 mm). Resting-state functional MRI data were acquired using gradient-echo echo-planar imaging sequences (TR = 2000 ms, TE = 30 ms, FA = 90°, matrix = 64 × 64, FOV = $24 \times 24 \, \text{cm}^2$, slice thickness/gap = 4 mm/0.4 mm), with an eight channel-phased array head coil. A total of 255 volumes were collected from each participant.

2.4. fMRI Preprocessing. Data preprocessing was performed using SPM8 (statistical parametric mapping, http://www.fil.ion.ucl.ac.uk/spm/). The first ten volumes were discarded for the magnetization equilibrium from all fMRI scans. Then, the remaining images were slice-timing corrected and realigned (motion-corrected). The transition and rotation parameters were checked, and given the relatively large head motion of the children or teenagers during fMRI scanning, we increased the motion threshold to 3 mm for head movement and 3° for head rotation as the exclusion standard just as other studies did with adolescent participants [41–43]. Group comparison was performed for the individual mean framewise displacement (FD) calculated by averaging the relative displacement from every time point for each subject [44], and no difference was found between the groups (one-way ANOVA, $P = 0.2439$). The formula to calculate the FD is

$$\text{FD} = \frac{1}{M-1} \sum_{i=2}^{M} \sqrt{\left|\Delta t_{x_i}\right|^2 + \left|\Delta t_{y_i}\right|^2 + \left|\Delta t_{z_i}\right|^2 + \left|\Delta d_{x_i}\right|^2 + \left|\Delta d_{y_i}\right|^2 + \left|\Delta d_{z_i}\right|^2},$$

(1)

where M is the length of the time courses; x_i, y_i, and z_i are translations/rotations at the ith time point in the x, y, and z directions, respectively; Δt represents the framewise displacement translation; Δd represents the framewise displacement rotation; and $\Delta d_{x_i} = x_i - x_{i-1}$, similar for Δd_{yi}, Δd_{zi}, Δt_{xi}, Δt_{yi}, and Δt_{zi}.

Spatial normalization was performed using the T1-based transformation. The individual T1 images were coregistered to the functional images and then segmented and normalized to the Montreal Neurologic Institute (MNI) space by a 12-parameter nonlinear transformation. Additionally, we used a cost-function modification to exclude the lesion area avoiding bias during spatial normalization [45]. The process has been implemented in SPM8 and adopted in other brain imaging studies with lesions in our lab [46]. The transformation parameters were applied to functional images. Then, functional data were resampled to $3 \times 3 \times 3 \, \text{mm}^3$ voxels after spatial normalization. Moreover, the images were spatially smoothed through convolution with a 6 mm full-width half-maximum (FWHM) Gaussian kernel.

2.5. Lesion Mapping. In this study, we constructed a lesion overlap image of CP. First, a radiologist marked the gray matter lesions on individual 3D T1 images. The lesions in this study mainly covered some voxels in the occipital region for one child and basal ganglia region for four children. Then,

the union of all individual lesions was used to construct a group lesion mask after the spatial normalization process. At last, a specific group mask was generated from the gray matter template excluding the patients' group lesion mask for the next ICA analysis.

2.6. Independent Component Analysis. As a data-driven statistical analysis technique, ICA processing yields independent components (ICs) which represent a group of brain regions with a unique pattern of synchronized neural activity. Components with special spatial pattern can be selected as resting-state networks. For all CP children and healthy controls, group ICA analysis was performed to decompose the data into ICs using GIFT software [38] (version 2.0e; http://mialab.mrn.org/software/gift/). The specific group mask excluding the CP lesion mask was used in the group ICA. Principal component analysis (PCA) was adopted for the reduction of data dimensionality. The number of ICs was determined according to the minimum description length (MDL) [47]. In ICASSO (http://research.ics.tkk.fi/ica/icasso), the infomax algorithm was repeated 20 times as an independent component estimation. Then, the dual-regression (DR) approach was used in the back reconstruction step to back reconstruct the individual participant components [48]. Thus, IC time courses and spatial maps were acquired for each participant, and the participant-specific maps were converted to Z-score. In addition, for the validation of the selection of the separated ICs, we implemented the ICA using different independent component numbers (model order) and severally conducted the following analysis (i.e., within RSN analysis and FNC analysis) for seven times.

2.7. Within RSN Analysis. Among the 39 components resulting from ICA, 14 components were selected as non-artifactual RSNs through visual inspection in accordance with previously published results [49–52]. For each of the RSNs, Z-maps in each group were firstly gathered using the one-sample t-test for revealing group main effects, and the resulting statistical map was thresholded at $P < 0.05$ using the false discovery rate (FDR) correction. Then, group comparison was conducted for the Z-maps of the RSN using one-way ANOVA restricted to the voxels within a union mask, which was defined by the one-sample t-test results in three groups. Between-group effects were thresholded at $P < 0.05$ with voxel-wise FDR correction, and the minimum cluster size was 25 voxels. Regions (3*3*3 voxels) with high significant difference in ANOVA were chosen from each RSN and used in the post hoc analysis. During the one-way ANOVA and post hoc analysis, age and sex, as well as head-motion variables, were treated as unconcerned covariates.

2.8. FNC Analysis between RSNs. After ICA, the individual-level time courses of the identified RSNs were derived from the spatial-temporal dual regression. In order to investigate the relationship between time courses of different RSNs, FNC analysis was performed. First, temporal band-pass filter (band pass 0.01–0.1 Hz) was used to reduce the effects of low-frequency drift and high-frequency physiological noise on the time courses. Then, correlations were computed between the time courses of any two of the RSNs for each participant. Thus, individual potential internetwork connections (91 connections) were generated. After Fisher Z-translation of the correlation coefficients, one-sample t-test ($P = 0.05$, corrected by FDR) was applied to examine the significant temporal interactions between any two RSNs in DCP, SCP, and HC groups, respectively. To better understand the group difference of FNC, one-way ANOVA was performed for all potential connections between RSNs, with the significance cutoff $P < 0.05$ corrected by FDR to control for multiple comparisons. Then, the post hoc comparison ($P < 0.01$) was used to the connections with statistical significance in the ANOVA between groups. During the one-way ANOVA and post hoc analysis, age and sex, as well as head-motion variables, were treated as unconcerned covariates.

2.9. Correlations with Clinical Measurement. Correlations were calculated between the functional connectivity in RSNs/FNC and the clinical measurements of CP. For each RSN, the regions ($3*3*3$ voxels) with a peak F value in the ANOVA were selected as regions of interest (ROIs), and the coordinates of the ROIs were extracted. Then, the mean Z-scores within the ROI was used for the following correlation calculation. In addition, the coefficients of FNC with high significance in ANOVA were also used to calculate the correlation with the GMFCS and ADL scores.

2.10. Statistical Analyses. Before statistical analyses, normality of the data distribution was tested using the Lilliefors test, including the age, ADL scores, Z-map of RSNs for each voxel, and FNC connections. Then, to investigate the group difference for demographic and clinical data, chi-square test was applied to the categorical data including gender and GMFCS scores; one-way ANOVA and two-sample t-test were used for age and ADL scores, respectively. For RSN and FNC analysis, group comparison among the three groups was performed using one-way ANOVA. Significant differences revealed by ANOVA ($P < 0.05$, corrected by FDR) were further analyzed for multiple comparisons using Tukey's post hoc test. In addition, relationship between functional connectivity and clinical scores was examined using Pearson correlation for ADL and Spearman correlation for GMFCS, with statistical significance level $P < 0.05$ corrected by FDR. The voxel-level statistical analysis of RSNs was conducted using SPM8 (statistical parametric mapping), and the other statistical analysis, including the FNC group comparison and the correlation, was conducted using MATLAB functions (MATLAB 2015).

3. Results

3.1. Participants and Clinical and Radiological Findings. After the fMRI data head-motion checking, the final cohort in this study consisted of 16 DCP, 18 SCP, and 18 HC children. No significant difference was found for age and gender among the three groups (one-way ANOVA for age, $P = 0.818$; chi-square test for gender, $P = 0.907$). Comparing to SCP, DCP showed higher GMFCS (chi-square test, $P = 0.003$) and lower ADL (two-sample t-test, $P < 0.001$), indicating more severe

motor and daily activity disability in the DCP group. Cerebral abnormalities were evaluated by two radiologists according to the high-resolution T1 (3D FSPGR) and T2 (OAx T2 FLAIR) images. Among 36 children, 5 children have gray matter lesions involving 1 child with small occipital lesion and 4 children with basal ganglia abnormality, mainly located in the bilateral putamen. 21 children have predominant white mater lesion types consisting of periventricular leukomalacia, ventricular enlargement, and other local white matter lesions. Demographic and clinical data of the sample were shown in Table 1.

3.2. RSN Identifications. Fourteen components were selected as the resting-state relevant networks from the group ICA in accordance with the previously published results [35, 51]. No clusters in each RSN fell within the lesion of any of the children. The spatial maps of the 14 RSNs are illustrated in Figure 1. These networks are labeled as follows: *cerebellum*: the spatial patterns primarily encompassed the cerebellum posterior lobe and declive; *SMN1*: sensorimotor network included the paracentral lobule, the supplementary motor area, and the pre- and postcentral gyrus; *SMN2*: sensorimotor network focused at the bilateral primary somatosensory cortex, including pre- and postcentral gyrus areas; *DAN*: dorsal attention network mainly included the bilateral intraparietal sulcus, frontal eye field, and middle temporal lobe; *antDMN*: the anterior part of default mode network (DMN) (antDMN) included the superior frontal gyrus and middle frontal gyrus; *postDMN*: the posterior part of DMN involved the posterior cingulate cortex (PCC), precuneus, and bilateral angular gyrus; *SRN*: the self-referential network mainly included the anterior cingulate and bilateral medial-ventral prefrontal cortex; *primVN*: the primary visual network showed the spatial patterns consisting of the cuneus, calcarine, and lateral lingual gyrus; *extraVN*: the extrastriate visual network encompassed the bilateral fusiform gyrus, middle temporal, and middle occipital areas; *AN*: the auditory network primarily encompassed middle temporal gyrus and superior temporal gyrus corresponding to the auditory system; *LFPN*: the left lateral frontoparietal network involved the left middle frontal gyrus, inferior parietal lobule, superior parietal lobule, and angular gyrus; *RFPN*: the right lateral frontoparietal network showed the similar spatial patterns with LFPN. LFPN and RFPN were the only maps strongly lateralized and left-right mirrors of each other; *SN*: the salience network showed spatial patterns mainly consisting of dorsal anterior cingulate (dACC) and orbital frontoinsular cortices, as well as part of prefrontal areas; *CEN*: the central executive network showed spatial patterns comprising the superior and middle frontal cortices, anterior cingulate, and paracingulate gyri. The group-level spatial maps of 14 RSNs for HC, SCP, and DCP were shown in Supplementary Material Figure S1.

3.3. Group Comparisons of Functional Connectivity within RSNs. Group comparison of functional connectivity within RSNs was performed using one-way ANOVA. Significant difference among the DCP, SCP, and HC groups was found within four RSNs ($P < 0.05$, corrected by FDR),

TABLE 1: Demographic and clinical data of the sample.

	DCP	SCP	HC	P value
Number of participants (N)	16	18	18	
Age (mean years ± std)	9.6 ± 5.0	8.9 ± 3.1	9.5 ± 2.2	0.818
Gender	10 M, 6 F	10 M, 8 F	11 M, 7 F	0.907
GMFCS	II: 3, III: 7, IV: 5, V: 1	I: 9, II: 5, III: 4		0.003
ADL (mean scores ± std)	38.44 ± 18	82.55 ± 3.4		<0.001
Neuroimage finding (N)				
White matter lesion	6	15		
Cortical gray matter abnormality	1	0		
Basal ganglia/thalamus abnormality	3	1		
Normal (N)	6	2		

M: male; F: female; std: standard deviation; N: number of participants. P value: comparisons for age and gender among the three groups: the variable gender was analyzed using chi-square test, while the age was analyzed using ANOVA; comparisons for GMFCS and ADL between DCP and SCP: the variable GMFCS was analyzed using chi-square test, while the ADL were analyzed using two-sample t-test.

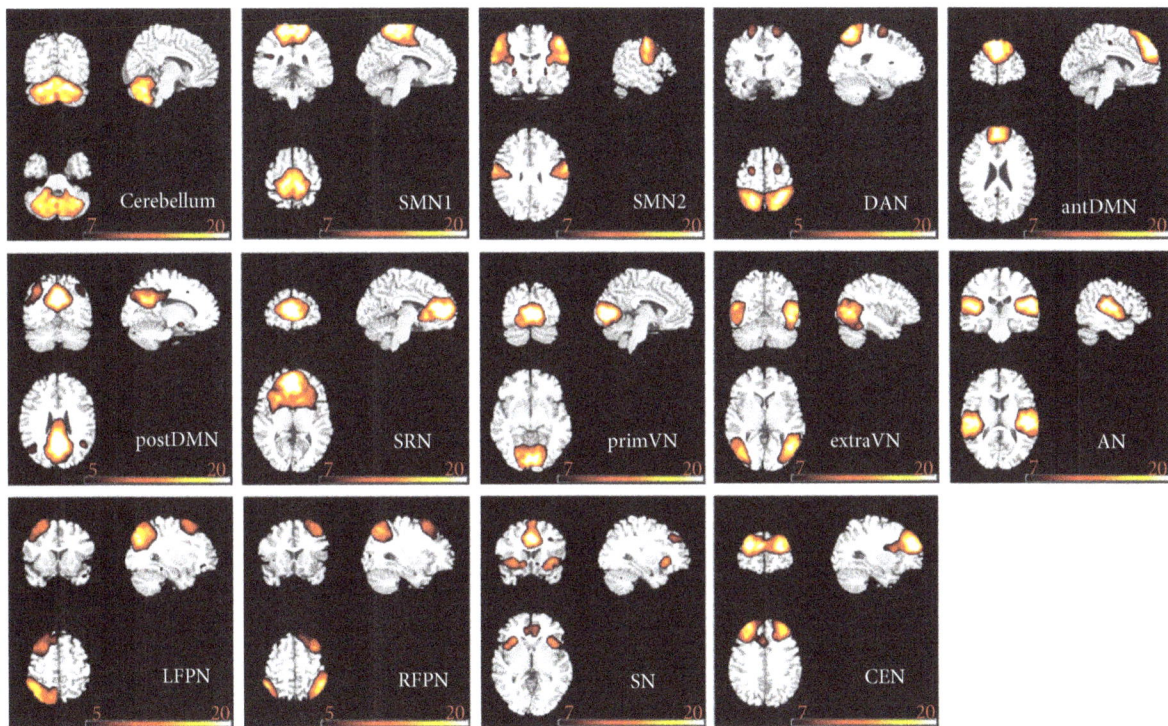

FIGURE 1: The spatial patterns of 14 RSNs identified according to the group ICA in all children. SMN: sensorimotor network; DAN: dorsal attention network; antDMN: the anterior part of default mode network; postDMN: the posterior part of default mode network; SRN: the self-referential network; primVN: the primary visual network; extraVN: the extrastriate visual network; AN: the auditory network; LFPN: the left lateral frontoparietal network; RFPN: the right lateral frontoparietal network; SN: the salience network; CEN: the central executive network.

including the cerebellum network, SMN2, LFPN, and SN (Table 2). Post hoc analysis between the groups was performed within the regions where significant difference was observed in the three groups (Table 3, Table 4). Figure 2 showed differences between the groups. Compared with HC, both DCP and SCP illustrated decreased functional connectivity within the cerebellum network, SMN2, and LFPN. Moreover, the SN revealed not only the reduced functional connectivity in middle frontal and superior frontal gyrus but also the increased functional connectivity in the anterior cingulum (ACC) in CP. No significant difference was found for functional connectivity within RSNs between the DCP and SCP group. In addition, according to the validation analysis using different independent component numbers in ICA processing, the results of functional connectivity within RSNs were mostly repeated in calculations seven times (details shown in Supplementary Material Figure S2).

TABLE 2: Significant differences of functional connectivity within four RSNs in one-way ANOVA comparison among the three groups (ANOVA, $P < 0.05$ FDR-corrected).

Networks	AAL regions	MNI coordinates			Peak F value	Cluster voxels
		x	y	z		
	Cerebelum_Crus1_R	27	−78	−36	31.3056	63
	Cerebelum_Crus2_R	33	−70	−38	19.3594	76
Cerebellum	Cerebelum_8_R	28	−65	−45	20.8600	54
	Cerebelum_Crus2_L	−15	−78	−33	19.4947	49
	Cerebelum_Crus1_L	−20	−74	−34	17.5934	43
SMN2	Postcentral_L	−54	−6	27	24.0388	25
	Parietal_Inf_L	−36	−72	39	21.8592	80
LFPN	Angular_L	−38	−66	43	16.813	37
	Occipital_Mid_L	−38	−69	41	19.2070	20
	Cingulum_Ant_L	−6	30	15	20.2391	47
SN	Frontal_Mid_R	33	36	30	17.3654	58
	Frontal_Sup_L	−18	39	36	22.8588	43
	Frontal_Mid_L	−30	34	37	14.0513.	39

MNI: Montreal Neurologic Institute; AAL: anatomical automatic labeling.

TABLE 3: Significant differences of functional connectivity within four RSNs between DCP and HC ($P < 0.001$).

Networks	AAL regions	MNI coordinates			Peak T value	Cluster voxels
		x	y	z		
	Cerebelum_Crus1_R	27	−78	−36	−6.9746	65
	Cerebelum_Crus2_R	22	−74	−39	−5.2359	74
Cerebellum	Cerebelum_8_R	21	−69	−40	−5.5828	47
	Cerebelum_Crus2_L	−15	−78	−33	−5.8267	47
	Cerebelum_Crus1_L	−20	−73	−34	−5.1369	54
SMN2	Postcentral_L	−51	−9	27	−6.5683	25
LFPN	Parietal_Inf_L	−36	−71	42	−5.0843	54
	Angular_L	−39	−66	42	−5.6904	36
	Frontal_Mid_R	30	36	27	−6.3314	48
SN	Frontal_Sup_L	−18	39	36	−7.1288	38
	Frontal_Mid_L	−30	34	38	−4.3143	39

MNI: Montreal Neurologic Institute; AAL: anatomical automatic labeling.

TABLE 4: Significant differences of functional connectivity within four RSNs between SCP and HC ($P < 0.001$).

Networks	AAL regions	MNI coordinates			Peak T value	Cluster voxels
		x	y	z		
	Cerebelum_Crus1_R	24	−75	−33	−5.5275	26
Cerebellum	Cerebelum_Crus2_R	29	−66	−41	−5.2380	27
	Cerebelum_8_R	28	−66	−44	−5.4002	42
SMN2	Postcentral_L	−51	−6	30	−5.722	25
LFPN	Parietal_Inf_L	−45	−54	51	−6.7446	78
	Cingulum_Ant_L	−3	33	15	6.9291	47
SN	Frontal_Mid_R	33	36	36	−5.3502	49
	Frontal_Sup_L	−24	39	36	−5.9748	30

MNI: Montreal Neurologic Institute; AAL: anatomical automatic labeling.

(a)

(b)

(c)

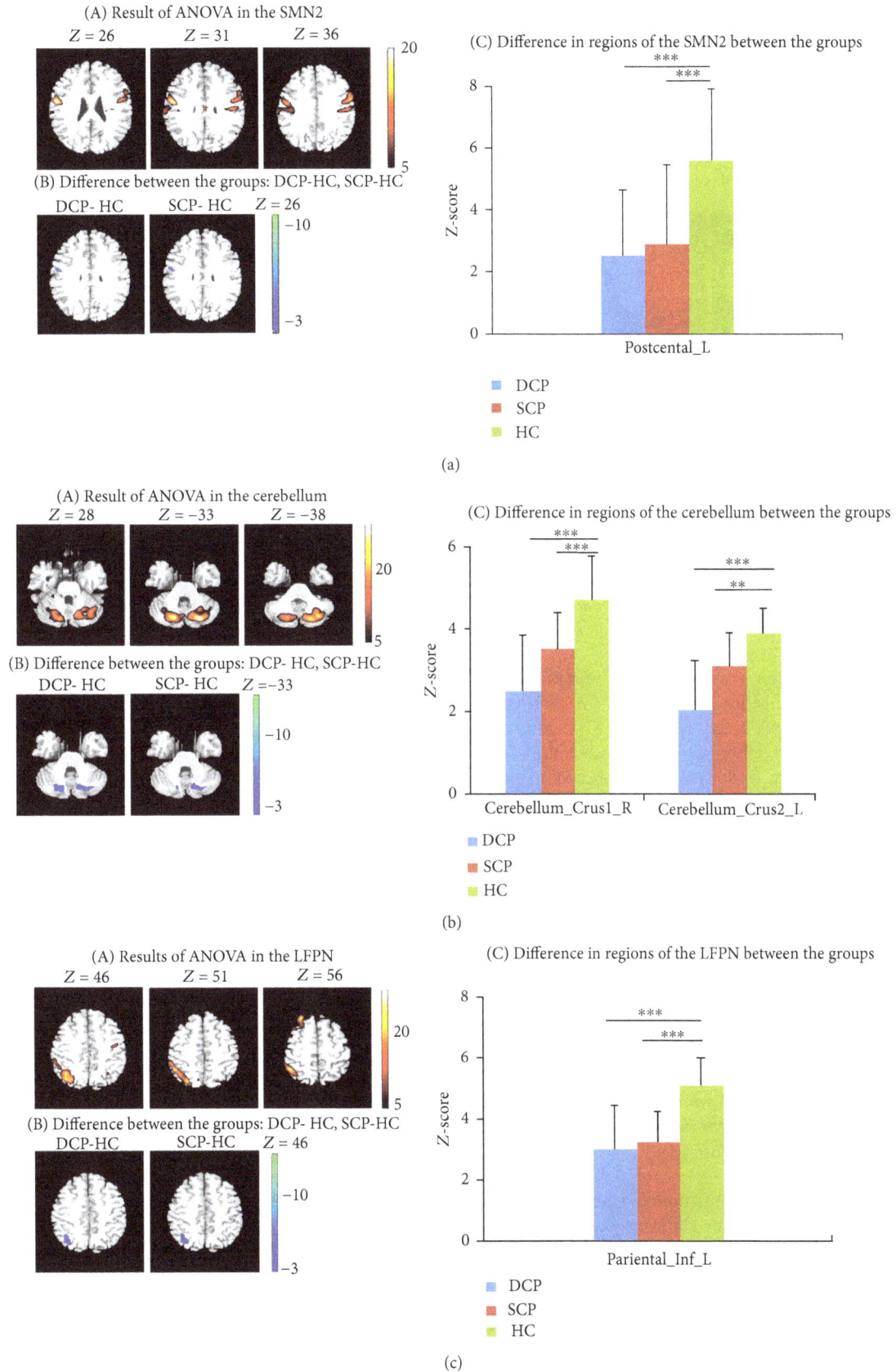

FIGURE 2: Continued.

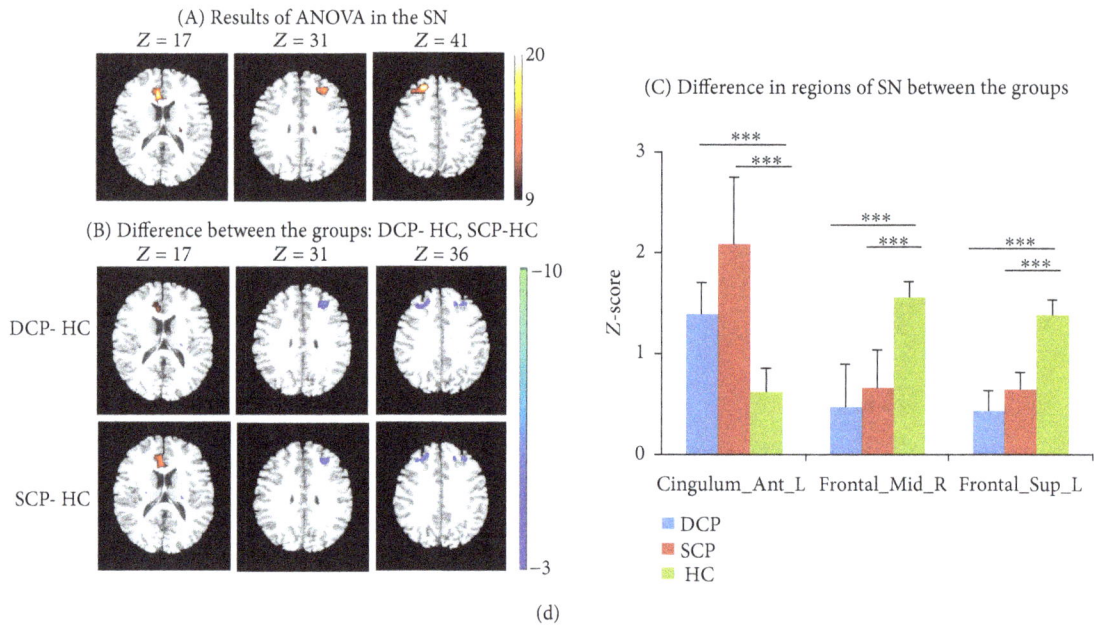

FIGURE 2: (a–d) Group comparison within four RSNs (SMN2, cerebellum, LFPN, and SN). (a) Significant difference was found in RSNs among the three groups. This result was achieved by performing one-way ANOVA on the maps of the three groups, with a threshold of corrected $P < 0.05$. (b) Differences were obtained between the DCP and HC group, as well as between the SCP and HC group, by performing post hoc test on the RSN maps ($P < 0.001$). (c) The bar maps present the between-group differences in the regions showing significant group difference. In the bar maps, $^{**}P < 0.01$, $^{***}P < 0.001$.

3.4. *FNC Analysis between Groups.* For FNC analysis, significant internetwork connections were found for each group based on the one-sample t-test ($P < 0.05$, FDR-corrected) (Figure 3(a)). A large number of positive associations were detected between RSNs, and a small number of negative connectivity existed. Then, one-way ANOVA showed significant difference among the groups, and six connections were found to be significantly altered ($P < 0.05$, FDR-corrected), including the primVN-extraVN connection, primVN-RFPN connection, RFPN-cerebellum connection, antDMN-SRN connection, postDMN-LFPN connection, and postDMN-SN connection. Moreover, in the DCP group, all of the six connections were impaired (correlation coefficient approaching zero) compared with HC, while in the SCP group, only four out of the six disconnections existed. Comparing to SCP, DCP gave rise to more serious deficiency in the RFPN-cerebellum connection and antDMN-SRN connection. The altered FNCs were mostly involved in the validation analysis using different IC numbers (details shown in Supplementary Material Figure S3).

3.5. *Relationship between Functional Connectivity and Clinical Scores.* Comparisons for clinical scores between the DCP and SCP group showed that GMFCS scores in the DCP group were significantly higher than those in the SCP group, and ADL scores in the DCP group were significantly lower than those in the SCP group. Correlations were performed between the mean Z-scores of seven ROIs in the four RSNs (Figure 2) and clinical scores, and significant negative correlations were found between the cerebellum crus and GMFCS (Figure 4(a)). Then, correlations were performed between the FNC coefficients (6 connections) and the clinical

measurement in the CP group. Three out of the six connections, including primVN-extraVN and postDMN-SN, as well as antDMN-SRN, were found having negative correlations with GMFCS. Moreover, three connections including primVN-RFPN, RFPN-cerebellum, and antDMN-SRN were found having significant positive correlations with ADL scores (Figures 4(b)–4(c)). Besides the correlations in the whole group, relationship between functional connectivity and clinical scores was also investigated in the subgroups (Supplementary Material Figure S4).

4. Discussion

In this study, we investigated the functional connectivity intra- and inter-RSNs in CP. Compared with HC, altered functional connectivity was found within the cerebellum, SMN2, LFPN, and SN networks for both the SCP and DCP groups. For FNC analysis, four functional disconnection inter-RSNs were observed in SCP, while six functional disconnection inter-RSNs were observed in DCP. The DCP and SCP groups showed different levels of aberrant connectivity. Furthermore, correlations between the functional disconnection and GMFCS/ADL scores were found. These findings indicate functional connectivity impairment, and altered integration widely exists in children with CP, and exploring the common and distinct functional connectivity patterns may contribute to our understanding of the neuropathophysiological mechanism of different CP subtypes.

Functional connectivity analysis alteration within RSNs may elucidate the abnormal intrinsic interaction in a certain spatial pattern [34, 53]. In this study, decreased functional connectivity was showed within two motor-related networks,

(a) FNC in the three groups

(b) Comparison results of FNC among the groups

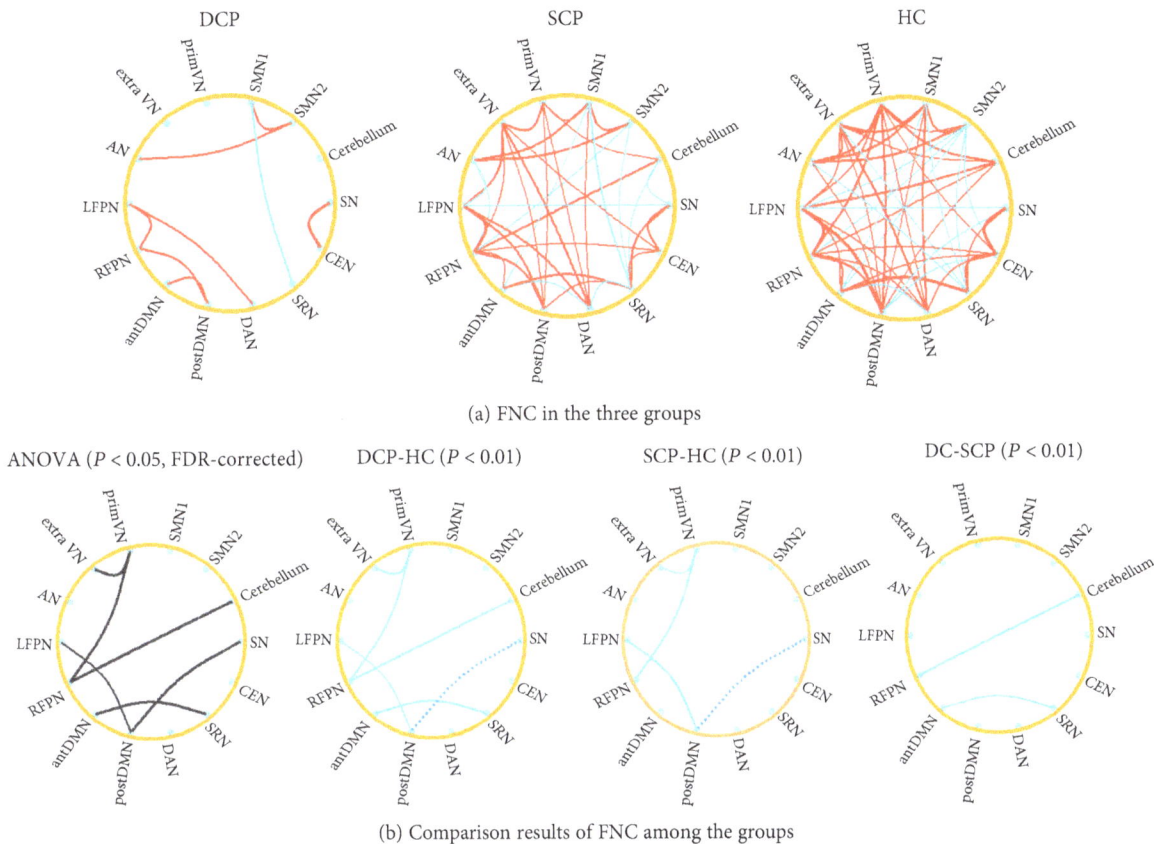

FIGURE 3: (a) The functional network connectivity in the DCP, SCP, and HC group. The red line represents the connection with positive correlation, and the blue line represents the connection with negative correlation. The results were obtained by the one-sample t-test with a threshold of corrected $P < 0.05$. (b) The comparison results of the functional network connectivity between the groups. The black line in the ANOVA result represents the altered connection among the three groups. Differences of functional network connectivity between DCP and HC and between SCP and HC, as well as between DCP and SCP, were observed. The blue solid line represents the connection with decreased positive FNC in CP children; and the blue dotted line represents the connection with decreased negative FNC in CP children.

that is, the cerebellum and SMN2 in children with CP. The role of the cerebellum has been well known to be involved in both motor learning and cognitive processing, and cerebellar injury might bring about posture and movement impairment [54–56]. Previous studies have demonstrated that children with CP had smaller volumes of the cerebellar hemispheres compared to controls [57]. Chronic cerebellar stimulation applied to the superomedial cortex has been used to reduce generalized cerebral spasticity, athetoid movements, and seizures [58]. Negative correlation between the cerebellum network and GMFCS in the current study suggested that decreased functional connectivity in the cerebellum would aggravate motor dysfunction in children with CP. As part of sensorimotor-related network, SMN2 focused on the primary motor and somatosensory areas, which were vulnerable regions in CP. Disrupted sensorimotor integration has been considered as a key factor that underlies motor function in CP and other movement disorders [22, 59, 60]. In this study, the decreased connectivity near the central sulcus indicated that defective sensorimotor organization could be a relevant pathophysiological element resulting to motor dysfunction in CP.

The LFPN and SN are two functional networks referred to the task activation ensemble. Frontoparietal network is an important network in spatial attention [61], and LFPN has been mentioned to correspond well to cognition-language paradigms [31]. Studies about mortality and adverse neurological outcome in preterm infants with periventricular hemorrhagic infarction (PVHI) found that extended frontoparietal lesions were associated with the development of cerebral palsy [62, 63]. Therefore, the dysfunction within the frontoparietal network might contribute to the cognitive impairment in CP. The salience network (SN) is a large-scale paralimbic network with coactivation in response to signal for behavioral change need [64, 65]. As part of the SN, prefrontal cortex (PFC) plays an important role in goal-relevant top-down control, and a previous study has reviewed that PFC was engaged in the executive control adaption [66, 67]. In addition, the ACC has been proposed to serve in monitoring and detecting conflict, as well as error compensation, which was one useful drivers to adjust the level of executive control [66, 68]. As evidences pointed to executive function impairment in children with CP [30], the reduced connectivity within the prefrontal cortex in this

(a) Relationship between the RSN and GMFCS

(b) Relationship between the FNC and GMFCS

(c) Relationship between the FNC and ADL

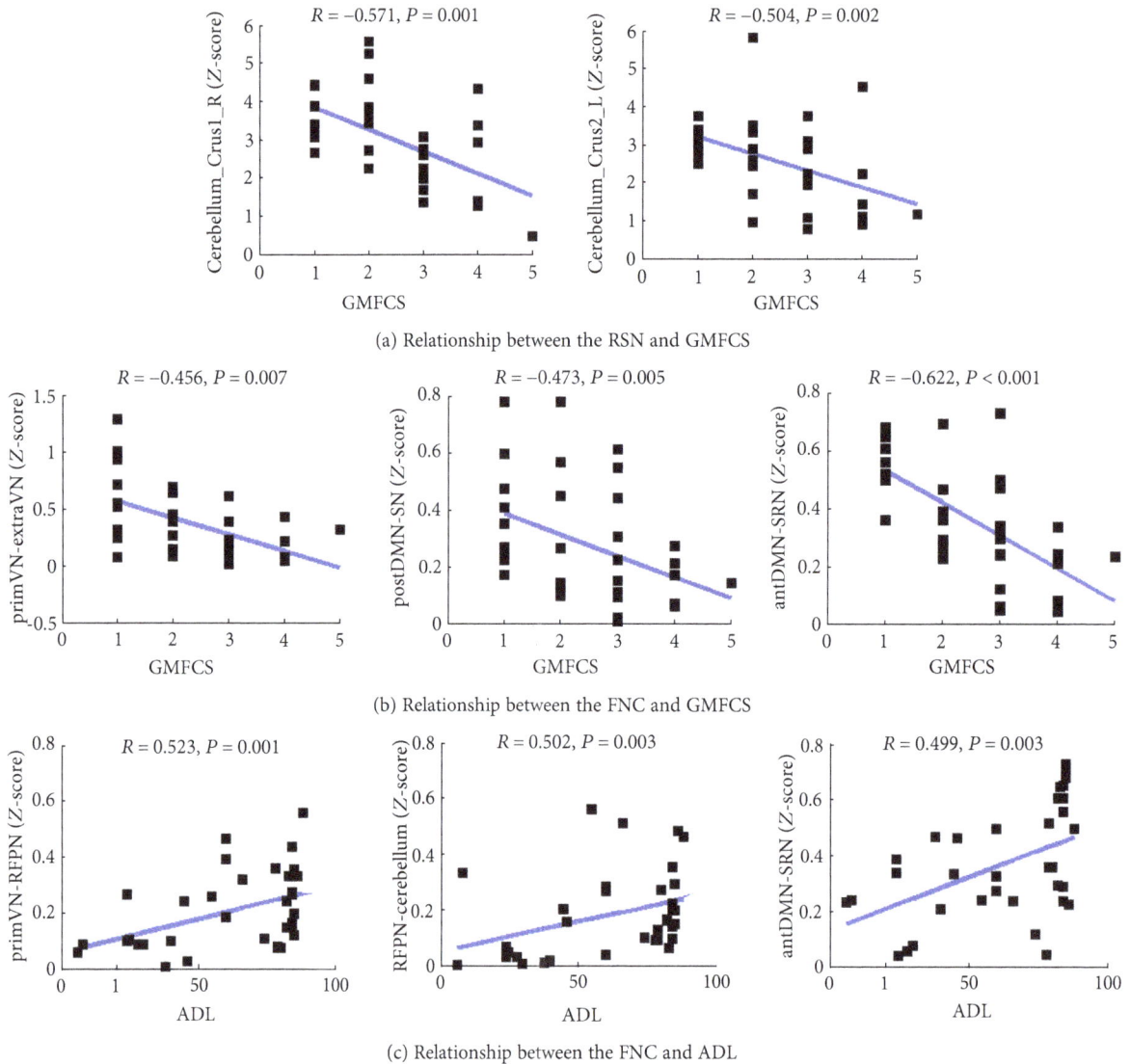

FIGURE 4: (a) Relationship between cerebellum network and GMFCS scores. (b) Relationship between primVN-extraVN, postDMN-SN, antDMN-SRN connection, and GMFCS scores. (c) Relationship between primVN-RFPN, RFPN-cerebellum, antDMN-SRN connection, and ADL scores.

study may correlate with the impaired executive function in CP, while the increased connectivity in the ACC may be the result of plasticity and compensation mechanism during development.

In the current study, common FNC alteration in DCP and SCP was revealed. Disrupted connectivity for primVN-extraVN, as well as primVN-RFPN connection, was found both in DCP and SCP. Visual perception dysfunction reflects an impairment of the capacity to process visual information, which frequently occurs in cerebral palsy and preterm children [10, 69]. As the frontoparietal network is an important network in visual-spatial attention [61], the disconnection of primVN-RFPN pathway might be one factor of visual perception impairment in CP. Moreover, decreased connectivity was exhibited in postDMN-SN and postDMN-LFPN in both DCP and SCP. The DMN, which has been studied extensively, has a set of brain regions that typically activate at rest

but deactivate during performance of cognitive tasks [52, 70]. SN and LFPN are both described as task-positive networks, with activation in corresponding areas during cognitive task performance [64]. The interaction among DMN, SN, and LFPN might be related to the low-frequency toggling between the introspective and extrospective states that ensures that the individual is attentive to the unexpected or novel environmental events [71].The decreased functional connectivity between the DMN and SN/LFPN implicated the inefficient balance and regulation among these networks, which may suggest network inhibition or network unbalance as a plausible mechanism for cognitive abnormality in children with CP.

Two distinct functional disconnections were found in the DCP group compared with the SCP group, that is, cerebellum-RFPN and antDMN-SRN connections. RFPN is a network related to visual-spatial attention and somesthetic perception, while the cerebellum is the center of motor planning and motor control. Their connection, as one part of motor pathway in the brain [22], may be a vulnerable link related with the dystonic DCP. As both DMN and SRN are associated with the psychological functions of introspective and self-referential processing [52, 71, 72], the discoupling between the antDMN and SRN might relate to the disrupted cognitive self-regulation in children with DCP [73, 74]. Moreover, negative correlation between the antDMN-SRN and GMFCS, as well as positive correlations between RFPN-cerebellum, antDMN-SRN, and ADL scores, suggested that these disconnections also contribute to motor and daily activities' dysfunction in children with CP.

In this study, some children in the CP group had gray matter abnormality, and children with DCP recruited in our study tended to have more severe motion and cognitive disability compared to the SCP group. In order to investigate the effect of gray matter lesions, we took the ratio of the gray matter volume of each RSN to the TIV into consideration as covariance and reconducted the post hoc t-test to examine the group difference between DCP and SCP in FNC analysis. The same disconnections (cerebellum-RFPN and antDMN-SRN connection) were found in the DCP group compared with SCP. These results suggested that gray matter volume did not have a negative impact on the functional connectivity values in this study, mainly due to the strict inclusion criteria that the children with serious brain loss or lesions have been excluded.

Structure effect is one common concern in CP functional studies. Severe lesions will certainly distort the brain functional connectivity and have adverse effect in group analysis. Although children with severe brain lesions and complex clinical features were excluded in this study, potential structural effect may be inevitable. In this study, two valid measures were applied in order to weaken the effect of lesion structure to functional connectivity. On one hand, gray template mask without lesion was applied. One the other hand, ICA detects interacting networks of regions and offers the advantage to diminish the effect of abnormal signal of voxel level. During the dual-regression (temporal and spatial) back reconstruction, abnormal time courses of lesions would have slight contribution to the individual IC networks [75]. Furthermore, the FNC comparison between two CP groups, using the ratio of the gray matter volume of each network to the TIV as covariance, demonstrated slight influence of gray matter volume variation. The result suggested that the combination of participant exclusion criterion, the methodology, and reasonable template without lesions was capable to weaken the adverse impact of structural lesions during fMRI studies.

5. Limitations

However, there do exist some methodological issues and limitations that may affect our results. Firstly, there are a variety of brain lesions in the CP group. We chose the participants mainly according to the clinical diagnosis and MRI structure images, and there may be potential structural effect. In this study, some children with DCP have lesions in the putamen,

and the lesions are excluded in the following analysis. However, the basal ganglia is an important motor-related network; the negligence of relative region in this study limited the functional connectivity analysis for the basal ganglia [17, 73]. Secondly, as most of the children with CP are accompanied by involuntary and uncontrolled movement, it is hard for them to keep still during MRI scanning for a relatively long time. Therefore, we have to scan these children under sedation state in this study. The sedation effect on the resting-state brain is inevitable. The widely recognized effects of drug-induced sedation on RSNs were the increased connectivity within motor network and visual network and the decreased connectivity in the DMN and SN [76–78]. Although our study showing inconsistent results revealed decreased connectivity in the SMN2 and increased connectivity in the ACC of the SN for CP children under sedation condition, the influence of sedation drug on functional connectivity cannot be ignored. Also, as there were only GMFCS and ADL measurement in this study, no specificity in motion and cognitive scores was applied. In the future study, more and refined related clinical scores should be adopted. Moreover, the sample size is small in this study, and future studies should include larger sample size to determine the mechanism underlying the abnormal functional connectivity found in the current study. Finally, ICA is an unsupervised method, which remains an indirect limitation when applying to identify the RSNs. The number of independent components and the reliability of IC maps are still open questions. Although we implemented ICA at different model orders and got a relatively stable result, the individual patient-specific network combined with the seed-based functional connectivity analysis and cluster analysis might provide complementary information in the comparisons.

6. Conclusions

This study demonstrated the functional network alteration in children with spastic and dyskinetic cerebral palsy based on resting-state fMRI. It provided a valid tool to help elucidate the abnormal functional connectivity patterns in different CP subtypes. Aberrant functional connectivity in CP groups was found, particularly within the cerebellum, SMN, LFPN, and SN networks, covering the motor- and cognitive-related networks. For FNC analysis, altered visual pathway and the covariance of DMN with other networks may be important factors of the visual perception and cognitive impairment in CP. In addition, distinct disconnections were revealed in DCP between the cerebellum and RFPN, as well as between the antDMN and SRN, which may act as an objective indicator of the clinical response in DCP. Exploring the common and distinct functional connectivity alteration is therefore beneficial for understanding the underlying mechanism of different CP subtypes and may contribute to more appropriate interventions.

Abbreviations

CP: Cerebral palsy
SCP: Spastic cerebral palsy

DCP: Dyskinetic cerebral palsy
RSNs: Resting-state networks
FNC: Functional network connectivity
GMFCS: Gross Motor Function Classification System
ADL: Everyday activities of daily living
SMN1: Sensorimotor network 1, included the paracentral lobule, the supplementary motor area, and pre- and postcentral gyrus
SMN2: Sensorimotor network 2, focused at the lateral primary somatosensory cortex, including pre- and postcentral gyrus areas
primVN: The primary visual network
extraVN: The extrastriate visual network.

Conflicts of Interest

None of the authors has any conflict of interests to disclose.

Authors' Contributions

Yun Qin, Hui He, Cheng Lu, and Chengyan Sun conceived and designed the work. Rui Peng, Yanan Li, and Jianfu Li acquired the data. Yun Qin, Hui He, Cheng Lu, and Bo Sun analyzed the data. Yun Qin and Tao Zhang wrote the paper. All authors revised the work for important intellectual content. All of the authors have read and approved the manuscript.

Acknowledgments

This work was supported by grants from the National Nature Science Foundation of China (Grant nos. 81330032, 81771822), Special-Funded Program on National Key Scientific Instruments and Equipment Development of China (no. 2013YQ490859), the Chinese Fundamental Research Funding for the Central Universities in the University of Electronic Science and Technology of China (ZYGX2015J091, ZYGX2016J124), and the Project of Science and Technology Department of Sichuan Province (2017HH0001 and 2017SZ0004). Thanks are due to the two radiologists for the neuroimaging evaluation and to Benjamin Klugah-Brown for the English language improvement.

Supplementary Materials

The group-level spatial maps of 14 RSNs for HC, SCP, and DCP and the relationships between RSN/FNC and clinical scores in the subgroups. (Supplementary Materials)

References

[1] I. Novak, M. Hines, S. Goldsmith, and R. Barclay, "Clinical prognostic messages from a systematic review on cerebral palsy," Pediatrics, vol. 130, no. 5, pp. e1285–e1312, 2012.

[2] M. Oskoui, F. Coutinho, J. Dykeman, N. Jetté, and T. Pringsheim, "An update on the prevalence of cerebral palsy: a systematic review and meta-analysis," Developmental Medicine & Child Neurology, vol. 55, no. 6, pp. 509–519, 2013.

[3] M. Bax, M. Goldstein, P. Rosenbaum et al., "Proposed definition and classification of cerebral palsy, April 2005," Developmental Medicine and Child Neurology, vol. 47, no. 8, pp. 571–576, 2005.

[4] P. Rosenbaum, "The definition and classification of cerebral palsy: are we any further ahead in 2006?," NeoReviews, vol. 7, no. 11, pp. e569–e574, 2006.

[5] P. I. Tomlin, The StaticEncephalopathies, Times-Wolfe International, London, 1995.

[6] M. Bax, C. Tydeman, and O. Flodmark, "Clinical and MRI correlates of cerebral palsy," JAMA, vol. 296, no. 13, pp. 1602–1608, 2006.

[7] C. Cans, H. Dolk, M. Platt, A. Colver, A. Prasauskene, and I. K. Rägeloh-Mann, "Recommendations from the SCPE collaborative group for defining and classifying cerebral palsy," Developmental Medicine & Child Neurology, vol. 49, pp. 35–38, 2007.

[8] T. D. Sanger, D. Chen, D. L. Fehlings et al., "Definition and classification of hyperkinetic movements in childhood," Movement Disorders, vol. 25, no. 11, pp. 1538–1549, 2010.

[9] L. Bottcher, E. M. Flachs, and P. Uldall, "Attentional and executive impairments in children with spastic cerebral palsy," Developmental Medicine & Child Neurology, vol. 52, no. 2, article e42, e47 pages, 2010.

[10] A. Ego, K. Lidzba, P. Brovedani et al., "Visual-perceptual impairment in children with cerebral palsy: a systematic review," Developmental Medicine and Child Neurology, vol. 57, pp. 46–51, 2015.

[11] D. S. Reilly, M. H. Woollacott, P. van Donkelaar, and S. Saavedra, "The interaction between executive attention and postural control in dual-task conditions: children with cerebral palsy," Archives of Physical Medicine and Rehabilitation, vol. 89, no. 5, pp. 834–842, 2008.

[12] C. Papadelis, B. Ahtam, M. Nazarova et al., "Cortical somatosensory reorganization in children with spastic cerebral palsy: a multimodal neuroimaging study," Frontiers in Human Neuroscience, vol. 8, p. 725, 2014.

[13] K. Himmelmann and P. Uvebrant, "Function and neuroimaging in cerebral palsy: a population-based study," Developmental Medicine & Child Neurology, vol. 53, no. 6, pp. 516–521, 2011.

[14] S. Yoshida, K. Hayakawa, K. Oishi et al., "Athetotic and spastic cerebral palsy:anatomic characterization based on diffusion-tensor imaging," Radiology, vol. 260, no. 2, pp. 511–520, 2011.

[15] A. Okumura, T. Kato, K. Kuno, F. Hayakawa, and K. Watanabe, "MRI findings in patients with spastic cerebral palsy. II: correlation with type of cerebral palsy," Developmental Medicine & Child Neurology, vol. 39, no. 6, pp. 369–372, 1997.

[16] M. Hadders-Algra, "Early diagnosis and early intervention in cerebral palsy," Frontiers in Neurology, vol. 5, 2014.

[17] B. R. Aravamuthan and J. L. Waugh, "Localization of basal ganglia and thalamic damage in dyskinetic cerebral palsy," Pediatric Neurology, vol. 54, pp. 11–21, 2016.

[18] I. Krägeloh-Mann and C. Cans, "Cerebral palsy update," Brain & Development, vol. 31, no. 7, pp. 537–544, 2009.

[19] A. H. Hoon, W. T. Lawrie, E. R. Melhem et al., "Diffusion tensor imaging of periventricular leukomalacia shows affected

sensory cortex white matter pathways," *Neurology*, vol. 59, no. 5, pp. 752–756, 2002.

[20] B. Thomas, M. Eyssen, R. Peeters et al., "Quantitative diffusion tensor imaging in cerebral palsy due to periventricular white matter injury," *Brain*, vol. 128, no. 11, pp. 2562–2577, 2005.

[21] R. Trivedi, S. Agarwal, V. Shah et al., "Correlation of quantitative sensorimotor tractography with clinical grade of cerebral palsy," *Neuroradiology*, vol. 52, no. 8, pp. 759–765, 2010.

[22] J. D. Lee, H. J. Park, E. S. Park et al., "Motor pathway injury in patients with periventricular leucomalacia and spastic diplegia," *Brain*, vol. 134, no. 4, pp. 1199–1210, 2011.

[23] A. M. Pagnozzi, K. Shen, J. D. Doecke et al., "Using ventricular modeling to robustly probe significant deep gray matter pathologies: application to cerebral palsy," *Human Brain Mapping*, vol. 37, no. 11, pp. 3795–3809, 2016.

[24] S. M. Reid, C. D. Dagia, M. R. Ditchfield, and D. S. Reddihough, "Grey matter injury patterns in cerebral palsy: associations between structural involvement on MRI and clinical outcomes," *Developmental Medicine and Child Neurology*, vol. 57, no. 12, pp. 1159–1167, 2015.

[25] J. Accardo, H. Kammann, and A. H. Hoon Jr, "Neuroimaging in cerebral palsy," *The Journal of Pediatrics*, vol. 145, no. 2, pp. S19–S27, 2004.

[26] E. Chinier, S. N'Guyen, G. Lignon, A. ter Minassian, I. Richard, and M. Dinomais, "Effect of motor imagery in children with unilateral cerebral palsy: fMRI study," *PLoS One*, vol. 9, no. 4, article e93378, 2014.

[27] K. Lidzba, M. Staudt, M. Wilke, and I. Krageloh-Mann, "Visuospatial deficits in patients with early left-hemispheric lesions and functional reorganization of language: consequence of lesion or reorganization?," *Neuropsychologia*, vol. 44, no. 7, pp. 1088–1094, 2006.

[28] J. G. Ojemann, R. C. McKinstry, P. Mukherjee, T. S. Park, and H. Burton, "Hand somatosensory cortex activity following selective dorsal rhizotomy: report of three cases with fMRI," *Child's Nervous System*, vol. 21, no. 2, pp. 115–121, 2005.

[29] J. R. Wingert, R. J. Sinclair, S. Dixit, D. L. Damiano, and H. Burton, "Somatosensory-evoked cortical activity in spastic diplegic cerebral palsy," *Human Brain Mapping*, vol. 31, no. 11, pp. 1772–1785, 2010.

[30] L. Bottcher, "Children with spastic cerebral palsy, their cognitive functioning, and social participation: a review," *Child Neuropsychology*, vol. 16, no. 3, pp. 209–228, 2010.

[31] S. M. Smith, P. T. Fox, K. L. Miller et al., "Correspondence of the brain's functional architecture during activation and rest," *Proceedings of the National Academy of Sciences of the United States of America*, vol. 106, no. 31, pp. 13040–13045, 2009.

[32] H. Burton, S. Dixit, P. Litkowski, and J. R. Wingert, "Functional connectivity for somatosensory and motor cortex in spastic diplegia," *Somatosensory & Motor Research*, vol. 26, no. 4, pp. 90–104, 2010.

[33] X. Mu, Z. Wang, B. Nie et al., "Altered regional and circuit resting-state activity in patients with occult spastic diplegic cerebral palsy," *Pediatrics & Neonatology*, 2017.

[34] M. de Luca, C. F. Beckmann, N. de Stefano, P. M. Matthews, and S. M. Smith, "fMRI resting state networks define distinct modes of long-distance interactions in the human brain," *NeuroImage*, vol. 29, no. 4, pp. 1359–1367, 2006.

[35] M. D. Fox and M. E. Raichle, "Spontaneous fluctuations in brain activity observed with functional magnetic resonance imaging," *Nature Reviews Neuroscience*, vol. 8, no. 9, pp. 700–711, 2007.

[36] M. J. Jafri, G. D. Pearlson, M. Stevens, and V. D. Calhoun, "A method for functional network connectivity among spatially independent resting-state components in schizophrenia," *NeuroImage*, vol. 39, no. 4, pp. 1666–1681, 2008.

[37] A. Abou Elseoud, H. Littow, J. Remes et al., "Group-ICA model order highlights patterns of functional brain connectivity," *Frontiers in Systems Neuroscience*, vol. 5, p. 37, 2011.

[38] V. D. Calhoun, T. Adali, G. D. Pearlson, and J. J. Pekar, "A method for making group inferences from functional MRI data using independent component analysis," *Human Brain Mapping*, vol. 14, no. 3, pp. 140–151, 2001.

[39] R. J. Palisano, P. Rosenbaum, D. Bartlett, and M. H. Livingston, "Content validity of the expanded and revised gross motor function classification system," *Developmental Medicine & Child Neurology*, vol. 50, no. 10, pp. 744–750, 2008.

[40] B. R. van Zelst, M. D. Miller, R. N. Russo, S. Murchland, and M. Crotty, "Activities of daily living in children with hemiplegic cerebral palsy: a cross-sectional evaluation using the assessment of motor and process skills," *Developmental Medicine & Child Neurology*, vol. 48, no. 9, pp. 723–727, 2006.

[41] L. An, Q. J. Cao, M. Q. Sui et al., "Local synchronization and amplitude of the fluctuation of spontaneous brain activity in attention-deficit/hyperactivity disorder: a resting-state fMRI study," *Neuroscience Bulletin*, vol. 29, no. 5, pp. 603–613, 2013.

[42] X. Bai, M. Vestal, R. Berman et al., "Dynamic time course of typical childhood absence seizures: EEG, behavior, and functional magnetic resonance imaging," *Journal of Neuroscience*, vol. 30, no. 17, pp. 5884–5893, 2010.

[43] M. Dinomais, G. Lignon, E. Chinier, I. Richard, A. ter Minassian, and S. N.'. G. T. Tich, "Effect of observation of simple hand movement on brain activations in patients with unilateral cerebral palsy: an fMRI study," *Research in Developmental Disabilities*, vol. 34, no. 6, pp. 1928–1937, 2013.

[44] J. D. Power, K. A. Barnes, A. Z. Snyder, B. L. Schlaggar, and S. E. Petersen, "Spurious but systematic correlations in functional connectivity MRI networks arise from subject motion," *NeuroImage*, vol. 59, no. 3, pp. 2142–2154, 2012.

[45] M. Brett, A. P. Leff, C. Rorden, and J. Ashburner, "Spatial normalization of brain images with focal lesions using cost function masking," *NeuroImage*, vol. 14, no. 2, pp. 486–500, 2001.

[46] M. Yang, J. Li, Y. Li et al., "Altered intrinsic regional activity and interregional functional connectivity in post-stroke aphasia," *Scientific Reports*, vol. 6, no. 1, article 24803, 2016.

[47] Y.-O. Li, T. Adalı, and V. D. Calhoun, "Estimating the number of independent components for functional magnetic resonance imaging data," *Human Brain Mapping*, vol. 28, no. 11, pp. 1251–1266, 2007.

[48] H. Zhang, X. N. Zuo, S. Y. Ma, Y. F. Zang, M. P. Milham, and C. Z. Zhu, "Subject order-independent group ICA (SOI-GICA) for functional MRI data analysis," *NeuroImage*, vol. 51, no. 4, pp. 1414–1424, 2010.

[49] N. U. F. Dosenbach, D. A. Fair, F. M. Miezin et al., "Distinct brain networks for adaptive and stable task control in humans," *Proceedings of the National Academy of Sciences of the United States of America*, vol. 104, no. 26, pp. 11073–11078, 2007.

[50] M. D. Fox, A. Z. Snyder, J. L. Vincent, M. Corbetta, D. C. Van Essen, and M. E. Raichle, "The human brain is intrinsically

organized into dynamic, anticorrelated functional networks," *Proceedings of the National Academy of Sciences of the United States of America*, vol. 102, no. 27, pp. 9673–9678, 2005.

[51] C. Luo, Q. Li, Y. Lai et al., "Altered functional connectivity in default mode network in absence epilepsy: a resting-state fMRI study," *Human Brain Mapping*, vol. 32, no. 3, pp. 438–449, 2011.

[52] C. Luo, C. Qiu, Z. Guo et al., "Disrupted functional brain connectivity in partial epilepsy: a resting-state fMRI study," *PLoS One*, vol. 7, no. 1, article e28196, 2012.

[53] C. F. Beckmann, M. Deluca, J. T. Devlin, and S. M. Smith, "Investigations into resting-state connectivity using independent component analysis," *Philosophical Transactions of the Royal Society B: Biological Sciences*, vol. 360, no. 1457, pp. 1001–1013, 2005.

[54] M. Allin, H. Matsumoto, A. M. Santhouse et al., "Cognitive and motor function and the size of the cerebellum in adolescents born very pre-term," *Brain*, vol. 124, no. 1, pp. 60–66, 2001.

[55] M. Rapoport, R. van Reekum, and H. Mayberg, "The role of the cerebellum in cognition and behavior: a selective review," *Journal of Neuropsychiatry & Clinical Neurosciences*, vol. 12, no. 2, pp. 193–198, 2000.

[56] W. T. Thach, "What is the role of the cerebellum in motor learning and cognition?," *Trends in Cognitive Sciences*, vol. 2, no. 9, pp. 331–337, 1998.

[57] W. Kułak and W. Sobaniec, "Magnetic resonance imaging of the cerebellum and brain stem in children with cerebral palsy," *Advances in Medical Sciences*, vol. 52, Supplement 1, pp. 180–182, 2007.

[58] R. Davis, "Cerebellar stimulation for cerebral palsy spasticity, function, and seizures," *Archives of Medical Research*, vol. 31, no. 3, pp. 290–299, 2000.

[59] G. Abbruzzese and A. Berardelli, "Further progress in understanding the pathophysiology of primary dystonia," *Movement Disorders*, vol. 26, no. 7, pp. 1185-1186, 2011.

[60] H. Tsao, K. Pannek, R. N. Boyd, and S. E. Rose, "Changes in the integrity of thalamocortical connections are associated with sensorimotor deficits in children with congenital hemiplegia," *Brain Structure and Function*, vol. 220, no. 1, pp. 307–318, 2015.

[61] M. Corbetta, "Frontoparietal cortical networks for directing attention and the eye to visual locations: identical, independent, or overlapping neural systems?," *Proceedings of the National Academy of Sciences of the United States of America*, vol. 95, no. 3, pp. 831–838, 1998.

[62] H. Bassan, C. B. Benson, C. Limperopoulos et al., "Ultrasonographic features and severity scoring of periventricular hemorrhagic infarction in relation to risk factors and outcome," *Pediatrics*, vol. 117, no. 6, pp. 2111–2118, 2006.

[63] E. Roze, "Risk factors for adverse outcome in preterm infants with periventricular hemorrhagic infarction," *Pediatrics*, vol. 122, no. 1, pp. e46–e52, 2008.

[64] V. Bonnelle, T. E. Ham, R. Leech et al., "Salience network integrity predicts default mode network function after traumatic brain injury," *Proceedings of the National Academy of Sciences of the United States of America*, vol. 109, no. 12, pp. 4690–4695, 2012.

[65] W. W. Seeley, V. Menon, A. F. Schatzberg et al., "Dissociable intrinsic connectivity networks for salience processing and executive control," *The Journal of Neuroscience*, vol. 27, no. 9, pp. 2349–2356, 2007.

[66] F. A. Mansouri, T. Egner, and M. J. Buckley, "Monitoring demands for executive control: shared functions between human and nonhuman primates," *Trends in Neurosciences*, vol. 40, no. 1, pp. 15–27, 2017.

[67] E. K. Miller and J. D. Cohen, "An integrative theory of prefrontal cortex function," *Annual Review of Neuroscience*, vol. 24, no. 1, pp. 167–202, 2001.

[68] C. S. Carter, A. M. Macdonald, M. Botvinick et al., "Parsing executive processes: strategic vs. evaluative functions of the anterior cingulate cortex," *Proceedings of the National Academy of Sciences of the United States of America*, vol. 97, no. 4, pp. 1944–1948, 2000.

[69] E. Fazzi, S. Bova, A. Giovenzana, S. Signorini, C. Uggetti, and P. Bianchi, "Cognitive visual dysfunctions in preterm children with periventricular leukomalacia," *Developmental Medicine and Child Neurology*, vol. 51, no. 12, pp. 974–981, 2009.

[70] M. E. Raichle, A. M. MacLeod, A. Z. Snyder, W. J. Powers, D. A. Gusnard, and G. L. Shulman, "A default mode of brain function," *Proceedings of the National Academy of Sciences of the United States of America*, vol. 98, no. 2, pp. 676–682, 2001.

[71] S. J. Broyd, C. Demanuele, S. Debener, S. K. Helps, C. J. James, and E. J. S. Sonuga-Barke, "Default-mode brain dysfunction in mental disorders: a systematic review," *Neuroscience and Biobehavioral Reviews*, vol. 33, no. 3, pp. 279–296, 2009.

[72] A. D'Argembeau, F. Collette, M. van der Linden et al., "Self-referential reflective activity and its relationship with rest: a PET study," *NeuroImage*, vol. 25, no. 2, pp. 616–624, 2005.

[73] K. Himmelmann, "The quest for patterns in dyskinetic cerebral palsy," *Developmental Medicine & Child Neurology*, vol. 58, no. 2, pp. 112–112, 2016.

[74] K. Himmelmann, G. Hagberg, L. M. Wiklund, M. N. Eek, and P. Uvebrant, "Dyskinetic cerebral palsy: a population-based study of children born between 1991 and 1998," *Developmental Medicine & Child Neurology*, vol. 49, no. 4, pp. 246–251, 2007.

[75] X. N. Zuo, C. Kelly, J. S. Adelstein, D. F. Klein, F. X. Castellanos, and M. P. Milham, "Reliable intrinsic connectivity networks: test-retest evaluation using ICA and dual regression approach," *NeuroImage*, vol. 49, no. 3, pp. 2163–2177, 2010.

[76] A. G. Hudetz, "General anesthesia and human brain connectivity," *Brain Connectivity*, vol. 2, no. 6, pp. 291–302, 2012.

[77] P. Liang, H. Zhang, Y. Xu, W. Jia, Y. Zang, and K. Li, "Disruption of cortical integration during midazolam-induced light sedation," *Human Brain Mapping*, vol. 36, no. 11, pp. 4247–4261, 2015.

[78] M. Qiu, D. Scheinost, R. Ramani, and R. T. Constable, "Multi-modal analysis of functional connectivity and cerebral blood flow reveals shared and unique effects of propofol in large-scale brain networks," *NeuroImage*, vol. 148, pp. 130–140, 2017.

3

Effects of Transcranial Alternating Current Stimulation on Repetitive Finger Movements in Healthy Humans

Andrea Guerra,[1] Matteo Bologna [1,2] Giulia Paparella,[2] Antonio Suppa [1,2] Donato Colella,[2] Vincenzo Di Lazzaro [3] Peter Brown,[4,5] and Alfredo Berardelli[1,2]

[1]Neuromed Institute IRCCS, Pozzilli, Italy
[2]Department of Human Neurosciences, Sapienza University of Rome, Rome, Italy
[3]Unit of Neurology, Neurophysiology, Neurobiology, Department of Medicine, University Campus Bio-Medico, Rome, Italy
[4]Nuffield Department of Clinical Neurosciences, John Radcliffe Hospital, University of Oxford, Oxford, UK
[5]Medical Research Council Brain Network Dynamics Unit, Department of Pharmacology, University of Oxford, Mansfield Road, Oxford, UK

Correspondence should be addressed to Matteo Bologna; matteo.bologna@uniroma1.it

Academic Editor: Stuart C. Mangel

Transcranial alternating current stimulation (tACS) is a noninvasive neurophysiological technique that can entrain brain oscillations. Only few studies have investigated the effects of tACS on voluntary movements. We aimed to verify whether tACS, delivered over M1 at beta and gamma frequencies, has any effect on repetitive finger tapping as assessed by means of kinematic analysis. Eighteen healthy subjects were enrolled. Objective measurements of repetitive finger tapping were obtained by using a motion analysis system. M1 excitability was assessed by using single-pulse TMS and measuring the amplitude of motor-evoked potentials (MEPs). Movement kinematic measures and MEPs were collected during beta, gamma, and sham tACS and when the stimulation was off. Beta tACS led to an amplitude decrement (i.e., progressive reduction in amplitude) across the first ten movements of the motor sequence while gamma tACS had the opposite effect. The results did not reveal any significant effect of tACS on other movement parameters, nor any changes in MEPs. These findings demonstrate that tACS modulates finger tapping in a frequency-dependent manner with no concurrent changes in corticospinal excitability. The results suggest that cortical beta and gamma oscillations are involved in the motor control of repetitive finger movements.

1. Introduction

A growing number of studies on humans have shown that the two main natural rhythms of the primary motor cortex (M1), namely, beta (13–30 Hz) and gamma (30–100 Hz), play a role in motor control. Beta oscillatory activity increases during tonic contraction and decreases during movement preparation and execution [1–6]. By contrast, gamma oscillatory activity increases during movement preparation and execution [3, 7–9]. The contrasting functional effects of the two frequency bands of activity are supported by the effects of electrical stimulation on healthy subjects [10–12] and by the changes observed in patients with Parkinson's disease (PD). In this condition, untreated patients have elevated beta activity in basal ganglia-cortical circuits and slowed movement [13], whereas dyskinetic treated patients have elevated gamma activity at about 70 Hz and have excessive movement [14, 15].

Transcranial alternating current stimulation (tACS) is a recent noninvasive neurophysiological technique that entrains brain oscillations by inducing coherent changes in the firing and timing of populations of neurons [16]. The resulting neuronal synchronization may affect the activity of different cortical areas in a frequency-specific manner, resulting in the so-called "resonance principle." Namely, the ability of tACS to modify brain rhythms especially when the externally superimposed oscillation is close to the natural frequency of the cortical area is stimulated [17, 18].

Accordingly, tACS can transiently entrain beta or gamma rhythms and modify the neuronal activity of M1 [19–22]. Beta and gamma tACS over M1 can also modulate voluntary movement performance in healthy subjects. Beta tACS delivered during a visually cued arm movement reduces movement velocity [10]. Similarly, the initial and peak force rates of the hand grip are both reduced when beta tACS is applied during a cued go/no-go task [11]. By contrast, gamma tACS improves initial and peak force generation in a hand grip task [11] and increases hand movement velocity and acceleration in a visually guided motor task [23].

Only one previous study has assessed the effects of tACS on fast finger tapping in healthy subjects [12]. Beta tACS was continuously delivered over M1 for 10 minutes, and motor performance was assessed 0, 30, and 60 minutes after stimulation was discontinued. The authors found that beta tACS slowed movement execution only at 0 min [12]. The effects of tACS were not assessed during the 10 minutes of stimulation. It is worth noting, however, that some effects of tACS delivered to M1 occur during, but not after, stimulation [21]. Moreover, not only did the study by Wach et al. not investigate the effects of gamma tACS, but the analysis of finger tapping was limited to tapping intervals used as an indirect measure of movement velocity and accuracy [12]. To investigate the effects of tACS on repetitive finger tapping is relevant for several reasons. First, repetitive finger movements are largely dependent upon M1 activation [24, 25], so we predict that these movements can be better modulated by noninvasive stimulation of cortical motor areas than proximal arm movements. Second, it is still not clear whether or not the oscillatory activity of M1 has a role in the generation of repetitive finger movements. Finally, repetitive finger tapping is one of the tests most commonly used in the clinical assessment of patients with parkinsonian syndromes. Namely, specific kinematic abnormalities of finger tapping, that is, the amplitude decrement (also known as the sequence effect) are hallmarks of PD [25–28]. Thus, a better knowledge of the effectiveness of tACS on motor control is essential for future studies in pathological conditions [29].

In the present study, we tested the effects of beta and gamma tACS on repetitive finger tapping. We performed a comprehensive kinematic analysis of various movement parameters (i.e., amplitude, velocity, and rhythm, as well as progressive amplitude and velocity changes associated with movement repetition) known to reflect different physiological mechanisms [26]. The results were also compared with those obtained during sham tACS. Lastly, in order to ascertain whether the effects of tACS on finger movements are due to concomitant changes in corticospinal excitability, we recorded motor-evoked potentials (MEPs) during tACS.

2. Material and Methods

2.1. Participants. The study enrolled 18 right-handed healthy subjects (7 females, age: 26.4 ± 3.5 (mean $\pm$ SD) years) with no history of neurological and psychiatric diseases or medication intake. None of the participants had any contraindications to non-invasive brain stimulation, as described in the latest international guidelines [30].

2.2. Motor Task and Kinematic Recordings. The motor task was adopted from previous studies [26–28, 31]. Repetitive finger movements were recorded using an optoelectronic motion system (Smart Motion System, BTS Engineering, Milan, Italy). This system comprises three infrared cameras (sampling rate, 120 Hz) that follow the 3D displacement of reflective markers taped to the participant's hand. We used five reflective markers (5 mm in diameter) of negligible weight. One marker was placed on the tip of the index finger, and another was put on the tip of the thumb. Three additional reflective markers were placed on the hand to define a reference plane that was used to mathematically exclude possible contamination due to unwanted hand movements from the index finger tapping recordings [26, 32].

To quantify repetitive finger movement kinematics, we used linear regression techniques to determine the intercept, which reflects the initial movement amplitude (degree) and initial velocity (degree/s), and the slope, which reflects the amplitude and velocity decrement during the movement repetition. Movement rhythm was also measured by the coefficient of variation (CV) of the intertap intervals (with higher values representing a lower regularity of repetitive movements). These analyses were performed on the first ten movements of the sequence as well as on the entire sequence, that is, 15 seconds of repetitive movements, as adopted in our previous study [26]. The focus on the initial movements was also motivated by the modified Movement Disorder Society UPDRS [33] which proposes a 10-tap trial in the assessment of finger tapping.

2.3. Brain Stimulation and Electromyographic Recordings. tACS was delivered through conductive rubber electrodes enclosed in saline-soaked sponges using BrainSTIM (EMS, Italy), with the stimulating electrodes (5 × 5 cm) placed over M1 and Pz, as detailed elsewhere [20]. Both the electrodes were secured in place using rubber strips around the head. The set-up was optimized in order to ensure that the impedance for stimulation, as measured by the stimulation device, would be <10 kΩ. tACS was delivered at two different frequencies: 20 Hz (beta) and 70 Hz (gamma). For gamma tACS, the frequency of 70 Hz was used as in previous studies investigating the effects of tACS on motor behaviour [11, 23]. Also, previous magnetoencephalographic studies in healthy subjects showed that the average peak frequency of movement-related gamma synchronization occurs at 70–75 Hz [9, 21, 34]. A sham tACS stimulation was used as a control. Similar to previous studies [23, 35], for sham tACS the stimulator was turned on only for 7 seconds (3 seconds of ramp-up, 1 second of stimulation, and 3 seconds of ramp-down). The frequency used for sham was 20 Hz, applied at the individual intensity used for beta tACS. Sine wave stimulation was delivered with no direct current offset and a peak-to-peak amplitude of 1 mA. If the participants complained unpleasant sensation (e.g., visual or skin discomfort), the stimulation intensity was lowered in steps of 0.05 mA until the discomfort was no longer perceived [11, 21, 35]. Thus, the mean stimulation intensity for beta tACS was 0.61 mA, while the intensity did not need to be adjusted for gamma tACS in any participant. This procedure ensured that subjects could also not be able to distinguish among the different stimulation conditions (including sham). Also, it allowed us to reasonably exclude the occurrence of any placebo or attentional effects due to perception of the stimulation.

Transcranial magnetic stimulation (TMS) was performed by using a MAGSTIM 200 (Magstim Company Limited, Whitland, South West Wales) connected to a standard figure-of-eight 70 mm coil delivering monophasic pulses. The TMS coil was held with the handle angled at 45° to the midsagittal line, pointing posteriorly and laterally. The precise area of cortical representation ("hotspot") of the first dorsal interosseous (FDI) muscle of the right hand was targeted as the point from which stimuli at the minimal excitability threshold of TMS triggered MEPs of maximal amplitude and minimal latency in the target muscle. The MEPs were recorded through a pair of surface electrodes placed on the FDI muscle of the right hand in a belly/tendon montage. The resting motor threshold (RMT), that is, the stimulator's output able to elicit MEPs of $\geq 50\,\mu$V peak-to-peak amplitude in at least 5 out of 10 consecutive stimuli, was determined, as was the minimum intensity needed to reliably produce MEPs of about 1 mV in size (MT1mV).

Electromyographic (EMG) signals were amplified by means of a Digitimer D360 amplifier (Digitimer Ltd., Welwyn Garden City, UK), digitized at 5 kHz (CED 1401 laboratory interface, Cambridge Electronic Design, Cambridge, UK), and stored on a laboratory computer for off-line analysis with dedicated software (Signal software version 5.08, Cambridge Electronic Design).

2.4. Experimental Design. Participants were comfortably seated in a chair during the experimental procedures. We first applied single-pulse TMS before movement recordings in order to identify the FDI "hotspot" on the scalp. We then centered the tACS electrode on the FDI "hotspot" and recorded the finger tapping movements during tACS. Four conditions were tested in a random order: 20 Hz (beta tACS), 70 Hz (gamma tACS), sham tACS, and no stimulation (baseline). The motor task consisted of 12 trials in total. We recorded one trial for each condition in 3 separate, consecutive blocks. Each trial consisted of 15 seconds of finger tapping, performed at the maximal voluntary rate. During the motor task, the participants were continuously encouraged to tap with as large and fast movements as possible. A 5-minute and 10-minute rest period was provided between each trial and between each block, respectively, to avoid fatigue between trials and across blocks (Figure 1). Of note, the motor task started about 10 seconds after the beginning of the stimulation, so that for the sham condition, the motor task was performed while the stimulation was off. One practice trial was allowed before the kinematic recordings started to allow the subjects to become familiar with the experimental procedure.

The participants underwent a TMS assessment at the end of the kinematic recordings. The FDI "hotspot" targeting was repeated over the sponge of the stimulating electrode, and the site was marked with a felt-tip pen to allow the coil to be repositioned more easily during collection of the MEPs. The MT1mV was then determined. Twenty single-pulse MEPs were recorded at rest during beta, gamma, sham, and off tACS. The four conditions were randomized and performed at 5-minute intervals.

The participants were blinded to the stimulation conditions and unable to distinguish them. The experimenter who analyzed the kinematic measures and the MEPs was also blinded to the stimulation paradigm. There was only one operator who was not blinded to the experimental procedure, that is, the researcher who applied tACS and set up the stimulation frequencies.

2.5. Statistical Analysis. To evaluate the effects of tACS on finger tapping kinematics, we performed a repeated measures analysis of variance (ANOVA) using CONDITION (four levels: beta, gamma, sham, and baseline) and SEQUENCE (two levels: first ten movements and whole sequence) as within-subject factors. Different kinematic variables were analyzed in separate ANOVAs. To evaluate the effects of tACS on MEP amplitude, we performed a repeated measures analysis of variance (ANOVA) using CONDITION (four levels: beta, gamma, sham, and baseline) as the within-subject factor. Fisher's pairwise least significant difference test was used for post hoc analyses in ANOVAs.

Pearson's product-moment correlation was used to evaluate possible associations between the effects of tACS on movement kinematics and M1 excitability. For this purpose, we normalized the kinematic and TMS values recorded during beta and gamma tACS to their respective baselines (no stimulation).

Unless otherwise stated, all the results are shown as mean values ± standard error of the mean (SEM). The level of significance was set at $P < 0.05$ in all the tests. Data were analyzed using Statistica® (StatSoft Inc.).

3. Results

3.1. Effects of tACS on Finger Tapping Kinematics. The kinematic variables of repetitive finger tapping in the four tACS conditions are shown in Figure 2. Two-way repeated measures ANOVA revealed a significant effect of CONDITION for the amplitude decrement $(F(3, 51) = 3.00, P = 0.03)$; the post hoc analysis revealed higher values during gamma tACS and lower values during beta tACS $(P < 0.01)$. Most importantly, the analysis on the amplitude decrement detected a significant CONDITION × SEQUENCE interaction $(F(3, 51) = 3.42, P = 0.02)$. The post hoc analysis showed that the effects of tACS occurred in the early phase, that is, during the first ten movements of the motor task, with higher values being observed during gamma tACS $(P = 0.01)$ and lower values during beta tACS $(P = 0.04)$ in comparison with those of the unstimulated baseline tapping performance. Moreover, there was no difference between sham tACS and baseline tapping performance $(P = 0.31)$. In addition, the analysis of the amplitude decrement did not detect any effect of SEQUENCE $(F(1, 17) = 0.13, P = 0.72)$. The analysis did not reveal any effect of CONDITION, for the other finger tapping kinematics (all $P > 0.05$).

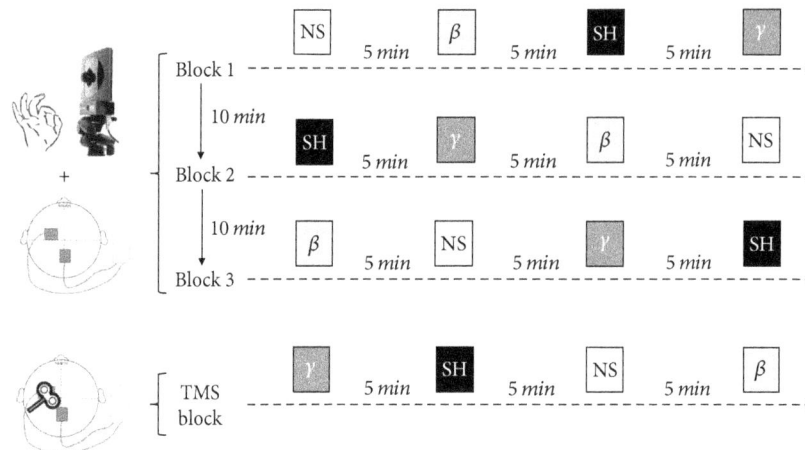

FIGURE 1: Experimental design. Finger tapping movements were recorded during no stimulation (NS), sham (SH), beta (β), and gamma (γ) tACS using an optoelectronic motion system. The four conditions were tested in a random order. We recorded one trial for each condition in 3 separate, consecutive blocks (total of 12 trials). Each trial consisted of 15 seconds of finger tapping. A 5-minute and 10-minute rest period was provided between each trial and between each block, respectively, to avoid fatigue. At the end of the kinematic recordings, the participants underwent a TMS assessment. Twenty single-pulse MEPs were recorded at rest during NS, SH, β, and γ tACS. The four conditions were randomized and performed at 5-minute intervals.

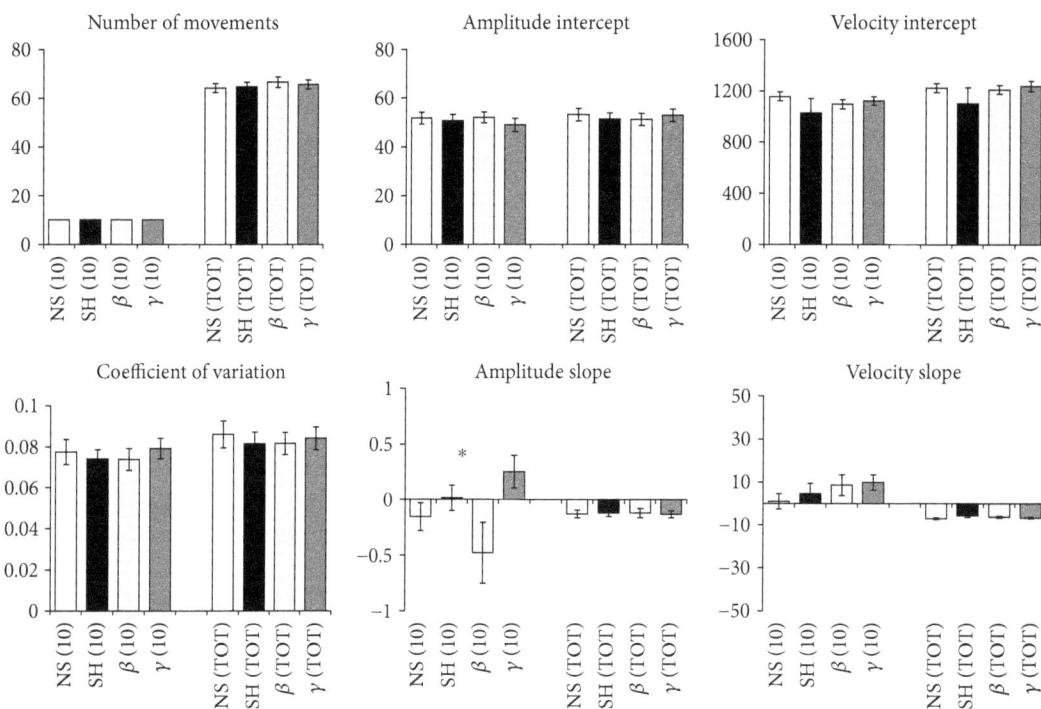

FIGURE 2: Kinematic variables. (10) refers to the first ten movements and (TOT) refers to the whole motor sequence. NS, SH, β, and γ refer to no stimulation, sham, beta, and gamma tACS, respectively. The asterisk denotes a significant CONDITION × SEQUENCE interaction in a repeated measures ANOVA. Error bars indicate the standard error of the mean.

The remaining results are represented in Table 1 and indicate the main effect of SEQUENCE on the slope and intercept of tapping velocity. The former was a consequence of a drop in velocity (negative velocity slope) across the whole trial (physiological fatigue) as opposed to a drop in velocity within the first 10 movements, over which there was a slight increase in velocity (Figure 2). The change in the intercept of tapping velocity between the first 10 movements and the whole series of movements was a product of the linear

regression technique, given these small differences in slopes. Importantly, however, these effects were independent of stimulation.

Further analyzing our data, rather than estimating the intercepts and slopes, we calculated the average amplitude and velocity for the first 10 movements of the motor task and for the whole sequence of 15 seconds. These measures were analyzed by a repeated measures ANOVA using CONDITION (four levels: beta, gamma, sham, and baseline)

Table 1: Effect of CONDITION (four levels: beta, gamma, sham, and baseline), SEQUENCE (two levels: first ten movements and whole sequence), and their interaction on movement kinematics. Significant effects are shown in bold. Post hoc tests confirmed that the main effect of CONDITION and the CONDITION × SEQUENCE interaction for amplitude slope was due to a frequency-dependent modulation of the amplitude slope estimated over the first 10 movements, but not over the whole trial. In contrast, the main effect of sequence on the slope and intercept of tapping velocity reflected a drop in velocity across the whole trial as opposed to a drop in velocity within the first 10 movements, over which there was a slight increase in velocity (Figure 2). Importantly, however, the longer-term physiological fatigue-related effects on velocity were independent of stimulation condition.

	CONDITION			SEQUENCE			CONDITION × SEQUENCE		
	F	d, f	P	F	d, f	P	F	d, f	P
N Movements*	0.57	3.51	0.63	—	—	—	—	—	—
CV	0.66	3.51	0.57	2.64	1.17	0.12	0.17	3.51	0.91
Amplitude intercept	0.85	3.51	0.47	3.26	1.17	0.09	4.52	3.51	0.07
Velocity intercept	1.28	3.51	0.29	62.13	1.17	**<0.001**	1.43	3.51	0.24
Amplitude slope	3.00	3.51	**0.03**	0.13	1.17	0.72	3.42	3.51	**0.02**
Velocity slope	1.97	3.51	0.12	44.30	1.17	**<0.001**	0.89	3.51	0.45

*shown are only the results of CONDITION, since the number of movements considered in the early part of the motor task is always 10.

and SEQUENCE (two levels: first ten movements and whole sequence) as within-subject factors. This analysis showed a significant effect of SEQUENCE for both parameters (average amplitude: $F(1, 17) = 34.68$, $P < 0.001$; average velocity: $F(1, 17) = 6.82$, $P = 0.01$). Post hoc analysis indicated higher values for both measures during the first ten movements (average amplitude: $46.57 \pm 1.41°$; average velocity: $438.62 \pm 16.71°/\text{sec}$) in comparison to those measured for the whole sequence (average amplitude: $43.88 \pm 1.18°$; average velocity: $418.43 \pm 13.96°/\text{sec}$). This analysis, however, showed no significant effect of CONDITION and no CONDITION × SEQUENCE interaction for both parameters (all $P > 0.05$). The results were therefore consistent with physiological fatigue across the whole trial, irrespective of the trial type.

Also, since tACS affected the slope of tap amplitudes over the first ten movements of the tapping task and yet velocity remained unchanged, we checked whether there were any changes in tapping frequency during tACS over the first ten movements. We calculated the average frequency and intercept and slope of the linear regression of the instantaneous tapping frequency versus the tap number over the first ten movements of the motor sequence. Then, we performed three separate repeated measures ANOVAs using CONDITION (four levels: beta, gamma, sham, and baseline) as the within-subject factor. The analyses showed no significant results (frequency average: $F(3, 51) = 2.26$, $P = 0.09$; frequency intercept: $F(3, 51) = 0.65$, $P = 0.59$; and frequency slope: $F(3, 51) = 1.12$, $P = 0.35$).

We finally explored whether fatigue might accrue during the experimental recordings or whether the rest periods provided between the four (intrablock) stimulation conditions and the three recording blocks (Figure 1) were sufficient to prevent this. We therefore assessed the occurrence of intrablock fatigue using a repeated measures ANOVA using CONDITION ORDER (four levels: 1st, 2nd, 3rd, and 4th condition) and SEQUENCE (two levels: first ten movements and whole sequence) as within-subject factors. We also assessed the occurrence of fatigue across consecutive blocks using a repeated measures ANOVA using BLOCK ORDER (three levels: 1st, 2nd, and 3rd block) and SEQUENCE (two levels:

first ten movements and whole sequence) as within-subject factors. The two ANOVAs did not reveal any significant effects of the main factors of analysis, nor any significant interaction between them (all $P > 0.05$, lowest $P = 0.12$).

In summary, the results indicate that the participants' performance was frequency-dependently modulated by tACS. Beta tACS led to an early amplitude decrement while gamma tACS had the opposite effect during the first ten movements of the motor sequence (Figure 3). Other measures of movement amplitude and velocity were similar in all four tACS conditions examined. Lastly, the results also provide evidence of longer-term physiological fatigue in terms of a drop in average amplitude and velocity across all taps when compared to the first 10 taps. However, this was unaffected by stimulation or stimulation condition order and did not carry over between blocks.

3.2. Effects of tACS on MEP. Relative MEP amplitude was not modulated by M1 tACS delivered at different frequencies (no stimulation/baseline: 0.97 ± 0.03; beta: 0.96 ± 0.04; gamma: 1.01 ± 0.05; and sham: 0.99 ± 0.04 mV). A repeated measures ANOVA on MEP values did not reveal any significant effect of the main factor CONDITION ($F(3, 51) = 1.24$, $P = 0.30$), thereby indicating that tACS delivered in different conditions did not modify M1 excitability. These findings suggest that tACS did not modulate corticospinal excitability at the current intensities used.

3.3. Intensity-Dependent Effects of Beta tACS. Since the stimulation intensity of beta tACS (0.61 ± 0.05 mA) was on average significantly lower than that of gamma tACS (1.00 ± 0.00 mA), we also investigated possible intensity-dependent effects of beta tACS on movement kinematics and MEP amplitude. We applied the median split procedure for this purpose [21]. We divided the participants into two groups according to the intensity of stimulation for beta tACS: a low-beta-intensity group (9 subjects, 0.37 ± 0.04 mA) and a high-beta-intensity group (9 subjects, 0.84 ± 0.05 mA). Kinematic data and MEP values during beta tACS were normalized to their corresponding baseline (no

Beta tACS

Gamma tACS

Baseline (no stimulation)

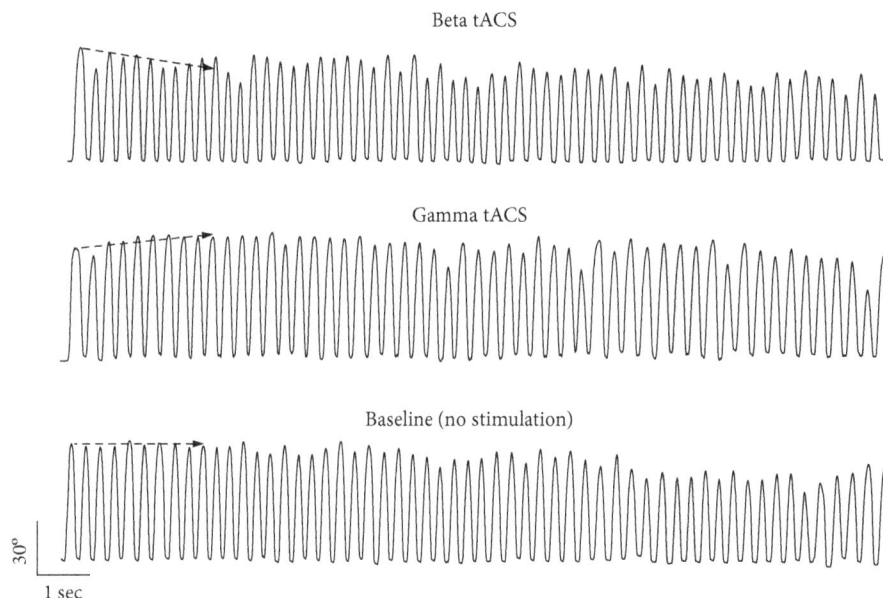

FIGURE 3: Paradigmatic example of kinematic recordings of finger tapping during beta and gamma tACS. The participant's performance was frequency-dependently modulated by tACS. Namely, beta tACS led to an early amplitude decrement during repetitive finger tapping while gamma tACS had the opposite effect.

stimulation). We then conducted separate ANOVAs, using the between-group factor INTENSITY (two levels: high versus low beta) and the within-group factor SEQUENCE (two levels: first ten movements and whole sequence). The analysis on amplitude slope did not reveal any significant effects of INTENSITY ($F(1, 16) = 0.20$, $P = 0.65$) or SEQUENCE ($F(1, 16) = 1.68$, $P = 0.21$), nor any INTENSITY $\times$ SEQUENCE interaction ($F(1, 16) = 0.35$, $P = 0.55$). No significant effects were observed for the main factors and their interaction term for either of the other kinematic parameters (all $P > 0.05$). Similarly, beta tACS intensity did not have any effect on normalized MEP (high beta subgroup: 0.97 ± 0.04 mV versus low beta subgroup: 1.09 ± 0.07 mV ($P = 0.12$) by unpaired t-test). Lastly, we also investigated possible correlations between the stimulation intensity during beta tACS and the normalized amplitude slope and other kinematic variables (both during the first ten movements and during the whole sequence), none of which were found to be statistically significant (r values ranged between -0.01 and 0.20 and the P value was always >0.05). Similarly, no significant correlation emerged between the beta tACS intensity and the MEP amplitude ratio ($r = -0.14$; $P = 0.57$).

3.4. Correlations between Movement Kinematics and MEP. In this analysis, we aimed to verify whether the kinematic variable modulation of repetitive finger movements correlated, at the individual level, with the MEP amplitude recorded during beta and gamma tACS. We did not detect any correlation between kinematic variables during the first ten movements of the sequence and M1 excitability changes either during beta tACS (r values ranged between -0.25 and 0.19 and the P value was always >0.05) or during gamma tACS (r values ranged between -0.01 and 0.38 and the P values were always

>0.05). Similarly, we did not detect any correlation between kinematic variables measured on the whole 15-second sequence and M1 excitability changes either during beta tACS (r values ranged between -0.12 and 0.19 and the P value was always >0.05) or during gamma tACS (r values ranged between -0.15 and 0.48 and the P values were always >0.05). These data further suggest that the frequency-dependent effects of tACS on movement kinematics were unrelated to individual M1 excitability changes.

4. Discussion

In the present study, we demonstrate that in healthy humans, beta tACS leads to an early and progressive reduction in amplitude (amplitude decrement) during repetitive finger tapping while gamma tACS has the opposite effect. These frequency-dependent stimulation effects are observed during the first ten movements of the motor sequence. As the tapping sequence continues still, further physiological fatigue sets in [23], but this is unaffected by tACS. tACS, as applied here, does not significantly affect other movement parameters, including overall movement amplitude, velocity, and rhythm which are mediated by distinct physiological mechanisms [26–28]. Finally, tACS does not induce any changes in MEP amplitude.

Since the amplitude, velocity, and rhythm of finger tapping in our study were similar in all four tACS conditions examined, the effects of beta and gamma tACS on the early amplitude decrement cannot be ascribed to varying levels of motor performance. Moreover, the changes in initial amplitude slope during beta and gamma tACS are unlikely to be due to any effect of physiological fatigue because the presentation of conditions was randomized and successive blocks were performed at least ten minutes apart. Accordingly, the effects of fatigue carrying over successive blocks were excluded by means of a specific statistical analysis on consecutive measurements. We can also rule out the possibility that the effects of beta and gamma tACS on the amplitude decrement are due to nonspecific factors (e.g., scalp or visual sensations) because we lowered the stimulation intensity of tACS to a level at which these effects were not present. We may thus speculate that the effects of tACS on the amplitude decrement result from an interaction between the modulation of motor resonant brain rhythms induced by stimulation and the physiological mechanisms involved in repetitive finger tapping. This would be in line with evidence that tACS at appropriate frequencies may entrain local oscillations, and, where these are the product of circuit resonances, amplify such rhythms [8–12].

Previous studies have shown that oscillatory activity in the beta frequency range varies with motor behaviour. In physiological conditions, beta activity is considered to have an antikinetic effect; that is, it is enhanced during movement suppression and depressed during voluntary movement execution [4, 36, 37]. The early but short-lived progressive amplitude decrement during repetitive finger tapping seen during beta tACS may be therefore explained by the entrainment of beta activity in M1, with or without amplitude amplification through resonance effects. In contrast, gamma tACS led to an early but short-lived progressive increment in tapping amplitude. Synchronized oscillations in the gamma frequency band are also functionally relevant in human M1. A rapid increase in the power of gamma oscillations occurs before and during movement execution as well as during rapid action stopping [2, 7, 38–41]. Gamma activity in M1 has been considered to be a prokinetic rhythm [42, 43] or to underlie flexible motor control [41]. Therefore, by entraining neuronal activity in the gamma frequency band, gamma tACS may exert prokinetic effects on repetitive finger movements and promote the dynamic control of motor output. Due to the limited topographical specificity of the electric stimulation, another possible explanation for prokinetic effects of gamma tACS on M1 is the concurrent modulation of the somatosensory cortex (S1). High gamma cortical activity is also a natural rhythm of S1 [44–47], and high gamma tACS on S1 is known to modulate central sensory processing [47]. Therefore, the improvement of motor performance at the beginning of the tapping sequence could be due to changes in sensory processing. A further possibility for the effects of tACS on repetitive finger movements is the modulation of frontal areas other than M1. Among these, the anterior cingulate cortex (ACC) has a role in planning and executing motor sequences [48, 49]. Entrainment of the gamma and beta rhythm might then facilitate or interfere with converging motor input from upstream areas, like the ACC, to M1. The fact that both the effects of beta and gamma tACS were only evident early on during movement sequences raises the possibility that their functional effects rapidly saturate. Indeed over time, they are compounded by the effects of physiological fatigue which overtake repetitive movement sequences irrespective of the stimulation state. Another possible explanation is the occurrence of a ceiling effect for gamma tACS and the activation of compensatory mechanisms counteracting the detrimental effect of beta tACS in physiological conditions.

The absence of tACS-related changes in movement velocity observed in our study is at odds with observations in previous studies [10, 11, 23], but we did not focus on repetitive finger movements and tested more proximal arm movements or alternative tasks, such as the hand force grip. In addition, while we evaluated internally generated voluntary movements, Pogosyan et al. [10], Joundi et al. [11], and Moisa et al. [23] tested externally cued motor tasks, which are known to be generated by different brain networks [50–52].

Another result of our study is that beta and gamma tACS did not modify the level of corticospinal excitability, as measured by changes in MEP amplitude following single-pulse TMS. This is in line with previous studies reporting similar findings in healthy subjects [20, 21, 35, 53], although other studies imply otherwise [19, 22, 54–56]. We have also found that there was no correlation between MEP change and early amplitude slope modulation during tACS on M1. This result suggests that modifications in cortical oscillations rather than changes in the global level of M1 excitability are responsible for the amplitude decrement of repetitive finger movements.

The present results may provide a background for future studies investigating voluntary movements in physiological conditions and movement abnormalities, like bradykinesia, in patients. The term bradykinesia is clinically defined as slowness and reduced amplitude of voluntary movement that is exacerbated by repetitive actions [57, 58]. Several studies have suggested that changes in the oscillatory activity in the basal ganglia or coupling between cortical and subcortical rhythms are all putative mechanisms involved in various hand movement abnormalities in PD patients [41, 59–63]. The observation that tACS delivered in the beta range leads to an early amplitude decrement may suggest that one of the mechanisms that underlies amplitude decrement in PD is an excess of beta oscillations in M1 and its connections.

The present study has a number of limitations that warrant consideration. Due to a lack of data allowing a direct estimation of tACS effects on brain oscillations, the interpretation of the mechanisms underlying our results remains speculative. Most importantly, the effects of tACS on movement kinematics may be relatively specific to finger control. It may not be possible to extrapolate the results we obtained in our study by testing repetitive finger movements to repetitive movements of other body segments, which may differ both in terms of inertia of the moving part and of the segment's underlying physiological mechanisms. In addition, despite the existing controversies on non-invasive electrical stimulation (e.g., topographical specificity and intensity-related effects) [64], several studies have demonstrated significant effects on the cortical areas being targeted [20, 21, 65] and no additional advantages in using stronger stimulation intensities once these reach about 1 mA [66]. In this regard, our results also demonstrate that the effects of stimulation, namely, beta tACS, are not influenced by the different intensities applied. Also, we did not use a navigation system for the TMS procedure. Finally, although we examined corticospinal excitability using single-pulse TMS, we cannot exclude that other physiological mechanisms known to be affected by beta and gamma tACS, such as cortical interneuronal excitability, [20, 21, 67] contributed to our results. The assessment of the possible relationship between tACS-dependent behavioural changes and concurrent changes of interneuronal activity is beyond the present study, and future studies are needed to explore this issue.

In conclusion, this study provides novel information on the effects of tACS, delivered at functionally relevant frequencies, on motor behaviour in healthy human subjects. Our findings point to a physiological role of cortical beta and gamma oscillations in the organisation and execution of repetitive finger movements. The novel finding of the study is the demonstration of differential effects of gamma and beta tACS on repetitive finger movements, specifically on the amplitude decrement. This could help in better understanding the role of cortical oscillations in the generation and modulation of sequence effect. The results also have pathophysiological implications and suggest that the amplitude decrement observed in PD may be due to exaggerated endogenous oscillatory activity in the beta band in M1 and its connections. The hope is that it may be possible to ameliorate movement abnormalities in PD through frequency-specific tACS, as already evidenced in tremor [29]. Further studies are needed to fully understand the behavioural effects of tACS in healthy subjects and in patients with movement disorders, as well as the clinical implications of tACS for therapeutic purposes in patients.

Conflicts of Interest

None of the authors have any potential conflicts of interest to disclose.

Authors' Contributions

Andrea Guerra and Matteo Bologna contributed equally to this work.

References

[1] A. K. Engel and P. Fries, "Beta-band oscillations–signalling the status quo?," *Current Opinion in Neurobiology*, vol. 20, no. 2, pp. 156–165, 2010.

[2] S. D. Muthukumaraswamy, "Functional properties of human primary motor cortex gamma oscillations," *Journal of Neurophysiology*, vol. 104, no. 5, pp. 2873–2885, 2010.

[3] W. Gaetz, J. C. Edgar, D. J. Wang, and T. P. L. Roberts, "Relating MEG measured motor cortical oscillations to resting γ-aminobutyric acid (GABA) concentration," *NeuroImage*, vol. 55, no. 2, pp. 616–621, 2011.

[4] J. M. Kilner, S. N. Baker, S. Salenius, V. Jousmäki, R. Hari, and R. N. Lemon, "Task-dependent modulation of 15-30 Hz coherence between rectified EMGs from human hand and forearm muscles," *The Journal of Physiology*, vol. 516, no. 2, pp. 559–570, 1999.

[5] J. M. Kilner, S. N. Baker, S. Salenius, R. Hari, and R. N. Lemon, "Human cortical muscle coherence is directly related to specific motor parameters," *The Journal of Neuroscience*, vol. 20, no. 23, pp. 8838–8845, 2000.

[6] R. Kristeva, L. Patino, and W. Omlor, "Beta-range cortical motor spectral power and corticomuscular coherence as a mechanism for effective corticospinal interaction during steady-state motor output," *NeuroImage*, vol. 36, no. 3, pp. 785–792, 2007.

[7] N. Crone, D. L. Miglioretti, B. Gordon, and R. P. Lesser, "Functional mapping of human sensorimotor cortex with electrocorticographic spectral analysis. II. Event-related synchronization in the gamma band," *Brain*, vol. 121, no. 12, pp. 2301–2315, 1998.

[8] T. Ball, E. Demandt, I. Mutschler et al., "Movement related activity in the high gamma range of the human EEG," *NeuroImage*, vol. 41, no. 2, pp. 302–310, 2008.

[9] D. Cheyne, S. Bells, P. Ferrari, W. Gaetz, and A. C. Bostan, "Self-paced movements induce high-frequency gamma oscillations in primary motor cortex," *NeuroImage*, vol. 42, no. 1, pp. 332–342, 2008.

[10] A. Pogosyan, L. D. Gaynor, A. Eusebio, and P. Brown, "Boosting cortical activity at beta-band frequencies slows movement in humans," *Current Biology*, vol. 19, no. 19, pp. 1637–1641, 2009.

[11] R. A. Joundi, N. Jenkinson, J.-S. Brittain, T. Z. Aziz, and P. Brown, "Driving oscillatory activity in the human cortex enhances motor performance," *Current Biology*, vol. 22, no. 5, pp. 403–407, 2012.

[12] C. Wach, V. Krause, V. Moliadze, W. Paulus, A. Schnitzler, and B. Pollok, "Effects of 10 Hz and 20 Hz transcranial alternating current stimulation (tACS) on motor functions and motor cortical excitability," *Behavioural Brain Research*, vol. 241, pp. 1–6, 2013.

[13] J.-S. Brittain, A. Sharott, and P. Brown, "The highs and lows of beta activity in cortico-basal ganglia loops," *European Journal of Neuroscience*, vol. 39, no. 11, pp. 1951–1959, 2014.

[14] F. Alonso-Frech, I. Zamarbide, M. Alegre et al., "Slow oscillatory activity and levodopa-induced dyskinesias in Parkinson's disease," *Brain*, vol. 129, no. 7, pp. 1748–1757, 2006.

[15] N. C. Swann, C. de Hemptinne, S. Miocinovic et al., "Gamma oscillations in the hyperkinetic state detected with chronic human brain recordings in Parkinson's disease," *The Journal of Neuroscience*, vol. 36, no. 24, pp. 6445–6458, 2016.

[16] A. Antal and W. Paulus, "Transcranial alternating current stimulation (tACS)," *Frontiers in Human Neuroscience*, vol. 7, 2013.

[17] D. J. L. G. Schutter and R. Hortensius, "Brain oscillations and frequency-dependent modulation of cortical excitability," *Brain Stimulation*, vol. 4, no. 2, pp. 97–103, 2011.

[18] F. Fröhlich and D. A. McCormick, "Endogenous electric fields may guide neocortical network activity," *Neuron*, vol. 67, no. 1, pp. 129–143, 2010.

[19] M. Feurra, G. Bianco, E. Santarnecchi, M. Del Testa, A. Rossi, and S. Rossi, "Frequency-dependent tuning of the human motor system induced by transcranial oscillatory potentials," *The Journal of Neuroscience*, vol. 31, no. 34, pp. 12165–12170, 2011.

[20] A. Guerra, A. Pogosyan, M. Nowak et al., "Phase dependency of the human primary motor cortex and cholinergic inhibition cancelation during beta tACS," *Cerebral Cortex*, vol. 26, no. 10, pp. 3977–3990, 2016.

[21] M. Nowak, E. Hinson, F. van Ede et al., "Driving human motor cortical oscillations leads to behaviorally relevant changes in

local GABAA inhibition: a tACS-TMS study," *The Journal of Neuroscience*, vol. 37, no. 17, pp. 4481–4492, 2017.

[22] M. Feurra, P. Pasqualetti, G. Bianco, E. Santarnecchi, A. Rossi, and S. Rossi, "State-dependent effects of transcranial oscillatory currents on the motor system: what you think matters," *The Journal of Neuroscience*, vol. 33, no. 44, pp. 17483–17489, 2013.

[23] M. Moisa, R. Polania, M. Grueschow, and C. C. Ruff, "Brain network mechanisms underlying motor enhancement by transcranial entrainment of gamma oscillations," *The Journal of Neuroscience*, vol. 36, no. 47, pp. 12053–12065, 2016.

[24] R. Agostino, A. Currà, M. Giovannelli, N. Modugno, M. Manfredi, and A. Berardelli, "Impairment of individual finger movements in Parkinson's disease," *Movement Disorders*, vol. 18, no. 5, pp. 560–565, 2003.

[25] M. Bologna, A. Guerra, G. Paparella et al., "Neurophysiological correlates of bradykinesia in Parkinson's disease," *Brain*, 2018.

[26] M. Bologna, G. Leodori, P. Stirpe et al., "Bradykinesia in early and advanced Parkinson's disease," *Journal of the Neurological Sciences*, vol. 369, pp. 286–291, 2016.

[27] A. J. Espay, D. E. Beaton, F. Morgante, C. A. Gunraj, A. E. Lang, and R. Chen, "Impairments of speed and amplitude of movement in Parkinson's disease: a pilot study," *Movement Disorders*, vol. 24, no. 7, pp. 1001–1008, 2009.

[28] A. J. Espay, J. P. Giuffrida, R. Chen et al., "Differential response of speed, amplitude, and rhythm to dopaminergic medications in Parkinson's disease," *Movement Disorders*, vol. 26, no. 14, pp. 2504–2508, 2011.

[29] J.-S. Brittain, P. Probert-Smith, T. Z. Aziz, and P. Brown, "Tremor suppression by rhythmic transcranial current stimulation," *Current Biology*, vol. 23, no. 5, pp. 436–440, 2013.

[30] P. M. Rossini, D. Burke, R. Chen et al., "Non-invasive electrical and magnetic stimulation of the brain, spinal cord, roots and peripheral nerves: basic principles and procedures for routine clinical and research application. An updated report from an I.F.C.N. Committee," *Clinical Neurophysiology*, vol. 126, no. 6, pp. 1071–1107, 2015.

[31] H. Ling, L. A. Massey, A. J. Lees, P. Brown, and B. L. Day, "Hypokinesia without decrement distinguishes progressive supranuclear palsy from Parkinson's disease," *Brain*, vol. 135, no. 4, pp. 1141–1153, 2012.

[32] M. Bologna, F. Di Biasio, A. Conte, E. Iezzi, N. Modugno, and A. Berardelli, "Effects of cerebellar continuous theta burst stimulation on resting tremor in Parkinson's disease," *Parkinsonism & Related Disorders*, vol. 21, no. 9, pp. 1061–1066, 2015.

[33] C. G. Goetz, B. C. Tilley, S. R. Shaftman et al., "Movement Disorder Society-sponsored revision of the Unified Parkinson's Disease Rating Scale (MDS-UPDRS): scale presentation and clinimetric testing results," *Movement Disorders*, vol. 23, no. 15, pp. 2129–2170, 2008.

[34] W. Gaetz, M. Macdonald, D. Cheyne, and O. C. Snead, "Neuromagnetic imaging of movement-related cortical oscillations in children and adults: age predicts post-movement beta rebound," *NeuroImage*, vol. 51, no. 2, pp. 792–807, 2010.

[35] A. Guerra, A. Suppa, M. Bologna et al., "Boosting the LTP-like plasticity effect of intermittent theta-burst stimulation using gamma transcranial alternating current stimulation," *Brain Stimulation*, vol. 11, no. 4, pp. 734–742, 2018.

[36] T. Gilbertson, E. Lalo, L. Doyle, V. Di Lazzaro, B. Cioni, and P. Brown, "Existing motor state is favored at the expense of new movement during 13-35 Hz oscillatory synchrony in the human corticospinal system," *The Journal of Neuroscience*, vol. 25, no. 34, pp. 7771–7779, 2005.

[37] Y. Zhang, X. Wang, S. L. Bressler, Y. Chen, and M. Ding, "Prestimulus cortical activity is correlated with speed of visuomotor processing," *Journal of Cognitive Neuroscience*, vol. 20, no. 10, pp. 1915–1925, 2008.

[38] G. Pfurtscheller and F. H. Lopes da Silva, "Event-related EEG/MEG synchronization and desynchronization: basic principles," *Clinical Neurophysiology*, vol. 110, no. 11, pp. 1842–1857, 1999.

[39] D. O. Cheyne, "MEG studies of sensorimotor rhythms: a review," *Experimental Neurology*, vol. 245, pp. 27–39, 2013.

[40] W. Gaetz, C. Liu, H. Zhu, L. Bloy, and T. P. L. Roberts, "Evidence for a motor gamma-band network governing response interference," *NeuroImage*, vol. 74, pp. 245–253, 2013.

[41] P. Fischer, A. Pogosyan, D. M. Herz et al., "Subthalamic nucleus gamma activity increases not only during movement but also during movement inhibition," *eLife*, vol. 6, 2017.

[42] X. Jia and A. Kohn, "Gamma rhythms in the brain," *PLoS Biology*, vol. 9, no. 4, article e1001045, 2011.

[43] A. Oswal, P. Brown, and V. Litvak, "Synchronized neural oscillations and the pathophysiology of Parkinson's disease," *Current Opinion in Neurology*, vol. 26, no. 6, pp. 662–670, 2013.

[44] S. M. Arnfred, L. K. Hansen, J. Parnas, and M. Mørup, "Proprioceptive evoked gamma oscillations," *Brain Research*, vol. 1147, pp. 167–174, 2007.

[45] N. Kanayama, A. Sato, and H. Ohira, "The role of gamma band oscillations and synchrony on rubber hand illusion and cross-modal integration," *Brain and Cognition*, vol. 69, no. 1, pp. 19–29, 2009.

[46] A. M. Cebolla, C. de Saedeleer, A. Bengoetxea et al., "Movement gating of beta/gamma oscillations involved in the N30 somatosensory evoked potential," *Human Brain Mapping*, vol. 30, no. 5, pp. 1568–1579, 2009.

[47] M. Feurra, W. Paulus, V. Walsh, and R. Kanai, "Frequency specific modulation of human somatosensory cortex," *Frontiers in Psychology*, vol. 2, p. 13, 2011.

[48] E. Lee, J. E. Lee, K. Yoo et al., "Neural correlates of progressive reduction of bradykinesia in de novo Parkinson's disease," *Parkinsonism & Related Disorders*, vol. 20, no. 12, pp. 1376–1381, 2014.

[49] T. C. Blanchard and B. Y. Hayden, "Neurons in dorsal anterior cingulate cortex signal postdecisional variables in a foraging task," *The Journal of Neuroscience: The Official Journal of the Society for Neuroscience*, vol. 34, no. 2, pp. 646–655, 2014.

[50] M. Jahanshahi, I. H. Jenkins, R. G. Brown, C. D. Marsden, R. E. Passingham, and D. J. Brooks, "Self-initiated versus externally triggered movements: I. An investigation using measurement of regional cerebral blood flow with PET and movement-related potentials in normal and Parkinson's disease subjects," *Brain*, vol. 118, no. 4, pp. 913–933, 1995.

[51] C. Gerloff, J. Richard, J. Hadley, A. E. Schulman, M. Honda, and M. Hallett, "Functional coupling and regional activation of human cortical motor areas during simple, internally paced and externally paced finger movements," *Brain*, vol. 121, no. 8, pp. 1513–1531, 1998.

[52] S. M. Papa, J. Artieda, and J. A. Obeso, "Cortical activity preceding self-initiated and externally triggered voluntary movement," *Movement Disorders*, vol. 6, no. 3, pp. 217–224, 1991.

[53] A. Antal, K. Boros, C. Poreisz, L. Chaieb, D. Terney, and W. Paulus, "Comparatively weak after-effects of transcranial alternating current stimulation (tACS) on cortical excitability in humans," *Brain Stimulation*, vol. 1, no. 2, pp. 97–105, 2008.

[54] S. Zaghi, L. de Freitas Rezende, L. M. de Oliveira et al., "Inhibition of motor cortex excitability with 15Hz transcranial alternating current stimulation (tACS)," *Neuroscience Letters*, vol. 479, no. 3, pp. 211–214, 2010.

[55] A. Cancelli, C. Cottone, G. Zito, M. Di Giorgio, P. Pasqualetti, and F. Tecchio, "Cortical inhibition and excitation by bilateral transcranial alternating current stimulation," *Restorative Neurology and Neuroscience*, vol. 33, no. 2, pp. 105–114, 2015.

[56] D. Cappon, K. D'Ostilio, G. Garraux, J. Rothwell, and P. Bisiacchi, "Effects of 10 Hz and 20 Hz transcranial alternating current stimulation on automatic motor control," *Brain Stimulation*, vol. 9, no. 4, pp. 518–524, 2016.

[57] W. R. Gibb and A. J. Lees, "The relevance of the Lewy body to the pathogenesis of idiopathic Parkinson's disease," *Journal of Neurology, Neurosurgery & Psychiatry*, vol. 51, no. 6, pp. 745–752, 1988.

[58] R. B. Postuma, D. Berg, M. Stern et al., "MDS clinical diagnostic criteria for Parkinson's disease," *Movement Disorders*, vol. 30, no. 12, pp. 1591–1601, 2015.

[59] A. Anzak, H. Tan, A. Pogosyan et al., "Subthalamic nucleus activity optimizes maximal effort motor responses in Parkinson's disease," *Brain*, vol. 135, no. 9, pp. 2766–2778, 2012.

[60] C. de Hemptinne, E. S. Ryapolova-Webb, E. L. Air et al., "Exaggerated phase-amplitude coupling in the primary motor cortex in Parkinson disease," *Proceedings of the National Academy of Sciences of the United States of America*, vol. 110, no. 12, pp. 4780–4785, 2013.

[61] H. Tan, A. Pogosyan, A. Anzak et al., "Frequency specific activity in subthalamic nucleus correlates with hand bradykinesia in Parkinson's disease," *Experimental Neurology*, vol. 240, pp. 122–129, 2013.

[62] H. Tan, A. Pogosyan, A. Anzak et al., "Complementary roles of different oscillatory activities in the subthalamic nucleus in coding motor effort in Parkinsonism," *Experimental Neurology*, vol. 248, pp. 187–195, 2013.

[63] H. Tan, A. Pogosyan, K. Ashkan et al., "Subthalamic nucleus local field potential activity helps encode motor effort rather than force in parkinsonism," *The Journal of Neuroscience*, vol. 35, no. 15, pp. 5941–5949, 2015.

[64] M. Vöröslakos, Y. Takeuchi, K. Brinyiczki et al., "Direct effects of transcranial electric stimulation on brain circuits in rats and humans," *Nature Communications*, vol. 9, no. 1, p. 483, 2018.

[65] R. F. Helfrich, T. R. Schneider, S. Rach, S. A. Trautmann-Lengsfeld, A. K. Engel, and C. S. Herrmann, "Entrainment of brain oscillations by transcranial alternating current stimulation," *Current Biology*, vol. 24, no. 3, pp. 333–339, 2014.

[66] K.-A. Ho, J. L. Taylor, T. Chew et al., "The effect of transcranial direct current stimulation (tDCS) electrode size and current intensity on motor cortical excitability: evidence from single and repeated sessions," *Brain Stimulation*, vol. 9, no. 1, pp. 1–7, 2016.

[67] V. Di Lazzaro, J. Rothwell, and M. Capogna, "Noninvasive stimulation of the human brain: activation of multiple cortical circuits," *The Neuroscientist*, vol. 24, no. 3, pp. 246–260, 2018.

4

Guiding Lights in Genome Editing for Inherited Retinal Disorders: Implications for Gene and Cell Therapy

Carla Sanjurjo-Soriano[1,2] and Vasiliki Kalatzis [1,2]

[1]*Inserm U1051, Institute for Neurosciences of Montpellier, Montpellier, France*
[2]*University of Montpellier, Montpellier, France*

Correspondence should be addressed to Vasiliki Kalatzis; vasiliki.kalatzis@inserm.fr

Academic Editor: Melissa R. Andrews

Inherited retinal dystrophies (IRDs) are a leading cause of visual impairment in the developing world. These conditions present an irreversible dysfunction or loss of neural retinal cells, which significantly impacts quality of life. Due to the anatomical accessibility and immunoprivileged status of the eye, ophthalmological research has been at the forefront of innovative and advanced gene- and cell-based therapies, both of which represent great potential as therapeutic treatments for IRD patients. However, due to a genetic and clinical heterogeneity, certain IRDs are not candidates for these approaches. New advances in the field of genome editing using Clustered Regularly Interspaced Short Palindromic Repeats (CRISPR) and CRISPR-associated protein (Cas) have provided an accurate and efficient way to edit the human genome and represent an appealing alternative for treating IRDs. We provide a brief update on current gene augmentation therapies for retinal dystrophies. Furthermore, we discuss recent advances in the field of genome editing and stem cell technologies, which together enable precise and personalized therapies for patients. Lastly, we highlight current technological limitations and barriers that need to be overcome before this technology can become a viable treatment option for patients.

1. Introduction

The eye, and more specifically the retina, as an extension of the central nervous system (CNS), provides a powerful and unique "window" to study neuronal diseases. The retina shares anatomical and developmental characteristics with the brain [1]. For example, it is relatively immunoprivileged and has specialized immune responses similar to the ones found in the brain and spinal cord [2, 3]. In addition, it is surrounded by the inner blood-retinal barrier (BRB), which is composed of the same nonfenestrated endothelial cells as those found in the blood-brain barrier (BBB) [4]. Due to the accessibility of the eye by modern techniques of vitreoretinal surgery, it is not surprising that major research and understanding in the context of the CNS has emerged from studies of the retina and the optic nerve [5–11]. Furthermore, the significant compartmentalization of the eye, and specifically the retina, has allowed it to become a prototype for the development of innovative therapies and has brought ocular diseases to the forefront of clinical translation for gene- and cell-based therapies. Here, we will specifically review current progress in these therapeutic strategies for diseases of the posterior retina (namely the neuronal photoreceptor cells). Optic neuropathies affecting the anterior retina (retinal ganglion cells (RGCs)) and optic nerve are beyond the scope of this review.

2. The Retina

The retina is an embryonic extension of the prosencephalon [12]. It lines the back of the eye and consists of multiple cell layers that are responsible for the detection and processing of visual information. The retina has a highly structured architecture that can be divided into a posterior pigmented monolayer and an anterior multilayered neuroretina. The posterior layer, the retinal pigment epithelium (RPE), plays an important role in protection (excess light absorption, phagocytosis, water and ion transport) and support (growth

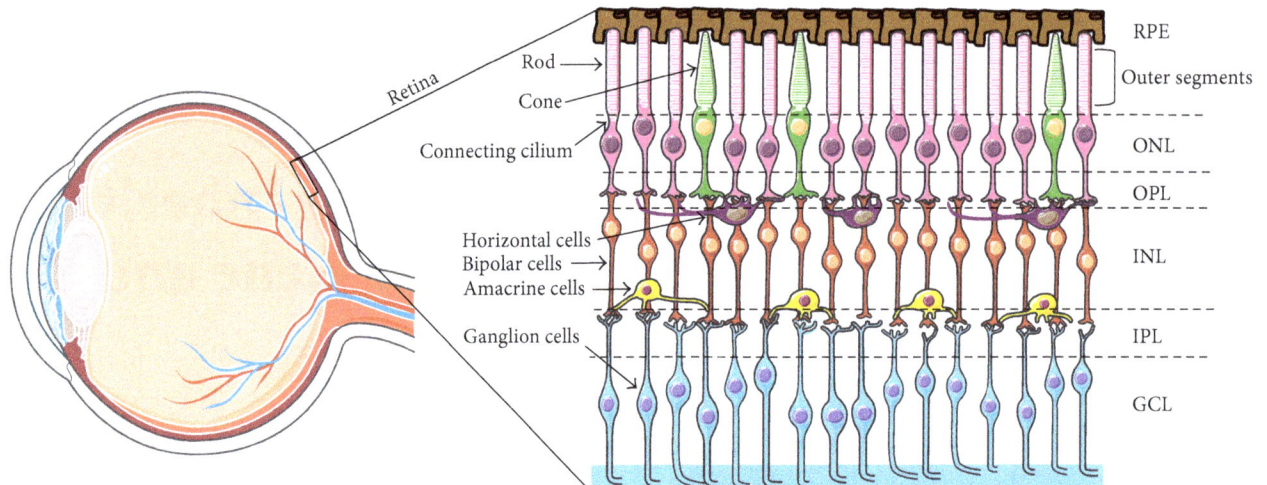

FIGURE 1: Schematic representation of the retina and the retinal cell layers. The retina is a layered structure lining the back of the eye consisting of a pigmented layer, the RPE, and a multilayered neuroretina. The RPE is in close contact with the outer segments of the photosensitive rod and cone cells of the neuroretina. The connecting cilium connects the photoreceptor outer segments with the cell bodies, which constitute a layer known as the outer nuclear layer (ONL). The axons of the photoreceptors synapse with the neuronal (bipolar, amacrine, and horizontal) cells of the inner nuclear layer (INL) via the outer plexiform layer (OPL). The axons of the INL cells in turn synapse with the ganglion cell layer (GCL) via the inner plexiform layer (IPL). The axons of the ganglion cells converge to form the optic nerve.

factor section, nutrient transport) of the photoreceptor layer [13, 14]. The neuroretina is highly stratified, and it is composed of three layers of specialized neurons that are interconnected by two synaptic layers (Figure 1). The first layer comprises the photosensitive rod and cone photoreceptor cells with their characteristic outer segments, within which the phototransduction process that follows light interaction takes place. Light intensity dictates which photoreceptor cells are used. In bright light, it is the centrally prevalent cones, and in low light, it is the peripherally prevalent rods. The photoreceptors then synapse with interneurons within the second layer, which transmit the electrical signal arriving from the photoreceptors to the RGCs in the third layer [15]. The axons of the RGCs form a nerve fibre layer, which becomes the optic nerve, and hence, the signal is transmitted from the eye to the brain for image interpretation. The inability to convert the light signal and transmit the electrical signal to the brain is the primary cause of visual impairment in the developing world. A large proportion of cases is due to dysfunction and/or loss of photoreceptors caused by a series of risk factors including age, diabetes, and genetics [16]. The latter gives rise to a specific subset of conditions referred to as inherited retinal dystrophies.

3. Inherited Retinal Dystrophies

Inherited retinal dystrophies (IRDs) are a genetically and clinically heterogeneous group of neurodegenerative disorders that lead to progressive visual impairment [16, 17]. They affect approximately 1 in 2000 individuals worldwide [18]. IRDs have been associated with mutations in more than 250 genes (see http://www.sph.uth.tmc.edu/Retnet), affecting the development, function and/or survival of the photoreceptors, and RPE [19], and with autosomal dominant,

recessive, or X-linked transmission [16]. Furthermore, complex, multifactorial, and heterogeneous diseases such as age-related macular degeneration (AMD) are also considered retinal dystrophies.

IRDs can be divided into nonsyndromic forms, characterized by an isolated retinal phenotype, or syndromic forms, in which another organ in addition to the eye is affected. Nonsyndromic IRDs can be further broken down into subgroups based on the disease progression and the region of the retina that is affected. Firstly, progressive conditions affecting exclusively the central retina (macula), leading to central vision loss, are known as macular dystrophies. The most common example is Stargardt disease with a prevalence of 1/10000, which is due to mutations in the gene ABCA4 [20]. Secondly, progressive conditions affecting the retina more widely can be classified depending on the type of photoreceptor that degenerates initially. Rod-cone dystrophies, where the rods are first affected, are characterized initially by night blindness and subsequently by peripheral vision loss; the most prevalent example (1/4000) is retinitis pigmentosa (RP), caused by mutations in over 80 genes [21]. By contrast, in cone-rod dystrophies, the cones are first affected, leading to decreased sharpness of visual acuity and blind spots in the center of the visual field; ABCA4 mutations also account for the majority of these cases [22].

When both the macula and the peripheral retina are affected and there is a rapid retinal degeneration from birth, the condition is known as Leber congenital amaurosis (LCA; prevalence of 1/50000), of which 18 types are recognized. In addition, if the retinal changes are associated with a degeneration of the choroid, a highly vascular, pigmented tissue underlying the retina, these diseases are referred to as chorioretinopathies. Choroideremia (CHM) is the most common example (prevalence of 1/50000) in this group. The most common form of syndromic IRD is the heterogeneous Usher syndrome group (prevalence of 1/20000), which is characterized by RP and hearing loss [23]. Usher syndrome is further subdivided into three subtypes depending on the severity and progression of the hearing loss and the age of onset of the RP. Usher syndrome type 1 (USH1) is the most severe; Usher syndrome type 2 (USH2) is the most common presenting moderate to severe symptoms. Lastly, Usher syndrome type 3 (USH3) presents a moderate phenotype and variable progression and onset of the disease.

The monogenic nature of IRDs coupled to the accessibility and immunoprivileged nature of the human eye has led to the advancement of pioneer gene therapies that hold promise for the development of future treatments. Most predominantly, IRDs have been targets for gene augmentation therapy [24]. More recently, gene correction of the causative gene, either by inactivation of the autosomal dominant allele or by correction of the recessive or X-linked alleles, has been explored as a possible treatment strategy. Currently, there is no standardized therapeutic option in the clinic for IRDs, due to the challenges of a diverse genetic landscape, fluctuating disease prevalence, variable age of onset and clinical course, and the specificity of the therapeutic products.

4. Gene Augmentation Therapy for IRDs

Gene augmentation therapy provides a normal copy of a mutated gene into native cells and hence is applicable for the treatment of haploinsufficiency or loss-of-function mutations. Most commonly, but not exclusively, the genes are vehicled by viral vectors, a pertinent example being adeno-associated viral (AAV) vectors [25]. AAV vectors present specific characteristics such as low immunogenicity and toxicity, lack of pathogenicity, long-term transgene expression, and relative ease in manipulating genetic elements, making them the safest and most effective viral vector platform for gene delivery into the retina to date [26]. Delivery can be achieved by subretinal injection, where the vector is administered into the subretinal space between the photoreceptors and RPE, which can result in the transduction of both cell types depending on the serotype used [27]. Other methods, such as intravitreal delivery, are less invasive and thus result in fewer complications postsurgery, but the delivery of the therapeutic genes, particularly to the posterior retina, is less effective [28].

A major milestone in gene augmentation therapy for IRDs was achieved in 2001 using a canine model for LCA2 due to mutations in the gene $RPE65$ ($RPE65^{-/-}$). AAV2/2-mediated delivery of $RPE65$ led to the long-term restoration of vision in treated dogs [29]. Following this study, multiple phase 1/2 clinical gene therapy trials assessed the effects of subretinal administration of AAV-RPE65 and demonstrated improved vision in some patients with no adverse effects of the vector [30–34]. A phase 3 clinical trial for LCA2, in which the therapeutic vector was administrated in both eyes, was subsequently launched. The vision of the treated group significantly increased compared to the control group, and this became the first ocular clinical trial in which both eyes were treated successfully [35]. As a consequence, the

corresponding vector has been recently commercialized as a drug under the name of voretigene neparvovec (Luxturna).

Hot on the heels of the AAV-RPE65 trial, phase 1/2 clinical trials for the X-linked chorioretinopathy choroideremia were initiated [36, 37] following preclinical studies in $Chm^{null/WT}$ mice [38]. These trials are also using an AAV2/2 vector, administered subretinally, to vehicle the causative CHM gene into both photoreceptors and the RPE. However, preclinical studies have shown that other AAV serotypes such as AAV2/5 [39] and AAV2/8 [40] are also effective for choroideremia. Lastly, a phase 1 clinical trial to treat RP was performed using an AAV2/2 vector to vehicle the causative gene $MERTK$ [41] confirming the safety profile of this vector serotype. A variety of other clinical trials have been initiated worldwide for other IRD genes using alternative AAV serotypes, but the results are still forthcoming.

Despite its numerous advantages, AAV vectors are limited by their cloning capacity (<4.7 kb) [42–44]. To overcome this limitation, efforts have turned to the use of equine infectious anemia virus- (EIAV-) based lentiviral vectors, which although integrative are nonpathogenic to humans. An EIAV vector was first tested in the case of the $ABCA4$ gene, which has a 6.8 kb coding sequence. Preclinical studies in the mouse $Abca4^{-/-}$ model showed a reduction in toxic A2E accumulation in the RPE of treated mice as compared to controls [45]. Following biodistribution and safety studies of the corresponding EIAV ABCA4-carrying vector [46], a clinical trial was begun in 2011, but the results are still pending. Similarly, an EIAV vector, carrying the $MYO7A$ gene (6.5 kb), was tested for its efficiency in the treatment of RP associated with Usher syndrome 1B [47]. Proof-of-concept studies in the mouse $Myo7A^{-/-}$ model suggested that the vector was able to prevent light-induced retinal degeneration [48]; however, the results of the clinical trial begun in 2012 are also pending. The outcome of these two EIAV clinical trials is essential to assess the suitability of lentiviral-based vectors for therapy of IRDs due to large causative genes.

Since the landmark canine LCA2 study by Acland et al., the progress in precision medicine research has continued to develop. However, several challenges remain to be overcome. Despite variations in visual improvements among treated patients in the LCA2 trials, long-term follow-up studies showed that the retinal structure continued to degenerate [49, 50]. This could be attributed to the advanced disease course at the time of treatment at which point the degeneration process could no longer be halted [51–53]. Advanced stages of retinal degeneration are incompatible with gene augmentation therapy, which, to be successful, requires that the nonfunctional target cells are still alive. Such patients might benefit better from cell-based transplantation therapy, which has the potential to restore visual function as detailed later.

An alternative explanation for the continual degeneration posttreatment could be inefficient vector transduction [52, 54]. Achieving correct levels of gene expression is essential for a robust and significant rescue of the phenotype [50, 55, 56]. This may be improved by the use of alternative [39, 57, 58] or modified [59] AAV serotypes, which have been shown to have a higher transduction efficiency than

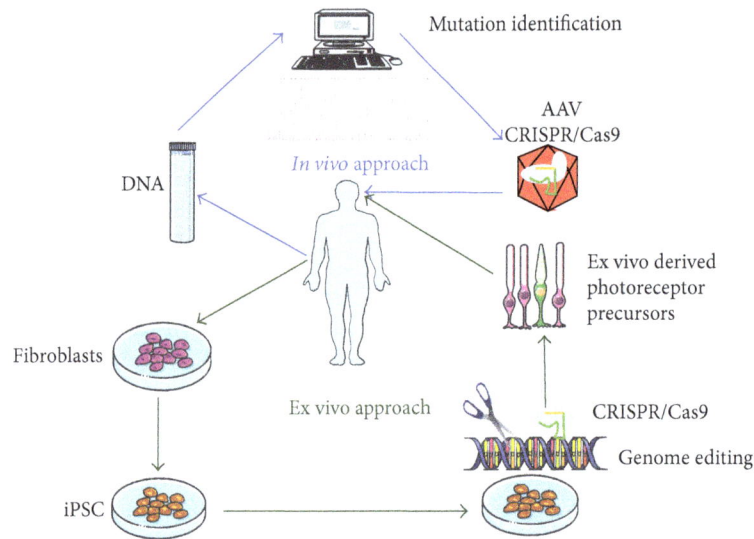

FIGURE 2: Therapeutic approaches for treating retinal dystrophies. For an *in vivo* approach (indicated in blue), the patient's DNA is isolated, and genetic screening is carried out to identify the pathogenic mutation causing the retinal phenotype. Delivery of the CRISPR/Cas9 components to correct the pathogenic mutation *in vivo* is achieved via AAV vectors administrated directly to the retina of the patients. For an ex vivo approach (in green), patient's fibroblasts with a known mutation in an IRD gene are isolated and reprogrammed to patient-specific iPSC. Genome editing of iPSCs is carried out using the CRISPR/Cas9 system. The corrected iPSCs are further differentiated into retinal cells, which can then be reimplanted into the patient's retina.

AAV2/2 in multiple species, or optimized promoter and/or codon-optimized cDNA sequences, which can stabilize transcript expression and hence increase protein levels [60, 61]. Finally, gene augmentation strategies are not convenient approaches for treating dominant or dominant-negative mutations, in which the mutated allele causing the disease needs to first be inactivated so that it does not interfere with the wild-type copy [62]. This is generally most easily accomplished by dual (wild-type and mutant) allele silencing prior to gene augmentation [63–66]. Therefore, despite the limited benefit demonstrated in clinical trials using AAV-mediated retinal gene augmentation therapy for the treatment of recessive mutations, other approaches for treating IRDs are being investigated with promising results.

5. Genome Editing for the Treatment of IRDs

Providing a wild-type copy of the mutated allele to restore a phenotype does not directly impact the pathogenic host gene. In contrast, a genome-editing approach has the potential of correcting the mutation directly in the patient's DNA. This approach could thus fill the void left by gene augmentation therapy in the case of large causative genes or dominant mutations. There are potentially two different approaches in the case of genome editing: an *in vivo* approach whereby the disease-causing mutations are corrected directly in the retina and an ex vivo approach in which the mutation is corrected in the patient's cells in view of future cell transplantation (Figure 2). The advances and current progress for both strategies will be summarized here. In addition to correcting pathogenic mutations, genome editing has also been used in a variety of preclinical models to further understand disease pathogenesis and to determine feasible treatment options.

Genome editing has advanced at an exceptionally rapid rate, creating huge impacts on biotechnology and biomedicine. The genome-editing era was initially triggered by the use of engineered meganucleases and zinc finger nucleases (ZFN) to specifically target a genomic sequence. Later, the development of transcription activator-like effector nucleases (TALEN) and more recently, the Clustered Regularly Interspaced Short Palindromic Repeats (CRISPR) and CRISPR-associated genes (Cas) system have led to a scientific genome-editing revolution.

5.1. ZFNs and TALENs. Efficient genome editing, regardless of which tool is used, is based upon the introduction of a double-strand break (DSB) at a precise point in the genome, which rapidly stimulates one of the two DNA repair pathways of the cell [67, 68]. The nonhomologous end-joining (NHEJ) pathway is the default method of repair, introducing insertions and deletions (INDELs) that normally will result in a nonfunctional genetic product [69]. Alternatively, homology-directed repair (HDR) uses the sister chromatids from a homologous chromosome as a template, or, in the case of directed genome editing, a donor template containing the desired sequence [70] (Figure 3). HDR occurs much less frequently than NHEJ, since homologous recombination naturally occurs in the late S and G2 phases of cellular division [71].

To induce a DSB, ZFNs and TALENs need to be guided to the target sequence by a protein DNA-binding domain. They therefore rely on the engineering of new proteins for each target, which has made genome editing difficult, laborious, and challenging [72]. Zinc finger proteins are a class of transcription factors that bind DNA through Cys2-His2 zinc finger domains [73]. ZFNs consist of a modifiable zinc finger domain designed to bind and target specific sequences in the

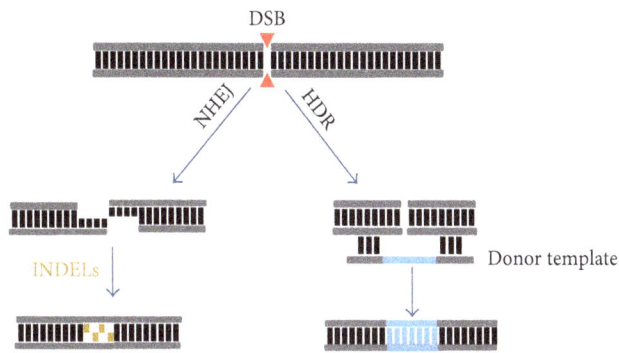

FIGURE 3: Schematic representation of a double-stranded break (DSB; red arrowheads), which can be repaired through nonhomologous end-joining (NHEJ) or homology-directed repair (HDR) pathways. The introduction of a double-strand break in the DNA will typically undergo the error-prone NHEJ repair pathway, which results in insertions and deletions (INDELs) of variable length that will lead to premature stop codon formation. HDR, an error-free repair pathway, occurs using a wild-type donor template with homology to the target site, which serves as a template for precise gene correction of the host's DNA.

genome and a cleavage domain consisting of the FokI nuclease [74, 75]. The cleavage of the DNA at the desired site is triggered by the dimerization of FokI; thus, two sets of ZFN on either side of the cleavage site are needed for the introduction of the DSB [76]. Similarly, TALENs are engineered by fusing a TAL effector DNA-binding domain with a FokI nuclease cleavage domain [77, 78]. TAL proteins are made of tandem repeats binding to individual nucleotides, which is different to ZFNs in which a zinc finger domain can bind to three different nucleotides (Figure 4). TALENs emerged as an alternative to ZFNs, as they represented a quicker turnaround from design to implementation and a more affordable option. Nonetheless, TALENs are relatively large proteins and contain repetitive DNA sequences resulting in TALEN inactivation [79], making genome editing still very challenging for researchers. In addition, similar to ZFNs, engineering of novel proteins for each DNA target is required.

Despite the challenges, ZFNs have been used as a proof-of-concept treatment for retinal disease. Human embryonic retinoblast cells expressing the Pro23His mutation in the Rhodopsin (RHO) gene were targeted with ZFNs. An increase in homologous recombination events occurred when the ZFNs were transfected with a homologous donor template compared to delivery of the ZFNs alone [80]. Similarly, researchers achieved site-specific gene correction in HEK293 cells stably expressing a missense mutation in *Ush1c*, causing Usher syndrome 1C. The authors reported correction of the pathogenic mutation by homologous recombination triggered by ZFNs and a donor plasmid template, when both were transfected to the cells [81]. These studies were the first to demonstrate the feasibility of gene targeting for retinal dystrophies using ZFNs. The major limitation for the applicability of ZFN relies on the design of the zinc fingers to bind every combination of three base pairs present in the genome, which has not yet been achieved.

Thus, many sites cannot be targeted using these engineered nucleases [77]. TALEN engineering has also been applied to the retina for the correction of a mutation in the $Crb1^{rd8}$ mouse, a model for LCA8. The mouse oocytes were treated with mRNA-encoding TALENs targeting the $Crb1^{rd8}$ allele together with a single-stranded oligonucleotide (ssODN) to correct the pathogenic allele. HDR triggered by TALEN and ssODN repair template was observed in 27% of the treated mice embryos, which presented an improvement of the ocular defects [82].

5.2. CRISPR/Cas Systems. The CRISPR/Cas system represents a novel and efficient method for genome editing compared to ZFNs and TALENs. CRISPR were first noticed in the bacterial genome in 1987 and described as an "unusual structure" in the $3'$ region of the *iap* gene, containing 29-base pair repeats interspaced by 32 nonrepetitive nucleotides [83]. Later, similar repeats were found in numerous bacteria and archaea [84–86]. It was in 2000 when the acronym CRISPR was given to unify these repeats observed in the bacterial genome [87, 88]. In addition, researchers discovered several clusters of protein-coding genes adjacent to these repeats, and they were subsequently called CRISPR-associated genes or Cas genes [87]. Evidence emerged that CRISPR loci might be involved in bacterial immunity, but it was not until 2007 when it was demonstrated that the CRISPR/Cas system provides resistance against specific phages in the bacterial strain *Streptococcus thermophiles* [89].

CRISPR as a genome editing-system was first described in 2012 [90]. Jinek and colleagues found that the CRISPR/Cas system of *Streptomyces pyogenes* (spCas9) was capable of inducing a DSB when two RNA molecules were present, a CRISPR RNA (crRNA) and a *trans*-activating RNA (tracrRNA). In addition, the authors showed that the fusion of the crRNA and tracrRNA produces a single-guide RNA (gRNA), which is equally effective in binding to target DNA. At the $5'$ end of this fused gRNA, 20 nucleotides can be customized to target specific sequences, becoming the first requirement for site-specific genome editing using CRISPR technology [90]. A second requirement for precise genome editing is found at the $3'$ end directly downstream of the cleavage site, where the protospacer adjacent motif (PAM), a three-nucleotide sequence (NGG in the case of SpCas9), is an absolute requirement for Cas9 recognition (Figure 5) [91]. The combination of both, the gRNA and the PAM sequence, allows target-specific cleavage of the DNA triggered by the Cas9 endonuclease [92]. Not long after these developments, the system was used to provide efficient gene repair in cells and in numerous organisms [70, 93–97].

5.3. Developments and Advances in CRISPR/Cas Technology. Since the emergence of the CRISPR/Cas9 technology, researchers have focused on the development of more efficient Cas9-like nucleases, presenting similar on-target activity but reduced off-target activity. A limiting factor for the reduction of off-targets triggered by the Cas endonuclease is the cellular levels of Cas9 protein in the cells. It has been shown that high levels increase the likelihood of off-target cleavage, most likely due to the increase in mismatch

(a)

(b)

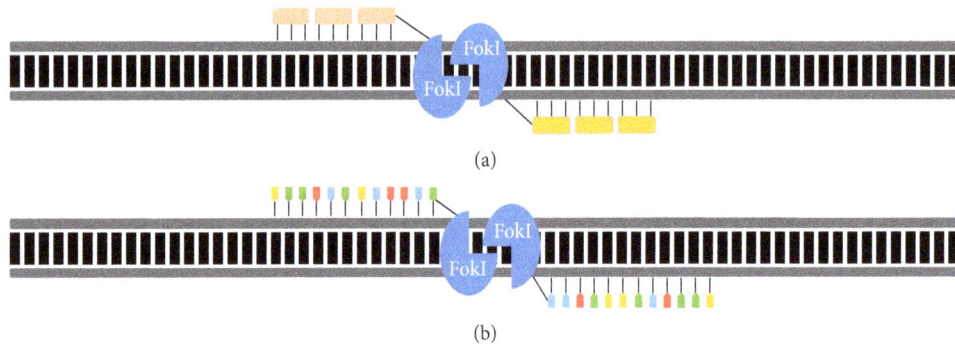

FIGURE 4: Schematic representation of the structure of a zinc finger nuclease (ZFN) and transcription activator-like effector nucleases (TALENs). (a) Cartoon of a ZFN dimer bound to DNA. ZFNs consist of two functional domains. A DNA-binding domain composed of three zinc finger modules, each one recognizing a unique triplet (3 bp) in the DNA. The DNA-cleaving domain composed of the FokI nuclease is attached to the zinc finger modules and induces the DSB in the DNA. (b) Cartoon of a TALEN dimer bound to DNA. TALENS bind DNA using the TAL effector recognizing individual nucleotides forming the DNA-binding domain. In addition, a DNA-cleaving domain comprised of the FokI nuclease is also present and will induce the DSB at the precise location in the DNA.

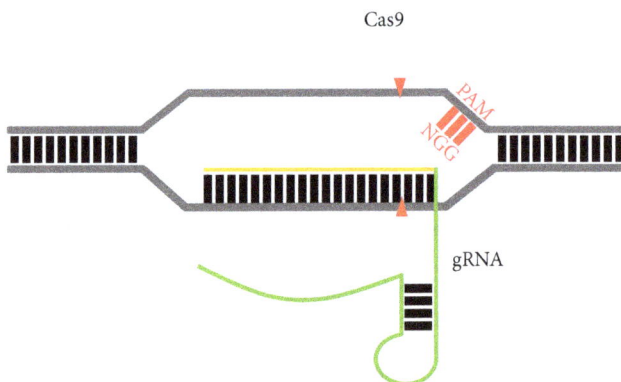

FIGURE 5: Schematic representation of the CRISPR/Cas9 system. The *Streptococcus pyogenes* Cas9 nuclease, with a "NGG" protospacer adjacent motif (PAM) sequence, has been targeted to a 20-nucleotide guide sequence in a specific region in the genome (yellow). The gRNA is complementary to the non-PAM strand. The green line represents the gRNA scaffold, which complexes with the Cas9 nuclease (light blue) and directs it to the desired site to induce a DSB (red arrowheads) in the DNA. Cas9 mediates the DSB 3 bp upstream of the PAM sequence.

tolerance between the gRNA and the DNA [98–100]. Successful efforts to overcome this limitation have been the delivery of Cas9 as a purified protein instead of using expression plasmids with strong promoters [101–105]. Alternatively, limiting the duration of Cas9 expression in the targeted cells has also been investigated. This approach has been successfully achieved in the retinal landscape as described below, presenting a huge advantage for future *in vivo* genome editing for eye diseases [106]. The use of two gRNA flanking the target region can also increase the on-target activity while reducing off-target events [92]. This strategy known as nickase Cas9 can be achieved by inactivation of one of the two nuclease domains of the Cas9, resulting in the cleavage of only one DNA strand. This strategy reduces the off-target DNA cleavage rate by 50- to 1500-fold as compared to a DSB performed at the same sequence [92]. Recent

advances have come with the development of Cas9 mutants, which decrease nonspecific DNA interactions. Two parallel studies developed rationally altered spCas9 mutants (eSpCas9 and "high-fidelity" Cas9) by modification of different amino acids to significantly reduce off-target effects [107, 108]. While these new mutants and other recent approaches are promising, off-target activity for each gRNA should be tested carefully before use in the clinic to avoid unintended mutagenesis in other regions of the genome [109].

Research has also focused on increasing the repertoire of host sequences that can be targeted by the CRISPR/Cas system, which is dictated by the recognition of the PAM sequence by Cas9. Ideally, the PAM sequence should be within 10 bp of the target sequence; thus, in some regions of the genome, there might be paucity of PAM sequences. Cas9 proteins of various bacterial species have different PAM motif requirements [70, 110–112], which can be naturally exploited to expand the CRISPR/Cas target space and increase the repertoire of accessible therapeutic targets. The most commonly used Cas9 is the SpCas9, which recognizes a short NGG PAM sequence, allowing it to be used across many genomic regions [90, 113]. Other Cas9 proteins, such as those of *S. thermophilus* and *Neisseria meningitides*, require the PAM motifs NNAGAAW and NNNGATT, respectively. In addition, *Streptococcus aureus* Cas9 that recognizes a NNGRRN PAM motif has a dual interest as it is also useful for AAV delivery *in vivo* due to its smaller (3.1 kb versus 4.2 kb for SpCas9) size [112, 114]. Along this line, the 2.9 kb Cas9 from *Campylobacter jejuni* (CjCas9) also offers an attractive option for gene delivery purposes [115]. CjCas9 has been packaged into an AAV2/9 vector along with a gRNA-targeting *Vegf* and delivered to the retina in a mouse model of choroidal neovascularization (CNV) [115]. This opens up the possibility that this strategy could be an alternative to repeated administration of pharmacological anti-VEGF treatment for AMD. Lastly, the CRISPR-Cpf1 system identified in *Acidaminococcus* and *Lachnospiraceae* bacteria, which requires the PAM motif TTTN, has a dual advantage for genome editing because, in addition to a novel PAM sequence [116], it induces staggered cuts away from the critical seed region thus preventing NHEJ and increasing the efficiency of HDR [117].

To increase the repertoire of genomic target sequences even further, recent work has been aimed at artificially engineering SpCas9 and SaCas9 with alternative PAM recognition sites [118, 119]. SpCas9 recognizing PAM target sites NGA and NGCG are known as "VQR" and "VRER", respectively; the modified SaCas9 known as "KKH" has a PAM recognition site NNNRRT. Since CRISPR/Cas9 technology was first used in 2012 for genome-editing purposes, significant advances have occurred to improve efficiency and specificity of the nucleases. The use and development of Cas9 nucleases with different PAM motifs may expand the use of CRISPR/Cas technology throughout the human genome.

6. *In Vivo* CRISPR/Cas Genome Editing

CRISPR/Cas genome editing in animal models has been useful for developing and testing possible therapeutic techniques that could represent sight-saving approaches in the future for patients. The biggest challenge researchers face is the delivery of the CRISPR system directly into the tissue or cells of interest in the retina. As mentioned above, AAV vectors are the most effective gene delivery method for a variety of retinal cells including photoreceptors and RPE [120]. However, their limited cloning capacity has not facilitated their application as a vehicle for CRISPR/Cas. CRISPR/Cas studies with AAV have been previously explored in the field of brain diseases [121] where the delivery of the SpCas9 and gRNA was divided between two vectors. Hung and colleagues applied a similar approach to the mouse retina whereby intravitreal administration of an AAV2/2 vector mediated the delivery of a CRISPR/Cas system designed to disrupt yellow fluorescent protein expression in a Thy1-YFP transgenic mouse model [122]. This resulted in an 84% reduction of YFP expression, providing for the first time proof of concept for CRISPR/Cas genome editing in the retina *in vivo*.

The use of dual AAV2/8 systems for the delivery of CRISPR-Cas9 components into the retina was also used to knock out the *Nrl* (neural retina-specific leucine zipper) gene in postmitotic photoreceptors. Subretinal injection of the dual AAV system prevented cone degeneration and restored the survival of rod photoreceptors in three different genetic mouse models of retinal degeneration ($Rho^{-/-}$ mice, Nrl-L-EGFP/Rd10 mice, and in RHO P347S transgenic mice) [123]. Similarly, subretinal injection of a dual AAV2/5 CRISPR/Cas9 system in mice deleted the wild-type mouse intron 25 of the causative LCA10 gene *CEP290* [106]. This intron is homologous to the human intron 26 that houses a variant, which is the most prevalent recurrent causative mutation of LCA10 [124, 125]. Hence, this *in vivo* study is a proof of concept for the potential treatment of patients by ablation of the intronic variant [106]. In addition, the authors developed a self-limiting CRISPR/Cas9 system by incorporating recognition sites for the gRNAs into the SpCas9 plasmid, limiting the expression time of the Cas9. This self-limiting Cas9 approach lowers the chance of undesirable

off-target events, potential toxicity, and SpCas9-specific cellular immune response [126].

The use of purified Cas9 ribonucleoproteins (RNP) has also been studied in the retina as an alternative delivery approach to AAV. This method reduces the time of Cas9 exposure potentially reducing off-targets, as the Cas9 RNP complex is degraded in the cell 24 h after delivery [102, 103]. Subretinal delivery of Cas9 RNP-targeting *Vegf* in a mouse model of CNV significantly reduced expression [105], thus providing preliminary evidence that this method could be used for an *in vivo* treatment of patients with AMD and more importantly expanding the possibilities for the treatment of retinal dystrophies using purified Cas9 proteins delivered directly into the retina. Further studies are needed in order to determine if the *in vivo* delivery of Cas9 RNP into the retinal cells is as efficient as viral vector-mediated delivery by subretinal injections.

These above *in vivo* studies used CRISPR/Cas9 technology to mediate NHEJ, which results in INDELs and gene inactivation. A major problem that still remains to be addressed is how to achieve effective and accurate genome editing in the retina, as photoreceptors are postmitotic cells and largely lack HDR repair mechanisms. Suzuki and colleagues developed a novel strategy called homology-independent targeted integration (HITI), which allows for targeted NHEJ knock-in in nondividing cells, such as the photoreceptors [127]. After subretinal injection of the AAV2/8- or 2/9-vehicled HITI system in a rat model of RP, correct knock-in preserved the thickness of the ONL and improved visual function. Therefore, this approach is a highly promising solution for postmitotic neurons, as it relies on the NHEJ mechanism, as opposed to HDR, for functional integration of a desired DNA sequence.

The use of CRISPR/Cas9 system and HDR in preclinical animal models has also been performed. Wu and colleagues used this technique to determine the causative variant for the RP phenotype found in the "rodless" (rd1) mouse model. The *rd1* mice carry two homozygous variants in *Pde6b*: a nonsense mutation (Y347X) in exon 7 and a murine leukemia virus insertion in intron 1. Following CRISPR-mediated correction of the nonsense variant, the retinal phenotype of the treated mice was restored demonstrating that the Y347X mutation was pathogenic [128]. Similarly, the pathogenicity of a novel missense variant in *REEP6*-causing RP, was proven by generating a mouse knock-in model of *Reep6* using CRISPR/Cas9 technology [129].

One of the biggest challenges before the CRISPR revolution was the treatment of autosomal dominant conditions, in which specific inactivation of the mutant allele is required to restore the phenotype. The treatment of these disorders was previously considered as complicated, as gene augmentation approaches did not directly target the pathogenic gene. The development of CRISPR technology has now changed the landscape of dominant disorders. One promising therapeutic approach is to decrease gene transcription through a strategy known as CRISPR interference (CRISPRi) [130]. In this strategy, Cas9 lacks nuclease activity, known as dead Cas9 (dCas9). Blockage of the transcriptional machinery occurs when dCas9 is coupled with a sequence-specific gRNA, preventing the RNA polymerase and transcription factors from transcribing genes. This strategy has been successfully achieved in eukaryotes and human cells [131–133]. Currently, this approach has not been applied to retinal dystrophies, but it carries a great potential due to the minimal off-target effects, which is an improvement to previous strategies involving RNA interference [134, 135].

Ablation of the mutant allele using CRISPR/Cas9 technology is another strategy that has been used in dominant forms for RP due to mutations in the gene encoding Rhodopsin (RHO). Bakondi and colleagues targeted an allele-specific PAM sequence present only in the Rho^{S334} mutant allele of an RP mouse model. Following subretinal administration and electroporation of the CRISPR components, the photoreceptor phenotype was rescued and visual acuity increased by 53% [136]. Similarly, Latella et al. performed a targeted knockout of a patient-derived mutant RHO P23H minigene in a transgenic mouse model. Subretinal electroporation of Cas9 and two gRNA targeting the 5' and the 3' regions of exon 1 resulted in reduced expression of the RHO gene [137]. These studies carry huge promise for the use of CRISPR/Cas systems to inactivate autosomal dominant pathogenic alleles in humans.

The rapid development of these technologies and the success achieved by proof-of-concept studies in vivo are speeding up the clinical translation of CRISPR technology. There is currently no CRISPR-based clinical trial for eye disease. Nonetheless, this may soon change as EDITAS medicine appears dedicated to bringing the aforementioned intron 26 skipping approach for CEP290 to LCA10 patients (https://www.allergan.com/news/news/thomson-reuters/allergan-and-editas-medicine-enter-into-strategic).

7. Ex Vivo Gene Correction and Cell-Based Therapy

While gene-based therapies may halt or at least slow down the progression of the disease by targeting dysfunctional cells, another promising approach in treating retinal dystrophies is stem cell-derived retinal cell transplantation. The retina develops from the neuroectoderm, thus, like any other CNS tissue, presents a low regeneration potential. Therefore, IRDs caused by degeneration or loss of photoreceptors could potentially benefit from cell-based therapies, which would restore a functional retina and reverse the ocular condition.

The first evidence showing functional photoreceptor replacement was achieved when freshly dissociated rod photoreceptors were transplanted into the subretinal space [138]. However, the number of transplanted cells could not be increased in vitro due to their postmitotic state. Thus, there was a need to increase the number of photoreceptors for efficient transplantation into the donor retina. Lamba and colleagues showed that human embryonic stem cells (ESCs) can be directed to a retinal cell fate and differentiated into retinal precursors [139]. The transplantation of these ESC-derived photoreceptors precursors into the subretinal space of an LCA mouse model resulted in restoration of the light response, establishing ESCs as a source for photoreceptor replacement [140]. ESCs present a high proliferative, self-renewal, and differentiation potential, which makes them an ideal tool to study human diseases in vitro.

However, the use of ESCs is associated with controversial and ethical considerations, thus severely impeding major progress towards exploiting their full potential. Takahashi et al. performed groundbreaking work in 2007, which overcame the major limitations associated with the use of human ESCs. Takahashi et al. demonstrated that it is possible to generate induced pluripotent stem cells (iPSCs) from adult human fibroblasts by a reprograming process, which involves expression of four transcription factors that revert the somatic cells to a pluripotent state [141]. These cells have the potential to replace patient's tissue and represent a large source of cells for the study of human disease [142, 143]. In addition, iPSC-derived cells have two major advantages in terms of cell transplantation: they avoid the ethical issues associated with the use of embryonic or fetal tissue and they offer the possibility of autologous transplantation avoiding risks of immune rejection.

Both ESCs and iPSCs have been used extensively in the area of stem cell-derived photoreceptor generation and transplantation. Sasai and colleagues revolutionized this field by showing that it is possible to mimic optic morphogenesis in 3D culture using murine [144] and human [145] ESCs and thus obtain a large source of appropriate-staged photoreceptor precursors. It was subsequently shown that, if present in sufficient numbers, both ESC-derived and donor photoreceptor precursors could restore visual function in preclinical retinal models [140, 146–149]. In addition, it was demonstrated that photoreceptor precursors [150–152] as well as functional [153] photoreceptors could also be obtained from iPSCs. Moreover, iPSC-derived photoreceptor precursors were transplantable and could also restore vision in preclinical models [154]. Human ESCs and iPSC will continue to have a huge impact on the study and the treatment of human eye disease, as more optimal and standardized differentiation protocols continue to be developed.

The coupling of iPSC and CRISPR/Cas genome-editing technologies to repair patient-specific mutations brings us to a new era of precise and personalized medicine for patients. Advances have already been made for the CRISPR/Cas-mediated correction of pathogenic mutations causing retinal dystrophies in patient's iPSCs. Bassuk and colleagues were the first to demonstrate the potential of this approach by correcting a missense mutation in RPGR responsible for X-linked RP [155]. Burnight and colleagues performed proof-of-concept studies for the correction of an exonic, deep intronic, and dominant gain of function variants: targeting an Alu insertion in exon 9 of MAK restored the retinal transcript and protein, NHEJ corrected a cryptic splice variant in CEP290-causing LCA10, and mutant allele-specific targeting invalidated the dominant Pro23His mutation in the RHO gene [156]. Further upstream, the most prevalent c.2299delG mutation in the USH2A gene, responsible for Usher syndrome type 2, was corrected in patient's fibroblasts using CRISPR/Cas9 and HDR [157]. These proof-of-concept studies support the development of personalized iPSC-based transplantation therapies for retinal disease. On a different note, CRISPR/Cas technology in iPSCs has been used for fluorescent reporter gene knock-in at the termination codon of the cone-rod homeobox (*Crx*) gene, a photoreceptor-specific transcription factor gene. This allows the real-time monitoring of photoreceptor differentiation [158], demonstrating the interest of this technology also for fundamental research.

Following on from the big and promising advances, which demonstrated that stem cell-derived photoreceptor transplantation can restore rod- and cone-mediated vision, recent studies demonstrated that these transplanted cells do not integrate into nondegenerative host retinas. Instead, postmitotic donor and host photoreceptors engage in the transfer of cellular material, such as RNA and proteins including Rhodopsin [149, 159–161]. The visual improvements observed after stem cell-derived photoreceptor transplantation were hypothesized to be the result of endogenous photoreceptors supplemented by donor cell-derived proteins. More recently, it was shown that both cell integration and cytoplasmic transfer can take place in degenerative hosts and that the relative contributions would depend on the local host environment [162]. Elucidation of the underlying mechanisms of this cellular material transfer could lead to novel therapeutic approaches in introducing functional proteins into dysfunctional photoreceptors as an alternative to gene replacement. In particular, it opens up the attractive possibility that Cas9 could be delivered as a purified protein for genome editing of viable photoreceptors.

The use of stem cell-derived photoreceptors is a powerful tool for the understanding of human retinal development and disease modeling and underlies a great potential for developing cell transplantation therapies. Such therapies are already underway in the clinic using hESC- [163–165] or hiPSC-derived [166] RPE. Initially, hESC-derived RPE was subretinally administered into AMD and Stargardt patients as dissociated cells. These cells safely persisted over time in the host retina and stably rescued visual acuity in a subset of patients [164]. Just recently, an RPE patch comprising a fully differentiated hESC-derived RPE monolayer on a coated, synthetic basement membrane was transplanted into AMD patients [165]. A one-year follow-up showed persistence of the sheet, which was associated with increased visual acuity and reading speed. It remains to be seen if these improvements will be stable over time. Lastly, the first ever, autologous transplantation for the retina was performed using a free hiPSC-derived RPE monolayer [166]. A one-year follow-up showed that the transplantation was safe and no immune response was provoked even in the absence of immunosuppression. This provides hope for the future autologous transplantation of genome-edited retinal cells in patients. Nonetheless, further work is required to establish robust and reproducible protocols for the generation of iPSC-derived photoreceptors. In addition, if such cells are transplanted following gene mutation repair, stringent quality control of the iPSCs before and after gene correction is extremely important. Furthermore, a detailed screening for possible off-target effects triggered by CRISPR/Cas

has to be performed prior to transplantation into the diseased host retina.

8. Future Challenges and Perspectives

The eye, more specifically the posterior retina, has proven to be a powerful model for the development of pioneer therapies, which could later be applied to other parts of the CNS. Despite the current success achieved by researchers and the relative ease and precise manipulation of the genome using the CRISPR/Cas system, improvements are being made. These are focused on the development of more efficient delivery methods, the identification and understanding of the off-target events, and increasing the efficiency of mutation correction. All these matters should be carefully addressed before this strategy can be safely applied in the clinic.

Potential delivery methods of the CRISPR/Cas components can be diverse. For an *in vivo* application, the ideal vehicle would be an AAV vector. The limitation of this method, in addition to size restrictions, is the constitutive expression of the Cas9 protein in the host organism, which increases the risk of unwanted off-target events in the genome [98–100]. The use of Cas9 RNP has been shown to be effective *in vivo* for reducing off-target events [101, 102, 167], although to our knowledge there has not been a study directly comparing the off-target effects of a given gRNA by AAV or RNP delivery. Thus, future research is needed in order to elucidate the most effective way, with high on-target activity and null off-target activity, to deliver CRISPR/Cas components *in vivo*.

A variety of methods aimed at testing for off-target mutations have been developed [168–170]. These methods are based on algorithms to computationally test homologous regions in the genome. However, currently, there is no gold standard, and it is not yet clear if Cas9 has the potential to alter other nonhomologous regions in the genome. Some studies have performed whole exome sequencing (WES) in CRISPR-treated cells and organisms [171, 172], providing an accurate and comprehensive way of testing off-target mutations. Such approaches should be taken into consideration following ex vivo gene correction in view of future transplantation into the patient.

In addition to improving the understanding of the off-target effects created by Cas9, much effort has focused on developing methods to enhance genome-editing efficiency. In cases where gene correction is required, the HDR repair pathway is needed, and this is incompatible with postmitotic photoreceptor targets. Exciting new developments in HDR-independent base-editing strategies have shown promise for gene correction in postmitotic cells. In these cases, Cas9 is fused to a cytidine deaminase to create a base-editor tool at the specific genome target [173, 174], thus circumventing the need for cell division. In addition, as mentioned above, the HITI approach also carries a great promise for precise gene correction in postmitotic cells by using the NHEJ pathway [127].

Overall, the future looks bright for the use of CRISPR/ Cas genome editing in ophthalmology, and it is likely that the studies presented here are just the beginning of what is to come.

Conflicts of Interest

The authors declare that they have no conflicts of interest.

Acknowledgments

The authors thank M. Diakatou for critical reading of the manuscript and helpful comments. The authors also thank the patient association SOS Retinite, which funded Carla Sanjurjo-Soriano.

References

[1] A. London, I. Benhar, and M. Schwartz, "The retina as a window to the brain—from eye research to CNS disorders," *Nature Reviews Neurology*, vol. 9, no. 1, pp. 44–53, 2013.

[2] J. W. Streilein, "Ocular immune privilege: therapeutic opportunities from an experiment of nature," *Nature Reviews Immunology*, vol. 3, no. 11, pp. 879–889, 2003.

[3] I. Benhar, A. London, and M. Schwartz, "The privileged immunity of immune privileged organs: the case of the eye," *Frontiers in Immunology*, vol. 3, p. 296, 2012.

[4] C. Kaur, W. Foulds, and E. Ling, "Blood–retinal barrier in hypoxic ischaemic conditions: basic concepts, clinical features and management," *Progress in Retinal and Eye Research*, vol. 27, no. 6, pp. 622–647, 2008.

[5] L. Benowitz and Y. Yin, "Rewiring the injured CNS: lessons from the optic nerve," *Experimental Neurology*, vol. 209, no. 2, pp. 389–398, 2008.

[6] M. Vidal-Sanz, G. M. Bray, M. P. Villegas-Perez, S. Thanos, and A. J. Aguayo, "Axonal regeneration and synapse formation in the superior colliculus by retinal ganglion cells in the adult rat," *The Journal of Neuroscience*, vol. 7, no. 9, pp. 2894–2909, 1987.

[7] P. Lingor, N. Teusch, K. Schwarz et al., "Inhibition of Rho kinase (ROCK) increases neurite outgrowth on chondroitin sulphate proteoglycan *in vitro* and axonal regeneration in the adult optic nerve *in vivo*," *Journal of Neurochemistry*, vol. 103, no. 1, pp. 181–189, 2007.

[8] A. London, E. Itskovich, I. Benhar et al., "Neuroprotection and progenitor cell renewal in the injured adult murine retina requires healing monocyte-derived macrophages," *Journal of Experimental Medicine*, vol. 208, no. 1, pp. 23–39, 2011.

[9] K. Kozar, M. A. Ciemerych, V. I. Rebel et al., "Mouse development and cell proliferation in the absence of D-cyclins," *Cell*, vol. 118, no. 4, pp. 477–491, 2004.

[10] C. Zaverucha-Do-Valle, F. Gubert, M. Bargas-Rega et al., "Bone marrow mononuclear cells increase retinal ganglion cell survival and axon regeneration in the adult rat," *Cell Transplantation*, vol. 20, no. 3, pp. 391–406, 2011.

[11] R. Shechter, A. Ronen, A. Rolls et al., "Toll-like receptor 4 restricts retinal progenitor cell proliferation," *Journal of Cell Biology*, vol. 183, no. 3, pp. 393–400, 2008.

[12] S. Hughes, H. Yang, and T. Chan-ling, "Vascularization of the human fetal retina: roles of vasculogenesis and angiogenesis," *Investigative Ophthalmology & Visual Science*, vol. 41, no. 5, pp. 1217–1228, 2000.

[13] J. Cai, K. C. Nelson, M. Wu, P. Sternberg Jr, and D. P. Jones, "Oxidative damage and protection of the RPE," *Progress in Retinal and Eye Research*, vol. 19, no. 2, pp. 205–221, 2000.

[14] X. Gu, N. J. Neric, J. S. Crabb et al., "Age-related changes in the retinal pigment epithelium (RPE)," *PLoS One*, vol. 7, no. 6, article e38673, 2012.

[15] M. A. Dyer and C. L. Cepko, "Regulating proliferation during retinal development," *Nature Reviews Neuroscience*, vol. 2, no. 5, pp. 333–342, 2001.

[16] W. Berger, B. Kloeckener-Gruissem, and J. Neidhardt, "The molecular basis of human retinal and vitreoretinal diseases," *Progress in Retinal and Eye Research*, vol. 29, no. 5, pp. 335–375, 2010.

[17] D. T. Hartong, E. L. Berson, and T. P. Dryja, "Retinitis pigmentosa," *The Lancet*, vol. 368, no. 9549, pp. 1795–1809, 2006.

[18] M. M. Sohocki, S. P. Daiger, S. J. Bowne et al., "Prevalence of mutations causing retinitis pigmentosa and other inherited retinopathies," *Human Mutation*, vol. 17, no. 1, pp. 42–51, 2001.

[19] L. S. Sullivan and S. P. Daiger, "Inherited retinal degeneration: exceptional genetic and clinical heterogeneity," *Molecular Medicine Today*, vol. 2, no. 9, pp. 380–386, 1996.

[20] P. Tanna, R. W. Strauss, K. Fujinami, and M. Michaelides, "Stargardt disease: clinical features, molecular genetics, animal models and therapeutic options," *British Journal of Ophthalmology*, vol. 101, no. 1, pp. 25–30, 2017.

[21] S. K. Verbakel, R. A. C. van Huet, C. J. F. Boon et al., "Nonsyndromic retinitis pigmentosa," *Progress in Retinal and Eye Research*, 2018.

[22] C. P. Hamel, "Cone rod dystrophies," *Orphanet Journal of Rare Diseases*, vol. 2, no. 1, p. 7, 2007.

[23] H. Kremer, E. van Wijk, T. Märker, U. Wolfrum, and R. Roepman, "Usher syndrome: molecular links of pathogenesis, proteins and pathways," *Human Molecular Genetics*, vol. 15, Supplement 2, pp. R262–R270, 2006.

[24] J. D. Sengillo, S. Justus, Y. T. Tsai, T. Cabral, and S. H. Tsang, "Gene and cell-based therapies for inherited retinal disorders: an update," *American Journal of Medical Genetics Part C: Seminars in Medical Genetics*, vol. 172, no. 4, pp. 349–366, 2016.

[25] K. H. Warrington Jr. and R. W. Herzog, "Treatment of human disease by adeno-associated viral gene transfer," *Human Genetics*, vol. 119, no. 6, pp. 571–603, 2006.

[26] S. Daya and K. I. Berns, "Gene therapy using adeno-associated virus vectors," *Clinical Microbiology Reviews*, vol. 21, no. 4, pp. 583–593, 2008.

[27] M. K. Lin, Y.-T. Tsai, and S. H. Tsang, "Emerging treatments for retinitis pigmentosa: genes and stem cells, as well as new electronic and medical therapies, are gaining ground," *Retinal Physician*, vol. 12, pp. 52–70, 2015.

[28] P. Yu-Wai-Man, "Genetic manipulation for inherited neurodegenerative diseases: myth or reality?," *British Journal of Ophthalmology*, vol. 100, no. 10, pp. 1322–1331, 2016.

[29] G. M. Acland, G. D. Aguirre, J. Ray et al., "Gene therapy restores vision in a canine model of childhood blindness," *Nature Genetics*, vol. 28, no. 1, pp. 92–95, 2001.

[30] J. W. B. Bainbridge, A. J. Smith, S. S. Barker et al., "Effect of gene therapy on visual function in Leber's congenital amaurosis," *The New England Journal of Medicine*, vol. 358, no. 21, pp. 2231–2239, 2008.

[31] A. M. Maguire, F. Simonelli, E. A. Pierce et al., "Safety and efficacy of gene transfer for Leber's congenital amaurosis," *The New England Journal of Medicine*, vol. 358, no. 21, pp. 2240–2248, 2008.

[32] A. V. Cideciyan, T. S. Aleman, S. L. Boye et al., "Human gene therapy for RPE65 isomerase deficiency activates the retinoid cycle of vision but with slow rod kinetics," *Proceedings of the National Academy of Sciences of the United States of America*, vol. 105, no. 39, pp. 15112–15117, 2008.

[33] J. Bennett, J. Wellman, K. A. Marshall et al., "Safety and durability of effect of contralateral-eye administration of AAV2 gene therapy in patients with childhood-onset blindness caused by *RPE65* mutations: a follow-on phase 1 trial," *The Lancet*, vol. 388, no. 10045, pp. 661–672, 2016.

[34] W. W. Hauswirth, T. S. Aleman, S. Kaushal et al., "Treatment of Leber congenital amaurosis due to *RPE65* mutations by ocular subretinal injection of adeno-associated virus gene vector: short-term results of a phase I trial," *Human Gene Therapy*, vol. 19, no. 10, pp. 979–990, 2008.

[35] S. Russell, J. Bennett, J. A. Wellman et al., "Efficacy and safety of voretigene neparvovec (AAV2-hRPE65v2) in patients with *RPE65*-mediated inherited retinal dystrophy: a randomised, controlled, open-label, phase 3 trial," *The Lancet*, vol. 390, no. 10097, pp. 849–860, 2017.

[36] R. E. MacLaren, M. Groppe, A. R. Barnard et al., "Retinal gene therapy in patients with choroideremia: initial findings from a phase 1/2 clinical trial," *The Lancet*, vol. 383, no. 9923, pp. 1129–1137, 2014.

[37] I. S. Dimopoulos, S. Chan, R. E. MacLaren, and I. M. MacDonald, "Pathogenic mechanisms and the prospect of gene therapy for choroideremia," *Expert Opinion on Orphan Drugs*, vol. 3, no. 7, pp. 787–798, 2015.

[38] T. Tolmachova, O. E. Tolmachov, A. R. Barnard et al., "Functional expression of Rab escort protein 1 following AAV2-mediated gene delivery in the retina of choroideremia mice and human cells ex vivo," *Journal of Molecular Medicine*, vol. 91, no. 7, pp. 825–837, 2013.

[39] N. Cereso, M. O. Pequignot, L. Robert et al., "Proof of concept for AAV2/5-mediated gene therapy in iPSC-derived retinal pigment epithelium of a choroideremia patient," *Molecular Therapy Methods & Clinical Development*, vol. 1, pp. 14011–14013, 2014.

[40] A. Black, V. Vasireddy, D. C. Chung et al., "Adeno-associated virus 8-mediated gene therapy for choroideremia: preclinical studies in *in vitro* and *in vivo* models," *The Journal of Gene Medicine*, vol. 16, no. 5-6, pp. 122–130, 2014.

[41] N. G. Ghazi, E. B. Abboud, S. R. Nowilaty et al., "Treatment of retinitis pigmentosa due to MERTK mutations by ocular subretinal injection of adeno-associated virus gene vector: results of a phase I trial," *Human Genetics*, vol. 135, no. 3, pp. 327–343, 2016.

[42] P. L. Hermonat, J. G. Quirk, B. M. Bishop, and L. Han, "The packaging capacity of adeno-associated virus (AAV) and the potential for *wild-type-plus* AAV gene therapy vectors," *FEBS Letters*, vol. 407, no. 1, pp. 78–84, 1997.

[43] Z. Wu, H. Yang, and P. Colosi, "Effect of genome size on AAV vector packaging," *Molecular Therapy*, vol. 18, no. 1, pp. 80–86, 2010.

[44] Y. Wang, C. Ling, L. Song et al., "Limitations of encapsidation of recombinant self-complementary adeno-associated viral genomes in different serotype capsids and their quantitation," *Human Gene Therapy Methods*, vol. 23, no. 4, pp. 225–233, 2012.

[45] J. Kong, S. R. Kim, K. Binley et al., "Correction of the disease phenotype in the mouse model of Stargardt disease by lentiviral gene therapy," *Gene Therapy*, vol. 15, no. 19, pp. 1311–1320, 2008.

[46] K. Binley, P. Widdowson, J. Loader et al., "Transduction of photoreceptors with equine infectious anemia virus lentiviral vectors: safety and biodistribution of StarGen for Stargardt disease," *Investigative Opthalmology & Visual Science*, vol. 54, no. 6, pp. 4061–4071, 2013.

[47] D. S. Williams and V. S. Lopes, "The many different cellular functions of MYO7A in the retina," *Biochemical Society Transactions*, vol. 39, no. 5, pp. 1207–1210, 2011.

[48] M. Zallocchi, K. Binley, Y. Lad et al., "EIAV-based retinal gene therapy in the *shaker1* mouse model for Usher syndrome type 1B: development of UshStat," *PLoS One*, vol. 9, no. 4, article e94272, 2014.

[49] A. V. Cideciyan, S. G. Jacobson, W. A. Beltran et al., "Human retinal gene therapy for Leber congenital amaurosis shows advancing retinal degeneration despite enduring visual improvement," *Proceedings of the National Academy of Sciences of the United States of America*, vol. 110, no. 6, pp. E517–E525, 2013.

[50] S. G. Jacobson, A. V. Cideciyan, A. J. Roman et al., "Improvement and decline in vision with gene therapy in childhood blindness," *The New England Journal of Medicine*, vol. 372, no. 20, pp. 1920–1926, 2015.

[51] R. J. Davis, C. W. Hsu, Y. T. Tsai et al., "Therapeutic margins in a novel preclinical model of retinitis pigmentosa," *The Journal of Neuroscience*, vol. 33, no. 33, pp. 13475–13483, 2013.

[52] K. J. Wert, J. Sancho-Pelluz, and S. H. Tsang, "Mid-stage intervention achieves similar efficacy as conventional early-stage treatment using gene therapy in a pre-clinical model of retinitis pigmentosa," *Human Molecular Genetics*, vol. 23, no. 2, pp. 514–523, 2014.

[53] J. B. Hurley and J. R. Chao, "It's never too late to save a photoreceptor," *The Journal of Clinical Investigation*, vol. 125, no. 9, pp. 3424–3426, 2015.

[54] C. L. Cepko and L. H. Vandenberghe, "Retinal gene therapy coming of age," *Human Gene Therapy*, vol. 24, no. 3, pp. 242–244, 2013.

[55] A. M. Maguire, K. A. High, A. Auricchio et al., "Age-dependent effects of RPE65 gene therapy for Leber's congenital amaurosis: a phase 1 dose-escalation trial," *The Lancet*, vol. 374, no. 9701, pp. 1597–1605, 2009.

[56] J. W. B. Bainbridge, M. S. Mehat, V. Sundaram et al., "Long-term effect of gene therapy on Leber's congenital amaurosis," *The New England Journal of Medicine*, vol. 372, no. 20, pp. 1887–1897, 2015.

[57] G. S. Yang, M. Schmidt, Z. Yan et al., "Virus-mediated transduction of murine retina with adeno-associated virus: effects of viral capsid and genome size," *Journal of Virology*, vol. 76, no. 15, pp. 7651–7660, 2002.

[58] L. H. Vandenberghe and A. Auricchio, "Novel adeno-associated viral vectors for retinal gene therapy," *Gene Therapy*, vol. 19, no. 2, pp. 162–168, 2012.

[59] F. M. Mowat, K. R. Gornik, A. Dinculescu et al., "Tyrosine capsid-mutant AAV vectors for gene delivery to the canine

retina from a subretinal or intravitreal approach," *Gene Therapy*, vol. 21, no. 1, pp. 96–105, 2014.

[60] A. Georgiadis, Y. Duran, J. Ribeiro et al., "Development of an optimized AAV2/5 gene therapy vector for Leber congenital amaurosis owing to defects in RPE65," *Gene Therapy*, vol. 23, no. 12, pp. 857–862, 2016.

[61] M. D. Fischer, M. E. McClements, C. Martinez-Fernandez de la Camara et al., "Codon-optimized RPGR improves stability and efficacy of AAV8 gene therapy in two mouse models of X-linked retinitis pigmentosa," *Molecular Therapy*, vol. 25, no. 8, pp. 1854–1865, 2017.

[62] G. J. Farrar, S. Millington-Ward, N. Chadderton, P. Humphries, and P. F. Kenna, "Gene-based therapies for dominantly inherited retinopathies," *Gene Therapy*, vol. 19, no. 2, pp. 137–144, 2012.

[63] A. Palfi, M. Ader, A. S. Kiang et al., "RNAi-based suppression and replacement of *rds*-peripherin in retinal organotypic culture," *Human Mutation*, vol. 27, no. 3, pp. 260–268, 2006.

[64] M. O'Reilly, A. Palfi, N. Chadderton et al., "RNA interference-mediated suppression and replacement of human rhodopsin in vivo," *The American Journal of Human Genetics*, vol. 81, no. 1, pp. 127–135, 2007.

[65] N. Chadderton, S. Millington-Ward, A. Palfi et al., "Improved retinal function in a mouse model of dominant retinitis pigmentosa following AAV-delivered gene therapy," *Molecular Therapy*, vol. 17, no. 4, pp. 593–599, 2009.

[66] S. Millington-Ward, N. Chadderton, M. O'Reilly et al., "Suppression and replacement gene therapy for autosomal dominant disease in a murine model of dominant retinitis pigmentosa," *Molecular Therapy*, vol. 19, no. 4, pp. 642–649, 2011.

[67] B. Pardo, B. Gómez-González, and A. Aguilera, "DNA repair in mammalian cells: DNA double-strand break repair: how to fix a broken relationship," *Cellular and Molecular Life Sciences*, vol. 66, no. 6, pp. 1039–1056, 2009.

[68] M. Yanik, B. Müller, F. Song et al., "*In vivo* genome editing as a potential treatment strategy for inherited retinal dystrophies," *Progress in Retinal and Eye Research*, vol. 56, pp. 1–18, 2017.

[69] M. Christian, T. Cermak, E. L. Doyle et al., "Targeting DNA double-strand breaks with TAL effector nucleases," *Genetics*, vol. 186, no. 2, pp. 757–761, 2010.

[70] L. Cong, F. A. Ran, D. Cox et al., "Multiplex genome engineering using CRISPR/Cas systems," *Science*, vol. 339, no. 6121, pp. 819–823, 2013.

[71] W.-D. Heyer, K. T. Ehmsen, and J. Liu, "Regulation of homologous recombination in eukaryotes," *Annual Review of Genetics*, vol. 44, no. 1, pp. 113–139, 2010.

[72] B. Schierling, N. Dannemann, L. Gabsalilow, W. Wende, T. Cathomen, and A. Pingoud, "A novel zinc-finger nuclease platform with a sequence-specific cleavage module," *Nucleic Acids Research*, vol. 40, no. 6, pp. 2623–2638, 2012.

[73] S. A. Wolfe, L. Nekludova, and C. O. Pabo, "DNA recognition by Cys2His2 zinc finger proteins," *Annual Review of Biophysics and Biomolecular Structure*, vol. 29, no. 1, pp. 183–212, 2000.

[74] Y. G. Kim, J. Cha, and S. Chandrasegaran, "Hybrid restriction enzymes: zinc finger fusions to Fok I cleavage domain," *Proceedings of the National Academy of Sciences of the United States of America*, vol. 93, no. 3, pp. 1156–1160, 1996.

[75] Y. G. Kim, Y. Shi, J. M. Berg, and S. Chandrasegaran, "Site-specific cleavage of DNA–RNA hybrids by zinc finger/FokI cleavage domain fusions," *Gene*, vol. 203, no. 1, pp. 43–49, 1997.

[76] J. Smith, M. Bibikova, F. G. Whitby, A. R. Reddy, S. Chandrasegaran, and D. Carroll, "Requirements for double-strand cleavage by chimeric restriction enzymes with zinc finger DNA-recognition domains," *Nucleic Acids Research*, vol. 28, no. 17, pp. 3361–3369, 2000.

[77] A. F. Gilles and M. Averof, "Functional genetics for all: engineered nucleases, CRISPR and the gene editing revolution," *EvoDevo*, vol. 5, no. 1, p. 43, 2014.

[78] D. Carroll, "Genome engineering with targetable nucleases," *Annual Review of Biochemistry*, vol. 83, no. 1, pp. 409–439, 2014.

[79] T. Gaj, C. A. Gersbach, and C. F. Barbas III, "ZFN, TALEN, and CRISPR/Cas-based methods for genome engineering," *Trends in Biotechnology*, vol. 31, no. 7, pp. 397–405, 2013.

[80] D. L. Greenwald, S. M. Cashman, and R. Kumar-Singh, "Engineered zinc finger nuclease-mediated homologous recombination of the human rhodopsin gene," *Investigative Ophthalmology & Visual Science*, vol. 51, no. 12, pp. 6374–6380, 2010.

[81] N. Overlack, T. Goldmann, U. Wolfrum, and K. Nagel-Wolfrum, "Gene repair of an Usher syndrome causing mutation by zinc-finger nuclease mediated homologous recombination," *Investigative Ophthalmology & Visual Science*, vol. 53, no. 7, pp. 4140–4146, 2012.

[82] B. E. Low, M. P. Krebs, J. K. Joung, S. Q. Tsai, P. M. Nishina, and M. V. Wiles, "Correction of the $Crb1^{rd8}$ allele and retinal phenotype in C57BL/6N mice via TALEN-mediated homology-directed repair," *Investigative Ophthalmology & Visual Science*, vol. 55, no. 1, pp. 387–395, 2014.

[83] Y. Ishino, H. Shinagawa, K. Makino, M. Amemura, and A. Nakata, "Nucleotide sequence of the iap gene, responsible for alkaline phosphatase isozyme conversion in *Escherichia coli*, and identification of the gene product," *Journal of Bacteriology*, vol. 169, no. 12, pp. 5429–5433, 1987.

[84] F. J. M. Mojica, C. Ferrer, G. Juez, and F. Rodriguez-Valera, "Long stretches of short tandem repeats are present in the largest replicons of the Archaea *Haloferax mediterranei* and *Haloferax volcanii* and could be involved in replicon partitioning," *Molecular Microbiology*, vol. 17, no. 1, pp. 85–93, 1995.

[85] H. P. Klenk, R. A. Clayton, J. F. Tomb et al., "The complete genome sequence of the hyperthermophilic, sulphate-reducing archaeon *Archaeoglobus fulgidus*," *Nature*, vol. 390, no. 6658, pp. 364–370, 1997.

[86] K. E. Nelson, R. A. Clayton, S. R. Gill et al., "Evidence for lateral gene transfer between Archaea and Bacteria from genome sequence of *Thermotoga maritima*," *Nature*, vol. 399, no. 6734, pp. 323–329, 1999.

[87] R. Jansen, J. D. A. v. Embden, W. Gaastra, and L. M. Schouls, "Identification of genes that are associated with DNA repeats in prokaryotes," *Molecular Microbiology*, vol. 43, no. 6, pp. 1565–1575, 2002.

[88] F. J. M. Mojica, C. Diez-Villasenor, E. Soria, and G. Juez, "Biological significance of a family of regularly spaced repeats in the genomes of Archaea, Bacteria and mitochondria," *Molecular Microbiology*, vol. 36, no. 1, pp. 244–246, 2000.

[89] R. Barrangou, C. Fremaux, H. Deveau et al., "CRISPR provides acquired resistance against viruses in prokaryotes," *Science*, vol. 315, no. 5819, pp. 1709–1712, 2007.

[90] M. Jinek, K. Chylinski, I. Fonfara, M. Hauer, J. A. Doudna, and E. Charpentier, "A programmable dual-RNA-guided DNA endonuclease in adaptive bacterial immunity," *Science*, vol. 337, no. 6096, pp. 816–821, 2012.

[91] J. A. Doudna and E. Charpentier, "The new frontier of genome engineering with CRISPR-Cas9," *Science*, vol. 346, no. 6213, article 1258096, 2014.

[92] F. A. Ran, P. D. Hsu, C. Y. Lin et al., "Double nicking by RNA-guided CRISPR cas9 for enhanced genome editing specificity," *Cell*, vol. 154, no. 6, pp. 1380–1389, 2013.

[93] P. Mali, L. Yang, K. M. Esvelt et al., "RNA-guided human genome engineering via Cas9," *Science*, vol. 339, no. 6121, pp. 823–826, 2013.

[94] N. Chang, C. Sun, L. Gao et al., "Genome editing with RNA-guided Cas9 nuclease in zebrafish embryos," *Cell Research*, vol. 23, no. 4, pp. 465–472, 2013.

[95] A. E. Friedland, Y. B. Tzur, K. M. Esvelt, M. P. Colaiácovo, G. M. Church, and J. A. Calarco, "Heritable genome editing in *C. elegans* via a CRISPR-Cas9 system," *Nature Methods*, vol. 10, no. 8, pp. 741–743, 2013.

[96] W. Jiang, H. Zhou, H. Bi, M. Fromm, B. Yang, and D. P. Weeks, "Demonstration of CRISPR/Cas9/sgRNA-mediated targeted gene modification in *Arabidopsis*, tobacco, sorghum and rice," *Nucleic Acids Research*, vol. 41, no. 20, article e188, 2013.

[97] J. E. DiCarlo, J. E. Norville, P. Mali, X. Rios, J. Aach, and G. M. Church, "Genome engineering in *Saccharomyces cerevisiae* using CRISPR-Cas systems," *Nucleic Acids Research*, vol. 41, no. 7, pp. 4336–4343, 2013.

[98] Y. Fu, J. A. Foden, C. Khayter et al., "High-frequency off-target mutagenesis induced by CRISPR-Cas nucleases in human cells," *Nature Biotechnology*, vol. 31, no. 9, pp. 822–826, 2013.

[99] P. D. Hsu, D. A. Scott, J. A. Weinstein et al., "DNA targeting specificity of RNA-guided Cas9 nucleases," *Nature Biotechnology*, vol. 31, no. 9, pp. 827–832, 2013.

[100] V. Pattanayak, S. Lin, J. P. Guilinger, E. Ma, J. A. Doudna, and D. R. Liu, "High-throughput profiling of off-target DNA cleavage reveals RNA-programmed Cas9 nuclease specificity," *Nature Biotechnology*, vol. 31, no. 9, pp. 839–843, 2013.

[101] S. W. Cho, J. Lee, D. Carroll, J. S. Kim, and J. Lee, "Heritable gene knockout in *Caenorhabditis elegans* by direct injection of Cas9–sgRNA ribonucleoproteins," *Genetics*, vol. 195, no. 3, pp. 1177–1180, 2013.

[102] S. Kim, D. Kim, S. W. Cho, J. Kim, and J. S. Kim, "Highly efficient RNA-guided genome editing in human cells via delivery of purified Cas9 ribonucleoproteins," *Genome Research*, vol. 24, no. 6, pp. 1012–1019, 2014.

[103] S. Lin, B. T. Staahl, R. K. Alla, and J. A. Doudna, "Enhanced homology-directed human genome engineering by controlled timing of CRISPR/Cas9 delivery," *eLife*, vol. 3, article e04766, 2014.

[104] X. Liang, J. Potter, S. Kumar, N. Ravinder, and J. D. Chesnut, "Enhanced CRISPR/Cas9-mediated precise genome editing by improved design and delivery of gRNA, Cas9 nuclease, and donor DNA," *Journal of Biotechnology*, vol. 241, pp. 136–146, 2017.

[105] K. Kim, S. W. Park, J. H. Kim et al., "Genome surgery using Cas9 ribonucleoproteins for the treatment of age-related macular degeneration," *Genome Research*, vol. 27, no. 3, pp. 419–426, 2017.

[106] G.-X. Ruan, E. Barry, D. Yu, M. Lukason, S. H. Cheng, and A. Scaria, "CRISPR/Cas9-mediated genome editing as a therapeutic approach for Leber congenital amaurosis 10," *Molecular Therapy*, vol. 25, no. 2, pp. 331–341, 2017.

[107] I. M. Slaymaker, L. Gao, B. Zetsche, D. A. Scott, W. X. Yan, and F. Zhang, "Rationally engineered Cas9 nucleases with improved specificity," *Science*, vol. 351, no. 6268, pp. 84–88, 2016.

[108] B. P. Kleinstiver, V. Pattanayak, M. S. Prew et al., "High-fidelity CRISPR–Cas9 nucleases with no detectable genome-wide off-target effects," *Nature*, vol. 529, no. 7587, pp. 490–495, 2016.

[109] S. Q. Tsai, Z. Zheng, N. T. Nguyen et al., "GUIDE-seq enables genome-wide profiling of off-target cleavage by CRISPR-Cas nucleases," *Nature Biotechnology*, vol. 33, no. 2, pp. 187–197, 2015.

[110] K. M. Esvelt, P. Mali, J. L. Braff, M. Moosburner, S. J. Yaung, and G. M. Church, "Orthogonal Cas9 proteins for RNA-guided gene regulation and editing," *Nature Methods*, vol. 10, no. 11, pp. 1116–1121, 2013.

[111] I. Fonfara, A. le Rhun, K. Chylinski et al., "Phylogeny of Cas9 determines functional exchangeability of dual-RNA and Cas9 among orthologous type II CRISPR-Cas systems," *Nucleic Acids Research*, vol. 42, no. 4, pp. 2577–2590, 2014.

[112] F. A. Ran, L. Cong, W. X. Yan et al., "*In vivo* genome editing using *Staphylococcus aureus* Cas9," *Nature*, vol. 520, no. 7546, pp. 186–191, 2015.

[113] W. Jiang, D. Bikard, D. Cox, F. Zhang, and L. A. Marraffini, "RNA-guided editing of bacterial genomes using CRISPR-Cas systems," *Nature Biotechnology*, vol. 31, no. 3, pp. 233–239, 2013.

[114] A. E. Friedland, R. Baral, P. Singhal et al., "Characterization of *Staphylococcus aureus* Cas9: a smaller Cas9 for all-in-one adeno-associated virus delivery and paired nickase applications," *Genome Biology*, vol. 16, no. 1, p. 257, 2015.

[115] E. Kim, T. Koo, S. W. Park et al., "*In vivo* genome editing with a small Cas9 orthologue derived from *Campylobacter jejuni*," *Nature Communications*, vol. 8, article 14500, 2017.

[116] B. Zetsche, J. S. Gootenberg, O. O. Abudayyeh et al., "Cpf1 is a single RNA-guided endonuclease of a class 2 CRISPR-Cas system," *Cell*, vol. 163, no. 3, pp. 759–771, 2015.

[117] R. D. Fagerlund, R. H. J. Staals, and P. C. Fineran, "The Cpf1 CRISPR-Cas protein expands genome-editing tools," *Genome Biology*, vol. 16, no. 1, pp. 251–253, 2015.

[118] B. P. Kleinstiver, M. S. Prew, S. Q. Tsai et al., "Broadening the targeting range of *Staphylococcus aureus* CRISPR-Cas9 by modifying PAM recognition," *Nature Biotechnology*, vol. 33, no. 12, pp. 1293–1298, 2015.

[119] B. P. Kleinstiver, M. S. Prew, S. Q. Tsai et al., "Engineered CRISPR-Cas9 nucleases with altered PAM specificities," *Nature*, vol. 523, no. 7561, pp. 481–485, 2015.

[120] T. P. Day, L. C. Byrne, D. V. Schaffer, and J. G. Flannery, "Advances in AAV vector development for gene therapy in the retina," *Advances in Experimental Medicine and Biology*, vol. 801, pp. 687–693, 2014.

[121] L. Swiech, M. Heidenreich, A. Banerjee et al., "*In vivo* interrogation of gene function in the mammalian brain

using CRISPR-Cas9," *Nature Biotechnology*, vol. 33, no. 1, pp. 102–106, 2015.

[122] S. S. C. Hung, V. Chrysostomou, F. Li et al., "AAV-mediated CRISPR/Cas gene editing of retinal cells in vivo," *Investigative Ophthalmology & Visual Science*, vol. 57, no. 7, pp. 3470–3476, 2016.

[123] W. Yu, S. Mookherjee, V. Chaitankar et al., "*Nrl* knockdown by AAV-delivered CRISPR/Cas9 prevents retinal degeneration in mice," *Nature Communications*, vol. 8, article 14716, 2017.

[124] A. I. den Hollander, R. K. Koenekoop, S. Yzer et al., "Mutations in the *CEP290 (NPHP6)* gene are a frequent cause of Leber congenital amaurosis," *The American Journal of Human Genetics*, vol. 79, no. 3, pp. 556–561, 2006.

[125] I. Perrault, N. Delphin, S. Hanein et al., "Spectrum of NPHP6/CEP290 mutations in Leber congenital amaurosis and delineation of the associated phenotype," *Human Mutation*, vol. 28, no. 4, p. 416, 2007.

[126] D. Wang, H. Mou, S. Li et al., "Adenovirus-mediated somatic genome editing of *Pten* by CRISPR/Cas9 in mouse liver in spite of Cas9-specific immune responses," *Human Gene Therapy*, vol. 26, no. 7, pp. 432–442, 2015.

[127] K. Suzuki, Y. Tsunekawa, R. Hernandez-Benitez et al., "In vivo genome editing via CRISPR/Cas9 mediated homology-independent targeted integration," *Nature*, vol. 540, no. 7631, pp. 144–149, 2016.

[128] W.-H. Wu, Y. T. Tsai, S. Justus et al., "CRISPR repair reveals causative mutation in a preclinical model of retinitis pigmentosa," *Molecular Therapy*, vol. 24, no. 8, pp. 1388–1394, 2016.

[129] G. Arno, S. A. Agrawal, A. Eblimit et al., "Mutations in *REEP6* cause autosomal-recessive retinitis pigmentosa," *The American Journal of Human Genetics*, vol. 99, no. 6, pp. 1305–1315, 2016.

[130] L. S. Qi, M. H. Larson, L. A. Gilbert et al., "Repurposing CRISPR as an RNA-guided platform for sequence-specific control of gene expression," *Cell*, vol. 152, no. 5, pp. 1173–1183, 2013.

[131] L. A. Gilbert, M. H. Larson, L. Morsut et al., "CRISPR-mediated modular RNA-guided regulation of transcription in eukaryotes," *Cell*, vol. 154, no. 2, pp. 442–451, 2013.

[132] M. L. Maeder, S. J. Linder, V. M. Cascio, Y. Fu, Q. H. Ho, and J. K. Joung, "CRISPR RNA–guided activation of endogenous human genes," *Nature Methods*, vol. 10, no. 10, pp. 977–979, 2013.

[133] L. A. Gilbert, M. A. Horlbeck, B. Adamson et al., "Genome-scale CRISPR-mediated control of gene repression and activation," *Cell*, vol. 159, no. 3, pp. 647–661, 2014.

[134] L. Jiang, T. Z. Li, S. E. Boye, W. W. Hauswirth, J. M. Frederick, and W. Baehr, "RNAi-mediated gene suppression in a GCAP1(L151F) cone-rod dystrophy mouse model," *PLoS One*, vol. 8, no. 3, article e57676, 2013.

[135] S. M. Cashman, E. A. Binkley, and R. Kumar-Singh, "Towards mutation-independent silencing of genes involved in retinal degeneration by RNA interference," *Gene Therapy*, vol. 12, no. 15, pp. 1223–1228, 2005.

[136] B. Bakondi, W. Lv, B. Lu et al., "In vivo CRISPR/Cas9 gene editing corrects retinal dystrophy in the S334ter-3 rat model of autosomal dominant retinitis pigmentosa," *Molecular Therapy*, vol. 24, no. 3, pp. 556–563, 2016.

[137] M. C. Latella, M. T. di Salvo, F. Cocchiarella et al., "*In vivo* editing of the human mutant *Rhodopsin* gene by electroporation of plasmid-based CRISPR/Cas9 in the mouse retina," *Molecular Therapy Nucleic Acids*, vol. 5, no. 11, article e389, 2016.

[138] R. E. MacLaren, R. A. Pearson, A. MacNeil et al., "Retinal repair by transplantation of photoreceptor precursors," *Nature*, vol. 444, no. 7116, pp. 203–207, 2006.

[139] D. A. Lamba, M. O. Karl, C. B. Ware, and T. A. Reh, "Efficient generation of retinal progenitor cells from human embryonic stem cells," *Proceedings of the National Academy of Sciences of the United States of America*, vol. 103, no. 34, pp. 12769–12774, 2006.

[140] D. A. Lamba, J. Gust, and T. A. Reh, "Transplantation of human embryonic stem cell-derived photoreceptors restores some visual function in *Crx*-deficient mice," *Cell Stem Cell*, vol. 4, no. 1, pp. 73–79, 2009.

[141] K. Takahashi, K. Tanabe, M. Ohnuki et al., "Induction of pluripotent stem cells from adult human fibroblasts by defined factors," *Cell*, vol. 131, no. 5, pp. 861–872, 2007.

[142] S. S. C. Hung, S. Khan, C. Y. Lo, A. W. Hewitt, and R. C. B. Wong, "Drug discovery using induced pluripotent stem cell models of neurodegenerative and ocular diseases," *Pharmacology & Therapeutics*, vol. 177, pp. 32–43, 2017.

[143] L. A. Wiley, E. R. Burnight, A. E. Songstad et al., "Patient-specific induced pluripotent stem cells (iPSCs) for the study and treatment of retinal degenerative diseases," *Progress in Retinal and Eye Research*, vol. 44, pp. 15–35, 2015.

[144] M. Eiraku, N. Takata, H. Ishibashi et al., "Self-organizing optic-cup morphogenesis in three-dimensional culture," *Nature*, vol. 472, no. 7341, pp. 51–56, 2011.

[145] T. Nakano, S. Ando, N. Takata et al., "Self-formation of optic cups and storable stratified neural retina from human ESCs," *Cell Stem Cell*, vol. 10, no. 6, pp. 771–785, 2012.

[146] R. A. Pearson, A. C. Barber, M. Rizzi et al., "Restoration of vision after transplantation of photoreceptors," *Nature*, vol. 485, no. 7396, pp. 99–103, 2012.

[147] E. L. West, A. Gonzalez-Cordero, C. Hippert et al., "Defining the integration capacity of embryonic stem cell-derived photoreceptor precursors," *Stem Cells*, vol. 30, no. 7, pp. 1424–1435, 2012.

[148] A. C. Barber, C. Hippert, Y. Duran et al., "Repair of the degenerate retina by photoreceptor transplantation," *Proceedings of the National Academy of Sciences of the United States of America*, vol. 110, no. 1, pp. 354–359, 2013.

[149] M. S. Singh, J. Balmer, A. R. Barnard et al., "Transplanted photoreceptor precursors transfer proteins to host photoreceptors by a mechanism of cytoplasmic fusion," *Nature Communications*, vol. 7, article 13537, 2016.

[150] Y. Hirami, F. Osakada, K. Takahashi et al., "Generation of retinal cells from mouse and human induced pluripotent stem cells," *Neuroscience Letters*, vol. 458, no. 3, pp. 126–131, 2009.

[151] J. S. Meyer, R. L. Shearer, E. E. Capowski et al., "Modeling early retinal development with human embryonic and induced pluripotent stem cells," *Proceedings of the National Academy of Sciences of the United States of America*, vol. 106, no. 39, pp. 16698–16703, 2009.

[152] S. Reichman, A. Terray, A. Slembrouck et al., "From confluent human iPS cells to self-forming neural retina and retinal pigmented epithelium," *Proceedings of the National Academy of Sciences of the United States of America*, vol. 111, no. 23, pp. 8518–8523, 2014.

[153] X. Zhong, C. Gutierrez, T. Xue et al., "Generation of three-dimensional retinal tissue with functional photoreceptors from human iPSCs," *Nature Communications*, vol. 5, p. 4047, 2014.

[154] B. A. Tucker, I. H. Park, S. D. Qi et al., "Transplantation of adult mouse iPS cell-derived photoreceptor precursors restores retinal structure and function in degenerative mice," *PLoS One*, vol. 6, no. 4, article e18992, 2011.

[155] A. G. Bassuk, A. Zheng, Y. Li, S. H. Tsang, and V. B. Mahajan, "Precision medicine: genetic repair of retinitis pigmentosa in patient-derived stem cells," *Scientific Reports*, vol. 6, no. 1, article 19969, 2016.

[156] E. R. Burnight, M. Gupta, L. A. Wiley et al., "Using CRISPR-Cas9 to generate gene-corrected autologous iPSCs for the treatment of inherited retinal degeneration," *Molecular Therapy*, vol. 25, no. 9, pp. 1999–2013, 2017.

[157] C. Fuster-García, G. García-García, E. González-Romero et al., "USH2A gene editing using the CRISPR system," *Molecular Therapy Nucleic Acids*, vol. 8, pp. 529–541, 2017.

[158] K. Homma, S. Usui, and M. Kaneda, "Knock-in strategy at 3′-end of Crx gene by CRISPR/Cas9 system shows the gene expression profiles during human photoreceptor differentiation," *Genes to Cells*, vol. 22, no. 3, pp. 250–264, 2017.

[159] R. A. Pearson, A. Gonzalez-Cordero, E. L. West et al., "Donor and host photoreceptors engage in material transfer following transplantation of post-mitotic photoreceptor precursors," *Nature Communications*, vol. 7, article 13029, 2016.

[160] T. Santos-Ferreira, S. Llonch, O. Borsch, K. Postel, J. Haas, and M. Ader, "Retinal transplantation of photoreceptors results in donor–host cytoplasmic exchange," *Nature Communications*, vol. 7, article 13028, 2016.

[161] S. Decembrini, C. Martin, F. Sennlaub et al., "Cone genesis tracing by the Chrnb4-EGFP mouse line: evidences of cellular material fusion after cone precursor transplantation," *Molecular Therapy*, vol. 25, no. 3, pp. 634–653, 2017.

[162] P. V. Waldron, F. di Marco, K. Kruczek et al., "Transplanted donor- or stem cell-derived cone photoreceptors can both integrate and undergo material transfer in an environment-dependent manner," *Stem Cell Reports*, vol. 10, no. 2, pp. 406–421, 2018.

[163] S. D. Schwartz, J. P. Hubschman, G. Heilwell et al., "Embryonic stem cell trials for macular degeneration: a preliminary report," *The Lancet*, vol. 379, no. 9817, pp. 713–720, 2012.

[164] S. D. Schwartz, C. D. Regillo, B. L. Lam et al., "Human embryonic stem cell-derived retinal pigment epithelium in patients with age-related macular degeneration and Stargardt's macular dystrophy: follow-up of two open-label phase 1/2 studies," *The Lancet*, vol. 385, no. 9967, pp. 509–516, 2015.

[165] L. da Cruz, K. Fynes, O. Georgiadis et al., "Phase 1 clinical study of an embryonic stem cell-derived retinal pigment epithelium patch in age-related macular degeneration," *Nature Biotechnology*, vol. 36, no. 4, pp. 328–337, 2018.

[166] M. Mandai, A. Watanabe, Y. Kurimoto et al., "Autologous induced stem-cell–derived retinal cells for macular degeneration," *The New England Journal of Medicine*, vol. 376, no. 11, pp. 1038–1046, 2017.

[167] M. A. DeWitt, J. E. Corn, and D. Carroll, "Genome editing via delivery of Cas9 ribonucleoprotein," *Methods*, vol. 121-122, pp. 9–15, 2017.

[168] X. H. Zhang, L. Y. Tee, X. G. Wang, Q. S. Huang, and S. H. Yang, "Off-target effects in CRISPR/Cas9-mediated genome engineering," *Molecular Therapy Nucleic Acids*, vol. 4, article e264, 2015.

[169] R. Peng, G. Lin, and J. Li, "Potential pitfalls of CRISPR/Cas9-mediated genome editing," *The FEBS Journal*, vol. 283, no. 7, pp. 1218–1231, 2016.

[170] J. K. Yee, "Off-target effects of engineered nucleases," *The FEBS Journal*, vol. 283, no. 17, pp. 3239–3248, 2016.

[171] K. Nakajima, A. A. Kazuno, J. Kelsoe, M. Nakanishi, T. Takumi, and T. Kato, "Exome sequencing in the knockin mice generated using the CRISPR/Cas system," *Scientific Reports*, vol. 6, no. 1, article 34703, 2016.

[172] S. W. Cho, S. Kim, Y. Kim et al., "Analysis of off-target effects of CRISPR/Cas-derived RNA-guided endonucleases and nickases," *Genome Research*, vol. 24, no. 1, pp. 132–141, 2014.

[173] A. C. Komor, Y. B. Kim, M. S. Packer, J. A. Zuris, and D. R. Liu, "Programmable editing of a target base in genomic DNA without double-stranded DNA cleavage," *Nature*, vol. 533, no. 7603, pp. 420–424, 2016.

[174] N. M. Gaudelli, A. C. Komor, H. A. Rees et al., "Programmable base editing of A•T to G•C in genomic DNA without DNA cleavage," *Nature*, vol. 551, no. 7681, pp. 464–471, 2017.

5

Botanicals as Modulators of Neuroplasticity: Focus on BDNF

Enrico Sangiovanni, Paola Brivio, Mario Dell'Agli, and Francesca Calabrese

Department of Pharmacological and Biomolecular Sciences, Università degli Studi di Milano, Milan, Italy

Correspondence should be addressed to Francesca Calabrese; francesca.calabrese@unimi.it

Academic Editor: Stuart C. Mangel

The involvement of brain-derived neurotrophic factor (BDNF) in different central nervous system (CNS) diseases suggests that this neurotrophin may represent an interesting and reliable therapeutic target. Accordingly, the search for new compounds, also from natural sources, able to modulate BDNF has been increasingly explored. The present review considers the literature on the effects of botanicals on BDNF. Botanicals considered were *Bacopa monnieri* (L.) Pennell, *Coffea arabica* L., *Crocus sativus* L., *Eleutherococcus senticosus* Maxim., *Camellia sinensis* (L.) Kuntze (green tea), *Ginkgo biloba* L., *Hypericum perforatum* L., *Olea europaea* L. (olive oil), *Panax ginseng* C.A. Meyer, *Rhodiola rosea* L., *Salvia miltiorrhiza* Bunge, *Vitis vinifera* L., *Withania somnifera* (L.) Dunal, and *Perilla frutescens* (L.) Britton. The effect of the active principles responsible for the efficacy of the extracts is reviewed and discussed as well. The high number of articles published (more than one hundred manuscripts for 14 botanicals) supports the growing interest in the use of natural products as BDNF modulators. The studies reported strengthen the hypothesis that botanicals may be considered useful modulators of BDNF in CNS diseases, without high side effects. Further clinical studies are mandatory to confirm botanicals as preventive agents or as useful adjuvant to the pharmacological treatment.

1. Introduction

One of the most complete forms of plasticity was described by Donald Hebb in 1949 who proposed an explanation for the adaptation of neurons during cognition and memory; this theory was later summarized by the famous sentence "neurons that fire together, wire together" [1]. Briefly, neuronal plasticity describes the versatility of neuronal connectivity and circuitry to which the nervous system responds and adapts to changing conditions of the body and the environment.

Among the genes involved in the modulation of neuronal activity, neurotrophic factors (NTFs), in particular the neurotrophin family of signaling proteins, play an important role in brain development [2, 3] and in adulthood modulating axonal and dendritic growth and remodeling, membrane receptor trafficking, neurotransmitter release, and synapse formation and function [4].

Brain-derived neurotrophic factor (BDNF) as well as nerve growth factor (NGF) is the most studied and best-characterized neurotrophins of the central nervous system (CNS), where they are involved in the development and

maintenance of physiological brain functions. The features of the BDNF system have been extensively reviewed elsewhere [5, 6]. Briefly, in rodents, the *BDNF* gene consists of nine $5'$ untranslated exons, each linked to individual promoter regions, and a $3'$ coding exon (IX), which codes for the BDNF preprotein amino acid sequence [7]. Similarly, the human *Bdnf* gene is also transcribed through multiple $5'$ exons spliced to a single coding exon [8]. The neurotrophin transcription is finely regulated by several intracellular signaling pathways and by different transcription factors [8–11].

Moreover, BDNF function is also highly dependent on translation and posttranslational changes. Indeed, BDNF is initially synthesized as a precursor form (proBDNF, 32 kDa) that can be cleaved into the mature neurotrophin (mBDNF, 14 kDa) or transported to the plasma membrane and released in an unprocessed manner. Upon release, the two forms of BDNF protein, as all the neurotrophins, bind with different receptors with multiple and opposite biological functions. The proBDNF binds with high-affinity p75^{NTR} leading to apoptosis, neurite retraction, and synaptic weakening and facilitating long-term depression, whereas mBDNF binds with TrkB receptors promoting cell survival, neurite extension, synaptic strengthening, and long-term potentiation (LTP) [4, 12, 13].

Alterations of NTF expression, including BDNF, are involved in the development of a variety of CNS diseases, including neurodegenerative disorders (Alzheimer's disease, Parkinson's disease, Huntington's disease, and amyotrophic lateral sclerosis) as well as psychiatric disorders (depression and schizophrenia) [14–16]. NTFs may be considered therapeutic targets, but their use has been limited so far by several, still unresolved, methodological problems aimed to guarantee their safety and efficacy [14, 15]. In particular, results from clinical studies using BDNF as a therapeutic agent have not been encouraging, possibly due to a failure of attaining relevant concentration of the trophic molecule at receptors. The two main problems seem to be related to the inability to deliver BDNF across the blood–brain barrier (BBB) and to the poor bioavailability of BDNF owing to its physiochemical properties [17].

For this reason, alternative options may be devoted to increase the endogenous content of BDNF. Accordingly, several drugs increase, indirectly, BDNF levels; however, considering the high number of nonresponder patients and the presence of serious side effects, the search for new strategies able to interfere with the mechanisms underlying CNS diseases would greatly benefit a high number of subjects. Botanicals are widely consumed all over the world as different types of products, including herbal medicinal products, plant food supplements, and functional foods. Nowadays, they are commonly used for promoting health and treating or preventing a variety of diseases even if, in most cases, clear evidence about their clinical efficacy is lacking. Emerging research provides substantial evidence to classify botanicals as modulators of markers, which are significantly altered during CNS dysfunction.

Some natural products are classified as antidepressants or anxiolytics according to the legislation of the countries in which they are sold [18, 19]. The ability of a variety of botanicals to positively modulate mood disorders and cognitive impairment resides on understanding that most of them are efficiently absorbed in humans. Recently, biologically active metabolites of botanicals able to interact with multiple targets associated with the promotion of resilience against mood disorders and cognitive impairment in response to stress have been discovered. Interventions with botanicals may benefit anxiety disorders by different mechanisms which include effects on the GABA system either via inducing ion channel transmission or through alteration of membrane structures [20]. A consistent number of botanicals, including *Ginkgo biloba* L., clinically improve cognitive impairment by ameliorating microvascular function in the brain whereas *Bacopa monnieri* (L.) Pennell has provided indications as a memory enhancer and protective agent in epilepsy [21].

The aim of the present review is to summarize the relevant literature concerning the role of botanicals as modulators of BDNF (Figure 1). Electronic literature searches were conducted in December 2016 taking into consideration also Epub articles and using Web of Science and PubMed databases. Search limit was the English language whereas no limit was applied for the year of publication. Research articles were searched for title and abstract using the following search terms: Latin name or common name or vernacular name of the plant matched with BDNF. Studies in the literature were found for the following botanicals: *Bacopa monnieri* (L.) Pennell, *Coffea arabica* L., *Crocus sativus* L., *Eleutherococcus senticosus* Maxim., *Camellia sinensis* (L.) Kuntze (green tea), *Ginkgo biloba* L., *Hypericum perforatum* L., *Olea europaea* L. (olive oil), *Panax ginseng* C.A. Meyer, *Rhodiola rosea* L., *Salvia miltiorrhiza* Bunge, *Vitis vinifera* L., *Withania somnifera* (L.) Dunal, and *Perilla frutescens* (L.) Britton.

This review emphasizes the part of the plant used, standardization of the active principles, and the protocol to manage studies in addition to the description of the behavioral test employed (Table 1). The effect of the pure compounds occurring in some plant able to modulate BDNF, such as salidroside, caffeine, epigallocatechin-3-*O*-gallate, and ginsenosides Rg1 and Rb1, will be reviewed as well whereas the effect of the pure compounds curcumin and resveratrol, which have been extensively studied as effective modulators of BDNF, will not be considered in the present review. In addition to the effect of the selected botanicals and/or their active compounds, papers describing biological effects of their association will be also considered.

2. *Bacopa monnieri* (L.) Pennell

Bacopa monnieri (L.) Pennell is a member of Scrophulariaceae traditionally used in Ayurvedic medicine for epilepsy and asthma. The best-characterized compounds occurring in the whole plant are dammarane-type triterpenoid saponins known as bacosides (mostly bacoside A), which are considered the main responsible for the biological activity [22].

2.1. In Vitro Studies. Two studies investigated the protective effect of *Bacopa monnieri* extract (BME) *in vitro*. In PC12 cells, pretreatment with a hydroalcoholic extract completely prevented the reduction of BDNF mRNA levels associated with cellular damage induced by scopolamine [23] or sodium nitroprusside [24].

2.2. In Vivo Studies. The effect of *Bacopa monnieri* was investigated, at preclinical levels, in eight studies using different animal models.

The unpredictable chronic mild stress (CMS), a well-established animal model of depression, was used to assess the ability of a compound to exert an antidepressant-like effect. Administration of BME by gavage (80 or 120 mg/kg) prevented the behavioral deficits and the reduction of 3′ UTR-long BDNF gene expression [25], as well as of the protein levels of the mature form in the hippocampus and frontal cortex of chronically stressed rats [26]. Similar effects were observed after treatment with the tricyclic antidepressant drug imipramine [25–27].

The cognition-enhancing properties of *Bacopa monnieri* were investigated in the scopolamine rodent model of "cholinergic amnesia" and in the olfactory bulbectomy (OBX), a model of cognitive and emotional dysfunction typical of neurodegenerative pathologies such as Alzheimer's disease [28].

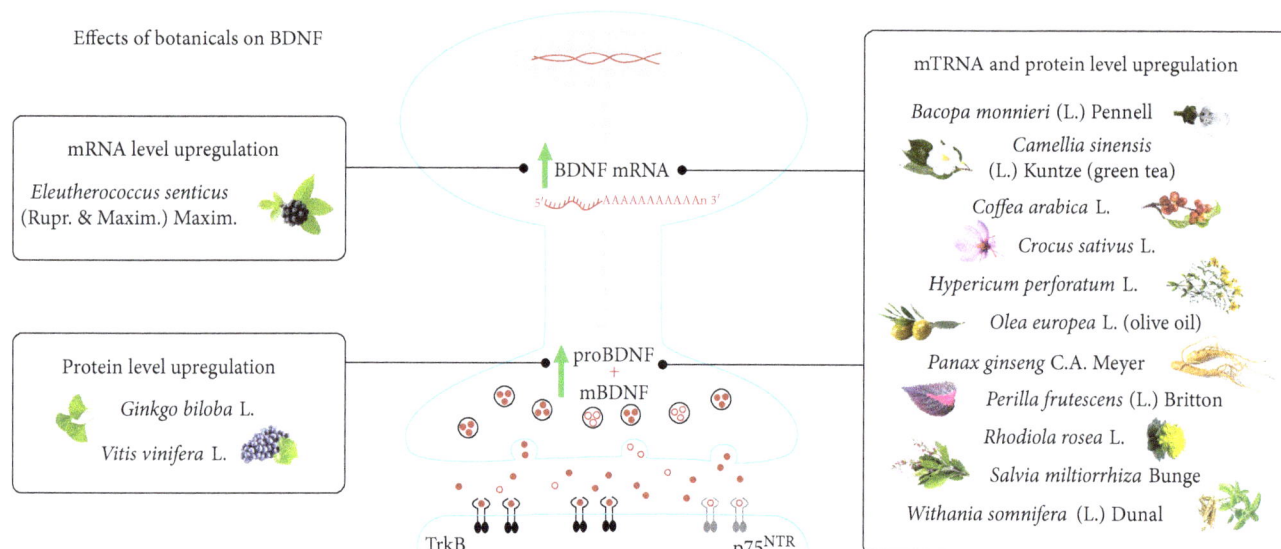

FIGURE 1: Effects of botanicals on BDNF mRNA and protein levels. The figure shows botanicals acting at transcriptional and translational levels.

Interestingly, chronic treatment (62 days) with an alcoholic BME (50 mg/kg in the drinking water) ameliorated the memory disturbance and completely normalized the reduction of hippocampal BDNF mRNA levels due to the OBX [29].

Moreover, 1 week of oral (os) treatment with the hydroalcoholic BME (10, 20, and 40 mg/kg) dose-dependently prevented the memory deficits induced by scopolamine and normalized the reduction of BDNF mRNA levels in the rat hippocampus [30]. A similar effect was found in young mice at postnatal day (PND) 30 [31] treated with CDRI-08 (BME standardized in bacoside A) (3 mg/kg, i.p., 7 days) before and after scopolamine injection. Both the protocols attenuated the decrease in proBDNF protein levels in the mouse cerebrum, caused by scopolamine administration. Furthermore, CDRI-08 per se induced an increase in BDNF gene and protein expression [31].

In a recent study, administration of CDRI-08 (80 mg/kg, i.p., 2 weeks) significantly increased the mRNA and the protein levels of proBDNF in the hippocampus of young rats (PND 32). Interestingly, this effect paralleled the upregulation of the unmethylated CpG islands 1 and improved the object recognition memory [32]. Using the same regime of treatment, CDRI-08 facilitated memory acquisition in the fear-conditioning paradigm and increased the expression of BDNF exon IV transcript in the hippocampus of PND 30 rats [33].

On this basis, even if clinical studies are needed, preclinical results indicate that *Bacopa monnieri* extract administration modulates a BDNF effect that may underline its ability as an antidepressant and procognitive agent.

3. *Coffea arabica* L.

The coffee plant, a woody perennial tree growing at higher altitudes, belongs to the family of Rubiaceae. Although beans are particularly rich in caffeine, other constituents are present

in a considerable amount, including tocopherols and caffeic acid derivatives, such as chlorogenic acid.

In the literature are present studies reporting the effect of caffeine on BDNF, whereas the effect of a *Coffea arabica* extract from fruits was investigated only in one clinical study.

3.1. In Vitro Studies. Three studies investigated the *in vitro* effect of caffeine on BDNF. In particular, caffeine upregulated the BDNF protein levels in mouse hippocampal slices (100 μM for 5 minutes) [34], increased the BDNF release in hippocampal neurons [35], and efficiently stimulated the BDNF isoform I and IV expression in the presence of KCl (10 mM) in cortical neurons [36].

3.2. In Vivo Studies. 15 studies investigated the effect of caffeine on BDNF *in vivo*. Treatment of zebrafish embryos with caffeine (100 μM) increased the BDNF mRNA levels specifically after 48 and 72 hours postfertilization [37].

Caffeine administration in naïve rats, during adulthood, counteracted the negative effect exerted by its intake in early life by increasing the protein levels of mBDNF [38]. Differently, administration of caffeine (1.0 g/L in drinking water) two weeks before mating, during pregnancy, and up to embryonic days 18–20 (E18 or E20) caused a decrease in BDNF protein levels in the whole cortex until E18, while an increase was found at E20 [39].

Caffeine intake during adolescence (from PND 28 to PND 53) by drinking water decreased both proBDNF and mBDNF in the hippocampus at 1.0 mg/mL, while an increase was found in the cerebral cortex at 0.3 and 1.0 mg/mL [40]. Interestingly, caffeine at 0.1 or 0.3 mg/mL improved recognition memory while the highest dose impaired the nonassociative memory [40].

During adulthood to old age, 30 consecutive days of free access to drinking water containing 1 mg/mL of caffeine solution reduced age-related memory impairment and increased proBDNF in the hippocampus of young adult (3 months old)

TABLE 1: Brief description of the behavioral test used in the studies reported.

	Test	Protocol	Parameters	Meaning	References
Depression					
Anhedonia	Sucrose consumption/intake	Animals can choose to drink water or 1% sucrose.	Amount of sucrose consumed and preference for water/sucrose	The anhedonic phenotype is characterized by a reduction of sucrose intake/preference.	[25, 26, 64, 99, 100, 102, 103, 119, 123]
Despair	Forced swimming test (FST)	Animals are put in a vessel filled with water.	Latency to floating, swimming time	Despair behavior is associated with shorter latency to float and with less swimming time.	[27, 55, 56, 64, 72, 87, 100–103, 105, 106, 123, 126, 130, 140]
	Tail suspension test (TST)	Animals are suspended by the tail.	Immobility time	Despair is correlated with an increase in the immobility time.	[27, 64, 100, 101, 105, 130]
Anxiety	Open field (OF) test	Animals are free to explore an empty arena.	Time of exploration and number of rearing	Anxiety behavior is correlated with a reduction of exploration and rearing.	[25, 26, 40, 63, 73, 74, 79, 100, 101, 118, 139, 140]
	Shuttle box escape test	Animal can avoid an electric shock by running in the other room of the apparatus.	Number of escapes	Anxiety is characterized by the increased number of escape failures.	[25, 27]
	Elevated plus maze	Animals are free to explore a maze with two open and two close arms.	Time spent in the open arms	The time spent in the open arms is inversely correlated with anxiety.	[73, 104, 106, 140]
	Novelty-induced hyponeophagia (NIH) test	After 48 h food deprivation, animals are put into a cage containing food in the center.	Latency to feeding	Increase latency is associated with an anxious phenotype.	[99, 101]
	Learned helplessness	Animals learn to associate an electric shock with a tone.	Freezing time	Time of freezing is directly correlated with anxiety.	[101]
Cognition	Novel object recognition (NOR) test	Animals must discriminate between a novel (n) and a familiar (F) object.	Time exploring the two objects and NOR index $(n - F)/(n + F) + 100$	To correctly perform it, the animals must spend more time exploring the novel object. Improvement of cognition is reflected by a higher NOR index, while worsening is reflected by a lower NOR index.	[29, 30, 40, 42, 43, 74, 78]
	Y maze	Animals are put in a maze (Y-shaped), and they must recognize the novel arm (which is closed in the trial phase).	Time exploring the new arm	An increase in time exploring the new arm is an index of a correct cognitive performance.	[29, 78, 113]
	Fear conditioning	Animals learn to associate a cue (context or tone) to an electric shock.	Freezing time when the cue is presented without a shock	Time of freezing is directly correlated with memory.	[29, 33, 77]
	Morris water maze (MWM)	The animals learn to escape onto a hidden platform using this swimming-based model.	Time spent in the target quadrant (where the platform is).	Preserved spatial memory corresponds to increased time in the correct quadrant.	[30, 45, 76, 77, 80, 90, 109, 110, 118, 121, 135, 145]
	Spontaneous alternation test	Animals are placed in the center of a four-arm maze and are free to explore.	Percentage of alternations in the entry of the different arms.	The spontaneous alternation is used as memory task.	[47, 90]
	Radial arm water maze (RAWM)	Animals must find a submerged platform at the end of one of the six arms of the maze, aided by the fixed visually cues on the walls of the room.	Number of errors	Reduction of errors is related to a better cognitive performance.	[52, 91, 139]

and middle-aged rats (12 months old); the treatment also prevented the age-related increase in the mature form in older rats [41].

Accordingly, prolonged treatment (12 months) with caffeine solution (1 mg/mL in drinking water) in 6-month-old mice counteracted the increase in mBDNF in the hippocampus of aged animals and prevented the age-associated memory decline [42]. Moreover, 4 consecutive days of caffeine treatment (10 mg/kg, i.p.) increased the protein levels of mBDNF in the same brain region and improved the performance in the object recognition task in adult mice [43].

In the hippocampus of a mouse model of Alzheimer's disease, induced by $AlCl_3$, cotreatment with caffeine (1.5 mg/day by gavage) partially prevented the decrease in BDNF gene expression, while the pretreatment completely normalized the impairment [44]. Accordingly, chronic caffeine treatment (0.75 mg/day or 1.5 mg/day for 8 weeks) dose-dependently increased the mBDNF protein levels in the hippocampus of APP/PS1 ($A\beta$ precursor protein/presenelin-1) double transgenic mice, another model of Alzheimer's disease, and reversed the memory impairment observed in the Morris water maze (MWM) test [45].

Chronic caffeine treatment (0.33 mg/L in drinking water) during 4 weeks of psychological stress (intruder model) restored the reduced BDNF protein levels found in the stressed group [46]. The i.p. injection of caffeine once a week was enough to normalize the deficit of BDNF protein levels induced by a high-fat diet. At behavioral level, caffeine fully prevented the diet-induced impairment and restored the spatial memory observed in control animals. Neither diet nor caffeine treatment affected motor activity [47].

Since sleep is a critical factor in memory consolidation and neural plasticity [48], the effect of the chronic caffeine treatment on sleep loss was investigated. Oral administration of caffeine (60 mg/kg) or the psychostimulant modafinil (100 mg/kg), at the onset of the light phase during 48 hours of sleep deprivation (SD), restored the normal levels of cell proliferation improving BDNF expression in the dentate gyrus [49]. Accordingly, 4 weeks of caffeine treatment in drinking water (0.3 g/L) prevented the SD-induced decrease in neurotrophin levels in the dentate gyrus and in the cornu ammonis-1 (CA1) of the hippocampus [50, 51] and alleviated the impairment in the spatial long-term memory observed in sleep-deprived rats, also through the modulation of BDNF protein levels [52].

In summary, caffeine affects BDNF protein levels with a specific temporal and dose profile in normal animals. While administration during adulthood or old age increased BDNF, caffeine intake at high doses in early life downregulated the neurotrophin concentration.

Moreover, even if few studies investigated the efficacy of caffeine in animal models of pathology, they provide promising results.

At behavioral levels, caffeine was evaluated as a cognitive enhancer with positive effects.

3.3. Clinical Studies. The clinical study by Reyes-Izquierdo et al. [53] investigated the effect of three different coffee fruit extracts (100 mg dose per os) on BDNF plasma levels in healthy subjects. Coffee fruit concentrate powder (WCFC) (0.7% caffeine) but neither green coffee caffeine (N677) (72.8% caffeine) nor green coffee bean extract (N625) (2% caffeine) increased the level of BDNF in blood suggesting that the effect of WFCF might be related to the amount of procyanidins rather than to caffeine [53].

4. *Crocus sativus* L.

Crocus sativus L. belongs to the Iridaceae family; stigmas are commonly known as saffron and are widely cultivated in Iran and used in modern and traditional medicines. The color of saffron is mostly due to the carotenoid named crocin, which is considered among the active principles mostly responsible for neuroprotective activity [54].

4.1. In Vivo Studies. Two in vivo studies investigated the effect of *Crocus sativus* on BDNF expression. Crocin administration (12.5 mg/kg, i.p.) for 21 days to naïve male Wistar rats exerted an antidepressant effect and significantly increased the transcription levels of BDNF in the hippocampus [55]. Similarly, chronic treatment with *C. sativus* aqueous extract (40, 80, or 160 mg/kg/day, i.p.), enhanced the gene and protein levels of BDNF in the rat hippocampus. Moreover, at 40 and 160 mg/kg/day, an antidepressant activity was also observed. Similar results were obtained following imipramine injection (10 mg/kg) [56].

5. *Eleutherococcus senticosus* (Rupr. & Maxim.) Maxim.

Eleutherococcus senticosus Maxim. or *Acanthopanax senticosus* Harms, also called "Siberian ginseng," is a small shrub from the Araliaceae family. *Eleutherococcus* consists of the whole or cut dried roots of the plant containing lignans, phenylpropanoids, and dicaffeoylquinic acids [57].

5.1. In Vitro Studies. One paper investigated in vitro the effect of *Eleutherococcus senticosus* on BDNF. A commercial dry aqueous extract of *Acanthopanax senticosus* stem bark (ASE) normalized the reduction of BDNF mRNA levels produced by the administration of corticosterone (200 μM) for 24 h in PC12 cells. Different concentrations of ASE (100, 200, and 400 μg/mL) significantly increased the mRNA expression of the neurotrophin in a concentration-dependent fashion [58].

Unfortunately, no in vivo or clinical studies are reported in the literature on the modulation of BDNF by *E. senticosus*, and no clear-cut conclusions can be drawn.

6. *Ginkgo biloba* L.

Ginkgo biloba is an ancient Chinese tree belonging to the family of Ginkgoaceae, cultivated for its health-promoting properties. Although both leaves and seeds are currently used as herbal medicine in China, in many countries, leaves are considered the unique source of active principles and dried green leaves are used for supplying pharmaceutical formulations or extracts as ingredients of food supplements. *Ginkgo biloba* and its constituents were evaluated on BDNF in three *in vitro*, eight *in vivo*, and one clinical studies.

6.1. In Vitro Studies. Ginkgo biloba leaf extract (EGb761, 100 μg/mL) restored the levels of BDNF protein (both pro and mature form) in cells stimulated with appropriate medium able to induce amyloid β-peptide Aβ expression.

Administration of individual EGb761 constituents, namely, ginkgolides A (GA), B (GB), C (GC), and J (GJ) and 10 μg/mL bilobalide, increased the levels of BDNF by following a similar pattern [59].

Accordingly, flavonol-enriched extract containing quercetin, kaempferol, and isorhamnetin (50 μg/mL) significantly restored BDNF protein expression in double transgenic APP/PS1 primary neurons [60].

Moreover, 100 μg/mL of YY162, a patented formula consisting of terpenoid-strengthened *Ginkgo biloba* and ginsenoside Rg3, prevented the reduction of BDNF protein levels induced by 48 h of Aroclor 1254 in SH-SY5Y neuroblastoma cell line [61].

6.2. In Vivo Studies. Ginkgo flavonols (50 mg/kg, per os, daily for 4 months) significantly normalized the deficit of BDNF protein levels in the hippocampus of transgenic APP/PS1 mice and improved spatial learning similar to the administration of the antidepressant SSRI (serotonin selective reuptake inhibitor) fluoxetine (10 mg/kg), while exerting an antidepressant effect on wild-type animals [60].

YY162 (200 mg/kg, per os, from PND 21 to PND 35) significantly attenuated the reduction of BDNF protein in the prefrontal cortex and ameliorated the ADHD- (attention deficit hyperactivity disorder-) like behavioral phenotype induced by Aroclor 1254 [61].

Intravenous (i.v.) injections of EGb761 (45 mg/kg), just before ischemia-reperfusion, induced a significant increase in BDNF positive neurons in the hippocampus with respect to the control group; the treatment significantly reduced the behavior grade measured by a postural reflex test at 24 h after reperfusion. The effect exerted by EGb761 was comparable to that exerted by the antihypertensive nimodipine (2 mg/kg) [62].

Chronic treatment with EGb761 (100 mg/kg/day via oral gavage for 30 days) increased the BDNF levels in plasma of both young and aged (18 months) rats, but the effect was not statistically significant; on the opposite, in the aged female group, treatment significantly increased the number of platform crossings in the aged female group in the open field test (OFT) [63].

Pretreatment with EGb761 (100 or 150 mg/kg/day, per os for 10 days) significantly inhibited the reduction of hippocampal BDNF protein due to LPS (lipopolysaccharide) injections (0.83 mg/kg, i.p.) and showed an antidepressant effect [64]. Furthermore, EGb761 treatment (50 mg/kg/day, by oral gavage for 5 weeks) normalized the reduction of BDNF protein levels induced by the first-generation antipsychotic haloperidol injection (2 mg/kg/day, i.p., 5 weeks) in the prefrontal cortex, striatum, substantia nigra, and globus pallidus and reduced the vacuous chewing movement scores over the withdrawal period [65]. Finally, 28 days of treatment with

EGb761 (40 mg/kg) increased the expression of BDNF and explored the behavior in stressed rats. The effect was comparable to that of the SNRI (serotonin noradrenaline reuptake inhibitor) antidepressant venlafaxine (15 mg/kg) [66]. Administration of bilobalide (10 mg/kg, i.p.) for 10 days enhanced the hippocampal protein levels in normal mice more efficiently than that of fluoxetine (10 mg/kg) [67].

Taken together, these preclinical results suggest that *Ginkgo biloba* L. administration may be efficacious in restoring BDNF in pathologies characterized by neurotrophin deficits. The main problem is that studies take into consideration different animal models mimicking different kinds of diseases, from Alzheimer's disease to stroke, thus making further results mandatory to confirm the supposed effect on BDNF.

6.3. Clinical Studies. In the unique clinical study, one hundred fifty-seven patients affected by tardive dyskinesia (TD) associated with long-term neuroleptic treatment were randomized to either EGb761 80 mg three times a day or placebo treatment. EGb761 significantly increased the BDNF protein plasma levels compared with placebo at week 12 in TD patients [68].

7. Green Tea (*Camellia sinensis* (L.) Kuntze)

Tea obtained from the dried leaves of *Camellia sinensis* (L.) Kuntze (Theaceae) is one of the most widely consumed beverages in the world. Green tea (GT) contains many bioactive compounds including amino acids (i.e., L-theanine), flavonoids (i.e., catechins), and their derivatives, which may constitute up to 30% of the dried weight [69].

7.1. In Vitro Studies. The potential neuroprotective effect of some constituents of green tea leaves, including catechins, was investigated in two *in vitro* studies.

L-Theanine pretreatment (500 μM) exerted a protective effect by significantly attenuating the downregulation of BDNF protein due to the treatment with two disease-related neurotoxicants (rotenone and dieldrin) in the human cell line SH-SY5Y [70].

Moreover, pretreatment with GT catechins, such as epicatechin (EC) and (+)-catechin, prevented the reduction of mBDNF and the increase in the precursor form induced by the toxic HIV (human immunodeficiency virus) protein Tat [71].

7.2. In Vivo Studies. 10 papers investigated the effects of GT on BDNF. Chronic administration of L-theanine at different doses (0.2, 0.4, and 10 mg/kg, i.p.) exerted an antidepressant activity and upregulated the protein levels of BDNF in the hippocampus, but not in the cortex of adult mice [72]. Moreover, daily consumption of the flavonol (−)-EC (4 mg/day in water for 14 weeks, ad libitum) in adult mice led to an anxiolytic-like effect and increased the pro and mBDNF levels in the hippocampus, while no effect was found in the cortex [73].

The effect of theanine administration during development was evaluated on rat pups receiving 0.3% theanine (through lactation before weaning and then directly by drinking water) showing increased exploratory activity and enhanced object recognition memory and levels of mBDNF protein in the hippocampus [74].

Assuncao et al. demonstrated that the decrease in BDNF protein levels in the rat hippocampus, associated with aging, was prevented by drinking GT-infused drink as the only drink available from 12 to 19 months of age [75]. Similarly, catechins (0.05% and 0.1%) mixed with drinking water for 6 months improved age-related spatial learning and memory decline of 14-month-old female mice and upregulated the hippocampal mature form of BDNF to levels comparable to those observed in young animals [76].

On the contrary, the addition of epigallocatechin-3-O-gallate (EGCG) (182 mg/kg/day) and β-alanine (417 mg/kg/day) to the diet for 4 months did not improve memory and did not alter the mRNA expression of BDNF in the hippocampus of 19-month-old male mice [77].

The GT effect has been studied in different animal models of learning impairments. Administration (1 g in 100 mL water for 5 min at 100°C, corresponding to 0.6–1 mg EGCG per day), from gestation to adulthood, corrected the lower BDNF mRNA levels in the hippocampus of mice overexpressing *DYRK1A* (dual-specificity tyrosine phosphorylation-regulated kinase 1A) but did not affect the performance in memory tasks [78].

In senescence-accelerated mice-prone 8 (SAMP8), a model characterized by the early onset of learning and memory deficits along with overproduction of soluble amyloid peptide in the brain, the chronic treatment with green tea catechins (GTC) (0.05% and 0.1% in drinking water for 6 months) restored the reduction of mBDNF levels in the hippocampus and prevented the learning impairment of SAMP8 mice [79]. Finally, 4 months of EC administration (50 mg/kg daily in drinking water) normalized the low levels of BDNF protein in the hippocampus of 8-month-old APP/PS1 mice, without affecting escape latency in MWM [80].

Teasaponin (10 mg/kg, i.p. for 21 days) rescued the upregulation of BDNF induced by the adipocyte-secreted hormone leptin in the prefrontal cortex of high-fat diet-fed mice. In addition, teasaponin (20 or 40 μM) reversed the effect of palmitic acid on the alteration induced by leptin in cultured cortical neurons [81].

To summarize, these studies provide robust evidence regarding the role of green tea as a modulator of BDNF and in improving cognitive performance at preclinical levels.

8. *Hypericum perforatum* L.

Hypericum perforatum L. (HYP), known as St John's wort, is a plant belonging to the family of Hypericaceae. Flowering aerial parts are used in many countries for their antidepressant activity, mostly ascribed to the active principles hyperforin, hypericin, and pseudohypericin [18, 57].

8.1. In Vivo Studies. The antidepressant activity of *Hypericum perforatum* was investigated at preclinical level in two *in vivo* studies using the CMS animal model. The chronic treatment with hydroalcoholic extract of HYP (350 mg/kg per os, 21 days) normalized the reduction of mRNA expression of

BDNF found in the hippocampus of stressed mice [82]. On the contrary, Butterweck et al. showed that the chronic administration of HYP methanolic extract (500 mg/kg, per os) did not prevent the stress-induced decrease in BDNF mRNA levels in the rat hippocampus, produced by the immobilization stress protocol (2 h once a day for 7 days) [83]. The different outcomes between these two preclinical studies could be due to the type of stressors or the protocol of treatment used.

8.2. Clinical Studies. In one large cohort of subjects, chronic HYP treatment restored the normal protein concentration of BDNF in the serum of depressed patients. This normalization was limited to HYP and serotonin reuptake inhibitors, whereas other classes of antidepressants, including the tricyclics and the noradrenergic and specific serotoninergic antidepressant, were ineffective. The limitation of this study is that the dose of the different drugs used is not clearly indicated [84].

9. Olive Oil (*Olea europaea* L.)

Olive oil is the main source of fat in the Mediterranean-style diet. Health benefit of olive oil consumption has been in part ascribed to minor phenol components (i.e., oleuropein, ligstroside aglycones, and hydroxytyrosol (HT)) whose composition varies qualitatively and quantitatively depending on the stage of fruit ripeness or the region of cultivation [85, 86].

9.1. In Vivo Studies. Five animal studies were performed to test the effect of olive oil components on BDNF. The administration of a mixture of olive oil polyphenols extracted from the olive residues (pomace) (10 mg/kg, i.p., 10 days) significantly increased the BDNF protein levels in the hippocampus and in the olfactory lobes, while decreasing the neurotrophin in the frontal cortex [87]. Moreover, this regime of treatment did not affect pain sensitivity in the hot-plate test or stress response in the FST in naïve animals [87].

Differently, if the blend of polyphenols was extracted from olive leaves (20 mg/kg, i.p. for 15 days), BDNF protein levels were downregulated in the hippocampus and striatum and upregulated in the olfactory lobes. Polyphenol administration significantly increased the concentration of BDNF protein in the mouse serum [88]. Interestingly, a diet enriched in olive oil components during prenatal life until weaning induced, at adulthood, an upregulation of the mRNA levels of the total BDNF and of the isoforms IV and VI in the prefrontal cortex but not in the hippocampus [89].

Before mating, the treatment with HT (10 or 50 mg/kg/day by gavage for 2 weeks), one of the most bioactive phenolic compound in olive oil, prevented the significant decrease in proBDNF and mBDNF due to prenatal stress exposure in male offspring and improved cognitive functions [90].

In Alzheimer's disease mouse model, HT chronic treatment (10 mg/day by gavage for 14 days) attenuated the spatio-cognitive deficits and normalized the hippocampal BDNF mRNA levels [91].

9.2. Clinical Studies. The effect of olive oil was investigated in two clinical studies. Taking Mediterranean diet supplemented with olive oil for 3 years did not alter the plasma BDNF protein levels in normal subjects [92]. Moreover, the administration of a blend of olive polyphenols (a tablet containing a total of 50 mg/day) extracted from the olive pomace and containing mostly HT and oleuropein for 15 consecutive days in alcoholic patients undergoing withdrawal induced a transient decrease in mBDNF protein levels in the serum after 3 days of treatment [93].

Even if not so many, *in vivo* studies provide positive results, while the effect in clinical studies (only 2) appears inconsistent or negligible.

10. *Panax ginseng* C.A. Meyer

Ginseng radix consists of the whole or cut dried root of *Panax ginseng* C.A. Meyer and contains not less than 0.4% of the sum of ginsenosides Rg1 (Rg1) and Rb1 (Rb1). Ginsenosides are triterpenoid saponins which are the main responsible for the biological activities of ginseng extracts [57].

10.1. In Vitro Studies. Five studies were performed *in vitro* to test the effect of ginseng or ginsenosides on BDNF. Rg1 treatment upregulated the mRNA expression and protein secretion of BDNF in primary cultured olfactory cells (Rg1, $40 \mu g/mL$ for 72 h) [94] and in Schwann cells (Rg1, $50 \mu M$ for 24 h) challenged with 0.2% H_2O_2 for 4 h [95]. The beneficial effect was also found in different "pathological conditions." Indeed, pretreatment of rat brain slices with Rg1 at different concentrations (60, 120, and $240 \mu M$ for 2 h), before okadaic acid administration, increased the BDNF protein expression in a dose-dependent fashion [96].

Red ginseng extract (RGE) (0.01–1.0 mg/mL applied for 1 h) dose-dependently increased the BDNF protein expression in primary cultures of rat hippocampal neurons exposed for 48 h to $100 \mu M$ kainic acid [97]. BDNF protein levels were significantly increased in PC12 cells subjected to oxygen glucose deprivation/reperfusion (OGD/R) for 4 h by ginsenoside Rd (Rd) at 50 and $100 \mu M$ [98].

10.2. In Vivo Studies. A total number of 25 studies were performed *in vivo*, mostly on pure ginsenosides.

Deficits induced at protein levels by the exposure to CMS were normalized by concomitant treatment with ginseng standardized in the saponin content (GTS) (50 and 100 mg/ kg) [99] or Rg1 (2.5, 5, 10, and 20 mg/kg, i.p.) [100] in the hippocampus and with ginsenoside Rb3 (Rb3) (30, 75, and 150 mg/kg, intragastrically) both in the prefrontal cortex and in the hippocampus [101]. At 40 mg/kg (i.p.), the effect, for Rg1, was also found in the lateral amygdala [102, 103]. Rg1 corrected the alteration found at translational level [100] similar to fluoxetine (10 mg/kg) [104, 105] and imipramine [100]. Moreover, all the compounds reverted the behavioral phenotype associated with this model [99–103].

A comparable effect was found after chronic restraint stress with Re (50 mg/kg) and fluoxetine (10 mg/kg) at transcriptional level in the hippocampus [106], while Rg1 (10 mg/kg) prevented the reduction of mBDNF in the prefrontal cortex [107]. Re produced an antidepressant and

anxiolytic effect [106], whereas Rg1 improved learning and memory [107].

The decreased expression of BDNF mRNA, found after the single prolonged stress, was significantly restored to normal level by chronic treatment with Rb1 (10 or 30 mg/kg, i.p., 14 days) or fluoxetine (10 mg/kg). Rb1 at 30 mg/kg normalized the percentage of time spent in the open arms in the elevated plus maze [104]. Rb1 (10 mg/kg), administered 30 min before acute immobilization stress, significantly inhibited the stress-mediated decline in BDNF mRNA level [108].

Accordingly, GTS (25 or 50 mg/kg/day), similar to fluoxetine (10 mg/kg), significantly upregulated the mRNA and protein levels of BDNF in the hippocampus of corticosterone-treated mice (20 mg/kg, once a day for 22 days) but not in that of normal animals and produced an antidepressant effect [105].

Panax ginseng extract or pure compounds exerted a positive effect also on the scopolamine animal model. Indeed, wild ginseng (WG) roots (200 mg/kg, i.p.) normalized the mRNA level of BDNF in the rat hippocampus of the scopolamine-treated group, as well as reducing the escape latency in the MWM test [109]. Accordingly, pretreatment with ginsenosides Rg5 (Rg5) and Rh3 (Rh3) (5, 10, and 20 mg/kg, per os) inhibited the reduction of mBDNF protein expression induced by scopolamine injection (1 mg/kg, i.p.) and reduced the latency time in MWM. The protective effect of Rh3 (5 and 10 mg/kg) on memory deficit was more potent than that of Rh5 and comparable with that of the acetyl cholinesterase inhibitor donepezil (5 mg/kg) used in the treatment of Alzheimer's disease [110].

Oral administration of Rg5 (5, 10, and 20 mg/kg) or donepezil (3 mg/kg) prevented the reduction of mBDNF induced by streptozotocin (STZ) (3 mg/kg intracerebroventricular administration) and enhanced the memory retention, the mean latency time, and the path length with respect to the STZ group in the MWM test [111].

Rd (10, 20, 40, and 80 mg/kg/day, i.p.) prevented the reduction of BDNF expression in both the cerebral cortex and lumbar spinal cord in an animal model of encephalomyelitis [112].

Rg1 (2.5, 5.0, and 10 mg/kg, i.p.) significantly increased, in a dose-dependent manner, the mBDNF protein level in SAMP8 mice and ameliorated the cognitive impairments observed in 9-month-old mice [113].

Similarly, chronic treatment with Rg1 (1 mg/kg or 10 mg/ kg, i.p. for 30 days) significantly enhanced the mBDNF expression in the hippocampal homogenate of middle-aged rats. Also, proBDNF was upregulated, but the effect was significant only for the 10 mg/kg-treated group. Furthermore, Rg1 administration significantly improved the memory in the fear-conditioning task [114].

The protective effect of Rg1 on memory performance and synaptic plasticity was assessed in a transgenic AD model constructed by overexpressing APP and PS1. The injection of 10 mg/kg Rg1 for 30 days (i.p.) upregulated the BDNF protein levels and ameliorated the memory in mice [115].

Moreover, in adult male rats, Rb1 infusion (40 mg/kg) significantly increased the BDNF protein expression from 3 h to 10 days after middle cerebral artery reperfusion, with a peak at 3 days [116]. On the opposite, treatment with Rb1 (7.5 mg/mL) by intragastric administration for three days, three times a day (12.5 mL/kg weight) before transient middle cerebral artery occlusion, did not prevent the increased levels of BDNF due to the damage. Indeed, BDNF protein levels were higher in the Rb1 group compared to the untreated animals [117].

Five- to 7-week-old male C57BL/6J mice were treated with Rd (10 or 30 mg/kg, i.p. for 21 days) fifteen days after bilateral carotid artery stenosis that induced chronic cerebral hypoperfusion (CCH). The dramatic decrease in BDNF protein and mRNA levels observed in the CCH model was reversed by Rd administration that also improved the memory task performance [118].

YY162 significantly reduced the BDNF protein decline in the prefrontal cortex and improved the ADHD behavioral phenotype [61].

Pretreatment for 3 days with Rg1 (10 or 30 mg/kg, i.p.) or the antibiotic minocycline (30 mg/kg, i.p.) significantly normalized the BDNF mRNA levels altered by a central injection of LPS (5 μg in 5 μL saline) in the cortex but not in the hippocampus.

Rg1 administration at both low and high doses alleviated the anorexic symptoms and increased the sucrose preference [119].

The effect of ginsenoside administration on naïve animals is conflicting. Indeed, injections of Rb1 5 mg/kg/day in 0.2 cc saline i.p. for 4 days did not modulate the BDNF mRNA levels in the hippocampus [120], while ginsenoside Rh1 (10 mg/kg/day for 3 months) significantly upregulated the BDNF protein levels in the hippocampus with respect to the control group. The Rh1-treated group (5 and 10 mg/kg) significantly promoted the spatial learning ability in the MWM test [121]. Finally, administration of gintonin (50 mg/kg per os, 7 days), a mixture of glycolipoproteins from *Panax ginseng*, significantly increased the BDNF protein levels [122].

Taken together, reviewed studies suggest that pure ginsenosides are effective modulators of neuroplasticity. The main criticism is the heterogeneity of the studies that evaluate the effect of each ginsenoside at a time.

11. *Perilla frutescens* (L.) Britton

Perilla frutescens (L.) Britton, also called *zi-su* in Chinese, is an annual herb belonging to the Lamiaceae family; stems, leaves, and seeds are widely used in traditional Chinese medicine or as food ingredients.

11.1. In Vivo Studies. Five papers investigated the effect of *Perilla frutescens* on in vivo models. Administration of essential oil from commercial *Perilla* leaf (EOPL) for 4 weeks, at 3 or 6 mg/kg, normalized the BDNF gene expression, while only the highest dose was effective at protein levels in the hippocampus of chronically stressed mice. Conversely, 3 weeks of EOPL was not enough to correct the molecular deficit observed. Moreover, EOPL produced an antidepressant-like effect in the sucrose preference test after 3 and 4 weeks at both concentrations and in the FST at 6 mg/kg after 3-week

treatment or at 3 mg/kg and 6 mg/kg after 4-week treatment, while no effect was observed on the locomotor activity. Interestingly, a similar effect was found in administering 20 mg/kg fluoxetine [123].

Male mice subjected to dietary restriction of α-linolenic acid (ALA) were fed with a diet supplemented with *Perilla* oil (5%) for 8 weeks. ALA restriction lowered the BDNF levels in the striatum, and *Perilla* oil significantly increased the BDNF protein levels [124, 125].

Six weeks of *Perilla* seed oil administration at 4% (*w/w*) in the diet to naïve Sprague-Dawley rats significantly upregulated the concentration of BDNF in the prefrontal cortex, while the immobility times were significantly shorter in the FST. A similar effect was observed after i.p. injection of imipramine (30 mg/kg) [126].

In a recent study, chronic treatment with *Perilla* oil (500 mg/kg/day by gastric gavage) normalized the decrease in BDNF protein levels in an animal model of Alzheimer's disease. The effect paralleled the anxiolytic-like effect and improved the cognitive performance measured in both the novel object recognition test and the MWM test [127].

On these bases, the few studies present in literature are encouraging, but other demonstrations are mandatory to draw clear-cut conclusions.

12. *Rhodiola rosea* L.

Rhodiola rosea L. (Crassulaceae) has a long history of use as a medicinal plant in several traditional medicines. *Rhodiola* root and rhizome increase the organism's resistance to physical, chemical, and biological stressors; the effect is mostly due to the active principle salidroside (SA, syn. rhodioloside) [128].

12.1. In Vitro Studies. One in vitro study evaluated the effect of SA on BDNF demonstrating that the pure compound induced mesenchymal stem cells to differentiate into dopaminergic neurons. Moreover, SA treatment (100 μg/mL) for 1–6 days significantly increased the BDNF mRNA levels while at 12 days, an opposite effect was found. Differently, the effect on the BDNF protein levels was more long lasting since it was still present after 12 days [129].

12.2. In Vivo Studies. In vivo, the treatment for 5 days (12 and 24 mg/kg, per os) with SA or fluoxetine prevented the development of the depression-like behavior and of the downregulation of BDNF protein levels in the hippocampus induced by a single injection of LPS [130].

13. *Salvia miltiorrhiza* Bunge

Salvia miltiorrhiza Bunge (Lamiaceae), also known as red sage, is a perennial plant; root and rhizome are widely used in China for the treatment of cardiovascular and cerebrovascular diseases [131].

13.1. In Vitro Studies. Two in vitro studies evaluated the effect of salvianolic acid B (SalB). Treatment with SalB (20 μg/mL, for 24 h) significantly increased the level of BDNF protein in bone marrow-derived neural stem cells [132].

Furthermore, SMND-309 (5, 10, and 20 μM for 24 h), the metabolite produced in the brain and heart of rats after SalB oral administration, restored the mBDNF protein expression in the human neuroblastoma cell line SH-SY5Y subjected for 2 h to OGD/R [133].

13.2. In Vivo Studies. *Salvia miltiorrhiza* extracts and pure compounds were also investigated in five *in vivo* studies. Hippocampal BDNF immunoreactivity was markedly decreased by the injection of the Aβ_{25-35} peptide in mice, and subchronic treatment with SalB (10 mg/kg, 7 days) reversed this reduction [134]. A similar effect was observed after oral treatment for 14 days (0.81 and 0.405 g/kg) with the formulation named Compound Danshen Tablet (CDT) (*Salvia miltiorrhiza*, *Panax notoginseng*, and borneol in a ratio 450 : 141 : 8). Indeed, CDT administered to mice at 0.81 g/kg or 0.405 g/kg normalized the hippocampal BDNF mRNA levels and improved the cognitive performance, while the lowest dose was effective also at the protein level [135].

Pretreatment with tanshinone I (10 mg/kg, i.p. for 3 days), a lipophilic diterpenoid occurring in the radix of *Salvia miltiorrhiza*, administered 5 minutes before ischemia-reperfusion by bilateral common carotid artery occlusion, corrected the reduced BDNF immunoreactivity in the CA1 of ischemic Mongolian gerbils [136]. Similarly, salvianolic acid A (100 μg/kg) administered intravenously 2 h after middle cerebral artery occlusion/reperfusion significantly reversed the protein levels of mBDNF in the ipsilateral ischemic brain hemisphere. Furthermore, the treatment significantly improved the reduction in tracking distance induced by stroke injury [137].

Salvianolate lyophilized injection (10.5, 21, and 42 mg/kg) ameliorated the deficits observed in diabetic rats after stroke normalizing the protein level of the mature form of BDNF [138].

14. *Vitis vinifera* L. (Red Wine)

Vitis vinifera L. is a plant belonging to the family of Vitaceae, native to the Mediterranean region and widely used to make wine or juice.

14.1. In Vivo Studies. Two *in vivo* studies were performed on male rats. Grape powder (including that of fresh red, green, and blue-black California grapes, seeded and seedless varieties) dissolved in tap water (15 g/L) for 3 weeks attenuated the reduction of BDNF protein levels induced by the oxidative stress mediator L-buthionine-(S,R)-sulfoximine in the amygdala, hippocampus, and cortex [139] or due to the exposure to a single prolonged stress [140]. Moreover, grape intake exerted an anxiolytic effect and a positive effect in the memory test [139, 140]. In addition to grape studies, few interesting papers investigated BDNF modulations by red wine or ethanol starting from 60 days before pregnancy up to pup weaning. Adult animals exposed to only ethanol showed disrupted levels of BDNF in several brain areas, including the hippocampus, and altered cognition and emotional behavior. Conversely, mice exposed to red wine had no changes in the behavior but a decrease

in hippocampal BDNF [141]. Another study investigated BDNF changes in old male mice following perinatal exposure to ethanol or red wine at the same ethanol concentration. The study demonstrates that ethanol alone is able to increase BDNF levels in limbic areas, whereas, in mice exposed to red wine, BDNF levels were comparable to those of control thus allowing one to hypothesize a protective role of wine polyphenols against the damaging effect of ethanol alone [142].

14.2. Clinical Studies. One clinical study was performed on 25 healthy fasted subjects treated with a single dose of grape seed extract (N31, 72% polyphenols). The participants were 18–55 years old and had a body mass index between 18.0 and 25.0 kg/m^2. N31 increased the BDNF levels in plasma by 30% with respect to the baseline, although the effect was not statistically significant [53].

15. *Withania somnifera* (L.) Dunal

Withania somnifera (L.) Dunal, also called Ashwagandha or Indian ginseng (Solanaceae), is a traditional Ayurvedic remedy reputed to be useful as an antistress and memory enhancer [143].

15.1. In Vivo Studies. Two papers investigated the effect of *Withania somnifera* on *in vivo* models. Pretreatment with an alcoholic extract of Ashwagandha leaves (100 mg, 200 mg, and 300 mg/kg for 7 days) significantly prevented the effects due to the scopolamine treatment (3 mg/kg) such as the reduction of the mRNA expression of BDNF transcript variant-1 and of proBDNF and mBDNF protein expression at all the concentrations tested. On the contrary, posttreatment at 200 mg/kg was ineffective [144].

Withanolide-enriched extract from the *Withania somnifera* root (methanol–water 25 : 75, *v/v*) was evaluated on induced hypobaric hypoxia in rats. Animals fed before and after hypobaric hypoxia with 200 mg/kg of the extract showed an increased expression of BDNF and a significant decrease in latency and path length in the MWM test [145].

16. Conclusions

In this review, we provide an upgrade of the current literature on the ability of some well-known botanicals to modulate BDNF expression in the brain. Recently, the strategy searching for new compounds, also from natural sources, able to modulate neurotrophin levels, has been increasingly explored. The growing interest in the use of botanicals as modulators of the CNS diseases is proved by the large amount of scientific papers we retrieved and reviewed on this topic (more than one hundred papers for 14 botanicals) (Figure 2). Results critically reviewed and discussed herein emphasize how botanicals modulate BDNF in different pathological conditions affecting the CNS, providing an alternative strategy to the conventional treatment. Indeed, most of the studies demonstrated that treatment with botanicals may prevent and/or normalize

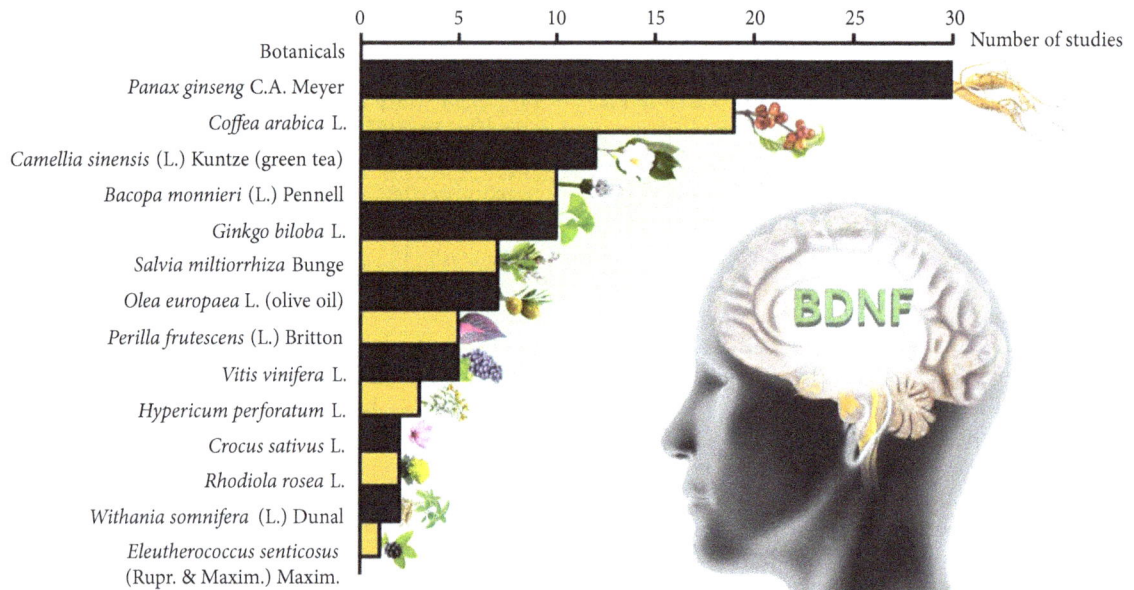

FIGURE 2: Number of studies investigating BDNF in the central nervous system for each botanical or active principle.

the alterations of BDNF caused by experimental handling (Table 2).

An added value of papers dealing with *in vivo* studies is that molecular analyses parallel the investigation of an animal model's behavior after treatment, thus allowing one to draw clear-cut conclusions on the functional outcome associated with the correction of the molecular deficits.

Indeed, despite a variety of different pathological conditions taken into consideration, from mood disorders to Alzheimer's disease and aging up to cerebral vascular damage, the common point is the impairment of cognition. Accordingly, among the behavioral phenotypes, the performance in learning and memory tasks was deeply explored as a common feature of different diseases occurring in the CNS and many botanicals considered have been demonstrated to have cognitive-enhancing properties such as *Bacopa monnieri*, *Coffea arabica*, *Ginkgo biloba*, green tea, olive oil, *Panax ginseng*, *Perilla frutescens*, *Salvia miltiorrhiza*, *Vitis vinifera*, and *Withania somnifera*.

This observation increases the meaning of the results summarized in the present review because the positive effect on a molecular target (BDNF) and on a functional deficit (in cognition) altered in several diseases makes the therapeutic ability of these compounds broad-spectrum.

Another point is that most studies compared the effect of botanicals with the effect obtained from a reference drug, showing similar efficacy. For example, *Bacopa monnieri*, *Crocus sativus*, *Ginkgo biloba*, green tea, *Panax ginseng*, *Perilla frutescens*, and *Rhodiola rosea* exert antidepressant-like effects in different behavioral tests compared to the classical drugs used in therapy. However, most of the clinical studies reported in the present review do not pay attention to the side effects following botanical treatment.

Moreover, even if promising results have been found on *Crocus sativus*, *Eleutherococcus senticosus* Maxim., *Hypericum perforatum*, *Rhodiola rosea*, *Salvia miltiorrhiza* Bunge,

Vitis vinifera, and *Withania somnifera* Dunal and BDNF modulation, the number of studies of these botanicals is too low for drawing conclusive results.

The current revision of the literature suggests that several issues need to be considered to draw consistent conclusions. Firstly, considering the complexity of the BDNF system, as briefly described in the introduction, a more refined analysis of the different elements both at transcription and translational levels is mandatory. Indeed, very few studies report the BDNF isoform or the form measured, and, in some cases, the molecular weight of the band examined does not correspond to either the mature or the precursor form.

Secondly, though not negligible, the number of clinical studies is very limited since few clinical trials have been found in literature. Among them, the first was carried out in schizophrenic patients following treatment with *Ginkgo biloba* L. extract [68] and the second was performed in depressed patients treated with *Hypericum perforatum* L. [84], whereas the others were performed in healthy subjects. Although the effect obtained from those studies was relevant, the paucity of clinical trials implies that botanicals discussed in the present review need to be carefully considered for human studies.

Standardization of the extract is an important prerequisite for efficacy of botanicals. Knowledge of the active principles is the first step for an adequate standardization. Results reported in literature show that ginsenosides are mostly responsible for BDNF modulation exerted by *Panax ginseng* C.A. Meyer whereas rhodioloside appears to be the main active principle occurring in *Rhodiola rosea* L. However, for other botanicals, the molecules driving the pharmacological effects are not clearly defined (i.e., *Vitis vinifera* L. or olive oil (*Olea europaea* L.)) and only speculations can be done at this regard. Thus, it is important to underline that most of the studies reviewed herein used standardized extracts,

TABLE 2: Summary of the experimental conditions employed to investigate the effect of botanical administration on BDNF expression.

Botanicals	Type of studies	Models	mRNA	Protein	References
Bacopa monnieri (L.)	In vitro	PC12	•		[23, 24]
	In vivo	Naïve animals	•	•	[32]
		Chronic stress	•	•	[25, 27]
				•	[26]
		Fear conditioning	•		[33]
		Olfactory bulbectomy	•		[29]
		Scopolamine	•		[30]
			•	•	[31]
Coffea arabica L.	In vitro	Hippocampal neurons		•	[34, 35]
		Cortical neurons	•		[36]
	In vivo	Naïve animals		•	[38–43]
			•		[37]
		Alzheimer's disease	•		[44]
				•	[45]
		Chronic stress		•	[46]
		Obesity (high-fat diet)		•	[47]
		Sleep deprivation	•		[49]
				•	[50–52]
	Clinical	Healthy subjects		•	[53]
Crocus sativus L.	In vivo	Naïve animals	•	•	[55, 56]
Eleutherococcus senticosus (Rupr. & Maxim.) Maxim.	In vitro	PC12	•		[58]
Ginkgo biloba L.	In vitro	N2a		•	[59]
		(APP/PS1) primary neurons		•	[60]
		SH-SY5Y		•	[61]
	In vivo	Naïve animals		•	[63, 67]
		Alzheimer's disease		•	[60]
		ADHD		•	[61]
		Cerebral ischemia-reperfusion		•	[62]
		Chronic stress		•	[66]
		Haloperidol		•	[65]
		LPS-induced depression		•	[64]
	Clinical	Tardive dyskinesia patients		•	[68]
Green tea (Camellia sinensis (L.) Kuntze)	In vitro	SH-SY5Y		•	[70]
		Cortical cultures		•	[71]
	In vivo	Naïve animals		•	[72–76]
			•		[77]
		Alzheimer's disease		•	[79, 80]
		DYRK1A transgenic mice	•		[78]
		Obesity (high-fat diet)		•	[81]
Hypericum perforatum L.	In vivo	Chronic stress	•		[82, 83]
	Clinical	Depressed patient		•	[84]
Olive oil (Olea europaea L.)	In vivo	Naïve animals		•	[87, 88]
			•		[89]
		Alzheimer's disease	•		[91]
		Prenatal stress		•	[90]
	Clinical	Healthy subjects		•	[92]
		Alcoholic patients		•	[93]

TABLE 2: Continued.

Botanicals	Type of studies	Models	mRNA	Protein	References
Panax ginseng C.A. Meyer	*In vitro*	OECs	•	•	[94]
		PC12		•	[98]
		Rat brain slices		•	[96]
		Rat hippocampal neurons		•	[97]
		SCs	•	•	[95]
	In vivo	Naïve animals		•	[114, 121, 122]
			•		[120]
		Acute stress	•	•	[108]
			•		[104]
		Alzheimer's disease		•	[115]
		ADHD		•	[61]
		Autoimmune encephalomyelitis		•	[112]
		Cerebral ischemia-reperfusion		•	[116, 117]
			•	•	[118]
		Chronic stress		•	[99, 101–103, 107]
			•		[106]
			•	•	[100]
		Corticosterone	•	•	[105]
		LPS-induced depression	•		[119]
		Scopolamine		•	[110]
			•		[109]
		SAMP8		•	[113]
		Streptozotocin		•	[111]
Perilla frutescens (L.) Britton	*In vivo*	Alzheimer's disease		•	[127]
		Chronic stress	•	•	[123]
		Dietary restriction of ALA		•	[124, 125]
		Naïve animals		•	[126]
Rhodiola rosea L.	*In vitro*	Mesenchymal stem cells	•	•	[129]
	In vivo	LPS-induced depression		•	[130]
Salvia miltiorrhiza Bunge	*In vitro*	BM-NSCs		•	[132]
		SH-SY5Y		•	[133]
	In vivo	Alzheimer's disease		•	[134]
			•	•	[135]
		Cerebral ischemia-reperfusion		•	[136, 137]
		Streptozotocin and cerebral ischemia-reperfusion		•	[138]
Vitis vinifera L.	*In vivo*	Naïve animals		•	[141, 142]
		Acute stress		•	[140]
		Oxidative stress		•	[139]
	Clinical	Healthy subjects		•	[53]
Withania somnifera (L.) Dunal	*In vivo*	Hypobaric hypoxia		•	[145]
		Scopolamine	•	•	[144]

Studies which measured the BDNF mRNA or protein levels are indicated with the symbol "•".

although few papers did not report properly the type of solvent used.

In conclusion, considering the key role of the marker in different pathological conditions affecting the CNS, BDNF may represent an important tool to counteract these conditions, as demonstrated by the studies reported herein. Botanicals may be considered useful candidates to modulate *in vivo* BDNF. If clinical studies confirm this evidence, these natural products may be used for preventing CNS dysfunction or as a useful adjuvant to the pharmacological treatment.

Conflicts of Interest

The authors declare no conflict of interest.

Acknowledgments

The publication costs are covered by "Piano di sviluppo di UNIMI—Linea 2, Azione A—Università degli Studi di Milano a giovani e talentuosi ricercatori (2016)."

References

[1] S. Lowel and W. Singer, "Selection of intrinsic horizontal connections in the visual cortex by correlated neuronal activity," *Science*, vol. 255, no. 5041, pp. 209–212, 1992.

[2] M. M. Poo, "Neurotrophins as synaptic modulators," *Nature Review Neuroscience*, vol. 2, no. 1, pp. 24–32, 2001.

[3] E. J. Huang and L. F. Reichardt, "Neurotrophins: roles in neuronal development and function," *Annual Review of Neuroscience*, vol. 24, no. 1, pp. 677–736, 2001.

[4] B. Lu, P. T. Pang, and N. H. Woo, "The yin and yang of neurotrophin action," *Nature Review Neuroscience*, vol. 6, no. 8, pp. 603–614, 2005.

[5] F. Calabrese, R. Molteni, G. Racagni, and M. A. Riva, "Neuronal plasticity: a link between stress and mood disorders," *Psychoneuroendocrinology*, vol. 34, Supplement 1, pp. S208–S216, 2009.

[6] R. B. Foltran and S. L. Diaz, "BDNF isoforms: a round trip ticket between neurogenesis and serotonin?," *Journal of Neurochemistry*, vol. 138, no. 2, pp. 204–221, 2016.

[7] T. Aid, A. Kazantseva, M. Piirsoo, K. Palm, and T. Timmusk, "Mouse and rat BDNF gene structure and expression revisited," *Journal of Neuroscience Research*, vol. 85, no. 3, pp. 525–535, 2007.

[8] P. Pruunsild, A. Kazantseva, T. Aid, K. Palm, and T. Timmusk, "Dissecting the human BDNF locus: bidirectional transcription, complex splicing, and multiple promoters," *Genomics*, vol. 90, no. 3, pp. 397–406, 2007.

[9] B. Lu, "BDNF and activity-dependent synaptic modulation," *Learn Memory*, vol. 10, no. 2, pp. 86–98, 2003.

[10] Z. L. Zhou, E. J. Hong, S. Cohen et al., "Brain-specific phosphorylation of MeCP2 regulates activity-dependent *Bdnf* transcription, dendritic growth, and spine maturation," *Neuron*, vol. 52, no. 2, pp. 255–269, 2006.

[11] R. Molteni, F. Calabrese, A. Cattaneo et al., "Acute stress responsiveness of the neurotrophin BDNF in the rat hippocampus is modulated by chronic treatment with the antidepressant duloxetine," *Neuropsychopharmacology*, vol. 34, no. 9, p. 2196, 2009.

[12] K. Martinowich, H. Manji, and B. Lu, "New insights into BDNF function in depression and anxiety," *Nature Neuroscience*, vol. 10, no. 9, pp. 1089–1093, 2007.

[13] B. Lu and K. Martinowich, "Cell biology of BDNF and its relevance to schizophrenia," *Novartis Foundation Symposia*, vol. 289, pp. 119–129, 2008.

[14] M. Mitre, A. Mariga, and M. V. Chao, "Neurotrophin signalling: novel insights into mechanisms and pathophysiology," *Clinical Science*, vol. 131, no. 1, pp. 13–23, 2017.

[15] A. H. Nagahara and M. H. Tuszynski, "Potential therapeutic uses of BDNF in neurological and psychiatric disorders," *Nature Review Drug Discovery*, vol. 10, no. 3, pp. 209–219, 2011.

[16] S. Yanev, "Neurotrophic and metabotrophic potential of nerve growth factor and brain-derived neurotrophic factor: linking cardiometabolic and neuropsychiatric diseases," *World Journal of Pharmacology*, vol. 2, no. 4, p. 92, 2013.

[17] B. Lu, G. H. Nagappan, X. M. Guan, P. J. Nathan, and P. Wren, "BDNF-based synaptic repair as a disease-modifying strategy for neurodegenerative diseases," *Nature Reviews Neuroscience*, vol. 14, no. 6, pp. 401–416, 2013.

[18] Q. X. Ng, N. Venkatanarayanan, and C. Y. X. Ho, "Clinical use of *Hypericum perforatum* (St John' wort) in depression: a meta-analysis," *Journal of Affective Disorders*, vol. 210, pp. 211–221, 2017.

[19] S. Bent, A. Padula, D. H. Moore, M. Patterson, and W. Mehling, "Valerian for sleep: a systematic review and meta-analysis," *Journal of General Internal Medicine*, vol. 20, p. 90, 2005.

[20] J. Sarris, E. McIntyre, and D. A. Camfield, "Plant-based medicines for anxiety disorders, part 1: a review of preclinical studies," *CNS Drugs*, vol. 27, no. 3, pp. 207–219, 2013.

[21] P. M. Kidd, "A review of nutrients and botanicals in the integrative management of cognitive dysfunction," *Alternative Medicine Review*, vol. 4, no. 3, pp. 144–161, 1999.

[22] S. Aguiar and T. Borowski, "Neuropharmacological review of the nootropic herb *Bacopa monnieri*," *Rejuvenation Research*, vol. 16, no. 4, pp. 313–326, 2013.

[23] M. D. Pandareesh and T. Anand, "Neuromodulatory propensity of *Bacopa monniera* against scopolamine-induced cytotoxicity in PC12 cells via down-regulation of AChE and up-regulation of BDNF and muscarnic-1 receptor expression," *Cellular and Molecular Neurobiology*, vol. 33, no. 7, pp. 875–884, 2013.

[24] M. D. Pandareesh and T. Anand, "Neuroprotective and anti-apoptotic propensity of *Bacopa monniera* extract against sodium nitroprusside induced activation of iNOS, heat shock proteins and apoptotic markers in PC12 cells," *Neurochemical Research*, vol. 39, no. 5, pp. 800–814, 2014.

[25] R. Banerjee, S. Hazra, A. K. Ghosh, and A. C. Mondal, "Chronic administration of Bacopa monniera increases BDNF protein and mRNA expressions: a study in chronic unpredictable stress induced animal model of depression," *Psychiatry Investigation*, vol. 11, no. 3, pp. 297–306, 2014.

[26] S. Hazra, S. Kumar, G. K. Saha, and A. C. Mondal, "Reversion of BDNF, Akt and CREB in hippocampus of chronic unpredictable stress induced rats: effects of phytochemical, *Bacopa Monnieri*," *Psychiatry Investigation*, vol. 14, no. 1, pp. 74–80, 2017.

[27] S. Kumar and A. C. Mondal, "Neuroprotective, neurotrophic and anti-oxidative role of *Bacopa monnieri* on CUS induced model of depression in rat," *Neurochemical Research*, vol. 41, no. 11, pp. 3083–3094, 2016.

[28] B. Czeh, E. Fuchs, O. Wiborg, and M. Simon, "Animal models of major depression and their clinical implications," *Progress in Neuro-Psychopharmacology and Biological Psychiatry*, vol. 64, pp. 293–310, 2016.

[29] X. T. Le, H. T. N. Pham, P. T. Do et al., "*Bacopa monnieri* ameliorates memory deficits in olfactory bulbectomized mice: possible involvement of glutamatergic and cholinergic systems," *Neurochemical Research*, vol. 38, no. 10, pp. 2201–2215, 2013.

[30] M. D. Pandareesh, T. Anand, and F. Khanum, "Cognition enhancing and neuromodulatory propensity of *Bacopa monniera* extract against scopolamine induced cognitive impairments in rat hippocampus," *Neurochemical Research*, vol. 41, no. 5, pp. 985–999, 2016.

[31] A. Konar, A. Gautam, and M. K. Thakur, "*Bacopa monniera* (CDRI-08) upregulates the expression of neuronal and glial plasticity markers in the brain of scopolamine induced amnesic mice," *Evidence-based Complementary and Alternative Medicine*, vol. 2015, Article ID 837012, 9 pages, 2015.

[32] J. Preethi, H. K. Singh, and K. E. Rajan, "Possible involvement of standardized *Bacopa monniera* extract (CDRI-08) in epigenetic regulation of *reelin* and brain-derived neurotrophic factor to enhance memory," *Frontiers in Pharmacology*, vol. 7, 2016.

[33] J. Preethi, H. K. Singh, J. S. Venkataraman, and K. E. Rajan, "Standardised extract of *Bacopa monniera* (CDRI-08) improves contextual fear memory by differentially regulating the activity of histone acetylation and protein phosphatases (PP1α, PP2A) in hippocampus," *Cellular and Molecular Neurobiology*, vol. 34, no. 4, pp. 577–589, 2014.

[34] C. Lao-Peregrin, J. J. Ballesteros, M. Fernandez et al., "Caffeine-mediated BDNF release regulates long-term synaptic plasticity through activation of IRS2 signaling," *Addiction Biology*, vol. 22, no. 6, pp. 1706–1718, 2016.

[35] A. Balkowiec and D. M. Katz, "Cellular mechanisms regulating activity-dependent release of native brain-derived neurotrophic factor from hippocampal neurons," *The Journal of Neuroscience*, vol. 22, no. 23, pp. 10399–10407, 2002.

[36] S. Connolly and T. J. Kingsbury, "Caffeine modulates CREB-dependent gene expression in developing cortical neurons," *Biochemical and Biophysical Research Communications*, vol. 397, no. 2, pp. 152–156, 2010.

[37] K. M. Capiotti, F. P. Menezes, L. R. Nazario et al., "Early exposure to caffeine affects gene expression of adenosine receptors, DARPP-32 and BDNF without affecting sensibility and morphology of developing zebrafish (*Danio rerio*)," *Neurotoxicology and Teratology*, vol. 33, no. 6, pp. 680–685, 2011.

[38] A. P. Ardais, A. S. Rocha, M. F. Borges et al., "Caffeine exposure during rat brain development causes memory impairment in a sex selective manner that is offset by caffeine consumption throughout life," *Behavioural Brain Research*, vol. 303, pp. 76–84, 2016.

[39] S. Mioranzza, F. Nunes, D. M. Marques et al., "Prenatal caffeine intake differently affects synaptic proteins during fetal brain development," *International Journal of Developmental Neuroscience*, vol. 36, pp. 45–52, 2014.

[40] A. P. Ardais, M. F. Borges, A. S. Rocha, C. Sallaberry, R. A. Cunha, and L. O. Porciuncula, "Caffeine triggers behavioral and neurochemical alterations in adolescent rats," *Neuroscience*, vol. 270, pp. 27–39, 2014.

[41] C. Sallaberry, F. Nunes, M. S. Costa et al., "Chronic caffeine prevents changes in inhibitory avoidance memory and hippocampal BDNF immunocontent in middle-aged rats," *Neuropharmacology*, vol. 64, pp. 153–159, 2013.

[42] M. S. Costa, P. H. Botton, S. Mioranzza, D. O. Souza, and L. O. Porciuncula, "Caffeine prevents age-associated recognition memory decline and changes brain-derived neurotrophic factor and tirosine kinase receptor (TrkB) content in mice," *Neuroscience*, vol. 153, no. 4, pp. 1071–1078, 2008.

[43] M. S. Costa, P. H. Botton, S. Mioranzza et al., "Caffeine improves adult mice performance in the object recognition task and increases BDNF and TrkB independent on phospho-CREB immunocontent in the hippocampus," *Neurochemistry International*, vol. 53, no. 3-4, pp. 89–94, 2008.

[44] F. M. Ghoneim, H. A. Khalaf, A. Z. Elsamanoudy et al., "Protective effect of chronic caffeine intake on gene expression of brain derived neurotrophic factor signaling and the immunoreactivity of glial fibrillary acidic protein and Ki-67 in Alzheimer's disease," *International Journal Clinical Experimental Pathology*, vol. 8, no. 7, pp. 7710–7728, 2015.

[45] K. Han, N. Jia, J. Li, L. Yang, and L. Q. Min, "Chronic caffeine treatment reverses memory impairment and the expression of brain BNDF and TrkB in the PS1/APP double transgenic mouse model of Alzheimer's disease," *Molecular Medicine Reports*, vol. 8, no. 3, pp. 737–740, 2013.

[46] K. H. Alzoubi, M. Srivareerat, A. M. Aleisa, and K. A. Alkadhi, "Chronic caffeine treatment prevents stress-induced LTP impairment: the critical role of phosphorylated CaMKII and BDNF," *Journal of Molecular Neuroscience*, vol. 49, no. 1, pp. 11–20, 2013.

[47] G. A. Moy and E. C. McNay, "Caffeine prevents weight gain and cognitive impairment caused by a high-fat diet while elevating hippocampal BDNF," *Physiology & Behavior*, vol. 109, pp. 69–74, 2013.

[48] J. S. Samkoff and C. H. M. Jacques, "A review of studies concerning effects of sleep deprivation and fatigue on residents' performance," *Academic Medicine*, vol. 66, no. 11, pp. 687–693, 1991.

[49] S. Sahu, H. Kauser, K. Ray, K. Kishore, S. Kumar, and U. Panjwani, "Caffeine and modafinil promote adult neuronal cell proliferation during 48 h of total sleep deprivation in rat dentate gyrus," *Experimental Neurology*, vol. 248, pp. 470–481, 2013.

[50] I. A. Alhaider, A. M. Aleisa, T. T. Tran, and K. A. Alkadhi, "Caffeine prevents sleep loss-induced deficits in long-term potentiation and related signaling molecules in the dentate gyrus," *European Journal of Neuroscience*, vol. 31, no. 8, pp. 1368–1376, 2010.

[51] K. A. Alkadhi and I. A. Alhaider, "Caffeine and REM sleep deprivation: effect on basal levels of signaling molecules in area CA1," *Molecular and Cellular Neuroscience*, vol. 71, pp. 125–131, 2016.

[52] I. A. Alhaider, A. M. Aleisa, T. T. Tran, and K. A. Alkadhi, "Sleep deprivation prevents stimulation-induced increases of levels of P-CREB and BDNF: protection by caffeine," *Molecular and Cellular Neuroscience*, vol. 46, no. 4, pp. 742–751, 2011.

[53] T. Reyes-Izquierdo, B. Nemzer, C. Shu et al., "Modulatory effect of coffee fruit extract on plasma levels of brain-derived neurotrophic factor in healthy subjects," *British Journal of Nutrition*, vol. 110, no. 03, pp. 420–425, 2013.

[54] M. R. Khazdair, M. H. Boskabady, M. Hosseini, R. Rezaee, and A. M. Tsatsakis, "The effects of *Crocus sativus* (saffron) and its constituents on nervous system: a review," *Avicenna Journal of Phytomedicine*, vol. 5, no. 5, pp. 376–391, 2015.

[55] F. V. Hassani, V. Naseri, B. M. Razavi, S. Mehri, K. Abnous, and H. Hosseinzadeh, "Antidepressant effects of crocin and its effects on transcript and protein levels of CREB, BDNF, and VGF in rat hippocampus," *Daru Journal of Pharmaceutical Sciences*, vol. 22, no. 1, p. 16, 2014.

[56] T. Ghasemi, K. Abnous, F. Vahdati, S. Mehri, B. M. Razavi, and H. Hosseinzadeh, "Antidepressant effect of *Crocus sativus* aqueous extract and its effect on CREB, BDNF, and

VGF transcript and protein levels in rat hippocampus," *Drug Research*, vol. 65, no. 07, pp. 337–343, 2015.

[57] *ESCOP Monographs*, Georg Thieme Verlag, Stuttgart, Germany, 2nd edition, 2009.

[58] F. Wu, H. Li, L. Zhao et al., "Protective effects of aqueous extract from *Acanthopanax senticosus* against corticosterone-induced neurotoxicity in PC12 cells," *Journal of Ethnopharmacology*, vol. 148, no. 3, pp. 861–868, 2013.

[59] Y. Xu, C. Cui, C. Pang, Y. Christen, and Y. Luo, "Restoration of impaired phosphorylation of cyclic AMP response element-binding protein (CREB) by EGb 761 and its constituents in Aβ-expressing neuroblastoma cells," *European Journal of Neuroscience*, vol. 26, no. 10, pp. 2931–2939, 2007.

[60] Y. Hou, M. A. Aboukhatwa, D. L. Lei, K. Manaye, I. Khan, and Y. Luo, "Anti-depressant natural flavonols modulate BDNF and beta amyloid in neurons and hippocampus of double TgAD mice," *Neuropharmacology*, vol. 58, no. 6, pp. 911–920, 2010.

[61] Y. Nam, E. J. Shin, S. W. Shin et al., "YY162 prevents ADHD-like behavioral side effects and cytotoxicity induced by Aroclor1254 via interactive signaling between antioxidant potential, BDNF/TrkB, DAT and NET," *Food and Chemical Toxicology*, vol. 65, pp. 280–292, 2014.

[62] Z. Zhang, D. Peng, H. Zhu, and X. Wang, "Experimental evidence of Ginkgo biloba extract EGB as a neuroprotective agent in ischemia stroke rats," *Brain Research Bulletin*, vol. 87, no. 2-3, pp. 193–198, 2012.

[63] M. Belviranli and N. Okudan, "The effects of *Ginkgo biloba* extract on cognitive functions in aged female rats: the role of oxidative stress and brain-derived neurotrophic factor," *Behavioral Brain Research*, vol. 278, pp. 453–461, 2015.

[64] Y. Zhao, Y. Zhang, and F. Pan, "The effects of EGb761 on lipopolysaccharide-induced depressive-like behaviour in C57BL/6J mice," *Central European Journal of Immunology*, vol. 1, no. 1, pp. 11–17, 2015.

[65] J. Shi, Y. L. Tan, Z. R. Wang et al., "*Ginkgo biloba* and vitamin E ameliorate haloperidol-induced vacuous chewingmovement and brain-derived neurotrophic factor expression in a rat tardive dyskinesia model," *Pharmacology Biochemistry and Behavior*, vol. 148, pp. 53–58, 2016.

[66] X. S. Qin, K. H. Jin, B. K. Ding, S. F. Xie, and H. Ma, "Effects of extract of *Ginkgo biloba* with venlafaxine on brain injury in a rat model of depression," *Chinese Medical Journal*, vol. 118, no. 5, pp. 391–397, 2005.

[67] F. Tchantchou, P. N. Lacor, Z. Cao et al., "Stimulation of neurogenesis and synaptogenesis by bilobalide and quercetin via common final pathway in hippocampal neurons," *Journal of Alzheimer's Disease*, vol. 18, no. 4, pp. 787–798, 2009.

[68] X. Y. Zhang, W. F. Zhang, D. F. Zhou et al., "Brain-derived neurotrophic factor levels and its Val66Met gene polymorphism predict tardive dyskinesia treatment response to Ginkgo biloba," *Biological Psychiatry*, vol. 72, no. 8, pp. 700–706, 2012.

[69] C. Di Lorenzo, M. Dell'Agli, E. Sangiovanni et al., "Correlation between catechin content and NF-κB inhibition by infusions of green and black tea," *Plant Foods Human Nutrition*, vol. 68, no. 2, pp. 149–154, 2013.

[70] H. S. Cho, S. Kim, S. Y. Lee, J. A. Park, S. J. Kim, and H. S. Chun, "Protective effect of the green tea component,

[71] S. Nath, M. Bachani, D. Harshavardhana, and J. P. Steiner, "Catechins protect neurons against mitochondrial toxins and HIV proteins via activation of the BDNF pathway," *Journal of Neurovirology*, vol. 18, no. 6, pp. 445–455, 2012.

[72] C. Wakabayashi, T. Numakawa, M. Ninomiya, S. Chiba, and H. Kunugi, "Behavioral and molecular evidence for psychotropic effects in L-theanine," *Psychopharmacology*, vol. 219, no. 4, pp. 1099–1109, 2012.

[73] T. P. Stringer, D. Guerrieri, C. Vivar, and H. van Praag, "Plant-derived flavanol (−)epicatechin mitigates anxiety in association with elevated hippocampal monoamine and BDNF levels, but does not influence pattern separation in mice," *Translational Psychiatry*, vol. 5, no. 1, article e493, 2015.

[74] A. Takeda, K. Sakamoto, H. Tamano et al., "Facilitated neurogenesis in the developing hippocampus after intake of theanine, an amino acid in tea leaves, and object recognition memory," *Cellular and Molecular Neurobiology*, vol. 31, no. 7, pp. 1079–1088, 2011.

[75] M. Assuncao, M. J. Santos-Marques, F. Carvalho, and J. P. Andrade, "Green tea averts age-dependent decline of hippocampal signaling systems related to antioxidant defenses and survival," *Free Radical Biology & Medicine*, vol. 48, no. 6, pp. 831–838, 2010.

[76] Q. Li, H. F. Zhao, Z. F. Zhang et al., "Long-term administration of green tea catechins prevents age-related spatial learning and memory decline in C57BL/6 J mice by regulating hippocampal cyclic amp-response element binding protein signaling cascade," *Neuroscience*, vol. 159, no. 4, pp. 1208–1215, 2009.

[77] T. E. Gibbons, B. D. Pence, G. Petr et al., "Voluntary wheel running, but not a diet containing (−)-epigallocatechin-3-gallate and β-alanine, improves learning, memory and hippocampal neurogenesis in aged mice," *Behavioural Brain Research*, vol. 272, pp. 131–140, 2014.

[78] F. Guedj, C. Sebrie, I. Rivals et al., "Green tea polyphenols rescue of brain defects induced by overexpression of *DYRK1A*," *PLoS One*, vol. 4, no. 2, 2009.

[79] Q. Li, H. F. Zhao, Z. F. Zhang et al., "Long-term green tea catechin administration prevents spatial learning and memory impairment in senescence-accelerated mouse prone-8 mice by decreasing a β_{1-42} oligomers and upregulating synaptic plasticity-related proteins in the hippocampus," *Neuroscience*, vol. 163, no. 3, pp. 741–749, 2009.

[80] Z. Y. Zhang, H. Wu, and H. C. Huang, "Epicatechin plus treadmill exercise are neuroprotective against moderate-stage amyloid precursor protein/presenilin 1 mice," *Pharmacognosy Magazine*, vol. 12, no. 46, pp. 139–146, 2016.

[81] Y. H. Yu, Y. Z. Wu, A. Szabo et al., "Teasaponin improves leptin sensitivity in the prefrontal cortex of obese mice," *Molecular Nutrition & Food Research*, vol. 59, no. 12, pp. 2371–2382, 2015.

[82] S. S. Patel, N. Mahindroo, and M. Udayabanu, "*Urtica dioica* leaves modulates hippocampal smoothened-glioma associated oncogene-1 pathway and cognitive dysfunction in chronically stressed mice," *Biomedicine & Pharmacotherapy*, vol. 83, pp. 676–686, 2016.

[83] V. Butterweck, H. Winterhoff, and M. Herkenham, "St John's wort, hypericin, and imipramine: a comparative analysis of mRNA levels in brain areas involved in HPA axis control following short-term and long-term administration in normal

and stressed rats," *Molecular Psychiatry*, vol. 6, no. 5, pp. 547–564, 2001.

[84] M. L. Molendijk, B. A. A. Bus, P. Spinhoven et al., "Serum levels of brain-derived neurotrophic factor in major depressive disorder: state-trait issues, clinical features and pharmacological treatment," *Molecular Psychiatry*, vol. 16, no. 11, pp. 1088–1095, 2011.

[85] M. Dell'agli and E. Bosisio, "Minor polar compounds of olive oil: composition, factors of variability and bioactivity," *Studies in Natural Products Chemistry*, vol. 27, pp. 697–734, 2002.

[86] E. Muto, M. Dell'Agli, E. Sangiovanni et al., "Olive oil phenolic extract regulates interleukin-8 expression by transcriptional and posttranscriptional mechanisms in Caco-2 cells," *Molecular Nutrition & Food Research*, vol. 59, no. 6, pp. 1217–1221, 2015.

[87] S. De Nicolo, L. Tarani, M. Ceccanti et al., "Effects of olive polyphenols administration on nerve growth factor and brain-derived neurotrophic factor in the mouse brain," *Nutrition*, vol. 29, no. 4, pp. 681–687, 2013.

[88] V. Carito, A. Venditti, A. Bianco et al., "Effects of olive leaf polyphenols on male mouse brain NGF, BDNF and their receptors TrkA, TrkB and p75," *Natural Product Research*, vol. 28, no. 22, pp. 1970–1984, 2014.

[89] C. S. Pase, A. M. Teixeira, K. Roversi et al., "Olive oil-enriched diet reduces brain oxidative damages and ameliorates neurotrophic factor gene expression in different life stages of rats," *The Journal of Nutritional Biochemistry*, vol. 26, no. 11, pp. 1200–1207, 2015.

[90] A. Zheng, H. Li, K. Cao et al., "Maternal hydroxytyrosol administration improves neurogenesis and cognitive function in prenatally stressed offspring," *The Journal of Nutritional Biochemistry*, vol. 26, no. 2, pp. 190–199, 2015.

[91] M. Arunsundar, T. S. Shanmugarajan, and V. Ravichandran, "3,4-Dihydroxyphenylethanol attenuates spatio-cognitive deficits in an Alzheimer's disease mouse model: modulation of the molecular signals in neuronal survival-apoptotic programs," *Neurotoxicity Research*, vol. 27, no. 2, pp. 143–155, 2015.

[92] A. Sanchez-Villegas, C. Galbete, M. A. Martinez-Gonzalez et al., "The effect of the Mediterranean diet on plasma brain-derived neurotrophic factor (BDNF) levels: the PREDIMED-NAVARRA randomized trial," *Nutritional Neuroscience*, vol. 14, no. 5, pp. 195–201, 2011.

[93] M. Ceccanti, V. Carito, M. Vitali et al., "Serum BDNF and NGF modulation by olive polyphenols in alcoholics during withdrawal," *Journal of Alcoholism & Drug Dependence*, vol. 3, no. 4, pp. 214–219, 2015.

[94] Z. F. Lu, Y. X. Shen, P. Zhang et al., "Ginsenoside Rg1 promotes proliferation and neurotrophin expression of olfactory ensheathing cells," *Journal of Asian Natural Products Research*, vol. 12, no. 4, pp. 265–272, 2010.

[95] J. Ma, J. Liu, Q. Wang, H. Yu, Y. Chen, and L. Xiang, "The beneficial effect of ginsenoside Rg1 on Schwann cells subjected to hydrogen peroxide induced oxidative injury," *International Journal of Biological Sciences*, vol. 9, no. 6, pp. 624–636, 2013.

[96] X. Li, M. Li, Y. Li, Q. Quan, and J. Wang, "Cellular and molecular mechanisms underlying the action of ginsenoside Rg1 against Alzheimer's disease," *Neural Regeneration Research*, vol. 7, no. 36, pp. 2860–2866, 2012.

[97] J. Y. Han, S. Y. Ahn, E. H. Oh et al., "Red ginseng extract attenuates kainate-induced excitotoxicity by antioxidative effects," *Evidence-based Complementary and Alternative Medicine*, vol. 2012, Article ID 479016, 10 pages, 2012.

[98] X. Y. Liu, X. Y. Zhou, J. C. Hou et al., "Ginsenoside Rd promotes neurogenesis in rat brain after transient focal cerebral ischemia via activation of PI3K/Akt pathway," *Acta Pharmacologica Sinica*, vol. 36, no. 4, pp. 421–428, 2015.

[99] H. Dang, Y. Chen, X. Liu et al., "Antidepressant effects of ginseng total saponins in the forced swimming test and chronic mild stress models of depression," *Progress in Neuro-Psychopharmacology and Biological Psychiatry*, vol. 33, no. 8, pp. 1417–1424, 2009.

[100] B. Jiang, Z. Xiong, J. Yang et al., "Antidepressant-like effects of ginsenoside Rg1 are due to activation of the BDNF signalling pathway and neurogenesis in the hippocampus," *British Journal of Pharmacology*, vol. 166, no. 6, pp. 1872–1887, 2012.

[101] J. Cui, L. Jiang, and H. Xiang, "Ginsenoside Rb3 exerts antidepressant-like effects in several animal models," *Journal of Psychopharmacology*, vol. 26, no. 5, pp. 697–713, 2012.

[102] X. Zhu, R. Gao, Z. Liu et al., "Ginsenoside Rg1 reverses stress-induced depression-like behaviours and brain-derived neurotrophic factor expression within the prefrontal cortex," *European Journal of Neuroscience*, vol. 44, no. 2, pp. 1878–1885, 2016.

[103] Z. Liu, Y. Qi, Z. Cheng, X. Zhu, C. Fan, and S. Y. Yu, "The effects of ginsenoside Rg1 on chronic stress induced depression-like behaviors, BDNF expression and the phosphorylation of PKA and CREB in rats," *Neuroscience*, vol. 322, pp. 358–369, 2016.

[104] B. Lee, B. Sur, S. G. Cho et al., "Ginsenoside Rb1 rescues anxiety-like responses in a rat model of post-traumatic stress disorder," *Journal of Natural Medicines*, vol. 70, no. 2, pp. 133–144, 2016.

[105] L. Chen, J. Dai, Z. Wang, H. Zhang, Y. Huang, and Y. Zhao, "Ginseng total saponins reverse corticosterone-induced changes in depression-like behavior and hippocampal plasticity-related proteins by interfering with GSK-3β-CREB signaling pathway," *Evidence-based Complementary and Alternative Medicine*, vol. 2014, Article ID 506735, 11 pages, 2014.

[106] B. Lee, I. Shim, H. Lee, and D. H. Hahm, "Effect of ginsenoside Re on depression- and anxiety-like behaviors and cognition memory deficit induced by repeated immobilization in rats," *Journal of Microbiology and Biotechnology*, vol. 22, no. 5, pp. 708–720, 2012.

[107] W. Kezhu, X. Pan, L. Cong et al., "Effects of ginsenoside Rg1 on learning and memory in a reward-directed instrumental conditioning task in chronic restraint stressed rats," *Phytotherapy Research*, vol. 31, no. 1, pp. 81–89, 2016.

[108] M. Kim, S. O. Kim, M. Lee et al., "Effects of ginsenoside Rb1 on the stress-induced changes of BDNF and HSP70 expression in rat hippocampus," *Environmental Toxicology and Pharmacology*, vol. 38, no. 1, pp. 257–262, 2014.

[109] B. Lee, J. Park, S. Kwon et al., "Effect of wild ginseng on scopolamine-induced acetylcholine depletion in the rat hippocampus," *Journal of Pharmacy and Pharmacology*, vol. 62, no. 2, pp. 263–271, 2010.

[110] E. J. Kim, I. H. Jung, T. K. Van Le, J. J. Jeong, N. J. Kim, and D. H. Kim, "Ginsenosides Rg5 and Rh3 protect scopolamine-

induced memory deficits in mice," *Journal of Ethnopharmacology*, vol. 146, no. 1, pp. 294–299, 2013.

[111] S. Chu, J. Gu, L. Feng et al., "Ginsenoside Rg5 improves cognitive dysfunction and beta-amyloid deposition in STZ-induced memory impaired rats via attenuating neuroinflammatory responses," *International Immunopharmacology*, vol. 19, no. 2, pp. 317–326, 2014.

[112] D. Zhu, M. Liu, Y. Yang et al., "Ginsenoside Rd ameliorates experimental autoimmune encephalomyelitis in C57BL/6 mice," *Journal of Neuroscience Research*, vol. 92, no. 9, pp. 1217–1226, 2014.

[113] Y. Q. Shi, T. W. Huang, L. M. Chen et al., "Ginsenoside Rg1 attenuates amyloid-β content, regulates PKA/CREB activity, and improves cognitive performance in SAMP8 mice," *Journal of Alzheimer's Disease*, vol. 19, no. 3, pp. 977–989, 2010.

[114] G. Zhu, Y. Wang, J. Li, and J. Wang, "Chronic treatment with ginsenoside Rg1 promotes memory and hippocampal long-term potentiation in middle-aged mice," *Neuroscience*, vol. 292, pp. 81–89, 2015.

[115] F. Li, X. Wu, J. Li, and Q. Niu, "Ginsenoside Rg1 ameliorates hippocampal long-term potentiation and memory in an Alzheimer's disease model," *Molecular Medicine Reports*, vol. 13, no. 6, pp. 4904–4910, 2016.

[116] X. Q. Gao, C. X. Yang, G. J. Chen et al., "Ginsenoside Rb1 regulates the expressions of brain-derived neurotrophic factor and caspase-3 and induces neurogenesis in rats with experimental cerebral ischemia," *Journal of Ethnopharmacology*, vol. 132, no. 2, pp. 393–399, 2010.

[117] Z. Jiang, Y. Wang, X. Zhang et al., "Preventive and therapeutic effects of ginsenoside Rb1 for neural injury during cerebral infarction in rats," *The American Journal of Chinese Medicine*, vol. 41, no. 02, pp. 341–352, 2013.

[118] Q. Wan, X. Ma, Z. J. Zhang et al., "Ginsenoside reduces cognitive impairment during chronic cerebral hypoperfusion through brain-derived neurotrophic factor regulated by epigenetic modulation," *Molecular Neurobiology*, vol. 54, no. 4, pp. 2889–2900, 2016.

[119] X. Zheng, Y. Liang, A. Kang et al., "Peripheral immunomodulation with ginsenoside Rg1 ameliorates neuroinflammation-induced behavioral deficits in rats," *Neuroscience*, vol. 256, pp. 210–222, 2014.

[120] K. N. Salim, B. S. McEwen, and H. M. Chao, "Ginsenoside Rb1 regulates ChAT, NGF and trkA mRNA expression in the rat brain," *Molecular Brain Research*, vol. 47, no. 1-2, pp. 177–182, 1997.

[121] J. Hou, J. Xue, M. Lee, J. Yu, and C. Sung, "Long-term administration of ginsenoside Rh1 enhances learning and memory by promoting cell survival in the mouse hippocampus," *International Journal of Molecular Medicine*, vol. 33, no. 1, pp. 234–240, 2014.

[122] S. Kim, M. S. Kim, K. Park et al., "Hippocampus-dependent cognitive enhancement induced by systemic gintonin administration," *Journal of Ginseng Research*, vol. 40, no. 1, pp. 55–61, 2016.

[123] L. T. Yi, J. Li, D. Geng et al., "Essential oil of *Perilla frutescens*-induced change in hippocampal expression of brain-derived neurotrophic factor in chronic unpredictable mild stress in mice," *Journal of Ethnopharmacology*, vol. 147, no. 1, pp. 245–253, 2013.

[124] D. Miyazawa, Y. Yasui, K. Yamada, N. Ohara, and H. Okuyama, "Biochemical responses to dietary α-linolenic acid restriction proceed differently among brain regions in mice," *Biomedical Research*, vol. 32, no. 4, pp. 237–245, 2011.

[125] D. Miyazawa, Y. Yasui, K. Yamada, N. Ohara, and H. Okuyama, "Regional differences of the mouse brain in response to an α-linolenic acid-restricted diet: neurotrophin content and protein kinase activity," *Life Sciences*, vol. 87, no. 15-16, pp. 490–494, 2010.

[126] H. C. Lee, H. K. Ko, B. E. Huang, Y. H. Chu, and S. Y. Huang, "Antidepressant-like effects of *Perilla frutescens* seed oil during a forced swimming test," *Food & Function*, vol. 5, no. 5, pp. 990–996, 2014.

[127] A. Y. Lee, J. M. Choi, J. Lee, M. H. Lee, S. Lee, and E. J. Cho, "Effects of vegetable oils with different fatty acid compositions on cognition and memory ability in $A\beta_{25-35}$-induced Alzheimer's disease mouse model," *Journal of Medicinal Food*, vol. 19, no. 10, pp. 912–921, 2016.

[128] A. Panossian, G. Wikman, and J. Sarris, "Rosenroot (*Rhodiola rosea*): traditional use, chemical composition, pharmacology and clinical efficacy," *Phytomedicine*, vol. 17, no. 7, pp. 481–493, 2010.

[129] H. B. Zhao, H. Ma, X. Q. Ha et al., "Salidroside induces rat mesenchymal stem cells to differentiate into dopaminergic neurons," *Cell Biology International*, vol. 38, no. 4, pp. 462–471, 2014.

[130] L. P. Zhu, T. T. Wei, J. Gao et al., "Salidroside attenuates lipopolysaccharide (LPS) induced serum cytokines and depressive-like behavior in mice," *Neuroscience Letters*, vol. 606, pp. 1–6, 2015.

[131] L. Bonaccini, A. Karioti, M. C. Bergonzi, and A. R. Bilia, "Effects of *Salvia miltiorrhiza* on CNS neuronal injury and degeneration: a plausible complementary role of Tanshinones and Depsides," *Planta Medica*, vol. 81, no. 12-13, pp. 1003–1016, 2015.

[132] N. Zhang, T. Kang, Y. Xia et al., "Effects of salvianolic acid B on survival, self-renewal and neuronal differentiation of bone marrow derived neural stem cells," *European Journal of Pharmacology*, vol. 697, no. 1–3, pp. 32–39, 2012.

[133] Y. Wang, J. Zhang, M. Han et al., "SMND-309 promotes neuron survival through the activation of the PI3K/Akt/CREB-signalling pathway," *Pharmaceutical Biology*, vol. 54, no. 10, pp. 1982–1990, 2016.

[134] Y. W. Lee, D. H. Kim, S. J. Jeon et al., "Neuroprotective effects of salvianolic acid B on an $A\beta_{25-35}$ peptide-induced mouse model of Alzheimer's disease," *European Journal of Pharmacology*, vol. 704, no. 1–3, pp. 70–77, 2013.

[135] Y. Teng, M. Q. Zhang, W. Wang et al., "Compound danshen tablet ameliorated $a\beta_{25-35}$-induced spatial memory impairment in mice via rescuing imbalance between cytokines and neurotrophins," *BMC Complementary and Alternative Medicine*, vol. 14, no. 1, p. 23, 2014.

[136] J. H. Park, O. K. Park, B. Yan et al., "Neuroprotection via maintenance or increase of antioxidants and neurotrophic factors in ischemic gerbil hippocampus treated with tanshinone I," *Chinese Medical Journal*, vol. 127, no. 19, pp. 3396–3405, 2014.

[137] M. Y. Chien, C. H. Chuang, C. M. Chern et al., "Salvianolic acid A alleviates ischemic brain injury through the inhibition of inflammation and apoptosis and the promotion of neurogenesis in mice," *Free Radical Biology & Medicine*, vol. 99, pp. 508–519, 2016.

[138] Q. He, S. Wang, X. Liu et al., "Salvianolate lyophilized injection promotes post-stroke functional recovery via the activation of VEGF and BDNF-TrkB-CREB signaling pathway," *International Journal of Clinical Experimental Medicine*, vol. 8, no. 1, pp. 108–122, 2015.

[139] F. Allam, A. T. Dao, G. Chugh et al., "Grape powder supplementation prevents oxidative stress-induced anxiety-like behavior, memory impairment, and high blood pressure in rats," *The Journal of Nutrition*, vol. 143, no. 6, pp. 835–842, 2013.

[140] N. Solanki, I. Alkadhi, F. Atrooz, G. Patki, and S. Salim, "Grape powder prevents cognitive, behavioral, and biochemical impairments in a rat model of posttraumatic stress disorder," *Nutrition Research*, vol. 35, no. 1, pp. 65–75, 2015.

[141] M. Fiore, G. Laviola, L. Aloe, V. di Fausto, R. Mancinelli, and M. Ceccanti, "Early exposure to ethanol but not red wine at the same alcohol concentration induces behavioral and brain neurotrophin alterations in young and adult mice," *Neurotoxicology*, vol. 30, no. 1, pp. 59–71, 2009.

[142] M. Ceccanti, R. Mancinelli, P. Tirassa et al., "Early exposure to ethanol or red wine and long-lasting effects in aged mice. A study on nerve growth factor, brain-derived neurotrophic factor, hepatocyte growth factor, and vascular endothelial growth factor," *Neurobiology of Aging*, vol. 33, no. 2, pp. 359–367, 2012.

[143] N. J. Dar, A. Hamid, and M. Ahmad, "Pharmacologic overview of *Withania somnifera*, the Indian ginseng," *Cellular and Molecular Life Sciences*, vol. 72, no. 23, pp. 4445–4460, 2015.

[144] A. Konar, N. Shah, R. Singh et al., "Protective role of Ashwagandha leaf extract and its component withanone on scopolamine-induced changes in the brain and brain-derived cells," *PLoS One*, vol. 6, no. 11, article e27265, 2011.

[145] I. Baitharu, V. Jain, S. N. Deep et al., "*Withania somnifera* root extract ameliorates hypobaric hypoxia induced memory impairment in rats," *Journal of Ethnopharmacology*, vol. 145, no. 2, pp. 431–441, 2013.

6

Laterality of Poststroke Cortical Motor Activity during Action Observation is Related to Hemispheric Dominance

Sook-Lei Liew ⓘ,[1] Kathleen A. Garrison,[2] Kaori L. Ito ⓘ,[1] Panthea Heydari,[1]
Mona Sobhani ⓘ,[1] Julie Werner ⓘ,[3,4] Hanna Damasio,[1] Carolee J. Winstein,[1]
and Lisa Aziz-Zadeh[1]

[1]*University of Southern California, Los Angeles, CA, USA*
[2]*Yale University, New Haven, CT, USA*
[3]*California State University, Dominguez Hills, Carson, CA, USA*
[4]*Children's Hospital Los Angeles, Los Angeles, CA, USA*

Correspondence should be addressed to Sook-Lei Liew; sliew@usc.edu

Academic Editor: Toshiyuki Fujiwara

Background. Increased activity in the lesioned hemisphere has been related to improved poststroke motor recovery. However, the role of the dominant hemisphere—and its relationship to activity in the lesioned hemisphere—has not been widely explored. *Objective.* Here, we examined whether the dominant hemisphere drives the lateralization of brain activity after stroke and whether this changes based on if the lesioned hemisphere is the dominant hemisphere or not. *Methods.* We used fMRI to compare cortical motor activity in the action observation network (AON), motor-related regions that are active both during the observation and execution of an action, in 36 left hemisphere dominant individuals. Twelve individuals had nondominant, right hemisphere stroke, twelve had dominant, left-hemisphere stroke, and twelve were healthy age-matched controls. We previously found that individuals with left dominant stroke show greater ipsilesional activity during action observation. Here, we examined if individuals with nondominant, right hemisphere stroke also showed greater lateralized activity in the ipsilesional, right hemisphere or in the dominant, left hemisphere and compared these results with those of individuals with dominant, left hemisphere stroke. *Results.* We found that individuals with right hemisphere stroke showed greater activity in the dominant, left hemisphere, rather than the ipsilesional, right hemisphere. This left-lateralized pattern matched that of individuals with left, dominant hemisphere stroke, and both stroke groups differed from the age-matched control group. *Conclusions.* These findings suggest that action observation is lateralized to the dominant, rather than ipsilesional, hemisphere, which may reflect an interaction between the lesioned hemisphere and the dominant hemisphere in driving lateralization of brain activity after stroke. Hemispheric dominance and laterality should be carefully considered when characterizing poststroke neural activity.

1. Introduction

Despite intensive research and clinical efforts, stroke remains a leading cause of physical disability worldwide [1], and there is an urgent need for improved poststroke rehabilitation strategies. Many studies have suggested that increased levels of activity in the ipsilesional hemisphere after stroke are associated with enhanced recovery [2–4]. Functional magnetic resonance imaging (fMRI) studies in individuals with stroke suggest that greater blood oxygen level-dependent (BOLD) activity in the contralateral (ipsilesional) hemisphere during a task with the impaired upper limb—a pattern consistent with typical motor control—is associated with better motor outcomes [4–6]. Poststroke therapeutic techniques have therefore aimed at promoting motor recovery by increasing activity in the ipsilesional hemisphere and decreasing activity in the contralesional hemisphere [7–10]. However, poststroke motor outcomes using such approaches remain variable, suggesting that other factors influence recovery beyond the level of brain activity in the ipsilesional hemisphere.

One factor that has been largely overlooked in stroke studies is the role of motor dominance relative to the lesioned hemisphere. Studies often discuss findings related to the ipsilesional or contralesional hemisphere, without distinguishing whether the ipsilesional hemisphere is the dominant or nondominant hemisphere prior to stroke. However, whether stroke occurs in the dominant or nondominant hemisphere can impact recovery in multiple ways, including impacting the pattern of brain activity achieved in poststroke therapy [11–13]. Research has shown clear hemispheric differences in the specialization of motor control, with differences in the performance of motor actions after stroke related to the lesioned hemisphere. Winstein and Pohl (1995) reported that individuals with left hemisphere stroke showed deficits in open-loop, motor planning aspects of movement, whereas individuals with right hemisphere stroke showed deficits in closed-loop, feedback-based aspects of movement [14]. Another study showed that in an arm-reaching task, individuals with left hemisphere stroke had difficulty controlling the direction of movement, whereas individuals with right hemisphere stroke had a tendency to overshoot their targets [11]. These studies and others suggest that there is hemispheric specialization in a distributed motor control scheme, where the left hemisphere is responsible for optimizing and predicting dynamic aspects of movement, and the right hemisphere is responsible for movement accuracy and stability [15]. There are thus likely differences in task-related brain activity depending on the dominance of the lesioned hemisphere. Better understanding the relationship between motor dominance, hemisphere of stroke, and brain activity is critical because it could enable greater personalization of interventions in stroke neurorehabilitation and allow us to better understand the neural mechanisms underlying deficits following stroke.

Here, we hypothesized that the motor dominant hemisphere might in fact drive poststroke brain activity during action observation more strongly than the side of the stroke lesion. We specifically evaluated brain activity in the action observation network (AON), as it is a brain network typically engaged through both the observation and performance of actions and is comprised of cortical motor regions in the premotor and parietal cortices [16]. Importantly, activity in the AON can be elicited simply through action observation, so even individuals with moderate to severe upper arm paresis can complete the task. Action observation therapy (AOT), in which individuals with stroke observe another person performing actions (e.g., through videos) before or during actual physical practice of those actions, has been proposed as a way to enhance the effects of occupational or physical therapy [17–20]. Behavioral studies examining outcomes of AOT with occupational or physical therapy show modest improvements in poststroke motor recovery when compared to traditional therapy alone [17–19, 21, 22]. Researchers hypothesize that action observation may enhance plasticity in the same motor pathways responsible for action execution [23]. The AON has also been shown to be active during action

observation in individuals after stroke [24]. In particular, activity in the AON was found to be lateralized to the ipsilesional, dominant hemisphere in individuals with motor dominant, left hemisphere stroke who observed actions being performed by the counterpart to their own paretic right arm [24]. However, since the left hemisphere was both the ipsilesional and motor dominant hemisphere, it was not possible to distinguish whether action observation drives activity in the ipsilesional hemisphere or in the motor dominant hemisphere.

The present study was designed with a primary aim of improving our understanding of the effects of motor dominance versus side of lesion on AON activity in individuals after stroke. We recruited individuals who were left hemisphere dominant (right handed) prior to stroke and had nondominant, right hemisphere stroke. Using the same fMRI protocol as in the earlier AON stroke study [24], we tested whether individuals with nondominant right hemisphere stroke had greater AON activity during action observation in the ipsilesional (right) hemisphere or in the dominant (left) hemisphere. We compared these data to the dominant left hemisphere stroke group and an age-matched control group from the earlier study [24]. We predicted that if action observation drives activity in the ipsilesional hemisphere, the right hemisphere stroke group should show greater activity in the right hemisphere, whereas if action observation drives activity in the motor dominant hemisphere, the right hemisphere stroke group should show greater activity in the left hemisphere.

2. Methods

2.1. Subjects. The current analysis included 36 individuals who were right-handed (left hemisphere motor dominant) as determined by the Edinburgh Handedness Inventory [25]. There were 24 participants with chronic stroke and moderate-to-severe upper extremity motor impairments and 12 nondisabled, age-matched controls. Both the nondisabled controls and 12 individuals with dominant left hemisphere stroke were included in an earlier study [24]. In the current study, 12 additional individuals with nondominant right hemisphere stroke were recruited from community centers. All participants gave informed consent in accordance with institutional guidelines approved by the University of Southern California Institutional Review Board. All individuals were right handed (prior to stroke), had normal or corrected-to-normal vision, and were safe for MRI. Additional inclusion criteria for individuals with stroke was chronic (>3 months since stroke onset), middle cerebral artery stroke, with no prior history of stroke, moderate-to-severe upper extremity impairment as determined by a phone screening form in which participants indicated difficulty moving their hand or arm for functional tasks, and no apraxia. For all participants, mean age (including nondisabled controls) was 63 ± 13 years and did not differ between groups ($F(2, 33) = 0.94$, $p = 0.40$). For participants with stroke, average time since stroke was 80 ± 58 months and did not differ between right and left

TABLE 1: Demographics of participants. Fugl-Meyer Assessment, Upper Extremity (FMA-UE; out of 66 points) and Wolf Motor Function Test (WMFT; out of 5 points). Stroke location was characterized as either internal capsule only (IC) or internal capsule plus cerebral cortex (C + IC). "−" indicates missing values.

Subject number	FMA-UE	WMFT	Age (years)	Sex	Time since stroke (months)	Location
			Right hemisphere stroke			
1	5	1	66	F	80	IC
2	17	1	65	F	22	IC
3	10	1	70	M	202	C + IC
4	8	1	59	F	46	C + IC
5	14	—	79	M	168	C + IC
6	16	2	56	F	6	IC
7	18	1.5	52	M	67	IC
8	31	1	33	M	10	C + IC
9	5	0	61	M	118	C + IC
10	31	3.25	71	M	74	IC
11	5	0	65	M	48	IC
12	18	1.25	35	F	21	IC
Mean	**14.83**	**1.18**	**59.33**	5 F	**71.83**	**7 IC**
SDEV	9.09	0.90	13.81		62.43	
			Left hemisphere stroke			
1	48	3.33	64	F	60	IC
2	13	0.5	64	F	180	C + IC
3	46	3.25	55	M	48	IC
4	18	2	74	M	204	IC
5	40	2	39	M	24	IC
6	13	0.67	73	M	48	IC
7	31	2.5	85	F	96	IC
8	14	0.25	51	F	72	C + IC
9	47	3.33	74	F	108	C + IC
10	15	0.75	68	F	72	C + IC
11	37	2.5	71	M	96	C + IC
12	35	4	71	M	48	C + IC
Mean	**29.75**	**2.09**	**65.75**	6 F	**88.00**	**6 IC**
SDEV	14.29	1.28	12.34		54.47	

hemisphere stroke groups ($t(22) = -0.17$, $p = 0.61$). Stroke characteristics are described in Table 1.

2.2. fMRI Data Acquisition. All scanning was completed on the same 3T Siemens Trio MRI scanner at the University of Southern California Dornsife Neuroimaging Center, using the scan parameters and task as described in Garrison et al. [24]. Functional images were acquired with a T2*-weighted gradient echo sequence (repetition time [TR]/echo time [TE] = 2000/30 ms, 37 slices, voxel size 3.5 mm isotropic voxels, and flip angle 90°); anatomical images were acquired with a T1-weighted magnetization-prepared rapid gradient-echo (MPRAGE) sequence (TR/TE = 2350/3.09 ms, 208 1 mm slices, 256 × 256 mm, and flip angle 10°).

The fMRI paradigm was a block design in which participants either observed either videos of right hand actions, videos of left hand actions, and images of a still hand (control condition) or rested. For the action

observation conditions, videos depicted a mean-age-matched nondisabled control actor grasp objects with either their right hand or their left hand, as previously described [24]. Actions were adapted from the Wolf Motor Function Test (WMFT, Wolf et al. [26]) and included (1) pick up pencil, (2) pick up paperclip, (3) stack checkers, and (4) flip cards (see Supplementary Figure S1 for an example). Each video was 3 s long, and each block consisted of four videos shown in a randomized order for a total block length of 12 s. The control condition (observation of a still hand) was also presented in 12 s blocks with 4 still images of either a left or a right hand shown for 3 s each in a randomized order. All blocks were repeated 15 times and randomized across three 6-minute runs.

Participants were instructed to remain still and watch the actions of the actor as they would be asked to imitate each action after the scanning session. To ensure attention, participants were asked questions about the videos at the end of each run (e.g., "In the last video you saw, which hand did the actor use?").

2.3. fMRI Analysis

2.3.1. Preprocessing and Analyses. Functional neuroimaging data analysis was carried out using FEAT (FMRI Expert Analysis Tool) Version 6, part of FSL (FMRIB's Software Library, http://www.fmrib.ox.ac.uk/fsl). Registration to high-resolution structural and standard space images was carried out using FLIRT [27, 28]. The following preprocessing steps were applied: semimanual skull stripping of the anatomical image using BET [29], motion correction using MCFLIRT [27], automated nonbrain removal of the fMRI data using BET [29], spatial smoothing using a Gaussian kernel of FWHM 5 mm, grand-mean intensity normalization of the entire 4D dataset by a single multiplicative factor, and high-pass temporal filtering (Gaussian-weighted least-squares straight line fitting, with sigma = 50 s). For each subject, a time-series statistical analysis was carried out using FILM GLM with local autocorrelation correction [30]. These Z (Gaussianized T/F) statistic images were then thresholded using clusters determined by $Z > 3.1$ and a (corrected) cluster significance threshold of $p < 0.05$ [31]. A second-level analysis for each subject was conducted, averaged across the three runs, and carried out using a fixed-effects model by forcing the random-effects variance to zero in FLAME (FMRIB's Local Analysis of Mixed Effects) [32–34]. At the group level, analyses were completed using a mixed-effects model that included both fixed effects and random effects from cross session/subject variance in FLAME. Again, Z (Gaussianized T/F) statistic images were then thresholded using clusters determined by $Z > 3.1$ and a (corrected) cluster significance threshold of $p < 0.05$. Whole brain analyses examined main effects of right hand action observation, main effects of left hand action observation, and contrasts of right hand action observation versus left hand action observation and left hand action observation versus right hand observation.

An additional aim of the current study was to directly compare new data from the right hemisphere stroke group to the data from the left hemisphere stroke group and nondisabled control group from the earlier study [24]. In order to do this, we reanalyzed all of the earlier data using the preprocessing steps described above to ensure that the same, up-to-date analysis techniques were used in all cohorts.

2.3.2. Region of Interest Analyses. A priori regions of interest (ROIs) included regions of the human AON: inferior frontal gyrus pars opercularis (IFGop) and pars triangularis (IFGtri), the supramarginal gyrus (SMG), and the precentral gyrus (PC) [35]. ROIs were defined anatomically using the probabilistic Harvard-Oxford Atlas included in FSL, with a probability threshold of greater than 25% applied for each ROI. The percent signal change (% SC) within each ROI was extracted for each task condition and each participant using Featquery in FSL.

2.3.3. Laterality Index. A laterality index (LI) was calculated to measure lateralization of brain activity during observation

of each hand (right, left) for each group (nondisabled control, right hemisphere stroke, and left hemisphere stroke). LI was calculated as the proportion of active voxels in the left versus right ROI averaged across multiple thresholds [36, 37]. We calculated LI using the proportion of active voxels, rather than percent signal change, based on previous work suggesting that this approach is more robust for lesioned brains (Jansen et al. [37]). The cluster tool in FSL was used to set the different threshold values ($Z = 1.0, 1.5, 2.3$); Fslstats was used to determine the number of active voxels. LI was calculated using the classic formula

$$LI = \frac{(left - right)}{(left + right)} \quad (1)$$

at each Z-threshold for each ROI [37], where LI is equal to left hemisphere activity minus right hemisphere activity divided by left hemisphere activity plus right hemisphere activity. The average of the three LIs at different Z-values was then calculated. LI scores range from +1 (all left hemisphere activation only) to −1 (all right hemisphere activation only) and were categorized as either bilateral ($|LI| \leq 0.1$), hemisphere dominant ($0.1 < |LI| < 0.2$), or hemisphere lateralized ($|LI| \geq 0.2$) [37]. Following previous work, the LI and standard error of the mean (SEM) are reported [24]. The complete LI values for each group at each threshold/ROI can be found in Supplementary Table 5 and for each individual at each threshold/ROI in Supplementary Tables 6–9.

2.3.4. ROI-Based Task by Hemisphere by Group Interactions. A three-way ANOVA was carried out in SPSS 22 (IBM Corp., Armonk, NY, USA) to determine the effects of hand observed (right, left), hemisphere of activity (right, left), and group (nondisabled control, right hemisphere stroke, and left hemisphere stroke) for each of our four regions of interest. We applied a Bonferroni correction for multiple comparisons. We also report any significant two-way interactions within the ANOVAs and subsequently tested for simple main effects where appropriate.

2.3.5. Lesion Analyses. Lesions were manually drawn by a trained research assistant following a detailed lesion tracing protocol [38, 39] using MRIcron [40]. Lesion masks were then smoothed using a 2 mm Gaussian kernel. For each subject, a small mask was manually created in the healthy white matter tissue of the contralesional hemisphere. The white matter mask was used to determine the mean and standard deviation of healthy white matter voxel intensities within each subject's anatomical image using fslstats. Each subject's anatomical image was then thresholded at one standard deviation away from the mean white matter intensity, such that voxels with a signal intensity within or above the normal range would be excluded from the final lesion mask. Finally, the volume of the lesion was calculated using fslstats. An independent-sample t-test was conducted to compare lesion size between the right hemisphere stroke group and the left hemisphere stroke group. For each ROI, Pearson product-moment correlations were tested between lesion size and LI for that ROI, for each stroke group.

2.3.6. Percent of Lesion Overlap with ROIs. To examine the percent of lesion overlap with each ROI, each individual's binarized lesion mask was normalized to standard space and masked with each ROI using fslmaths. The number of voxels in the overlapping area was obtained using fslstats. The number of voxels in the overlapping area was then divided by the total number of voxels within the ROI to calculate the percent of overlap between the lesion and the ROI for each subject.

2.4. Behavioral Assessments. Immediately after the scanning session, participants completed a series of behavioral assessments. Due to the small sample size, behavioral correlations with fMRI data were used as secondary, exploratory analyses. Participants were administered the Wolf Motor Function Test (WMFT) to test the function of the upper extremity in the motor domain [26]. Performance on the WMFT was videotaped and scored by a trained, blinded research assistant for a Functional Ability Scale (FAS) score, ranging from 0 to 5, where 0 = does not attempt movement and 5 = movement is normal. Individuals were also assessed with the Fugl-Meyer Assessment, Upper Extremity (FMA-UE) [41], a measure of poststroke motor impairment. Behavioral assessments were performed by graduate research assistants who were trained in the administration of both the WMFT and FMA-UE assessments.

For each ROI, Spearman's rho correlations were tested between ROI activity and motor scores for the WMFT and FMA-UE (both categorical variables) in SPSS 22. We note that these results are exploratory and report results, noting that correcting for multiple comparisons across ROIs results in a corrected p value of $p = 0.00625$ ($p = 0.05$ divided by 8 comparisons).

3. Results

In the current study, we aimed to understand whether individuals with nondominant right hemisphere stroke showed greater ipsilesional right hemisphere activity or greater motor dominant left hemisphere activity during action observation. In order to better generalize our findings, we also compared the nondominant right hemisphere stroke group with a dominant left hemisphere stroke group and a nondisabled control group from our earlier study [24].

3.1. Between-Group Behavioral Comparisons. Individuals with right hemisphere stroke had significantly lower Fugl-Meyer scores than individuals with left hemisphere stroke had ($t(22) = -0.67$, $p = 0.02$), indicating greater poststroke motor impairments of the upper extremity in the right hemisphere stroke group. Fugl-Meyer scores are reported in Table 1. Similarly, on the WMFT, individuals with right hemisphere stroke showed a trend towards lower FAS scores ($t(21) = 1.94$, $p = 0.06$) than did individuals with left hemisphere stroke, again indicating poorer motor performance. WMFT scores are reported in Table 1, along with all participant demographics.

3.2. Whole-Brain fMRI Analyses. Notably, overall, patterns of brain activity during right and left hand action observation

were similar between right and left hemisphere stroke groups, despite the groups having motor impairments in opposite hands. Contrasts of right versus left hand action observation, and vice versa, showed similar patterns in the stroke groups and a different pattern in the nondisabled group.

3.2.1. Right Hemisphere Stroke Group. For the right hemisphere stroke group, during *right (corresponding to nonparetic) hand action observation*, activity was found in the left premotor cortex, bilateral precentral gyri, bilateral superior parietal lobules, and bilateral occipital cortices, among other areas (Figure 1; Supplementary Table 1). During *left (corresponding to paretic) hand action observation*, activity was again found in the left supramarginal gyrus, bilateral precentral gyri, bilateral superior parietal lobules, and bilateral occipital cortices (Figure 1; Supplementary Table 2).

Comparing right and left hand action observation directly revealed the following: *Right* versus *left hand action observation* recruited greater activity in the left postcentral gyrus and superior parietal lobule and the right occipital pole. *Left* versus *right hand action observation* more strongly activated the right occipital pole and intracalcarine cortex (Figure 2; Supplementary Tables 3–4).

3.2.2. Left Hemisphere Stroke Group. Despite our reanalysis using a more stringent threshold, for the left hemisphere stroke group, we find results consistent with the findings reported in Garrison et al. [24]. During *right (corresponding to paretic) hand action observation*, activity was found in the left premotor cortex, bilateral precentral gyri, bilateral supramarginal gyri, and bilateral occipital cortices, among other areas, with greater activity in the left hemisphere (Figure 1; Supplementary Table 1).

During *left (corresponding to nonparetic) hand action observation*, a sparser pattern of activity was found in the left supramarginal gyrus, bilateral precentral gyri, bilateral superior parietal lobules, and bilateral occipital cortices among other areas (Figure 1; Supplementary Table 2).

Comparing right and left hand action observation directly revealed the following: *Right* versus *left hand action observation* recruited greater activity in left precentral gyrus and left postcentral gyrus. *Left* versus *right hand action observation* recruited greater activity in right occipital and occipitotemporal regions (Figure 2; Supplementary Figure S2; Supplementary Tables 3–4).

3.2.3. Nondisabled Control Group. Again, consistent with the findings reported in Garrison et al. [24] for the nondisabled control group, during *right (dominant) hand action observation*, activity was found in the right inferior frontal gyrus, right dorsal premotor cortex, right precentral gyrus, bilateral postcentral gyri, bilateral parietal cortices, and bilateral occipital cortices (Figure 3; Supplementary Table 1).

During *left (nondominant) hand action observation*, there was a similar pattern of activity, with activation in the right inferior frontal gyrus, right dorsal premotor cortex, bilateral precentral gyri, bilateral postcentral gyri, bilateral parietal

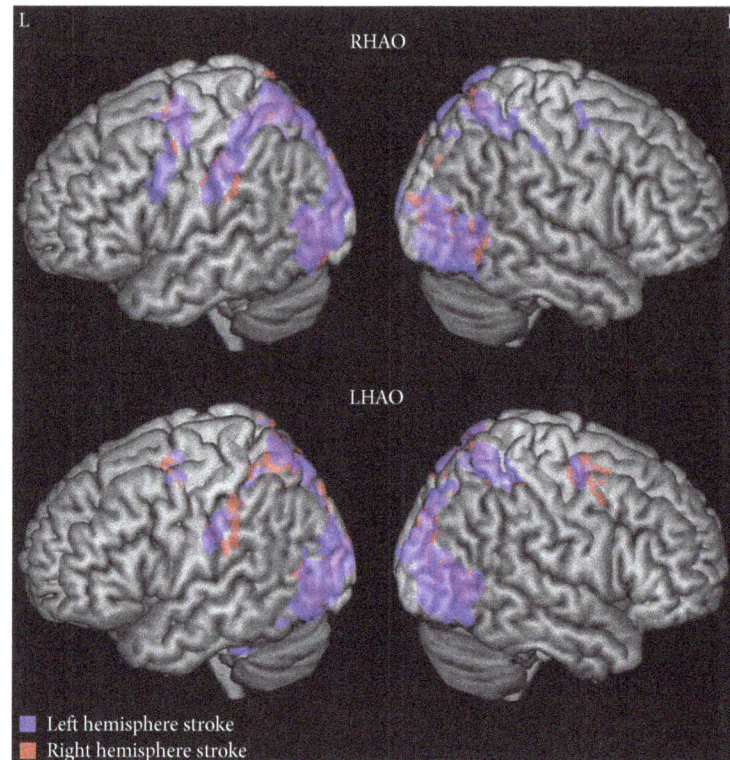

FIGURE 1: Whole brain activity during right and left action observation for individuals with stroke. While both stroke groups show bilateral activity during right and left hand action observation, activity in the left hemisphere was more extensive regardless of hemisphere of lesion. Top: right hand action observation (RHAO), bottom: left hand action observation (LHAO). Participants with left hemisphere stroke are represented in blue; participants with right hemisphere stroke are represented in red. Overlap between stroke groups is represented in purple. Thresholded at $Z > 3.1$, corrected for multiple comparisons at $p < 0.05$.

cortices, and bilateral occipital cortices, as well as the right posterior superior temporal sulcus at the temporoparietal junction (Figure 3; Supplementary Table 2).

Comparing right and left hand action observation directly revealed the following: *Right* versus *left hand action observation* revealed no significant activity (Figure 4; Supplementary Table 3). In contrast, *left* versus *right hand action observation* recruited more activity in the right hemisphere, particularly in the right postcentral gyrus, right superior parietal lobule, and right occipital cortex (Figure 4; Supplementary Table 4).

3.2.4. Interim Summary. Whole brain patterns in both stroke groups primarily showed greater left hemisphere activity during *right hand action observation*, while whole brain patterns in nondisabled controls were largely right lateralized during *left hand action observation*. Results here were reported at a relatively stringent threshold of $Z > 3.1$, cluster corrected at $p < 0.05$. Given our smaller group sample sizes and heterogeneity of lesion locations, we also wished to visualize this data at a more lenient threshold ($Z > 2.3$, cluster corrected at $p < 0.05$) to examine whether these laterality trends expanded. At this more lenient threshold, we found the same laterality patterns reported above, but they were extended to much wider regions of the AON (see Supplementary Figure S2).

3.3. Laterality Index. LI scores range from +1 (all left hemisphere activation only) to −1 (all right hemisphere activation only) and are typically categorized as either bilateral ($|LI| \leq 0.1$), hemisphere dominant ($0.1 < |LI| < 0.2$), or hemisphere lateralized ($|LI| \geq 0.2$; Jansen et al. [37]). Participants in both the right and left hemisphere stroke groups demonstrated a left hemisphere dominant/lateralized pattern of activation across ROIs during *right hand action observation*, independently of which limb was affected by stroke (Figure 5; Supplementary Tables 5–9). For participants with right hemisphere stroke, LI values were as follows: inferior frontal gyrus pars opercularis (LI = 0.33, SEM = 0.17), pars triangularis (LI = 0.16, SEM = 0.19), precentral gyrus (LI = 0.22, SEM = 0.09), and supramarginal gyrus (LI = 0.40, SEM = 0.08). For participants with left hemisphere stroke, LI values were as follows: inferior frontal gyrus pars opercularis (LI = 0.28, SEM = 0.17), pars triangularis (LI = 0.24, SEM = 0.21), precentral gyrus (LI = 0.15, SEM = 0.08), and supramarginal gyrus (LI = 0.32, SEM = 0.12).

Participants in both the right and left hemisphere stroke groups demonstrated a largely bilateral pattern of activation in most ROIs during *left hand action observation*, independent of the limb that was affected by stroke (Figure 5; Supplementary Tables 5–9). Participants with right hemisphere stroke showed bilateral results in the inferior frontal gyrus pars opercularis (LI = −0.10, SEM =

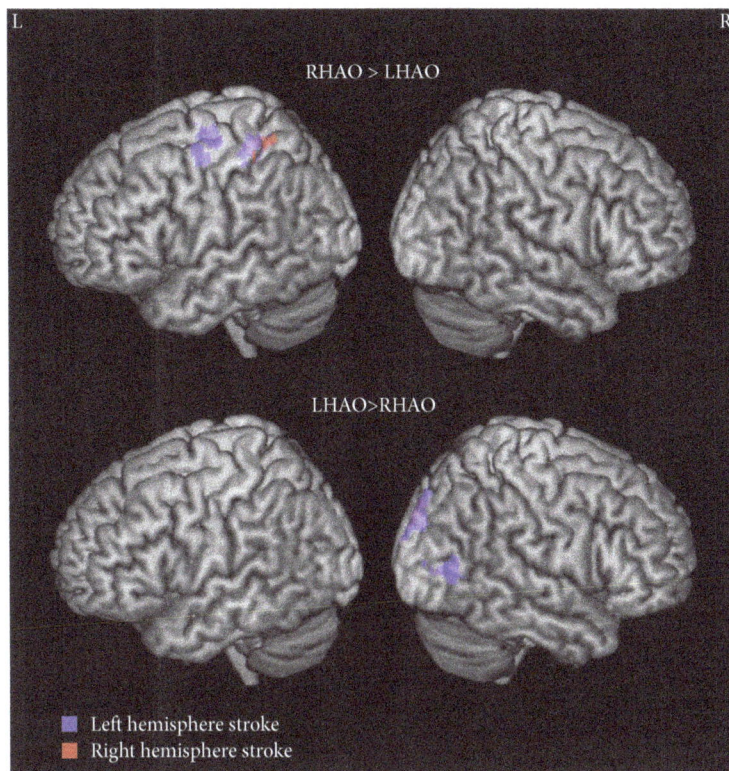

FIGURE 2: Whole brain activity contrasted between right and left action observation for individuals with stroke. Top: right hand action observation (RHAO) compared to left hand action observation (LHAO), bottom: Left hand action observation (LHAO) compared to right hand action observation (RHAO). Participants with left hemisphere stroke are represented in cool colors (blue); participants with right hemisphere stroke are represented in warm colors (red). Overlap between stroke groups is represented in purple. Thresholded at $Z > 3.1$, corrected for multiple comparisons at $p < 0.05$.

0.19), inferior frontal gyrus pars triangularis (LI = −0.08, SEM = 0.22), right hemisphere lateralization in the precentral gyrus (LI = −0.17, SEM = 0.10), and left hemisphere dominant in the supramarginal gyrus (LI = 0.21, SEM = 0.17). Participants with left hemisphere stroke showed bilateral results in the inferior frontal gyrus pars opercularis (LI = −0.05, SEM = 0.18), pars triangularis (LI = 0.01, SEM = 0.22), and supramarginal gyrus (LI = 0.07, SEM = 0.14) and right hemisphere lateralization in the precentral gyrus (LI = −0.23, SEM = 0.10; Figure 5; Supplementary Tables 5–9). We note that one difference in the LI pattern between stroke groups was that for the right hemisphere stroke group, activity in the supramarginal gyrus was left hemisphere dominant compared to bilateral in the left hemisphere stroke group.

For the nondisabled control group, regions in the AON demonstrated either right hemisphere dominant/lateralized or bilateral activity during both right and left hand action observation (Figure 5; Supplementary Tables 5–9). For *right hand action observation*, LI values are as follows: inferior frontal gyrus pars opercularis (LI = −0.15, SEM = 0.17), pars triangularis (LI = −0.21, SEM = 0.18), precentral gyrus (LI = −0.08, SEM = 0.11), and supramarginal gyrus (LI = −0.07, SEM = 0.14). For *left hand action observation*, LI values are as follows: inferior frontal gyrus pars opercularis

(LI = −0.17, SEM = 0.14), pars triangularis (LI = −0.11, SEM = 0.12), precentral gyrus (LI = −0.15, SEM = 0.04), and supramarginal gyrus (LI = 0.05, SEM = 0.09). Importantly, the laterality patterns seen in the nondisabled control group, particularly for right hand action observation, differ from those of the two stroke groups.

3.4. Task by Hemisphere by Group Interactions in ROI Activity

3.4.1. Right Hemisphere Stroke Group versus Nondisabled Controls. No three-way interactions were found between group (nondisabled control, right hemisphere stroke), hand observed (right, left), and hemisphere of activity (right, left) for any ROI. A significant two-way interaction was found for group (nondisabled control versus right hemisphere stroke) and hemisphere of activity (right, left) in the supramarginal gyrus ($F(1, 22) = 7.17$, $p = 0.01$, partial $\eta^2 = 0.25$; Bonferroni-corrected p value: $p = 0.04$). We then tested for simple main effects. For hemisphere of activity, there was a statistically significant difference between the left and right SMG in the right hemisphere stroke group ($F(1, 23) = 13.14$, $p = 0.001$, partial $\eta^2 = 0.36$), with greater activity in the left compared to right hemisphere (mean ± standard deviation reported for all analyses; left hemisphere: 0.20 ± 0.16, right hemisphere: 0.10 ± 0.19). There were no

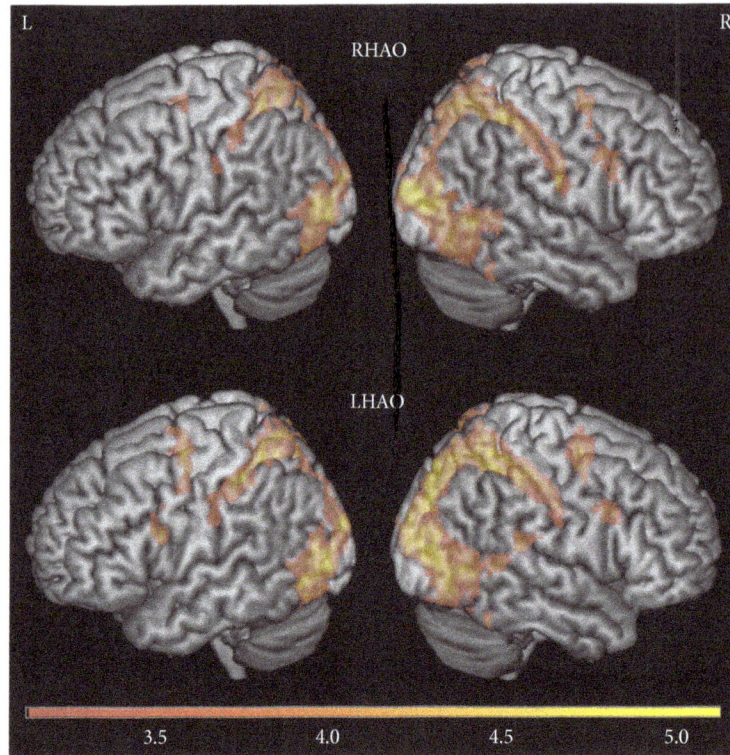

FIGURE 3: Whole brain activity during right and left action observation for the nondisabled control group. Unlike the two stroke groups, the nondisabled group did not show greater activity on the left hemisphere during right and left hand action observation. Top: right hand action observation (RHAO), bottom: left hand action observation (LHAO). Thresholded at $Z > 3.1$, corrected for multiple comparisons at $p < 0.05$.

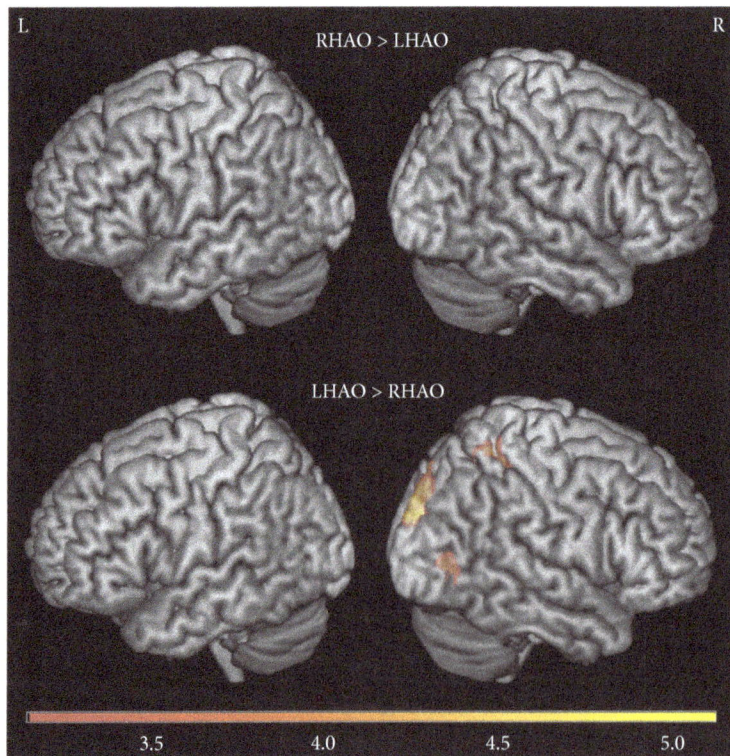

FIGURE 4: Whole brain activity contrasted between right and left action observation for the nondisabled control group. Top: right hand action observation (RHAO) compared to left hand action observation (LHAO), bottom: left hand action observation (LHAO) compared to right hand action observation (RHAO). Thresholded at $Z > 3.1$, corrected for multiple comparisons at $p < 0.05$.

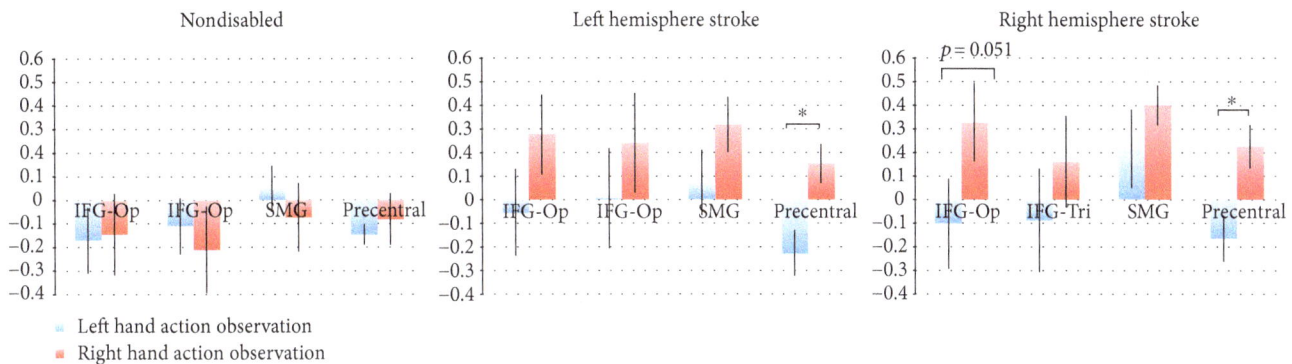

FIGURE 5: Laterality index in regions of interest. Left: nondisabled participants, middle: participants with left hemisphere stroke, right: participants with right hemisphere stroke; each during left hand (blue) and right hand (red) action observation; in the inferior frontal gyrus pars opercularis (IFG-Op), inferior frontal gyrus pars triangularis (IFG-Tri), supramarginal gyrus (SMG), and precentral gyrus (Precentral). $^*p < 0.05$. Positive values indicate left hemisphere laterality; negative values indicate right hemisphere laterality.

differences in left and right SMG activity in the ND group $(F(1, 23) = 2.35, p = 0.14)$. For group, there was a statistically significant difference between groups in the right SMG $(F(1, 46) = 6.60, p = 0.01, \text{partial } \eta^2 = 0.13)$, with greater activity for the nondisabled control group compared to the right hemisphere stroke group (nondisabled controls: 0.24 ± 0.19; right hemisphere stroke: 0.10 ± 0.19). No differences in activity were found between ND and RHS groups in the left SMG $(F(1, 46) = 0.04, p = 0.85)$. Put together, this suggests that the nondisabled control group had more activity in the right compared left supramarginal gyrus, whereas the right hemisphere stroke group had more activity in the left compared to right supramarginal gyrus.

A significant two-way interaction was also found for the hemisphere of activity (right, left) and side of hand observed (right, left) in the precentral gyrus $(F(1, 22) = 14.78, p = 0.001, \text{partial } \eta^2 = 0.40$; Bonferroni-corrected p value: $p = 0.004)$. We then tested for simple main effects. We did not find a simple main effect for hand observed (i.e., no difference in activity between right and left hand observation for either hemisphere (right hemisphere: $F(1, 23) = 0.19, p = 0.67$; left hemisphere: $F(1, 23) = 3.15, p = 0.09)$). We found a simple main effect of hemisphere of activity during right hand action observation, with greater activity in the left versus right precentral gyrus $(F(1, 23) = 7.3, p = 0.01$; left hemisphere: 0.09 ± 1.5, right hemisphere: 0.04 ± 0.13). Put another way, for both groups, during right hand action observation, activity was greater in the left precentral gyrus.

3.4.2. Right versus Left Hemisphere Stroke Group. We then compared the two stroke groups to one another directly. No three-way interactions were found between the side of the stroke (right, left), hand observed (right, left), and hemisphere of activity (right, left) in any ROI. A significant two-way interaction was found between the hemisphere of activity (right, left) and hand observed (right, left) in the precentral gyrus $(F(1, 22) = 18.73, p < 0.001, \text{partial } \eta^2 = 0.46$; Bonferroni-corrected p value: $p < 0.004$); this same interaction was also marginally significant in the inferior frontal gyrus pars opercularis after correcting for multiple

comparisons $(F(1), 22 = 5.74, p = 0.025, \text{partial } \eta^2 = 0.21$; Bonferroni-corrected p value: $p = 0.1)$. We then tested for simple main effects for each interaction. In the precentral gyrus, for effect of hand observed, there was a statistically significant difference in the left precentral gyrus, with greater activity during right hand action observation than during left hand action observation $(F(1, 23) = 13.78, p = 0.001$; partial $\eta^2 = 0.38$; left hand action observation: 0.01 ± 0.10, right hand action observation: 0.08 ± 0.11). There was no statistically significant main effect in the right precentral gyrus $(F(1, 23) = 0.37, p = 0.55)$. For simple main effect of hemisphere of activity, there was a statistically significant difference during right hand action observation $(F(1, 23) = 11.27, p = 0.003, \text{partial } \eta^2 = 0.33)$, with greater activity in the left compared to right precentral gyrus (left hemisphere: 0.08 ± 0.11, right hemisphere: 0.03 ± 0.13). There were no significant simple main effects for hemisphere during left hand action observation $(F(1, 23) = 3.14, p = 0.09)$.

For the inferior frontal gyrus pars opercularis, we found a similar simple main effect for hand observed in the left hemisphere with greater activity during right hand action observation compared to left hand action observation $(F(1, 23) = 8.1, p = 0.009, \text{partial } \eta^2 = 0.26$; right hand action observation: 0.08 ± 0.14, left hand action observation: 0.02 ± 0.14). There were no simple main effects for hand observed in the right hemisphere $(F(1, 23) = 0.002, p = 0.97)$ and no simple main effects for hemisphere during either right hand action observation $(F(1, 23) = 2.07, p = 0.16)$ or left hand action observation $(F(1, 23) = 1.17, p = 0.29)$. Overall, these results suggest there was more left hemisphere activity during right hand action observation for both stroke groups. Both stroke groups showed similar hemispheres by hand observed interactions, with brain activity lateralized toward the left motor dominant hemisphere, despite having lesions in different hemispheres.

3.5. Lesion Analyses

3.5.1. Lesion Volume Compared between Groups. No significant difference in lesion size was found between the right hemisphere stroke group ($M = 35593.08$ mm^3, SD = 55942.81) and the left hemisphere stroke group ($M = 23196.64$ mm^3, SD = 33296.69; $t(22) = -0.660$, $p = 0.52$). This suggests that, despite varying lesion sizes across individuals, reported results were not driven by a difference in overall lesion size between groups. Lesion overlap maps can be found in Supplementary Material Figures S3–S7.

3.5.2. ROI-Lesion Overlap. Overlap between the individual lesions and the AON ROIs (measured as greater than 5% overlap) occurred in only 4 of the individuals in the left hemisphere stroke group and 3 of the individuals in the right hemisphere stroke group. While we had considered also examining the relationship between lesion overlap and laterality index, to examine whether lesion overlap with critical AON regions influenced laterality results, the resulting sample of individuals with lesion overlap was too limited to make an accurate calculation.

3.6. Brain Behavior Analyses. Finally, as an exploratory analysis, we examined correlations between ROI activity and motor scores.

3.6.1. Correlations between ROI Activity and WMFT FAS Scores. For participants with right hemisphere stroke, there were no significant correlations between WMFT motor scores and ROI activity. For participants with left hemisphere stroke, nonsignificant trends showing negative correlations between WMFT scores and ROI activity during right hand action observation were found in the inferior frontal gyrus, pars opercularis ($\rho = -0.51$, $p = 0.091$), and pars triangularis ($\rho = -0.534$, $p = 0.074$). In addition, trends in negative correlations between WFMT scores and ROI activity during left hand action observation were found in the right inferior frontal gyrus ($\rho = -0.545$, $p = 0.067$) and precentral gyrus ($\rho = -0.517$, $p = 0.085$). Notably, however, none of these relationships meets the significance threshold after correcting for multiple comparisons ($p = 0.00625$).

3.6.2. Correlations between ROI Activity and Fugl-Meyer Scores. For participants with right hemisphere stroke, no significant correlations were found between Fugl-Meyer scores and ROI activity. For participants with left hemisphere stroke, activity in the right precentral gyrus during right hand action observation demonstrated a trend towards a negative correlation with Fugl-Meyer scores ($\rho = -0.53$, $p = 0.077$), although this again was not significant.

4. Discussion

In this study, our primary aim was to examine whether cortical motor activity in the action observation network was lateralized more towards the ipsilesional hemisphere or the motor dominant hemisphere during action observation after a stroke. In both individuals with nondominant right hemisphere stroke and individuals with dominant left hemisphere stroke, AON activity was lateralized toward the left motor dominant hemisphere. There were no significant differences in the lateralization of AON activity between the two stroke groups, despite having lesions in different

hemispheres. These results suggest that action observation after stroke may drive greater activity in the motor dominant rather than the ipsilesional hemisphere, at least in our sample of individuals who were right-handed prior to stroke. These findings also differed from our nondisabled control group, in which AON activity was either bilateral or slightly lateralized toward the right nondominant hemisphere.

As mentioned in the Introduction, hemispheric specialization could be an underlying cause of these results in stroke patients. That is, greater AON activity in the dominant left hemisphere may reflect hard-wired properties of the left hemisphere for motor control such as left hemisphere specialization for motor planning, and by extension, action observation, compared to the right hemisphere, regardless of which hemisphere is affected after stroke. This may mean that the motor dominant hemisphere may also play a role in the effectiveness of action observation therapy. While not tested here, it is possible that driving activity in the motor dominant hemisphere via action observation could help to promote motor recovery after stroke. Future studies could examine whether dominant hemisphere activation during action observation relates to changes in motor recovery following poststroke action observation therapy.

In addition, previous work has shown that the motor dominant hemisphere has greater descending motor pathways than the nondominant hemisphere has [42, 43]. Additionally, the typically motor dominant left precentral gyrus receives inputs from both the contralateral and ipsilateral hand, whereas the nondominant right precentral gyrus receives the majority of inputs solely from the contralateral left hand [44]. After a stroke, this imbalance in motor pathways may be accentuated to more strongly engage left-lateralized activity during right hand action observation and bilateral activity during left hand action observation. Likewise, individuals with dominant left hemisphere stroke have been shown to experience some motor deficits in both hands, whereas those with right hemisphere stroke typically only experience motor deficits in the contralateral left hand [45]. Again, while it remains to be tested in a future study, it is possible that individuals with nondominant right hemisphere stroke are able to continue to use their dominant (nonparetic) hand, and individuals with dominant left hemisphere stroke may place more emphasis on using their dominant (paretic) hand in spite of its impairments. Therefore, both groups may place greater emphasis on the dominant hand when asked to observe and later imitate actions, explaining the greater activation in the dominant left hemisphere in both groups.

Based on this logic, we might expect individuals with nondominant hand paresis to experience poorer motor recovery due to the ability to rely on the nonparetic dominant hand. Although results across studies vary, there is indeed evidence that individuals with right hemisphere stroke show poorer motor recovery of the affected nondominant left hand than those with left hemisphere stroke and an affected dominant right hand [46, 47]. Related, a limitation of the current study is the fact that the nondominant right hemisphere stroke group also had greater motor impairments (lower Fugl-Meyer and Wolf Motor Function Test scores) of the affected hand than the dominant left hemisphere stroke group, despite both groups falling within the eligibility range of moderate-to-severe motor impairments and having no differences in lesion volumes. While this may be reflective of trends in the general stroke population, this difference does introduce a potential confound, as the level of impairment could also drive patterns of cortical activity. However, importantly, there was no significant relationship between the level of impairment and brain activity within the right hemisphere stroke group, suggesting that the level of impairment for individuals with right hemisphere stroke does not influence AON activity. Given the small sample size, we further visually inspected the subject-level correlation data between brain activity and motor impairment, in case there were potential trends that were not significant. However, there were no relationships or trends between level of motor impairment and brain activity across this sample, such that individuals with less severe stroke did not show any differences in laterality index than individuals with more severe stroke. This suggests that between-group differences in level of motor impairment did not drive these left-lateralized results. Regardless, further research with a larger sample of nondominant, right hemisphere stroke patients, with a wider range from mild to severe impairments, is needed to confirm these findings.

In addition, although both right and left hemisphere stroke groups had *stronger* activations in the left hemisphere during action observation, it should be noted that there was still significant activity observed in the right hemisphere in all groups, including the two stroke groups (see Figure 1; Tables S1 and S2). General whole brain activity during action observation was bilateral for all groups, and the lateralization results emerged primarily when examining the laterality index, which calculates a ratio of left to right hemisphere activity. Thus, while we emphasize the role of the dominant left hemisphere because AON activity examined using the laterality index calculation was lateralized to the dominant left hemisphere more in both stroke groups compared to the control group, there is likely also a role of right hemisphere activity for all groups during action observation.

Finally, in line with this, we note that the healthy, age-matched control group showed bilateral or slightly right-lateralized activity. Although this is in line with many previous studies showing that AON activity in healthy right-handed individuals is typically bilateral [35, 48, 49], a previous study specifically examining the laterality index in healthy individuals showed left-lateralized AON patterns [50]. In reconciling our current findings with the previous literature, we first note that in that study, the laterality index was performed on entire lobes (e.g., LI of the frontal lobe was left-lateralized) whereas here we calculated the LI within specific AON nodes. This specificity may have affected results. In addition, a primary factor that may contribute to these disparate results is age. The previous study examining the laterality index of the AON in healthy individuals used healthy younger adults, while in our study, we used healthy older adults (age-matched to our stroke population). Research has shown that older adults typically recruit additional and broader

regions of the AON compared to younger adults [51–54]. While further research is needed to specifically examine the laterality of the AON in healthy younger versus older adults, it is possible that our healthy older adult control group shows more bilateral or slightly right-lateralized AON activity, instead of left-lateralized AON activity, due to age-related changes in the AON.

4.1. Limitations and Future Directions. Our results support the idea that hemispheric dominance affects patterns of neural activity induced by action observation after stroke. While the current sample size was small (12 participants per group), both right and left hemisphere stroke groups (24 participants in total) showed similar patterns of left-lateralized AON activity during observation of right hand actions and bilateral AON activity during observation of left hand actions, which was different from nondisabled individuals. However, as noted in the Discussion, the functional abilities of the two groups were significantly different. Notably, we did not find a relationship between the level of impairment and lateralization of AON activity within the right hemisphere group, suggesting that the differing functional levels were not associated with different brain activation patterns. However, we acknowledge that this group difference still provides a possible confounding factor as previous work has shown that degree of motor severity influences cortical recruitment [55]. In addition, previous work has shown that patients with greater corticospinal tract (CST) damage also show greater recruitment of cortical areas [56, 57]. Although lesion volumes were similar between groups, the current study did not specifically examine overlap of the lesion with the CST. Thus, a replication of these patterns in a larger, more diverse sample, with individuals across a range of motor impairment levels (mild, moderate, severe), and examining the overlap of the lesion with the CST, would improve our understanding of how the current findings relate to a diverse population of individuals after stroke.

Our findings support a possible specialization of the motor dominant hemisphere during action observation following stroke. However, the functional implications of this activation are unclear. An important question is whether and how these results, and recovery from nondominant (right hemisphere) stroke, may relate to real-world hand usage. Future studies might examine real-world hand usage during daily activities (e.g., using accelerometers [58, 59]), and relate that to laterality patterns in brain activity following stroke.

In addition, here we showed that action observation engages the motor dominant hemisphere in individuals who are right hemisphere dominant (left-handed) prior to stroke. Right hemisphere dominance is less common, and therefore, the population with stroke will be smaller and less is known about motor control in this group. However, given our findings' interpretations, we might expect AON activity to be lateralized toward the dominant right hemisphere in that group. A more complete understanding of the relationship between motor dominance, hemisphere of stroke, and AON activity should be studied to enable personalized interventions in stroke neurorehabilitation.

Finally, given the conventional wisdom that activity in the ipsilesional hemisphere promotes recovery of motor function after stroke [2–4], a logical next step is to evaluate what our findings may mean for stroke rehabilitation. Our findings, and those of others, suggest that optimal recovery of motor function may depend on the hemisphere of the lesion [20]. As such, parameters of AOT, such as whether individuals with stroke observe actions corresponding to their paretic limb only, versus observation of bilateral movements, may yield different results for different participants. While few stroke neuroimaging studies have been adequately powered to compare between right and left hemisphere stroke groups, it may be a critical difference that affects stroke rehabilitation and motor recovery. Future large-scale studies should examine whether and how the hemispheric dominance of the lesioned hemisphere affects neural activity during different types of therapy and subsequent motor recovery.

Disclosure

The contents of the study are solely the responsibility of the author and do not necessarily represent the official views of the NIH.

Conflicts of Interest

The authors have no conflicts of interest to declare.

Acknowledgments

The authors thank the research participants and Alicia Johnson and Matthew Konersman, DPT, for their contributions. This work was supported by the American Heart Association (10SDG3510062, 14CRP18200010, and 16IRG26960017), the National Institute on Drug Abuse (K12DA00167), the National Institutes of Health, Eunice Kennedy Shriver National Institute of Child Health and Human Development (R03HD067475 and K01HD091283), the National Institutes of Health (NIH) National Institute of Neurological Disorders and Stroke (NINDS) Intramural Competitive Fellowship Award, and the NIH Rehabilitation Research Career Development Program Grant K12 (HD055929).

Supplementary Materials

Figure S1: Example from video stimuli during fMRI. Figure S2: Whole brain activity contrasted between right and left action observation compared between stroke and control groups at a more lenient threshold. Figure S3: Lesion overlap heat map (whole group). Figure S4: Lesion overlap heat map for cortical left hemisphere strokes ($n = 6$). Figure S5: Lesion overlap heat map for subcortical left hemisphere strokes ($n = 6$). Figure S6: Lesion overlap heat map for cortical right hemisphere stroke ($n = 5$). Figure S7: Lesion overlap heat map for subcortical right hemisphere stroke ($n = 7$). Table S1: Main effect of right hand action observation. Table S2: Main effect of left hand action observation. Table S3: Brain activity during right hand action observation versus left hand action observation (RHAO > LHAO). Table S4: Brain activity during left hand action observation versus right hand action observation (LHAO > RHAO). Table S5: Group laterality index values. Table S6: Individual laterality index values—inferior frontal gyrus and pars opercularis. Table S7: Individual laterality index values—inferior frontal gyrus and pars triangularis. Table S8: Individual laterality index values—supramarginal gyrus. Table S9: Individual laterality index values—precentral gyrus. *(Supplementary Materials)*

References

[1] D. Mozaffarian, E. J. Benjamin, A. S. Go et al., "Heart disease and stroke statistics-2016 update a report from the American Heart Association," *Circulation*, vol. 133, no. 4, pp. e38–e360, 2016.

[2] R. S. Marshall, G. M. Perera, R. M. Lazar, J. W. Krakauer, R. C. Constantine, and R. L. DeLaPaz, "Evolution of cortical activation during recovery from corticospinal tract infarction," *Stroke*, vol. 31, no. 3, pp. 656–661, 2000.

[3] R. J. Nudo, "Mechanisms for recovery of motor function following cortical damage," *Current Opinion in Neurobiology*, vol. 16, no. 6, pp. 638–644, 2006.

[4] N. S. Ward and L. G. Cohen, "Mechanisms underlying recovery of motor function after stroke," *Archives of Neurology*, vol. 61, no. 12, pp. 1844–1848, 2004.

[5] N. S. Ward, M. M. Brown, A. J. Thompson, and R. S. J. Frackowiak, "Neural correlates of outcome after stroke: a cross-sectional fMRI study," *Brain*, vol. 126, no. 6, pp. 1430–1448, 2003.

[6] K. J. Werhahn, A. B. Conforto, N. Kadom, M. Hallett, and L. G. Cohen, "Contribution of the ipsilateral motor cortex to recovery after chronic stroke," *Annals of Neurology*, vol. 54, no. 4, pp. 464–472, 2003.

[7] F. Fregni, P. S. Boggio, C. G. Mansur et al., "Transcranial direct current stimulation of the unaffected hemisphere in stroke patients," *Neuroreport*, vol. 16, no. 14, pp. 1551–1555, 2005.

[8] S.-L. Liew, E. Santarnecchi, E. R. Buch, and L. G. Cohen, "Noninvasive brain stimulation in neurorehabilitation: local and distant effects for motor recovery," *Frontiers in Human Neuroscience*, vol. 8, p. 77, 2014.

[9] R. Lindenberg, V. Renga, L. L. Zhu, D. Nair, and G. Schlaug, "Bihemispheric brain stimulation facilitates motor recovery in chronic stroke patients," *Neurology*, vol. 75, no. 24, pp. 2176–2184, 2010.

[10] N. Takeuchi, T. Chuma, Y. Matsuo, I. Watanabe, and K. Ikoma, "Repetitive transcranial magnetic stimulation of contralesional primary motor cortex improves hand function after stroke," *Stroke*, vol. 36, no. 12, pp. 2681–2686, 2005.

[11] S. Mani, P. K. Mutha, A. Przybyla, K. Y. Haaland, D. C. Good, and R. L. Sainburg, "Contralesional motor deficits after unilateral stroke reflect hemisphere-specific control mechanisms," *Brain*, vol. 136, no. 4, pp. 1288–1303, 2013.

[12] R. L. Sainburg and S. V. Duff, "Does motor lateralization have implications for stroke rehabilitation?," *Journal of*

Rehabilitation Research and Development, vol. 43, no. 3, pp. 311–322, 2006.

[13] S. Y. Schaefer, K. Y. Haaland, and R. L. Sainburg, "Ipsilesional motor deficits following stroke reflect hemispheric specializations for movement control," *Brain*, vol. 130, no. 8, pp. 2146–2158, 2007.

[14] C. J. Winstein and P. S. Pohl, "Effects of unilateral brain damage on the control of goal-directed hand movements," *Experimental Brain Research*, vol. 105, no. 1, pp. 163–174, 1995.

[15] V. Yadav and R. L. Sainburg, "Limb dominance results from asymmetries in predictive and impedance control mechanisms," *PLoS One*, vol. 9, no. 4, article e93892, 2014.

[16] G. Rizzolatti and L. Craighero, "The mirror-neuron system," *Annual Review of Neuroscience*, vol. 27, no. 1, pp. 169–192, 2004.

[17] P. Celnik, B. Webster, D. M. Glasser, and L. G. Cohen, "Effects of action observation on physical training after stroke," *Stroke*, vol. 39, no. 6, pp. 1814–1820, 2008.

[18] D. Ertelt, S. Small, A. Solodkin et al., "Action observation has a positive impact on rehabilitation of motor deficits after stroke," *NeuroImage*, vol. 36, pp. T164–T173, 2007.

[19] M. Franceschini, M. G. Ceravolo, M. Agosti et al., "Clinical relevance of action observation in upper-limb stroke rehabilitation: a possible role in recovery of functional dexterity. A randomized clinical trial," *Neurorehabilitation and Neural Repair*, vol. 26, no. 5, pp. 456–462, 2012.

[20] P. Sale, M. G. Ceravolo, and M. Franceschini, "Action observation therapy in the subacute phase promotes dexterity recovery in right-hemisphere stroke patients," *BioMed Research International*, vol. 2014, Article ID 457538, 7 pages, 2014.

[21] S. Sarasso, S. Määttä, F. Ferrarelli, R. Poryazova, G. Tononi, and S. L. Small, "Plastic changes following imitation-based speech and language therapy for aphasia: a high-density sleep EEG study," *Neurorehabilitation and Neural Repair*, vol. 28, no. 2, pp. 129–138, 2014.

[22] K. Sugg, S. Müller, C. Winstein, D. Hathorn, and A. Dempsey, "Does Action Observation Training with Immediate Physical Practice Improve Hemiparetic Upper-Limb Function in Chronic Stroke?," *Neurorehabilitation and Neural Repair*, vol. 29, no. 9, pp. 807–817, 2015.

[23] K. A. Garrison, C. J. Winstein, and L. Aziz-Zadeh, "The mirror neuron system: a neural substrate for methods in stroke rehabilitation," *Neurorehabilitation and Neural Repair*, vol. 24, no. 5, pp. 404–412, 2010.

[24] K. A. Garrison, L. Aziz-Zadeh, S. W. Wong, S. L. Liew, and C. J. Winstein, "Modulating the motor system by action observation after stroke," *Stroke*, vol. 44, no. 8, pp. 2247–2253, 2013.

[25] R. C. Oldfield, "The assessment and analysis of handedness: the Edinburgh inventory," *Neuropsychologia*, vol. 9, no. 1, pp. 97–113, 1971.

[26] S. L. Wolf, P. A. Catlin, M. Ellis, A. L. Archer, B. Morgan, and A. Piacentino, "Assessing Wolf motor function test as outcome measure for research in patients after stroke," *Stroke*, vol. 32, no. 7, pp. 1635–1639, 2001.

[27] M. Jenkinson, P. Bannister, M. Brady, and S. Smith, "Improved optimization for the robust and accurate linear registration and motion correction of brain images," *NeuroImage*, vol. 17, no. 2, pp. 825–841, 2002.

[28] M. Jenkinson and S. Smith, "A global optimisation method for robust affine registration of brain images," *Medical Image Analysis*, vol. 5, no. 2, pp. 143–156, 2001.

[29] S. M. Smith, "Fast robust automated brain extraction," *Human Brain Mapping*, vol. 17, no. 3, pp. 143–155, 2002.

[30] M. W. Woolrich, B. D. Ripley, M. Brady, and S. M. Smith, "Temporal autocorrelation in univariate linear modeling of FMRI data," *NeuroImage*, vol. 14, no. 6, pp. 1370–1386, 2001.

[31] K. J. Worsley, "Statistical analysis of activation images," *Functional Magnetic Resonance Imaging*, vol. 14, pp. 251–270, 2001.

[32] C. F. Beckmann, M. Jenkinson, and S. M. Smith, "General multilevel linear modeling for group analysis in FMRI," *NeuroImage*, vol. 20, no. 2, pp. 1052–1063, 2003.

[33] M. Woolrich, "Robust group analysis using outlier inference," *NeuroImage*, vol. 41, no. 2, pp. 286–301, 2008.

[34] M. W. Woolrich, T. E. J. Behrens, C. F. Beckmann, M. Jenkinson, and S. M. Smith, "Multilevel linear modelling for FMRI group analysis using Bayesian inference," *NeuroImage*, vol. 21, no. 4, pp. 1732–1747, 2004.

[35] S. Caspers, K. Zilles, A. R. Laird, and S. B. Eickhoff, "ALE meta-analysis of action observation and imitation in the human brain," *NeuroImage*, vol. 50, no. 3, pp. 1148–1167, 2010.

[36] K. L. Ito and S.-L. Liew, "Calculating the laterality index using FSL for stroke neuroimaging data," *GigaScience*, vol. 5, Supplement 1, pp. 14-15, 2016.

[37] A. Jansen, R. Menke, J. Sommer et al., "The assessment of hemispheric lateralization in functional MRI-robustness and reproducibility," *NeuroImage*, vol. 33, no. 1, pp. 204–217, 2006.

[38] J. D. Riley, V. le, L. der-Yeghiaian et al., "Anatomy of stroke injury predicts gains from therapy," *Stroke*, vol. 42, no. 2, pp. 421–426, 2011.

[39] S.-L. Liew, J. M. Anglin, N. W. Banks et al., "A large, open source dataset of stroke anatomical brain images and manual lesion segmentations," *Scientific Data*, vol. 5, article 180011, 2018.

[40] C. Rorden and M. Brett, "Stereotaxic display of brain lesions," *Behavioural Neurology*, vol. 12, no. 4, pp. 191–200, 2000.

[41] A. R. Fugl-Meyer, L. Jääskö, I. Leyman, S. Olsson, and S. Steglind, "The post-stroke hemiplegic patient. 1. A method for evaluation of physical performance," *Scandinavian Journal of Rehabilitation Medicine*, vol. 7, no. 1, pp. 13–31, 1975.

[42] G. Hammond, "Correlates of human handedness in primary motor cortex: a review and hypothesis," *Neuroscience & Biobehavioral Reviews*, vol. 26, no. 3, pp. 285–292, 2002.

[43] J. Rademacher, U. Bürgel, S. Geyer et al., "Variability and asymmetry in the human precentral motor system: a cytoarchitectonic and myeloarchitectonic brain mapping study," *Brain*, vol. 124, no. 11, pp. 2232–2258, 2001.

[44] S. Kim, J. Ashe, K. Hendrich et al., "Functional magnetic resonance imaging of motor cortex: hemispheric asymmetry and handedness," *Science*, vol. 261, no. 5121, pp. 615–617, 1993.

[45] K. Y. Haaland and D. L. Harrington, "Hemispheric asymmetry of movement," *Current Opinion in Neurobiology*, vol. 6, no. 6, pp. 796–800, 1996.

[46] J. E. Harris and J. J. Eng, "Individuals with the dominant hand affected following stroke demonstrate less impairment than those with the nondominant hand affected," *Neurorehabilitation and Neural Repair*, vol. 20, no. 3, pp. 380–389, 2006.

[47] J. E. Ween, M. P. Alexander, M. D'Esposito, and M. Roberts, "Factors predictive of stroke outcome in a rehabilitation setting," *Neurology*, vol. 47, no. 2, pp. 388–392, 1996.

[48] L. Aziz-Zadeh, L. Koski, E. Zaidel, J. Mazziotta, and M. Iacoboni, "Lateralization of the human mirror neuron system," *Journal of Neuroscience*, vol. 26, no. 11, pp. 2964–2970, 2006.

[49] L. Aziz-Zadeh, F. Maeda, E. Zaidel, J. Mazziotta, and M. Iacoboni, "Lateralization in motor facilitation during action observation: a TMS study," *Experimental Brain Research*, vol. 144, no. 1, pp. 127–131, 2002.

[50] M. Cabinio, V. Blasi, P. Borroni et al., "The shape of motor resonance: right- or left-handed?," *NeuroImage*, vol. 51, no. 1, pp. 313–323, 2010.

[51] M. C. Costello and E. K. Bloesch, "Are older adults less embodied? A review of age effects through the lens of embodied cognition," *Frontiers in Psychology*, vol. 8, p. 267, 2017.

[52] N. Diersch, K. Mueller, E. S. Cross, W. Stadler, M. Rieger, and S. Schütz-Bosbach, "Action prediction in younger versus older adults: neural correlates of motor familiarity," *PLoS One*, vol. 8, no. 5, article e64195, 2013.

[53] E. Kuehn, M. B. Perez-Lopez, N. Diersch, J. Döhler, T. Wolbers, and M. Riemer, "Embodiment in the aging mind," *Neuroscience & Biobehavioral Reviews*, vol. 86, no. 4, pp. 207–225, 2017.

[54] G. Léonard and F. Tremblay, "Corticomotor facilitation associated with observation, imagery and imitation of hand actions: a comparative study in young and old adults," *Experimental Brain Research*, vol. 177, no. 2, pp. 167–175, 2007.

[55] A. K. Rehme, G. R. Fink, D. Y. von Cramon, and C. Grefkes, "The role of the contralesional motor cortex for motor recovery in the early days after stroke assessed with longitudinal FMRI," *Cerebral Cortex*, vol. 21, no. 4, pp. 756–768, 2010.

[56] N. S. Ward, J. M. Newton, O. B. C. Swayne et al., "The relationship between brain activity and peak grip force is modulated by corticospinal system integrity after subcortical stroke," *European Journal of Neuroscience*, vol. 25, no. 6, pp. 1865–1873, 2007.

[57] N. S. Ward, J. M. Newton, O. B. C. Swayne et al., "Motor system activation after subcortical stroke depends on corticospinal system integrity," *Brain*, vol. 129, no. 3, pp. 809–819, 2006.

[58] R. R. Bailey, J. W. Klaesner, and C. E. Lang, "An accelerometry-based methodology for assessment of real-world bilateral upper extremity activity," *PLoS One*, vol. 9, no. 7, article e103135, 2014.

[59] C. E. Lang, J. M. Wagner, D. F. Edwards, and A. W. Dromerick, "Upper extremity use in people with hemiparesis in the first few weeks after stroke," *Journal of Neurologic Physical Therapy*, vol. 31, no. 2, pp. 56–63, 2007.

7

Corticospinal and Spinal Excitabilities are Modulated during Motor Imagery Associated with Somatosensory Electrical Nerve Stimulation

E. Traverse ⓘ, **F. Lebon** ⓘ, **and A. Martin**

INSERM UMR1093-CAPS, UFR des Sciences du Sport, Université Bourgogne Franche-Comté, 21000 Dijon, France

Correspondence should be addressed to E. Traverse; elodie.traverse@u-bourgogne.fr

Academic Editor: Ambra Bisio

Motor imagery (MI), the mental simulation of an action, influences the cortical, corticospinal, and spinal levels, despite the lack of somatosensory afferent feedbacks. The aim of this study was to analyze the effect of MI associated with somatosensory stimulation (SS) on the corticospinal and spinal excitabilities. We used transcranial magnetic stimulation and peripheral nerve stimulation to induce motor-evoked potentials (MEP) and H-reflexes, respectively, in soleus and medialis gastrocnemius (MG) muscles of the right leg. Twelve participants performed three tasks: (1) MI of submaximal plantar flexion, (2) SS at 65 Hz on the posterior tibial nerve with an intensity below the motor threshold, and (3) MI + SS. MEP and H-reflex amplitudes were recorded before, during, and after the tasks. Our results confirmed that MI increased corticospinal excitability in a time-specific manner. We found that MI + SS tended to potentiate MEP amplitude of the MG muscle compared to MI alone. We confirmed that SS decreased spinal excitability, and this decrease was partially compensated when combined with MI, especially for the MG muscle. The increase of CSE could be explained by a modulation of the spinal inhibitions induced by SS, depending on the amount of afferent feedbacks.

1. Introduction

Motor imagery (MI) is the mental simulation of a movement without muscular activities [1]. MI activates the motor cortical network, such as the primary motor cortex (M1), the premotor cortex, the supplementary motor area, and the parietal cortex [2], a network also involved when the movement is actually executed [3]. Most transcranial magnetic stimulation (TMS) studies have reported an increase of the corticospinal excitability (CSE) during MI in comparison to the rest, as evidenced by an increase of the motor-evoked potential (MEP) amplitude [4, 5]. Recently, the subliminal motor command evoked during MI has been evidenced to reach the spinal level and to modify the excitability of inhibitory interneurons [4].

Most of the previous cited results have been observed using kinesthetic imagery modality, which consists in imagining the actual movement feelings associated with its realization. Indeed, this MI modality has been reported to induce greater CSE increase in comparison to the visual modality [6, 7]. This difference is most likely due to the activation of the somatosensory cortex during kinesthetic MI [8], which interacts with M1 [3]. Interestingly, no somatosensory feedbacks related to the imagined movement are available as no movement is produced during MI. Therefore, the understanding of the interaction between MI and somatosensory feedbacks induced artificially could promote the use of MI for motor performance improvement [9].

Few studies analyzed the interaction between MI and external somatosensory inputs, such as those induced by somatosensory electrical nerve stimulation (SS). Saito et al. [10] measured CSE during an imagined opposition finger task combined with SS (10 Hz, 1 ms pulse width for 20 seconds). They observed an increase of CSE in the thumb muscle when SS intensity was set at the motor threshold. Similarly, Kaneko et al. [11] found an increase of CSE during an imagined index abduction combined with SS (50 Hz, 1 ms pulse width for 2–4 seconds) when the intensity was above the motor threshold in comparison to MI alone. These studies demonstrated the additional influence of SS during MI on upper-limb CSE. However, the SS intensity was set at or above the motor threshold, inducing force development that can modulate MEP amplitude [12]. Indeed, the CSE increase, observed during the stimulation above the motor threshold, could be attributed to the direct activation of the alpha-motoneuron rather than the sole activation of the somatosensory afferent pathway. Indeed, peripheral somatosensory stimulation evoked near the motor threshold activates proprioceptive, sensory and cutaneous afferent fibers [13]. Repetitive activation of these fibers induces inhibitory and/or excitatory neurotransmitter release into the synaptic cleft that can modulate the excitability threshold, that is, the electrophysiological properties of the resting motor neuron membrane. Thus, when a cortical stimulation is induced, the motor neuron may not be in the same state and the MEP amplitude may be affected [14]. This phenomenon is accentuated as the stimulation intensity is high, due to the greater number of fibers activated. In summary, CSE change may be related to the modulation of cortical and/or spinal excitability when the peripheral somatosensory stimulation is near the motor threshold [15]. Therefore, to properly examine the neural impact of the solicitation of afferent fibers during MI, it appears necessary to analyze both corticospinal and spinal excitabilities with SS below the motor threshold that avoids the contamination of the efferent pathway.

In the current study, we conducted a couple of experiments aiming at determining whether the combination of MI and SS below the motor threshold exacerbated the effect of MI on corticospinal and spinal excitabilities. In the first experiment, the participants performed 3 tasks: (1) MI alone, (2) SS alone (65 Hz), and (3) MI combined with SS. We assessed corticospinal and spinal excitabilities at different time points to probe the effects and aftereffects of MI and SS. We hypothesized that MI associated with SS would potentiate to a greater extent corticospinal and spinal excitabilities. We investigated CSE by measuring MEP amplitude evoked by TMS over M1 and spinal excitability by measuring H-reflex amplitude evoked by peripheral electrical nerve stimulation (PNS) over the posterior tibial nerve. In our experimental setup, we applied several PNS with short interstimulus intervals (ranged between 5 s and 10 s) that can affect spinal excitability due to homonymous postactivation depression [16–18]. Therefore, we conducted a second experiment to quantify the effect of successive PNS on spinal excitability at rest and during MI for our specific setup.

2. Methods

2.1. Subjects. Twelve young healthy adults volunteered to participate in experiment 1 (10 males and 2 females; age 26 ± 8.6 years, height 175 ± 8.7 cm, and weight 72.3 ± 8.8 kg). Data analysis was performed on the data from 11 of the participants, as data from one participant were discarded due to data saving errors. Eight young healthy adults volunteered to participate in experiment 2 (7 males and 1 female; age 28 ± 10 years, height 175.5 ± 3.8 cm, and weight 72.3 ± 7.5 kg), three of them participating in both experiments. Participants had no history of neurological and musculoskeletal disorders. They were normally active and gave their written consent. They did not engage in any strenuous physical activity for at least 24 h before the experimental sessions. All protocols of the current investigation were approved by the University of Burgundy Committee on Human Research and were performed in accordance with the Declaration of Helsinki.

2.2. Experimental Setup

2.2.1. Mechanical Recording. Participants sat in a position with hip, knee, and ankle joints placed at a 90° angular position. Measurements were realized on the right calf muscles with the foot secured by two straps to the footplate of a dynamometer (Biodex, Shirley, NY, USA) with the motor axis aligned with the external malleolus of the ankle. Participants were securely stabilized by two crossover shoulder harnesses, and head movements were reduced by a cervical collar strapped to the headrest of the seat.

2.2.2. Electromyographic Recording. The electromyographic activity (EMG) was recorded from two muscles of the right sural triceps (soleus (SOL) and medialis gastrocnemius (MG)) using silver-chloride surface electrodes (8 mm diameter, Ag-AgCl, Mini KR, Contrôle-Graphique S.A., Brie-Comte-Robert, France). Bipolar surface electrodes (interelectrode center-to-center distance of 2 cm) were placed on the midmuscle belly for MG and along the middorsal line of the leg, about 2 cm below the insertion of the gastrocnemius on the Achilles tendon for SOL. The reference electrode was placed between two gastrocnemius muscles of the right leg, below the stimulation site. Before electrode placement, the skin was shaved and cleaned with alcohol to obtain low impedance (<5 kΩ). EMG signals were amplified with a bandwidth frequency ranging from 15 Hz to 1 kHz (gain = 1000) and digitized online at a sampling frequency of 5 kHz using TIDA software (HEKA Elektronik, Lambrecht/Pfalz, Germany).

2.2.3. Transcranial Magnetic Stimulation. A TMS figure-of-eight-shaped conic coil (70 mm loop diameter) was positioned over the left M1 with anteroposterior-directed current orientation to elicit MEPs in SOL and MG muscles of the right leg (Magstim 200, Magstim Company Ltd., Great Britain). To find the optimal site, we stimulated the M1 area of the triceps surae muscle by starting from 1 cm posterior and 1 cm lateral to the vertex of the participant's head and using the lowest stimulation intensity that evoked the greatest amplitude in the SOL and MG muscles. Once the optimal site was found, a mark was placed on the scalp to ensure consistency between stimulations. The coil was then secured by using a homemade tripod with a lockable articulated arm (Otello Factory, T&O brand, France). Then, we realized a recruitment curve at rest to determine the optimal stimulation intensity. The stimulation intensity was increased by steps of 5% of the maximum stimulator output (MSO), and four consecutive stimulations were applied at the same intensity. The optimal intensity was defined when evoking the greatest and the less variable MEP amplitudes on the ascending part of the recruitment curve of both muscles (variation coefficient < 5%). During exp. 1, mean TMS intensity was

$72 \pm 10\%$ MSO (range: 60 to 98% MSO) corresponding to $131 \pm 15\%$ and $124 \pm 16\%$ of the rest motor threshold for SOL and MG, respectively. These stimulation intensities are in the range of those classically used in the literature when analyzing the CSE [19].

2.2.4. Peripheral Nerve Stimulation (PNS). To evoke M and H waves, a single 1 ms rectangular pulse was applied to the posterior tibial nerve using a Digitimer stimulator (model DS7, Hertfordshire, UK). We first placed the cathode electrode stylus in the popliteal fossa and the anode electrode (5×10 cm, Medicompex SA, Ecublens, Switzerland) over the patellar tendon, to find the optimal stimulation site, that is, the greatest H-reflex amplitude or M-wave amplitude for the SOL with the lowest stimulation intensity. Once the optimal site was found, we replaced the stylus with a surface electrode (8 mm diameter, Ag-AgCl), secured with a rubber band. Then, we realized a recruitment curve at rest to determine the three optimal stimulation intensities that evoked (1) the lowest EMG response (defined as the rest motor threshold (rMT)), (2) the most reproducible H-reflex, and (3) the maximal M-wave (M_{max}). For each participant, the stimulation intensity was progressively increased, with a 0.5 mA step, to the M_{max} amplitude.

In exp. 1, the mean PNS intensity inducing an H-reflex of about 10–15% of M_{max} was 9.1 ± 4.9 mA. The mean PNS intensity was 52.3 ± 20.6 mA corresponding to M_{max} wave amplitude of 8.0 ± 4.5 mV. For the somatosensory stimulation (SS), we applied 1 ms monophasic rectangular electrical pulses at 65 Hz for 9 seconds using a second Digitimer stimulator (model DS7, Hertfordshire, UK). The SS intensity was set at 80% of the participants' rMT (mean: 4.9 ± 3.1 mA) to induce afferent inputs without contaminating efferent activation. Due to the electrical noise induced by SS contaminating background EMG, the current was stopped 4 seconds after the beginning of SS for 200 ms to elicit H-reflex or MEP 100 ms after the last SS pulse.

In exp. 2, the PNS intensity to evoke H-reflexes was set at 15% of the M_{max} amplitude, to avoid antidromic collisions and to reduce intersubject variability (mean intensity: 10.3 ± 5.1 mA). The PNS intensity to evoke an M_{max} wave was set at 54.2 ± 18.1 mA corresponding to an M_{max} amplitude of 7.4 ± 4.2 mV.

2.3. Experimental Protocol. The duration of both experiments was about two hours. An overview of exp. 1 is depicted in Figure 1. The first experiment was designed to study the effects of MI associated with SS on corticospinal and spinal excitabilities. To determine maximal plantar flexion force, the participants first performed two maximal voluntary contractions (MVC). If the difference between the two exceeded 5%, an additional trial was performed. The maximal performance was considered for the continuation of the experiment. Then, PNS was applied 4 times at rest to record M_{max}. To memorize the sensations associated with actual contractions, the participants performed several trials at 50% MVC. A visual feedback helped the participants to match the level of force. Then, we assessed corticospinal and spinal excitabilities during the three tasks: MI only, SS

only, and MI associated with SS (MI + SS). All tasks included 8 trials of 45-second duration, half with TMS to elicit MEPs and half with PNS to elicit H-reflexes. The low number of stimulations was chosen to limit the risk of discomfort. A preliminary experiment helped us in determining the number of trials: we found that for 20, 10, or 4 trials, the MEP variation was not significantly different for SOL and MG muscles with 20, 10, and 4 trials ($41 \pm 27\%$ and $38 \pm 16\%$ with 20 trials; $35 \pm 21\%$ and $34.0 \pm 18\%$ with 10 trials; and $31 \pm 28\%$ and $31 \pm 23\%$ with 4 trials, resp.). The order of the tasks and of the stimulation type was counterbalanced across participants. TMS and PNS were evoked at 0 s (Pre), 9 s (Per), 16 s, 24 s, and 34 s (Post 1, 2, and 3, resp.). In SS and MI + SS tasks, SS was applied for 9 s (5 s after the first stimulation, i.e., Pre stimulation). In MI and MI + SS tasks, participants imagined a plantar-flexion contraction at 50% of MVC for 9 s. To start and stop imagining, the experimenter gave auditory go (5 s after the Pre stimulation) and stop signals (9 s after the go signal). Therefore, in the MI + SS task, MI and SS were performed at the same time. During MI, participants were instructed to feel the contraction normally generated during actual contractions (kinesthetic modality) and to stay relaxed to avoid muscular contractions.

SS, TMS, and PNS were triggered automatically by the TIDA patch-clamp software (HEKA Elektronik, Lambrecht/Pfalz, Germany) and synchronized with EMG recordings. During the experimental protocol, 60 TMS, 60 PNS, and 16 SS trains were applied.

Exp. 2 was designed to control the effects of successive PNS on H-reflex amplitude at rest and during MI. The experimental setup was similar to exp. 1, without application of SS. As in exp. 1, participants were instructed to stay at rest or to imagine a 50% MVC plantar-flexion contraction. In total, two tasks were performed: (1) PNS induced at 0 s, 9 s, and 16 s during MI (MI Pre-Per-Post) and (2) PNS induced at 0 s, 9 s, and 16 s at rest (Rest Pre-Per-Post). Eight trials were recorded for each task. During the experimental protocol, 48 PNS were applied (24 at rest and 24 during MI).

In both experiments, after each imagined trial, the subjects rated the vividness of their MI using a 7-point Likert scale (from 1 = "very hard to feel" to 7 = "very easy to feel," 2–6 being intermediate quotes).

2.4. Data Analysis. To ensure that the evoked responses were not contaminated by any muscle contraction, the normalized root mean square (RMS) EMG signal was measured 100 ms before each stimulation artefact. When the RMS/M_{max} ratio was different from the mean $\pm$ 2 SD of the RMS baseline, that is, observed at rest before the first stimulation, the trial was discarded from the general analysis (3% of all trials). Peak-to-peak MEP, M_{max}, and H-reflex amplitudes were measured during each task for SOL and MG muscles. The ratios MEP/M_{max} and H/M_{max} were calculated and analyzed.

2.5. Statistics Analysis. All data were normalized to M_{max} and expressed by their mean $\pm$ standard deviation (SD). Data distribution was tested using the Shapiro-Wilk test to ensure the use of the classical analysis of variance for parametric values when appropriate. In exp. 1, all variables were not normally

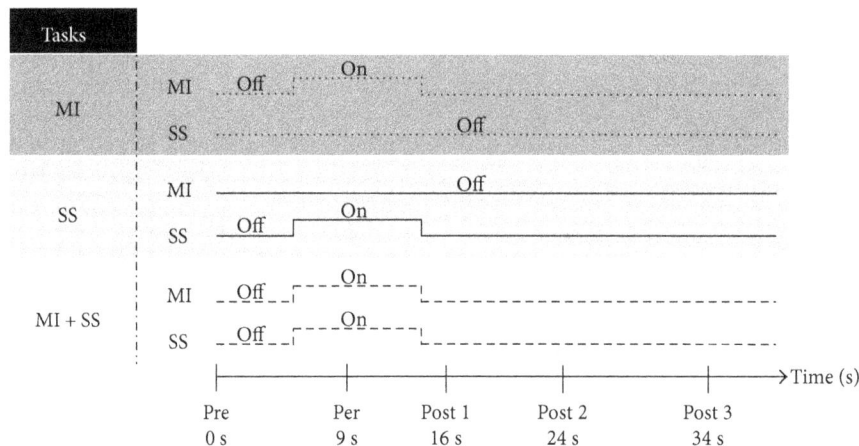

FIGURE 1: Experimental protocol of experiment 1. Transcranial magnetic stimulation and peripheral nerve stimulation were elicited at several stimulation times: 0, 9, 16, 24, and 34 seconds. Each trial lasted 45 seconds. During the motor imagery (MI) task, participants imagined a plantar-flexion contraction at 50% MVC for 9 s. During the somatosensory stimulation (SS) task, SS was applied for 9 s. During MI + SS, participants imagined the contraction when SS was applied.

distributed. The Likert scale score during MI and MI + SS was analyzed using a nonparametric Friedman ANOVA.

For both muscles, to ensure that muscles were relaxed, we used four nonparametric related samples Friedman's two-way ANOVAs by ranks with *stimulation* (Pre, Per, and Post 1) and *task* (MI, Rest) 100 ms before each stimulation artefact on EMG RMS/M_{max} ratios. We also analyzed MEP/M_{max} and H-reflex/M_{max} ratios with two nonparametric related samples Friedman's two-way ANOVAs by ranks with *stimulation* (Pre, Per, Post 1, Post 2, and Post 3) and *task* (MI, Rest). When appropriate, we used Wilcoxon's signed-rank tests for paired multiple comparisons applied with a Bonferroni correction.

For exp. 2, all variables were normally distributed for MG but not for SOL. We compared H-reflex ratios using nonparametric related samples Friedman's two-way ANOVAs by ranks for SOL. We used a two-way rmANOVA with *stimulation* (Pre, Per, and Post) and *task* (MI, Rest) for MG. When appropriate, we used Wilcoxon signed-rank tests or paired comparisons Bonferroni's tests, for SOL and MG muscles, respectively. Statistical analysis was performed with SPSS Statistics (2017 version, IBM). The level of significance was set at $p < 0.05$.

3. Results

3.1. Experiment 1. The vividness of MI, measured with a 7-point Likert scale, was not significantly different between all MI tasks ($\chi^2 = 6.94$, $p > 0.05$). The mean score was 5.3 ± 0.4 and 5.0 ± 0.2 for the MI and MI + SS tasks, respectively. This result ensured that modulations of MEP and H-reflex would not be attributed to the difficulty of task.

3.1.1. EMG Activity. The nonparametric related samples Friedman's two-way ANOVAs by ranks revealed an effect for SOL ($\chi^2 = 51.98$, $p < 0.01$ and $\chi^2 = 48.12$, $p < 0.01$ for TMS and PNS trials, resp.) and MG muscles ($\chi^2 = 35.88$, $p < 0.01$ and $\chi^2 = 33.27$, $p < 0.01$ for TMS and PNS trials,

resp.). During SS and MI + SS tasks, SS increased background EMG at Per (for all, $p < 0.01$ compared to Pre and Post stimulations), without an extra increase when imagining ($p > 0.05$). During the MI task, EMG ratios were similar to those at rest (for all, $p > 0.05$). These results ensured that modulations of MEP and H-reflex amplitude would not be attributed to muscle activities (see Table 1).

3.1.2. Corticospinal Excitability. The first stimulation (Pre), induced at the beginning of each trial, was not significantly different between all tasks for both muscles (for all, $p > 0.05$). For MI, SS, and MI + SS, MEP amplitude for the first stimulation was $1.9 \pm 1.0\%$, $2.1 \pm 1.0\%$, and $1.9 \pm 0.8\%$ of M_{max}, respectively, for the SOL muscle and $2.9 \pm 1.5\%$, $3.5 \pm 2.0\%$, and $2.9 \pm 1.4\%$ of M_{max}, respectively, for the MG muscle.

For the SOL muscle, a typical trace of one participant was represented in Figure 2. The main results were illustrated in Figure 3(a). The nonparametric related samples Friedman's two-way ANOVA by ranks revealed an effect ($\chi^2 = 29.72$, $p = 0.008$). The Wilcoxon signed-rank tests demonstrated that MEPs increased when imagining with or without SS in comparison to the Pre test value, that is, baseline (at Per: $+106 \pm 140\%$, $p = 0.013$ and $+81 \pm 78\%$, $p = 0.026$, resp.). After imagining, MEPs returned to baseline from Post 1 for the MI task but not for the MI + SS task. Indeed, MEPs at Post 3 were still above baseline in this task. Note that MEP amplitude was not modulated during the SS task (all, $p > 0.05$).

For the MG muscle, a typical trace of one participant was represented in Figure 2. The main results were illustrated in Figure 3(c). The nonparametric related samples Friedman's two-way ANOVA by ranks revealed an effect ($\chi^2 = 30.82$, $p = 0.006$). The Wilcoxon signed-rank tests demonstrated that MEPs significantly increased when imagining in comparison to baseline (MI task, $+41 \pm 64\%$, $p = 0.041$; MI + SS task, $+84 \pm 66\%$, $p = 0.004$). Interestingly, MEP increase during MI + SS was marginally greater than that during MI alone ($p = 0.062$). After imagining, MEPs returned to

TABLE 1: Normalized EMG RMS (±SD) in experiment 1. RMS/M_{max} ratio is multiplied by 100 and recorded in SOL and MG muscles before (Pre), during (Per), and after (Post 1) motor imagery (MI), somatosensory stimulation (SS), and MI combined with SS (MI + SS) tasks. EMG RMS was measured 100 ms before each stimulation artefact. At Per, during SS and MI + SS (gray boxes), values significantly increased compared to that at Pre and Post 1 ($p < 0.05$).

		SOL			MG		
		Pre	Per	Post 1	Pre	Per	Post 1
MI	TMS	0.79 ± 0.31	0.84 ± 0.37	0.84 ± 0.38	1.6 ± 0.51	1.6 ± 0.47	1.6 ± 0.34
	PNS	0.84 ± 0.38	0.86 ± 0.39	0.84 ± 0.39	1.7 ± 0.56	1.6 ± 0.56	1.7 ± 0.60
SS	TMS	0.75 ± 0.31	5.4 ± 6.2	0.75 ± 0.28	1.6 ± 0.55	13.3 ± 21.9	1.5 ± 0.38
	PNS	0.94 ± 0.69	5.5 ± 6.2	0.95 ± 0.70	1.7 ± 0.56	14.0 ± 25.0	1.7 ± 0.60
MI + SS	TMS	0.79 ± 0.31	5.5 ± 6.2	0.80 ± 0.34	1.6 ± 0.60	13.9 ± 23.8	1.6 ± 0.57
	PNS	0.82 ± 0.33	5.6 ± 6.4	0.82 ± 0.36	1.6 ± 0.56	14.6 ± 26.1	1.6 ± 0.54

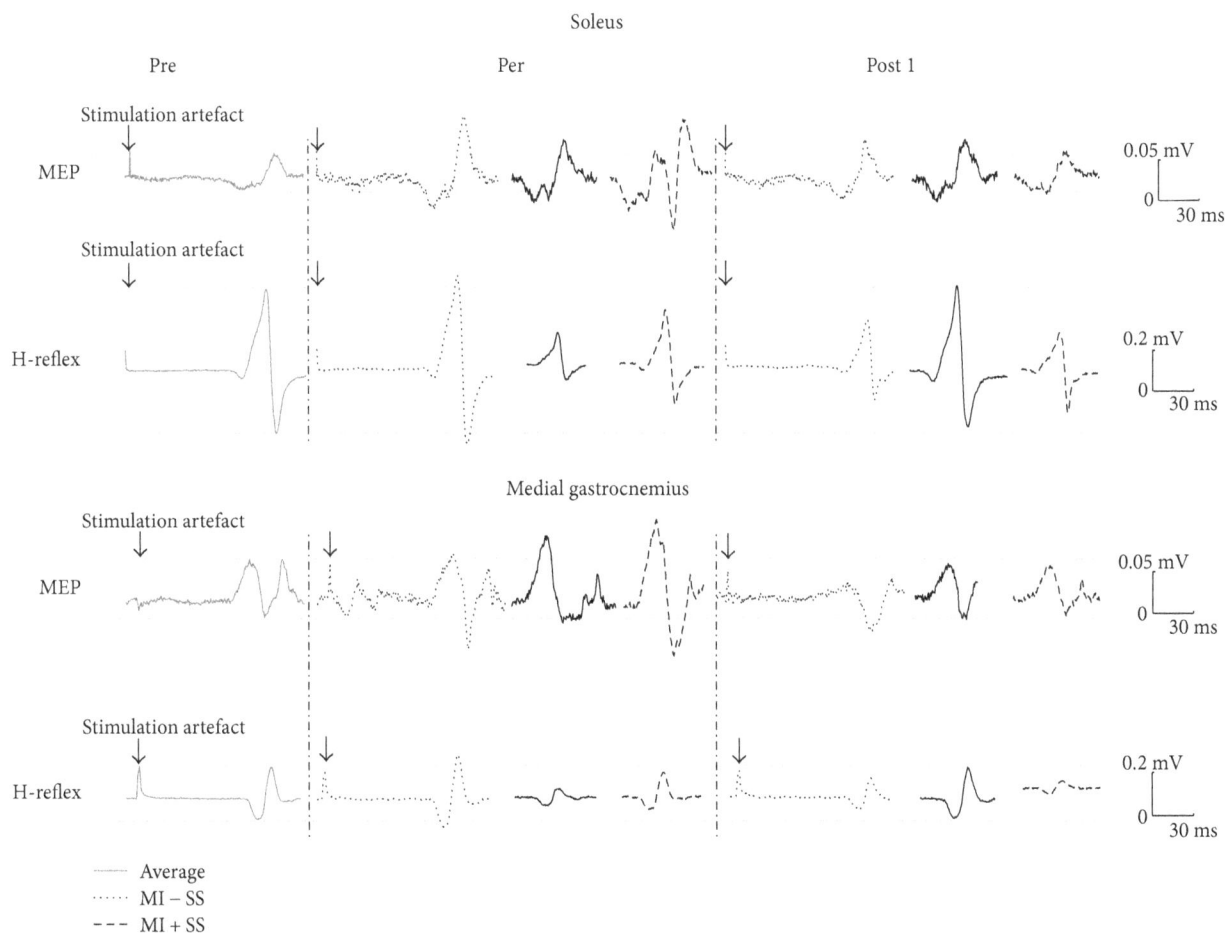

FIGURE 2: Typical subject. MEP and H-reflex mean responses at Pre, Per, and Post 1 stimulations during MI, SS, and MI + SS for SOL and MG muscles. For both muscles, MEP at Per, when imagining, were significantly greater in comparison to baseline. For MG muscle only, MEP amplitude tended to extra increase during MI + SS in comparison to MI alone. For both muscles, H-reflex at Per decreased during SS but not during the combination with MI.

baseline from Post 1 for the MI task (+15%±41%, $p > 0.05$) and at Post 3 for the MI + SS task (+13%±30%, $p > 0.05$). Note that MEP amplitude was not modulated during the SS task (all, $p > 0.05$).

3.1.3. Spinal Excitability. For both muscles, the first stimulation (Pre), applied at the beginning of each trial, did not differ between tasks (for all, $p > 0.05$). For MI, SS, and MI+SS tasks, H-reflex amplitude for the first stimulation was 12.7 ± 12.2%,

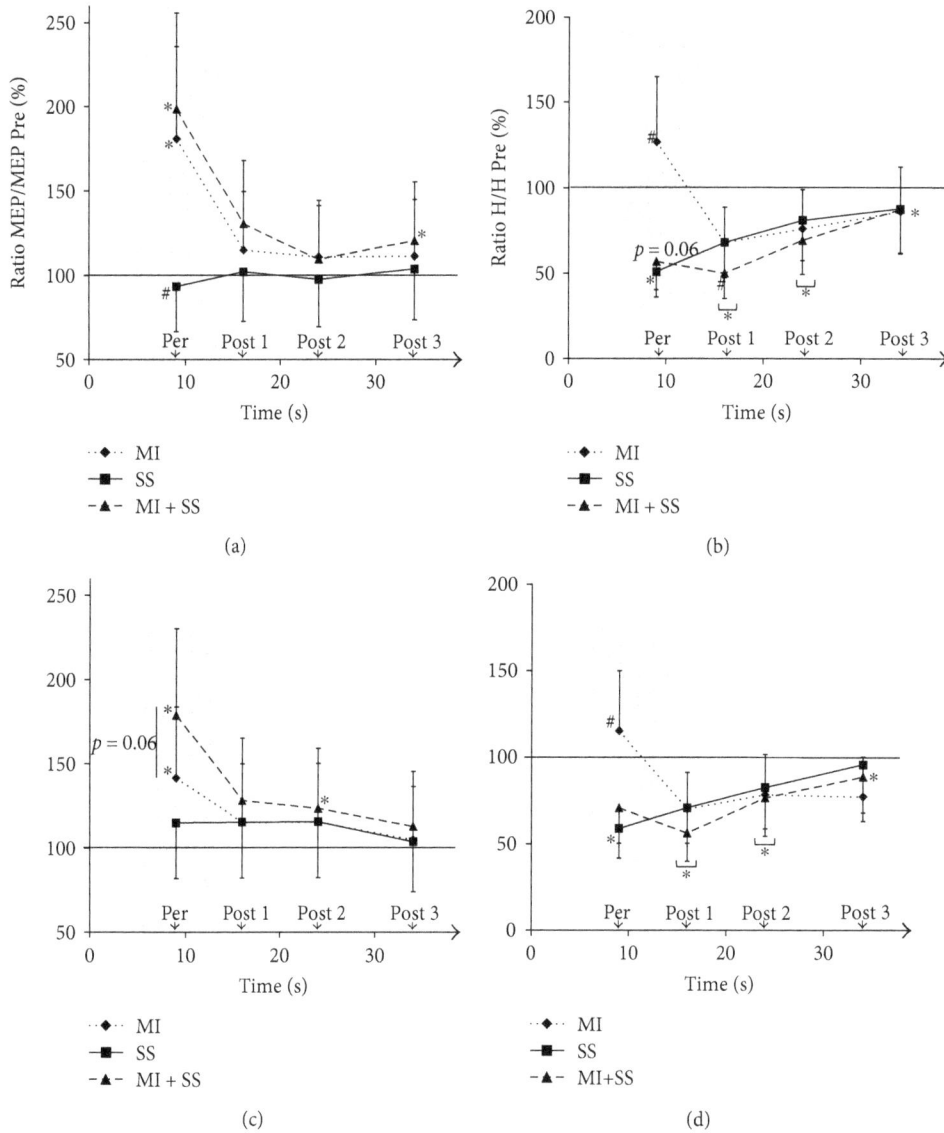

FIGURE 3: Normalized MEP and H-reflex amplitude. Values recorded in SOL (a and b) and MG (c and d) muscles. MEP amplitude increased when imagining (MI and MI + SS at Per). H-reflex amplitude decreased with SS (SS and MI + SS at Per) and progressively returned to baseline, except for MI + SS. *Significantly different from Pre test (baseline). #Significantly different from other conditions at the same stimulation time.

14.4 ± 10.0%, and 11.0 ± 6.1% of M_{max}, respectively, for the SOL muscle and 8.9 ± 8.9%, 8.4 ± 6.1%, and 6.9 ± 5.4% of M_{max}, respectively, for the MG muscle.

For the SOL muscle, a typical H-reflex trace of one participant was represented in Figure 2. The main results were illustrated in Figure 3(b). The nonparametric related samples Friedman's two-way ANOVA by ranks revealed an effect ($\chi^2 = 44.93$, $p < 0.001$). The Wilcoxon signed-rank tests demonstrated that H-reflex amplitude at Per was significantly depressed in comparison to baseline when SS was applied alone (SS task: −52 ± 54%, $p = 0.021$) and almost depressed when SS was combined with MI (MI + SS task: −47 ± 48%, $p = 0.062$). At Post 1 and 2, H-reflex was still depressed and returned to baseline at Post 3 for the SS task (−12 ± 27%, $p > 0.05$) but not for MI + SS

(−13% ± 20%, $p = 0.006$). Note that H-reflex amplitude was not modulated during MI ($p > 0.05$).

For the MG muscle, a typical H-reflex trace of one participant was represented in Figure 2. The main results were illustrated in Figure 3(d). The nonparametric related samples Friedman's two-way ANOVA by ranks revealed an effect ($\chi^2 = 32.67$, $p < 0.01$). The Wilcoxon signed-rank tests demonstrated that H-reflex amplitude at Per was depressed when SS was applied alone (SS task: −41 ± 42%, $p = 0.050$) but not when SS was combined with MI (MI + SS task: −30 ± 58%, $p > 0.05$). At Post 1 and 2, H-reflex was still depressed, but returned to baseline at Post 3 for SS (−4% ± 19%, $p > 0.05$) but not for MI + SS (−11% ± 26%, $p = 0.016$). Note that H-reflex amplitude was not modulated during MI ($p > 0.05$).

For both muscles, the results demonstrated a decrease of H-reflex amplitude at Post 1 in all conditions. For MI + SS and SS alone, this decrease may be due to the stimulation frequency, inducing homosynaptic post activation depression (HPAD) related to the repetitive stimulation of afferent fibers. However, after MI alone, this decrease may be related to a stimulation effect at Per and/or a condition effect. Experiment 2 was designed to examine the influence of successive PNS and condition effects on H-reflex amplitude.

3.2. Experiment 2. The main results of exp. 2 were illustrated in Figures 4(a) and 4(b), for the SOL and MG muscles, respectively.

For the SOL muscle, the nonparametric related samples Friedman's two-way ANOVA by ranks revealed an effect ($\chi^2 = 11.93$, $p < 0.05$). The Wilcoxon signed-rank tests showed that H-reflex amplitudes at Per and at Post were depressed in comparison to baseline when participants were at rest ($-11 \pm 10\%$, $p = 0.036$ and $-13 \pm 18\%$, $p = 0.017$, resp.). For the MI task, H-reflex at Per, that is, when imagining, almost increased compared to baseline ($+13 \pm 28\%$, $p = 0.069$) and was not different from baseline at Post ($-14\% \pm 19\%$, $p > 0.05$).

For the MG muscle, the rmANOVA revealed an interaction between *stimulation* and *task* ($F_{1,7} = 9.24$, $p = 0.003$). Bonferroni's post hoc test revealed that H-reflex amplitudes at Per, that is, when imagining, and at Post were not significantly modulated in comparison to baseline (MI task: $+12.8 \pm 13.9\%$, $p > 0.05$; $-8\% \pm 11\%$, $p > 0.05$, resp.). Note that H-reflex for the rest task was not modulated ($p > 0.05$).

4. Discussion

This study was designed to investigate how MI combined with SS modulated corticospinal and spinal excitabilities. The results confirmed that corticospinal excitability increased during MI and MI + SS but not during SS. During MI + SS, MEP amplitude was almost greater than that during MI alone, for MG muscle. On the contrary, spinal excitability was sensitive to SS, during which H-reflex was depressed. However, it was not modulated during MI associated or not with SS. Interestingly, the modulation of corticospinal and spinal excitabilities was muscle dependent.

4.1. Corticospinal Excitability. For both muscles, MEP amplitude only increased when participants imagined the plantar-flexion contractions, and not after imagining, which confirms that MI modulates CSE in a temporal-specific manner [20–23].

MEP amplitude during SS was similar to that at rest, showing that the excitatory afferent inputs induced by SS did not affect the corticomotoneuronal transmission efficacy. This result is in accordance with previous studies that applied a short SS duration below the motor threshold [24]. Other experiments using a longer SS duration showed an increase of MEP amplitude [25–28]. Therefore, it appears that the duration of SS seems to play a crucial role to modulate CSE.

MI associated with SS had a tendency to increase CSE to a greater extent in comparison to MI only for MG muscle. This

finding may be due to an increase of afferent inputs into M1 at the time of the stimulation. Indeed, through afferent inputs, SS activates the somatosensory cortex (S1), which can mediate the primary motor cortex (M1) activity leading to increased CSE [13, 29]. However, CSE was not modulated by the SS alone, suggesting that SS must be combined with MI to facilitate the interactions between M1 and S1. An alternative explanation would involve the interaction of MI and SS at the spinal level. Grosprêtre et al. [4] recently showed that MI induces a subliminal motor command that modulates the influence of the afferent input to motoneurons at the spinal level, via primary afferent depolarizing interneurons. This interaction likely modulates CSE. The tendency for CSE to increase was not observed for the SOL muscle, suggesting that the difference with the MG muscle could be explained by the amount of afferent inputs recruited during SS at the spinal level.

4.2. Spinal Excitability. For both muscles, our results confirmed that spinal excitability was not modulated when imagining [4].

During SS, spinal excitability was depressed. It was demonstrated that the repetition of stimulations decreased the H-reflex amplitude [17] due to a smaller neurotransmitter amount available at the Ia afferent-alpha motoneuron synapse [16]. These inhibitions may originate from the homosynaptic post activation depression effect, the primary afferent depolarization effect, and/or the refractory period of Ia-afferent neurons [30].

When associating MI and SS, the spinal excitability of MG was no longer depressed from baseline. For the SOL muscle, the spinal excitability was less reduced in comparison to SS alone. It seems likely that MI may compensate the inhibitory effects induced by SS. The different behavior between the two muscles could be explained by the amount of afferent inputs recruited during SS. This hypothesis is supported by a lower quantity of neuromuscular spindles in the MG than in the SOL muscle [31, 32] inducing less presynaptic inhibition at the spinal level when SS is applied [33, 34]. Therefore, the subliminal motor command generated during MI that reaches the spinal level [4, 31] may compensate to a greater extent the transmission efficiency between Ia-afferents and motoneurons in the MG muscle. This was observed by a greater reduction of inhibition during MI + SS in this muscle, in comparison to the SOL muscle (Figures 3(b) and 3(d)).

Note that spinal excitability was depressed at posttest right after each task and progressively returned to baseline values. This reduction may be due to successive stimulations elicited to induce H-reflexes and especially to the interstimulation interval, that is, less than 10 seconds inducing presynaptic inhibitions at the spinal level [17]. Indeed, the results of experiment 2 demonstrated that, while participants stayed at rest, the spinal excitability was depressed at Per and Post stimulations in comparison to baseline, with an interstimulus interval of 9 seconds and 7 seconds, respectively. Interestingly, we observed, in experiment 1, a greater decrease of spinal excitability for the MI + SS task at Post 1, that is, right after the task. This greater reduction in the amplitude of

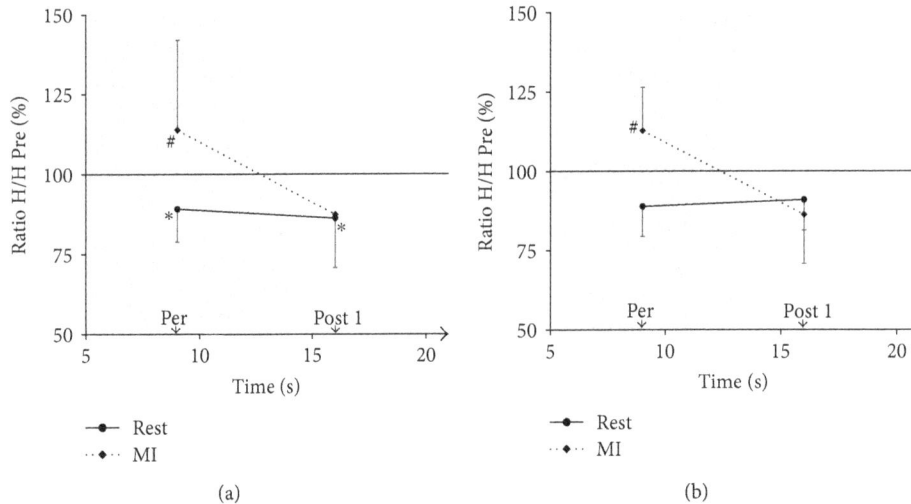

(a)   (b)

FIGURE 4: Normalized H-reflex amplitude. Values for SOL (a) and MG (b) muscles. At rest, H-reflex amplitude decreased at Per and Post 1 for the SOL but not for the MG. During the MI task, H-reflex amplitude was not modulated for both muscles. *Significantly different from Pre test (baseline). #Significantly different from other conditions at the same stimulation time.

the H-reflex after MI + SS may be related to the fact that MI compensates for SS-related inhibitions by reducing presynaptic inhibitions. This mechanism may induce a greater release of neurotransmitters, resulting in a reduction in the amount of neurotransmitters available to respond to Post 1 stimulation versus MI and SS tasks alone.

5. Conclusion

The combination of MI and SS exacerbated the effect of MI on corticospinal and spinal excitabilities depending on the afferent inputs elicited by SS at the spinal level. The results of this study were obtained during a single session when the participants were voluntarily engaged in the imagery task with or without SS. We know that MI training or repetitive somatosensory stimulation increases motor performance, specifically muscle strength. It would be of interest to test whether the repetition of the combination of MI and SS facilitates motor performance in comparison to MI and SS alone and to understand the underlying mechanisms.

Conflicts of Interest

The authors declare that they have no conflicts of interest.

References

[1] J. Decety, "The neurophysiological basis of motor imagery," *Behavioural Brain Research*, vol. 77, no. 1-2, pp. 45–52, 1996.

[2] E. Gerardin, A. Sirigu, S. Lehéricy et al., "Partially overlapping neural networks for real and imagined hand movements," *Cerebral Cortex*, vol. 10, no. 11, pp. 1093–1104, 2000.

[3] M. Lotze, P. Montoya, M. Erb et al., "Activation of cortical and cerebellar motor areas during executed and imagined hand movements: an fMRI study," *Journal of Cognitive Neuroscience*, vol. 11, no. 5, pp. 491–501, 1999.

[4] S. Grosprêtre, F. Lebon, C. Papaxanthis, and A. Martin, "New evidence of corticospinal network modulation induced by

motor imagery," *Journal of Neurophysiology*, vol. 115, no. 3, pp. 1279–1288, 2016.

[5] C. Ruffino, C. Papaxanthis, and F. Lebon, "Neural plasticity during motor learning with motor imagery practice: review and perspectives," *Neuroscience*, vol. 341, pp. 61–78, 2017.

[6] A. D. Fourkas, V. Bonavolontà, A. Avenanti, and S. M. Aglioti, "Kinesthetic imagery and tool-specific modulation of corticospinal representations in expert tennis players," *Cerebral Cortex*, vol. 18, no. 10, pp. 2382–2390, 2008.

[7] C. M. Stinear, W. D. Byblow, M. Steyvers, O. Levin, and S. P. Swinnen, "Kinesthetic, but not visual, motor imagery modulates corticomotor excitability," *Experimental Brain Research*, vol. 168, no. 1-2, pp. 157–164, 2006.

[8] N. Mizuguchi, M. Sakamoto, T. Muraoka et al., "Influence of somatosensory input on corticospinal excitability during motor imagery," *Neuroscience Letters*, vol. 514, no. 1, pp. 127–130, 2012.

[9] M. Reiser, D. Büsch, and J. Munzert, "Strength gains by motor imagery with different ratios of physical to mental practice," *Frontiers in Psychology*, vol. 2, p. 194, 2011.

[10] K. Saito, T. Yamaguchi, N. Yoshida, S. Tanabe, K. Kondo, and K. Sugawara, "Combined effect of motor imagery and peripheral nerve electrical stimulation on the motor cortex," *Experimental Brain Research*, vol. 227, no. 3, pp. 333–342, 2013.

[11] F. Kaneko, T. Hayami, T. Aoyama, and T. Kizuka, "Motor imagery and electrical stimulation reproduce corticospinal excitability at levels similar to voluntary muscle contraction," *Journal of NeuroEngineering and Rehabilitation*, vol. 11, no. 1, p. 94, 2014.

[12] V. Di Lazzaro and U. Ziemann, "The contribution of transcranial magnetic stimulation in the functional evaluation of microcircuits in human motor cortex," *Frontiers in Neural Circuits*, vol. 7, p. 18, 2013.

[13] M. P. Veldman, I. Zijdewind, S. Solnik et al., "Direct and crossed effects of somatosensory electrical stimulation on motor learning and neuronal plasticity in humans," *European Journal of Applied Physiology*, vol. 115, no. 12, pp. 2505–2519, 2015.

[14] D. F. Collins, D. Burke, and S. C. Gandevia, "Sustained contractions produced by plateau-like behaviour in human motoneurones," *The Journal of Physiology*, vol. 538, no. 1, pp. 289–301, 2002.

[15] J. Duclay, B. Pasquet, A. Martin, and J. Duchateau, "Specific modulation of corticospinal and spinal excitabilities during maximal voluntary isometric, shortening and lengthening contractions in synergist muscles," *The Journal of Physiology*, vol. 589, no. 11, pp. 2901–2916, 2011.

[16] C. Aymard, R. Katz, C. Lafitte et al., "Presynaptic inhibition and homosynaptic depression: a comparison between lower and upper limbs in normal human subjects and patients with hemiplegia," *Brain*, vol. 123, no. 8, pp. 1688–1702, 2000.

[17] E. P. Zehr, "Considerations for use of the Hoffmann reflex in exercise studies," *European Journal of Applied Physiology*, vol. 86, no. 6, pp. 455–468, 2002.

[18] J. Magladery and D. McDougal, "Electrophysiological studies of nerve and reflex activity in normal man. I. Identification of certain reflexes in the electromyogram and the conduction velocity of peripheral nerve fibres," *Bulletin of the Johns Hopkins Hospital*, vol. 86, no. 5, pp. 265–290, 1950.

[19] S. Bestmann and J. W. Krakauer, "The uses and interpretations of the motor-evoked potential for understanding behaviour," *Experimental Brain Research*, vol. 233, no. 3, pp. 679–689, 2015.

[20] S. Grosprêtre, C. Ruffino, and F. Lebon, "Motor imagery and cortico-spinal excitability: a review," *European Journal of Sport Science*, vol. 16, no. 3, pp. 317–324, 2015.

[21] L. Fadiga, G. Buccino, L. Craighero, L. Fogassi, V. Gallese, and G. Pavesi, "Corticospinal excitability is specifically modulated by motor imagery: a magnetic stimulation study," *Neuropsychologia*, vol. 37, no. 2, pp. 147–158, 1999.

[22] C. M. Stinear and W. D. Byblow, "Motor imagery of phasic thumb abduction temporally and spatially modulates corticospinal excitability," *Clinical Neurophysiology*, vol. 114, no. 5, pp. 909–914, 2003.

[23] F. Lebon, W. D. Byblow, C. Collet, A. Guillot, and C. M. Stinear, "The modulation of motor cortex excitability during motor imagery depends on imagery quality," *The European Journal of Neuroscience*, vol. 35, no. 2, pp. 323–331, 2012.

[24] T. Hortobagyi, J. L. Taylor, N. T. Petersen, G. Russell, and S. C. Gandevia, "Changes in segmental and motor cortical output with contralateral muscle contractions and altered sensory inputs in humans," *Journal of Neurophysiology*, vol. 90, no. 4, pp. 2451–2459, 2003.

[25] L. S. Chipchase, S. M. Schabrun, and P. W. Hodges, "Corticospinal excitability is dependent on the parameters of peripheral electric stimulation: a preliminary study," *Archives of Physical Medicine and Rehabilitation*, vol. 92, no. 9, pp. 1423–1430, 2011.

[26] M. C. Ridding, B. Brouwer, T. S. Miles, J. B. Pitcher, and P. D. Thompson, "Changes in muscle responses to stimulation of the motor cortex induced by peripheral nerve stimulation in human subjects," *Experimental Brain Research*, vol. 131, no. 1, pp. 135–143, 2000.

[27] M. C. Ridding, D. R. McKay, P. D. Thompson, and T. S. Miles, "Changes in corticomotor representations induced by prolonged peripheral nerve stimulation in humans," *Clinical Neurophysiology*, vol. 112, no. 8, pp. 1461–1469, 2001.

[28] D. McKay, R. Brooker, P. Giacomin, M. Ridding, and T. Miles, "Time course of induction of increased human motor cortex excitability by nerve stimulation," *Neuroreport*, vol. 13, no. 10, pp. 1271–1273, 2002.

[29] M. P. Veldman, N. A. Maffiuletti, M. Hallett, I. Zijdewind, and T. Hortobágyi, "Direct and crossed effects of somatosensory stimulation on neuronal excitability and motor performance in humans," *Neuroscience and Biobehavioral Reviews*, vol. 47, pp. 22–35, 2014.

[30] J. C. Dean, J. M. Clair-Auger, O. Lagerquist, and D. F. Collins, "Asynchronous recruitment of low-threshold motor units during repetitive, low-current stimulation of the human tibial nerve," *Frontiers in Human Neuroscience*, vol. 8, p. 1002, 2014.

[31] K. J. Tucker and K. S. Türker, "Muscle spindle feedback differs between the soleus and gastrocnemius in humans," *Somatosensory & Motor Research*, vol. 21, no. 3-4, pp. 189–197, 2004.

[32] K. J. Tucker, M. Tuncer, and K. S. Türker, "A review of the H-reflex and M-wave in the human triceps surae," *Human Movement Science*, vol. 24, no. 5-6, pp. 667–688, 2005.

[33] S. Grosprêtre and A. Martin, "H reflex and spinal excitability: methodological considerations," *Journal of Neurophysiology*, vol. 107, no. 6, pp. 1649–1654, 2012.

[34] J. Duclay and A. Martin, "Evoked H-reflex and V-wave responses during maximal isometric, concentric, and eccentric muscle contraction," *Journal of Neurophysiology*, vol. 94, no. 5, pp. 3555–3562, 2005.

8

Comparison of Adult Hippocampal Neurogenesis and Susceptibility to Treadmill Exercise in Nine Mouse Strains

Jong Whi Kim,[1] Sung Min Nam,[1,2] Dae Young Yoo,[1] Hyo Young Jung,[1] Il Yong Kim,[3] In Koo Hwang,[1,3] Je Kyung Seong,[1,3] and Yeo Sung Yoon[1,3]

[1]Department of Anatomy and Cell Biology, College of Veterinary Medicine, Research Institute for Veterinary Science, Seoul National University, Seoul 08826, Republic of Korea
[2]Department of Anatomy, College of Veterinary Medicine, Konkuk University, Seoul 05030, Republic of Korea
[3]KMPC (Korea Mouse Phenotyping Center), Seoul National University, Seoul 08826, Republic of Korea

Correspondence should be addressed to Je Kyung Seong; snumouse@snu.ac.kr and Yeo Sung Yoon; ysyoon@snu.ac.kr

Academic Editor: Clive R. Bramham

The genetic background of mice has various influences on the efficacy of physical exercise, as well as adult neurogenesis in the hippocampus. In this study, we investigated the basal level of hippocampal neurogenesis, as well as the effects of treadmill exercise on adult hippocampal neurogenesis in 9 mouse strains: 8 very commonly used laboratory inbred mouse strains (C57BL/6, BALB/c, A/J, C3H/HeJ, DBA/1, DBA/2, 129/SvJ, and FVB) and 1 outbred mouse strain (ICR). All 9 strains showed diverse basal levels of cell proliferation, neuroblast differentiation, and integration into granule cells in the sedentary group. C57BL/6 mice showed the highest levels of cell proliferation, neuroblast differentiation, and integration into granule cells at basal levels, and the DBA/2 mice showed the lowest levels. The efficacy of integration into granule cells was maximal in ICR mice. Treadmill exercise increased adult hippocampal neurogenesis in all 9 mouse strains. These results suggest that the genetic background of mice affects hippocampal neurogenesis and C57BL/6 mice are the most useful strain to assess basal levels of cell proliferation and neuroblast differentiation, but not maturation into granule cells. In addition, the DBA/2 strain is not suitable for studying hippocampal neurogenesis.

1. Introduction

Adult neurogenesis is a transient process for generating new neurons in the adult mammalian brain, which arise from the subgranular zone of the dentate gyrus and the subventricular zone of the lateral ventricles throughout adult life. Newly generated neural stem cells in the dentate gyrus pass through maturation stages, and the surviving neuroblasts migrate into the granular cell layer (GCL), where they finally become mature neurons [1–4]. Numerous studies have been conducted in adult hippocampal neurogenesis (AHN), including investigations into the pool of neural stem cells, the effects of neurotrophins, signaling pathways associated with AHN, the relationship of specific target genes with neural stem cells, and external conditions influencing AHN.

Major extrinsic factors influencing AHN are environmental enrichment, dietary moderation, antidepressant drugs, and exercise conditions [5, 6]. Physical exercise in particular has been shown to procure benefits for learning and memory and has also been shown to enhance long-term potentiation and AHN [7]. In addition, exercise training increases the size of the hippocampus and improves memory function in mice and aged humans [8, 9]. Exercise also has neuroprotective and therapeutic effects on neurodegenerative diseases, such as Parkinson's disease [10, 11], Huntington's disease [12], and Alzheimer's disease [13]. However, these studies have investigated AHN using a single inbred mouse strain or neurodegenerative disease models.

Strain-dependent genotypes and phenotypes from genetic background have been studied for decades. Using a genome sequencing approach, large differences in genome sequences were found among 17 inbred mouse strains, which could influence phenotypes, gene regulation, and functional variants [14]. In a study of genetic influence on hippocampal neurogenesis, the level of cell proliferation of neural progenitor cells in the subgranular zone of the dentate gyrus was different in 4 mouse strains: C57BL/6, BALB/c, CD1, and 129/SvJ. In another study, an analysis of 4 mouse strains, *Mus spretus*, A/J, C3H/HeJ, and DBA/2J, found that the inherent genetic background determined the basal level of AHN and the composition cell type [3, 15]. Furthermore, the 129/SvEms, 129.SvJ, C57, and C3H strains all showed different susceptibilities to kainic acid administration [16]. In addition, inbred strains performed differently on memory tasks, such as the Morris water maze and the contextual fear conditioning test [17]. More specifically, the 129S6/SvEv, 129T2/SvEmsJ, C57BL/6, and C57BL/10 strains performed well on the memory tests, whereas the BALB/c strain exhibited intermediate performance [17]. The DBA/2 strain, on the other hand, performed poorly, which is likely due to an impairment in hippocampal function, regardless of visual acuity [17]. Thus, differences in the background genes of mouse strains result in diverse phenotypes in hippocampus-dependent behavior and AHN [18, 19].

Among inbred mouse strains, markers for cell proliferation and neuroblast differentiation in AHN are expressed differentially in the C57BL/6, ICR, and BALB/c mouse strains [20], and genetic differences influence the population of neural stem cells in a strain-dependent manner. In our previous study, we showed that the C57BL/6 strain showed a high susceptibility to a high-fat diet as well as body weight gain and a significant reduction in cell proliferation and neuroblast differentiation, whereas the C3H/He strain is relatively resistant to a high-fat diet and body weight gain [21]. There is no established grade list, however, of the pool of neural stem cells and AHN in commonly used inbred strains, such as 129/SvJ, C57BL/6, BALB/c, A/J, and other *Mus musculus* subspecies.

In the present study, we investigated the basal level of cell proliferation, neuroblast differentiation, and cell survival in eight commonly used inbred mouse strains (C57BL/6, BALB/c, A/J, C3H/HeJ, DBA/1, DBA/2, 129/SvJ, and FVB) and one outbred mouse strain (ICR) to elucidate strain-specific differences in AHN. In addition, we also observed susceptibility to treadmill exercise and its enhancing effects on AHN in these 9 mouse strains to understand the phenotypic variation with genetic background and to determine the best mouse strain for use in AHN studies. Our data confirmed that there is diversity in the basal level of AHN in 9 different mouse strains, and also suggests avenues for future investigations into the mechanism of AHN, as well as the selection of proper mouse strains for genetically engineered mouse models.

2. Methods

2.1. Experimental Animals. Six-week-old male C57BL/6J, A/J, BALB/c, C3H/HeJ, FVB, 129/SvJ, DBA/1, DBA/2, and ICR mice were purchased from Japan SLC Inc. (Shizuoka, Japan). The animals were housed in a specific pathogen-free animal facility at 23°C with 60% humidity, a 12 h/12 h light/dark cycle, with ad libitum access to food and tap water. The handling and care of the animals conformed to guidelines established in compliance with current international laws and policies (NIH Guide for the Care and Use of Laboratory Animals, NIH Publication number 85-23, 1985, revised 1996) and were approved by the Institutional Animal Care and Use Committee (IACUC) of Seoul National University (SNU-120913-1-2). All experiments were conducted with an effort to minimize the number of animals used and the suffering caused by the procedures used in the study.

2.2. Exercise Condition. After a one-week acclimation to laboratory condition, each mouse strain was divided into 2 groups ($n = 5$ in each group): sedentary (SED) and exercise (EX) groups. The animals in the SED and EX groups were familiarized with treadmill exercise on a motorized treadmill (Model 1050 Exer3/6; Columbus Instruments, Columbus, OH, USA) for one week. In the EX group, running speed and durations were 10 m/min for 20 min on the first day, with an increase of 10 min/day until a total of 60 min/day was reached [22]. The animals in the SED group were placed on the treadmill without any running speed for the same period as the EX group. After familiarization, treadmill exercise was regularly practiced at 10 m/min for 60 min/day at 5 days/week for 4 weeks (Figure 1). This schedule was selected because a significant increase in proliferative activity and the production of new neurons in C57BL/6 and DBA/2J mice has been seen after 28 days of running, while only a small (not significant) and transient increase in proliferative activity was seen in these strains after 42 days of running [23].

2.3. Measurement of Body Weight and Food Intake. Body weight was measured at 10:00 AM every week on Wednesday and at the end of the experiment. Food intake was measured and corrected for spillage by weighing the jars containing food every week between 9:00 and 10:00 AM. Food intake was calculated from the average intake during the 4-week experimental period and expressed as g/mouse/week. Body weight gain was calculated as the difference in body weight between 12 weeks and 8 weeks.

2.4. Labeling of Newly Generated Cells. To label newly generated cells in the hippocampus, intraperitoneal injections of 5-bromo-2'-deoxyuridine (BrdU, 50 mg/kg, Sigma-Aldrich, St. Louis, MO, USA) were given to all mice twice daily (8:00, 20:00) for three days at the start of the exercise (when the mice were at eight weeks of age). Animals were euthanized at 12 weeks of age, one day after the last exercise (Figure 1).

2.5. Tissue Preparation. Animals ($n = 5$ in each group) were anesthetized by an intraperitoneal injection of 1 g/kg urethane (Sigma-Aldrich) and perfused transcardially with 0.1 M phosphate-buffered saline (PBS, pH 7.4) followed by 4% paraformaldehyde in 0.1 M PBS. The brains were then dissected and postfixed in the same fixative for 12 h. The brain tissues were cryoprotected by infiltration with 30% sucrose overnight. Thirty-micrometer-thick brain sections were serially sectioned in the coronal plane using a cryostat

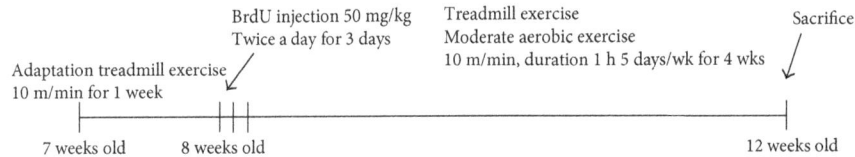

FIGURE 1: Experimental design of the present study. Treadmill exercise was adopted in 7-week-old mice for 1 week, and treadmill exercise was conducted for 4 weeks with 10 m/min speed for 1 h. During the first 3 days of exercise, BrdU was injected twice a day (at 8:00 AM and 8:00 PM) intraperitoneally to label newborn neural stem cells.

(Leica, Wetzlar, Germany) and collected in six-well plates containing PBS at −20°C for further processing.

2.6. Immunohistochemistry.

To obtain accurate data for immunohistochemistry, the free-floating sections from all animals were processed carefully under the same conditions. For each animal, tissue sections were selected from between 1.46 mm and 2.46 mm posterior to the bregma by referring to the mouse atlas by Franklin and Paxinos [24]. Ten sections, 90 μm apart, were sequentially treated with 0.3% hydrogen peroxide (H_2O_2) in PBS for 30 min and 10% normal goat or rabbit serum in 0.05 M PBS for 30 min. They were then incubated with a rabbit anti-Ki67 antibody (1:1000; Abcam, Cambridge, UK) or goat anti-DCX antibody (1:50; Santa Cruz Biotechnology, Santa Cruz, CA, USA) overnight at 25°C and subsequently treated with either a biotinylated goat anti-rabbit IgG or a rabbit anti-goat IgG and a streptavidin-peroxidase complex (1:200, Vector Labs, Burlingame, CA, USA). Sections were visualized by reaction with 3,3′-diaminobenzidine tetrachloride (Sigma) in 0.1 M Tris-HCl buffer (pH 7.2) and dehydrated and mounted in Canada balsam (Kanto Chemical, Tokyo, Japan) onto gelatin-coated slides.

2.7. Immunofluorescence.

For BrdU and NeuN double immunofluorescence, the sections were treated with 2 N HCl for 30 min at 37°C and were incubated with a mixture of mouse anti-NeuN (1:1000; Millipore, Temecula, CA, USA) and rat anti-BrdU (1:200; Abd Serotec, Bio-Rad Laboratories, Inc., Grand Island, NY, USA) for 2 h at 25°C, followed by overnight incubation at 4°C. After washing with PBS, the sections were subsequently incubated with secondary antibodies, FITC-conjugated goat anti-mouse IgG (1:100; Jackson ImmunoResearch, PA, USA), and Cy3-conjugated goat anti-rat IgG (1:100; Jackson ImmunoResearch, PA, USA), for 2 h. After that, the sections were mounted on silane-coated slides with DAPI-containing mounting medium (Vector Labs, CA, USA) for nuclei staining.

2.8. Microscopic Analysis.

Two independent masked investigators counted Ki67-, DCX-, BrdU-, or BrdU/NeuN-labeled cells in the dentate gyrus at 400x magnification under a light microscope (BX51, Olympus, Tokyo, Japan). All Ki67-, DCX-, BrdU-, or BrdU/NeuN-labeled cells were counted bilaterally in 10 sections (90 μm apart from each other) across the entire dentate gyrus between 1.46 mm and 2.46 mm posterior to the bregma by referring to the mouse atlas by Franklin and Paxinos [24].

2.9. Statistical Analysis.

Statistical analysis was performed using SPSS V.20.1 (IBM Corporation, Armonk, NY, USA). Experimental groups were compared using two-way analysis of variance (ANOVA), followed by a least significant difference (LSD) post hoc analysis.

3. Results

3.1. Effects of Strain and Exercise on Body Weight and Food Intake.

At eight weeks of age, each inbred mouse strain showed similar body weight, except for the outbred ICR strain, which had a significantly higher body weight than the inbred mice (Figure 2(a)). The body weight of the animals tended to increase with age by 12 weeks in both the SED and EX groups, with only the EX group of the 129/SvJ strain showing a significant increase in body weight compared to the SED group of the same strain (Figures 2(a) and 2(b)). Statistical analysis was also performed between-subjects effects in mouse strain, exercise, and mouse strain and exercise. F value and p value showed in Figures 2(a) and 2(b). Between-subjects effects of mouse strains, and exercise showed significance, but mouse strain and exercise have no significance. Among the inbred strains, there were significant differences in body weight gain between the EX and SED groups in the C57BL/6, 129/SvJ, and DBA/2 strains. There was a significant reduction in body weight gain in the C57BL/6 strain at the age of 12 weeks after exercise, whereas a significant increase in body weight gain was observed in the EX group of the 129/SvJ and DBA/2 mouse strains, as compared to that of the SED group (Figure 2(c)). To confirm the correlation of body weight gain with food intake, we analyzed food intake in the SED and EX groups. Between-subjects effects of mouse strains, exercise, and mouse strain and exercise showed significant, F value and p value showed in Figures 2(c) and 2(d). Exercise influenced food intake in some mouse strains; food intake significantly increased in the EX group of the C57BL/6, BALB/c, and DBA/1 strains compared to those in the SED group (Figure 2(d)). In contrast, the C57BL/6 strain showed a reverse correlation between exercise and body weight gain, and BALB/c and DBA/1 mice showed no significant change in body weight or food intake (Figures 2(c) and 2(d)).

3.2. Effects of Strain and Exercise on Cell Proliferation.

To observe the proliferation of hippocampal neural progenitor cells in the 9 mouse strains, as well as their susceptibility to the effects of 4 weeks of treadmill exercise, cells in the subgranular zone of the dentate gyrus were stained with the proliferation marker Ki67, and the mean number of

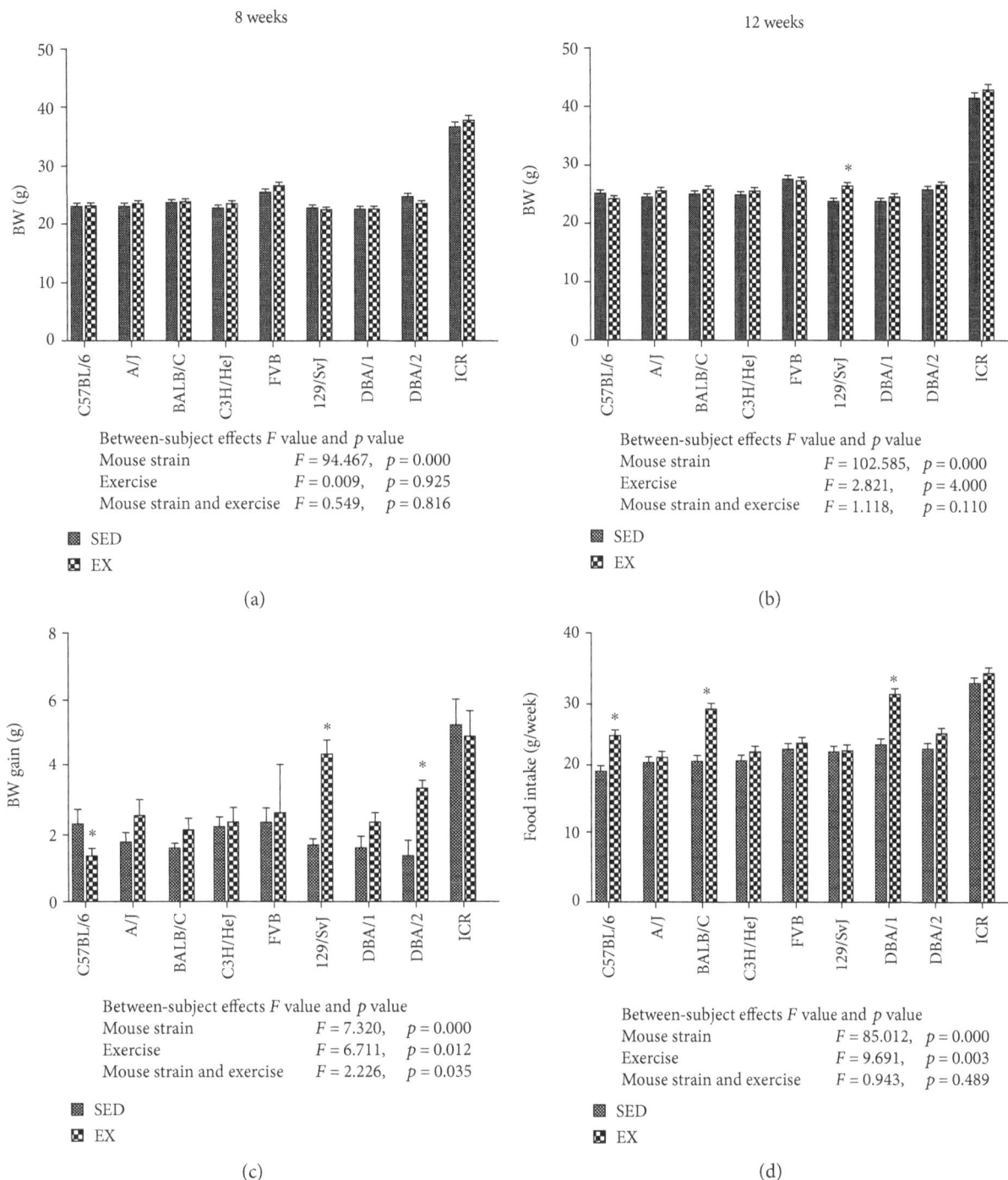

FIGURE 2: Body weight at the beginning (8 weeks of age) (a) and end (12 weeks of age) (b) of exercise and its control group ($n = 5$ per group). Body weight gains analysis was determined by calculating the difference in body weight at 12 weeks and 8 weeks (c). Food intake was calculated from the mean intake during the 4-week experimental period and expressed as g/mouse/week (d). F value and p value of between-subjects effects in mouse strain, exercise, and mouse strain and exercise showed in under the graph. ∗ indicates a significant difference between the sedentary and exercise groups ($p < 0.05$); data are shown as mean ± SEM.

Ki67 immunoreactive cells was calculated. In the SED groups, there were different population levels of Ki67-positive cells in the different mouse strains (Figure 3(b)). The number of Ki67-positive cells is shown in Table 1. Notably, the mean number of Ki67-positive cells was the highest in C57BL/6 mice (20.00 ± 1.58, Figures 3(a) and 3(b), Table 1) and the lowest in DBA/2 mice (2.40 ± 0.51,

Figures 3(a) and 3(b), Table 1). Similar numbers of Ki67-positive cells in the dentate gyrus were observed in other strains, including the AJ, 129/SvJ, C3H, ICR, FVB, and BALB/c strains (Table 1).

Compared to the SED group, the number of Ki67-positive cells was significantly increased in the dentate gyrus of the EX group in all mouse strains except for the DBA/2

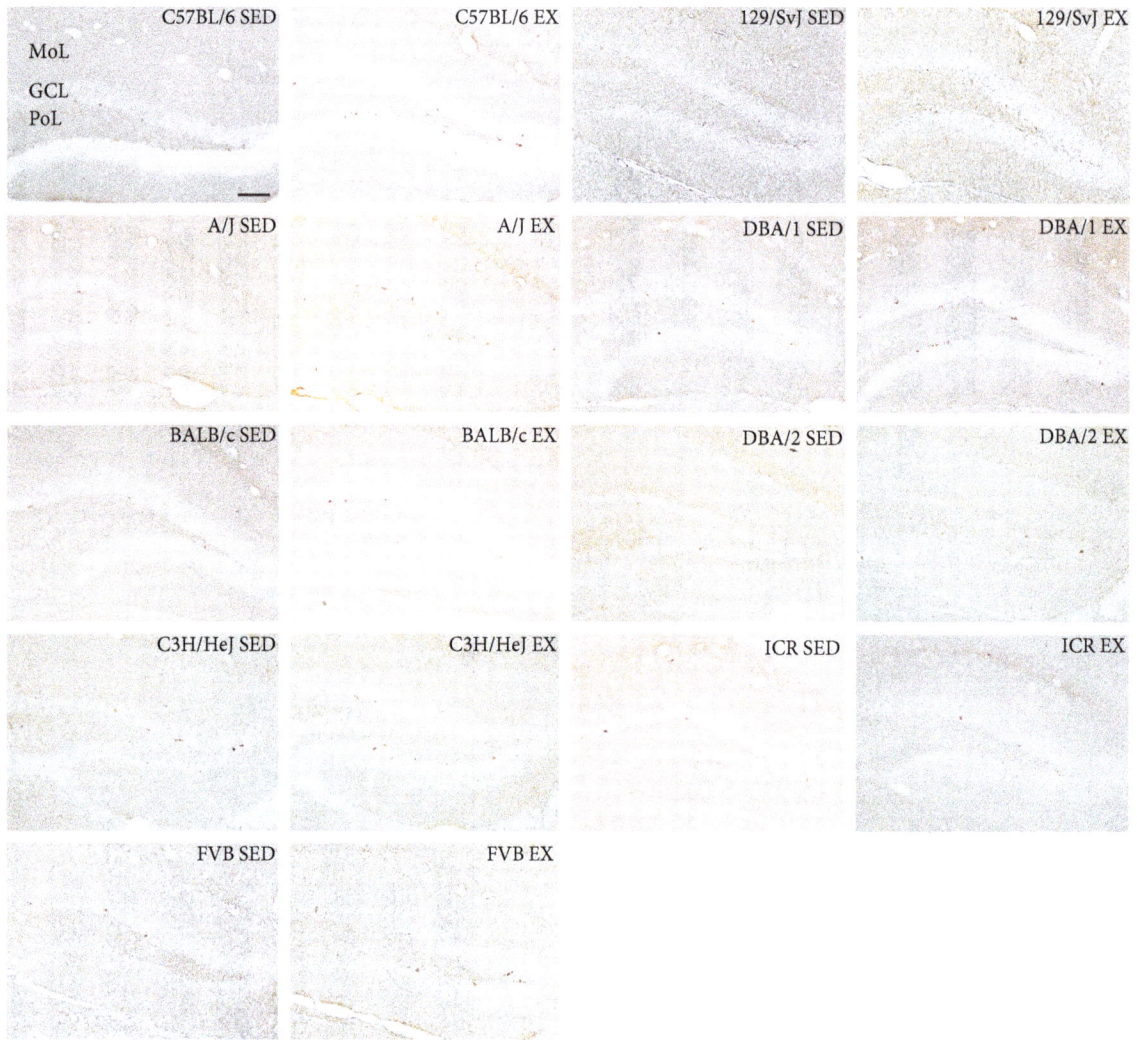

(a)

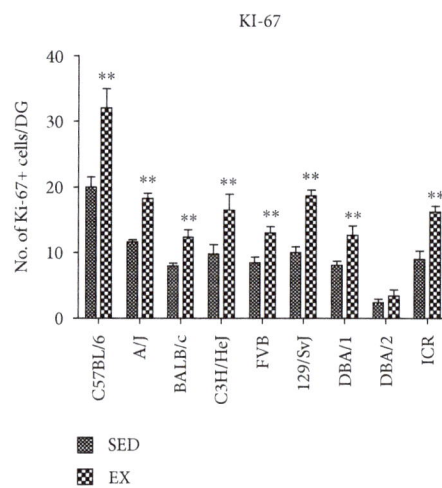

(b)

FIGURE 3: Immunohistochemistry for Ki67 in the dentate gyrus of sedentary and exercise mice of 9 different strains (a). GCL, granule cell layer; ML, molecular layer; PoL, polymorphic layer. Scale bar = 100 μm. Quantitative analysis of Ki67-positive nuclei per section in sedentary and exercise mice (b) ($n = 5$ per group); $**$ indicates a significant difference between the sedentary and exercise groups ($p < 0.01$). Data are shown as mean ± SEM.

TABLE 1: Summary of NSC proliferation, differentiation, and number of mature neurons across mouse strains, and efficacy of integration into mature neurons from proliferating NSCs and differentiating neuroblasts. (n = 5 per group); * indicates a significant difference between the sedentary and exercise groups ($p < 0.05$), and ** indicates a significant difference between the sedentary and exercise groups ($p < 0.01$). Data are shown as mean ± SEM. NSC: neural stem cells.

	Strains	CB7BL/6J Mean	SE	A/J Mean	SE	BALB/c Mean	SE	C3H/HeJ Mean	SE	FVB Mean	SE	129/Svj Mean	SE	DBA/1 Mean	SE	DBA/2 Mean	SE	ICR Mean	SE	Total increase %
Ki-67 Proliferation	SED	20.00	±1.58	11.60	±0.24	8.00	±0.32	9.80	±1.46	8.40	±0.93	10.00	±0.89	8.00	±0.71	2.40	±0.51	9.00	±1.22	
	EX	32.20	±2.97	18.20	±0.86	12.40	±1.03	16.40	±2.48	13.00	±0.95	18.60	±0.93	12.60	±1.44	3.40	±0.98	16.20	±0.86	
	Increase %	161.00	**	156.90	**	155.00	**	167.35	**	154.76	**	186.00	**	157.50	**	141.67	ns	180.00	**	162.24
DCX Differentiation	SED	122.80	±4.86	73.60	±2.91	47.20	±2.40	73.40	±1.12	60.00	±2.77	79.20	±5.34	45.40	±4.79	31.00	±4.18	71.60	±5.91	
	EX	210.2	±4.89	108.6	±2.94	68.4	±3.49	97.2	±7.44	82.2	±6.26	127.2	±2.48	73.00	±1.10	45.20	±4.31	97.8	±3.62	
	Increase %	171.17	**	147.55	**	144.92	**	132.43	**	137.00	**	160.61	**	160.79	**	145.81	*	136.59	**	148.54
BrdU/ NeuN +/+ Maturation & survival	SED	21.20	±1.81	8.00	±1.05	5.00	±0.55	6.40	±1.03	6.00	±0.55	7.80	±0.73	4.40	±1.25	2.20	±0.37	12.40	±0.51	
	EX	31.00	±2.18	15.60	±1.69	10.80	±1.50	11.60	±1.21	9.00	±0.55	12.80	±1.65	9.80	±0.58	4.00	±0.77	18.20	±1.74	
	Increase %	146.23	**	195.00	**	216.00	*	181.25	*	150.00	*	164.10	*	222.73	*	181.82	ns	146.77	*	160.39

		CB7BL/6J Mean	SE	A/J Mean	SE	Balb/c Mean	SE	C3H/HeJ Mean	SE	FVB Mean	SE	129/Svj Mean	SE	DBA/1 Mean	SE	DBA/2 Mean	SE	ICR Mean	SE
Efficacy of cell maturation	SED-BrdU + NeuN/Ki67	106.00	±16.61	69.09	±9.16	63.17	±7.70	72.99	±18.17	76.31	±11.45	78.14	±3.55	56.39	±16.57	125.00	±46.10	154.08	±32.48
	EX-BrdU + NeuN/Ki67	96.27	±13.39	85.32	±7.87	91.78	±16.63	75.12	±11.02	70.51	±5.91	69.09	±8.97	80.87	±7.48	136.43	±20.40	113.38	±11.96
	EX/SED %	90.82		123.49		145.28		102.93		92.40		88.42		143.41		109.14		73.59	
	SED-BrdU + NeuN/DCX	17.26	±1.34	11.04	±1.65	10.60	±0.98	8.70	±1.39	9.96	±0.70	9.79	±0.36	9.80	±2.84	7.80	±1.71	17.70	±1.31
	EX-BrdU + NeuN/DCX	14.75	±10.64	14.34	±1.48	16.10	±2.47	12.16	±1.40	11.12	±0.82	10.06	±1.32	14.63	±0.87	8.62	±0.87	18.78	±2.16
	EX/SED %	85.43		129.95		151.85		139.72		111.63		102.75		149.40		110.52		106.13	121.57

strain (Table 1). The increase in percentage of Ki67-positive cells in the EX group for each mouse strain is shown in Table 1. Proliferating cells were most prominently increased (186.00%) in the 129/SvJ strain after exercise and were least prominently increased (141.60%) in the DBA/2 strain. Across all strains, the average number of Ki67-positive cells in the dentate gyrus in the EX group was increased to 162.24% compared to those in the SED group (Table 1). p value in the Supplementary Table 1 obtained from LSD post hoc analysis was compared to the cross-matched group. Statistical analysis was also performed between-subjects effects in mouse strain, exercise, and mouse strain and exercise. Between-subjects effects of mouse strains, exercise, and mouse strain and exercise showed significant. F value and p value were showed in Supplementary Table 1.

3.3. Effects of Strain and Exercise on Neuroblast Differentiation.

Doublecortin (DCX) immunohistochemistry, which is a marker for differentiated neuroblasts found in the subgranular zone of the dentate gyrus, was used to examine the basal levels of neuroblast differentiation and the effects of 4 weeks of treadmill exercise on the differentiation of hippocampal neural progenitor cells. In the SED group, the mean number of DCX-immunoreactive neuroblasts was different in each mouse strain (Figures 4(a) and 4(b)). The mean number of DCX-immunoreactive neuroblasts was highest in the C57BL/6J strain (128.80 ± 4.86, Figures 4(a) and 4(b), Table 1) and lowest in the DBA/2 strain (31.00 ± 4.18, Figures 4(a) and 4(b), Table 1). We divided the animal strains into 2 groups: those with an intermediate number of DCX-immunoreactive neuroblasts and those with a lower number. The number of DCX-immunoreactive neuroblasts in the intermediate group was 60.00–79.20 cells and included the 129/SvJ, AJ, C3H, ICR, and FVB strains (Figure 4(b) and Table 1). In contrast, the BALB/c, DBA/1, and DBA/2 strains had 45.40–47.20 DCX-immunoreactive neuroblasts and were included in the lower group (Figure 4(b) and Table 1).

Exercise significantly increased the number of DCX-immunoreactive neuroblasts in the dentate gyrus of all mouse strains compared to that of the respective strains in the SED group, as shown in Table 1. The increase in the number of DCX-immunoreactive neuroblasts was the most prominent (171.17% increase) in the C57BL/6 strain and the lowest (132.43%) in the C3H/HeJ strain (Table 1). p value in the Supplementary Table 2 obtained from LSD post hoc analysis was compared to the cross-matched group. Statistical analysis was also performed between-subjects effects in mouse strain, exercise, and mouse strain and exercise. Between-subjects effects of mouse strains, exercise, and mouse strain and exercise showed significance. F value and p value were showed in Supplementary Table 2.

3.4. Effects of Strain and Exercise on Integration into Mature Granule Cells.

In this study, we quantified BrdU and NeuN double-positive cells in the GCL to evaluate integration into mature granule cells in the dentate gyrus, and the mean number of NeuN and BrdU double-positive cells was calculated to compare the effects of strain and exercise on neurogenesis. In the SED group, BrdU and NeuN double-positive cells were the most abundant in the C57BL6 strain (21.20 ± 1.93, Figure 5(a) and Table 1) compared to other mouse strains and were the least abundant in the DBA/2 strain (2.20 ± 0.37, Figure 5(a) and Table 1). The ICR strain also had a high number of BrdU and NeuN double-positive cells in the dentate gyrus, while other strains had an intermediate number of BrdU and NeuN double-positive cells (Figures 5(a) and 5(b), Table 1). In the EX group, the number of NeuN/BrdU double-positive cells was significantly increased compared to those in the SED group in all 9 mouse strains, (Table 1). The average number of NeuN/BrdU double-positive cells across all mouse strains was 160.39%, and the increase in NeuN/BrdU double-positive cells was most prominent in the DBA/1 and A/J strains and least prominent in the C57BL/6 and ICR mice (Table 1).

The ratio of BrdU and NeuN double-positive cells and DCX-immunoreactive neuroblasts (BrdU + NeuN/DCX) was also calculated and is shown in Table 1. The ratio of BrdU + NeuN/DCX was highest (17.70%) in the ICR mice and lowest (7.80%) in the DBA/2 mice. In the EX group, the ratio of BrdU + NeuN/DCX was most prominent (18.78%) in the ICR mice, and least prominent (8.62%) in the DBA/2 mice (Table 1). The other mouse strains did not show any significant differences in this ratio between groups (Table 1). p value in the Supplementary Table 3 obtained from LSD post hoc analysis was compared to the cross-matched group. Statistical analysis was also performed between-subjects effects in mouse strain, exercise, and mouse strain and exercise. Between-subjects effects of mouse strains, exercise showed significant and exercise, and mouse strain and exercise have no significant. F value and p value were showed in Supplementary Table 3.

4. Discussion

Our basic objectives were to investigate the differences in cell proliferation, neuroblast differentiation, and integration into mature granule cells in the dentate gyrus and evaluate the efficacy of treadmill exercise on the population of AHN in 9 mouse strains. In this study, we selected 9 mouse strains that are widely used in biomedical research, as well as mouse family tree groups, which were classified with informative single nucleotide polymorphism markers sorted by genetic relationship, resulting in the organization of 102 strains into 7 family tree groups [25]. On the basis of this report, the A/J, BALB/c, and C3H/HeJ strains were included in group 1, the FVB strain in group 2, the C57BL/6J strain in group 4, the 129X1/SvJ strain in group 5, and the DBA strains in group 6 [25]. We observed that the level of cell proliferation and neuroblast differentiation in normal mice was C57BL/6 > (A/J = 129X1/SvJ) > C3H/HeJ > ICR > FVB > BALB/c > DBA/1 > DBA/2. In addition, the efficacy of integration into mature neurons was C57BL/6 > ICR > (A/J = 129X1/SvJ) > C3H/HeJ > FVB > BALB/c > DBA/1 > DBA/2. These results suggest that the potential for neurogenesis is most prominent in the C57BL/6 and ICR strains and are the lowest in the DBA/2 strain. These results are consistent with previous reports that

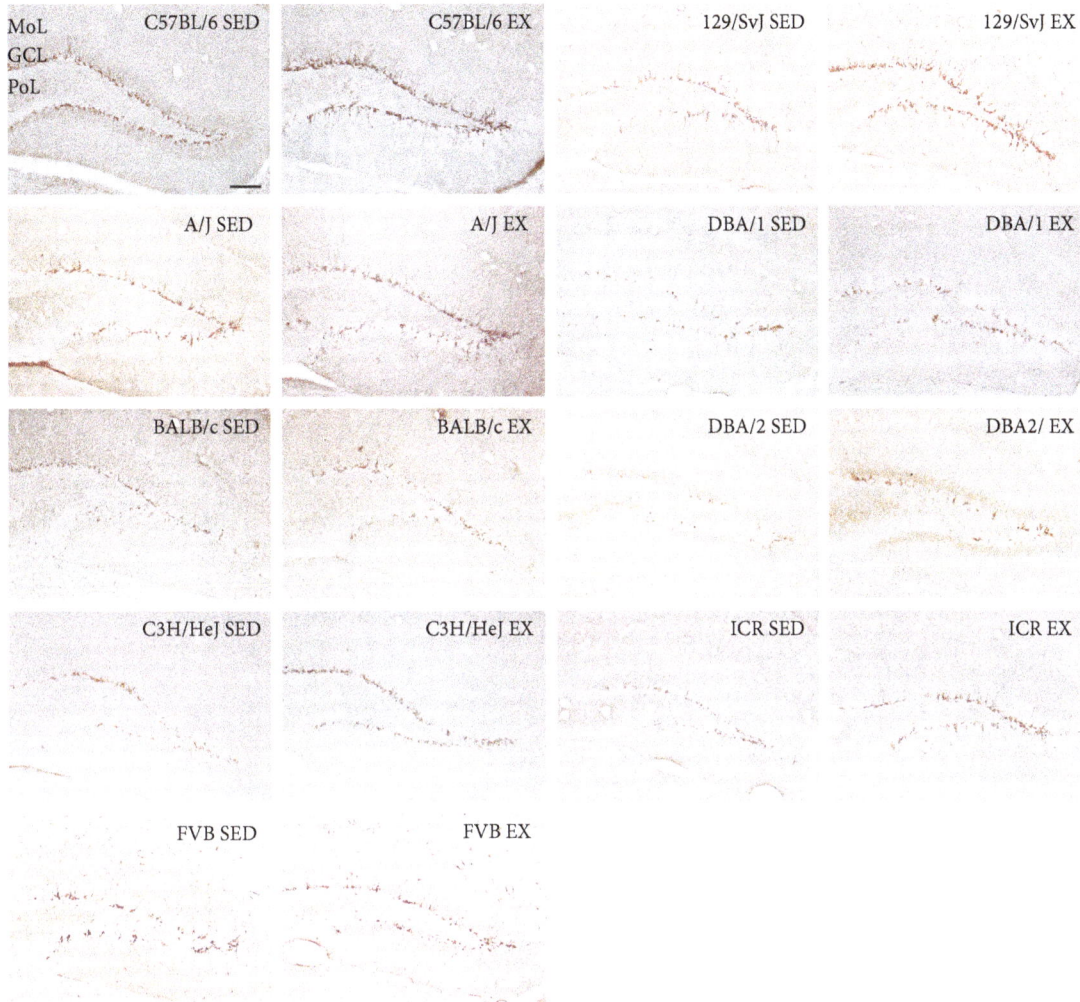

(a)

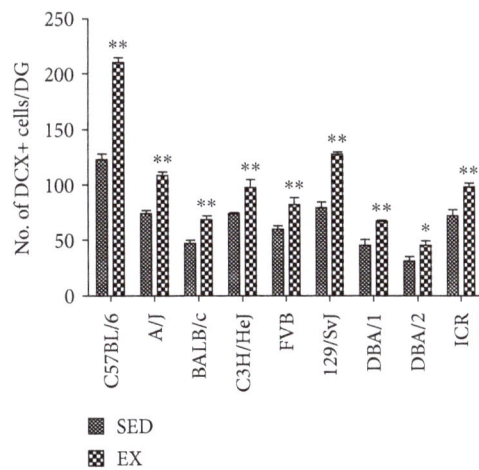

(b)

FIGURE 4: Immunohistochemistry for doublecortin (DCX) in the dentate gyrus of sedentary and exercise mice of 9 different strains (a). GCL, granule cell layer; ML, molecular layer; PoL, polymorphic layer. Scale bar = 100 μm. Quantitative analysis of DCX-immunoreactive neuroblasts per section in sedentary and exercise mice (b) ($n = 5$ per group); $*$ indicates a significant difference between the sedentary and exercise groups ($p < 0.05$), and $**$ indicates a significant difference between the sedentary and exercised groups ($p < 0.01$). Data are shown as mean ± SEM.

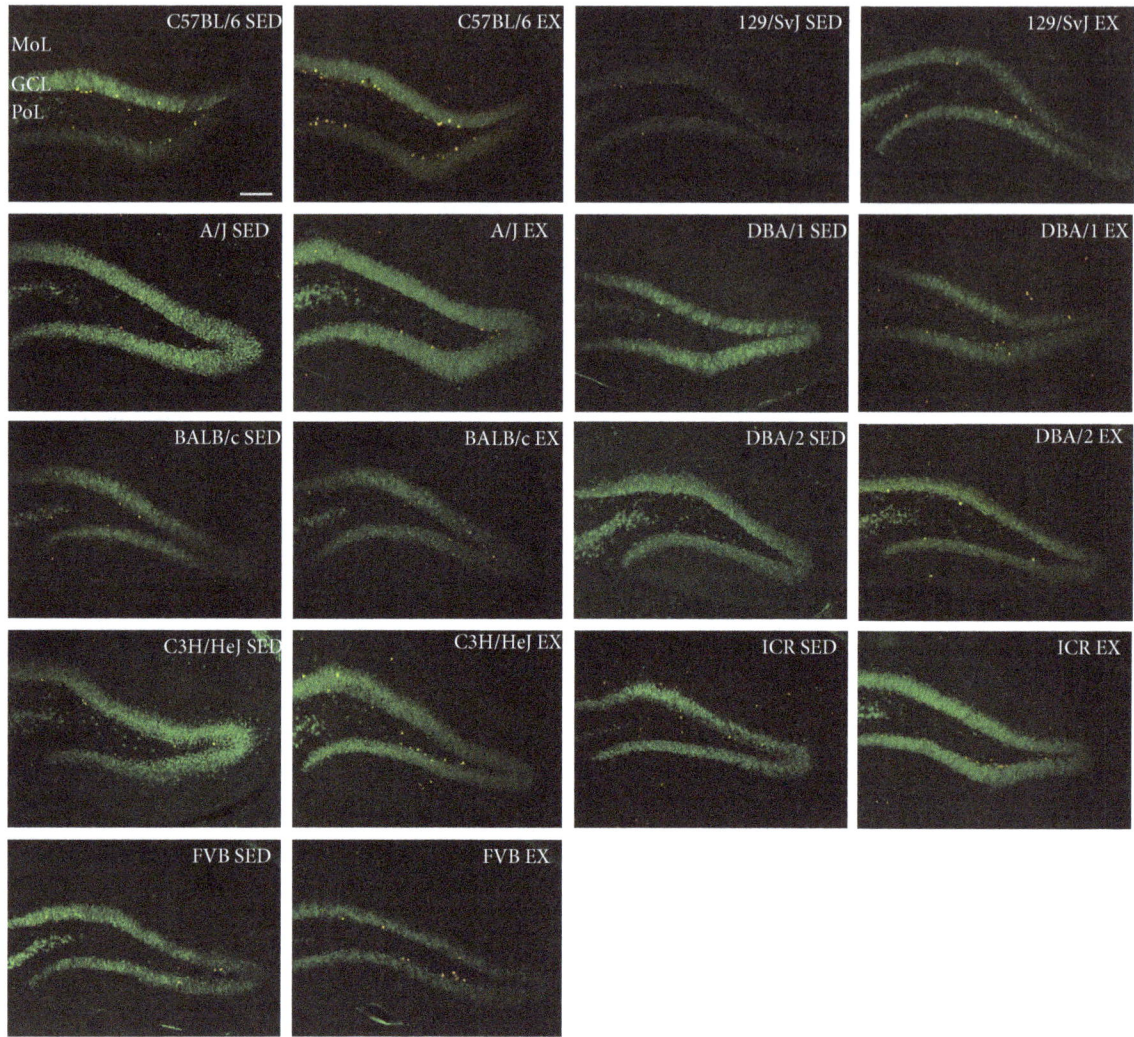

(a)

NeuN / BrdU +/+

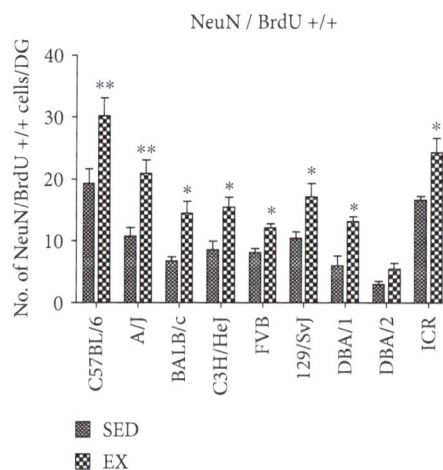

(b)

FIGURE 5: Double immunofluorescence staining for BrdU (red) and NeuN (green) in the dentate gyrus of sedentary and exercise mice of 9 different strains (a). GCL, granule cell layer; ML, molecular layer; PoL, polymorphic layer. Scale bar = 100 μm. Quantitative analysis of BrdU and NeuN double-labeled cells per section in sedentary and exercise mice (a) ($n = 5$ per group); quantitative cell number of BrdU (red) and NeuN (green) double-positive cells (b); $*$ indicates a significant difference between the sedentary and exercise groups ($p < 0.05$), and $**$ indicates a significant difference between the sedentary and exercise groups ($p < 0.01$). Data are shown as mean ± SEM.

precursor cell proliferation and net production of new neurons is strikingly higher in C57BL/6 strains [26–28]. On the other hand, we found that the DBA/1 and DBA/2 strains have a low capacity of cell proliferation and neuroblast differentiation in the dentate gyrus.

In the present study, ICR mice had a higher ratio of BrdU + NeuN/DCX positive cells than other strains. This result suggests that there is a higher efficacy for the integration of neuroblasts into mature neurons in ICR mice as compared to the other 8 inbred mouse strains. This result was consistent with a previous study that showed that proliferation was highest in the C57BL/6 strain, and the survival rate of newborn cells was highest in the ICR strain [3]. Other studies reported lower cell proliferation in FVB/NJ, ICR, and BALB/c mice compared to that in C57BL/6J strain [20, 29], with no differences in the number of surviving cells between C57BL/6J and FVB/NJ mice [29]. In addition, DCX-immunoreactive neuroblasts were more abundant in the C57BL/6 strain than in ICR and BALB/c mice [20]. However, they did not observe any significant differences in the number of Ki67- and DCX-immunoreactive cells between BALB/c and ICR mice [20]. This discrepancy with our data may be associated with differences in the experimental paradigm and the tissue processing methods that were used. In this study, we used our animals at 12 weeks of age and sectioned the tissue at $30\,\mu m$ thickness, while previous study used mice at 8 weeks of age and also sectioned with a thickness of $5\,\mu m$ and used paraffin embedding [20].

Several lines of evidence show that there are strain-dependent differences in various phenotypes, including hippocampus-dependent learning and memory and long-term potentiation (LTP) in the hippocampus. Electrophysiological and behavioral tests showed strain-dependent differences in LTP and hippocampal-dependent learning memory in C57BL/6, CBA/J, DBA/2J, and 129SvEms mice [30]. In particular, C57BL/6 mice exhibited long-lasting LPT, higher behavioral scores, and better long-term memory, while DBA/2J and CBA/J mice exhibited deficient long-term memory [30]. In the behavioral task in response to stimulation, phenotypic differences were observed across inbred mouse strains and was especially notable in the behavioral phenotypes of C57BL/6 and DBA/2 mice. In the open-field test and the Morris water maze task, C57BL/6 mice performed better than other inbred strains, and DBA/2 performed worse [30]. Other C57 substrains, such as C57BL/10, C57BR, and C57L, showed higher levels of spatial memory, longer-lasting LTP, and reduced anxiety behavior [30]. The observed behavioral and electrophysiological superiorities of C57BL/6 mice and the inferiorities of DBA/2 mice [30] are consistent with our data. Furthermore, our results showed that C57BL/6 mice have the largest NSC population and NSC lineage, while DBA/2 have a small NSC population and NSC lineage. Differences in AHN phenotype in 9 mouse strains are related to genuinely inherent genetic backgrounds, and differences in behavioral tests, LTP, and SNP markers may be correlated with our data in cell proliferation, differentiation, and survival.

There is evidence that newly generated neurons contribute to learning and memory function, synaptic formation,

and integration into the hippocampal network circuit [31–33]. New neurons in the hippocampus make distinctive contributions to hippocampal function; at different stages of maturation, cells of NSC lineage also play unique roles in hippocampal function [34]. Many studies have shown that newborn neurons in the hippocampus play potential roles in pattern separation and the erasure of memories [35]. Current studies have also suggested that adult born dentate granule neurons are involved in pattern separation and the reactivation of dentate granule neurons [36]. This series of studies indicates that AHN and the associated newly generated neurons, along with integrated neurons, contribute to hippocampal learning function. The previously mentioned strain-dependent differences in performance on behavioral tests, LTP [30], and basal levels of AHN might regulate hippocampal function and determine differences in hippocampus phenotype across mouse strains. Several hippocampal genes related to neurological phenotypes were different in eight inbred mouse strains (A/J, Balb/cByJ, C3H/HeJ, C57BL/6J, DBA/2J, FVB/NJ, SJL/J, and 129S1/SvImJ) [36]. These differences in gene expression could be related to phenotypic differences in the hippocampus [36]. In addition, the C57BL/6 strain performed well on memory tasks, including the Morris water maze and the contextual fear conditioning test, whereas the DBA/2 strain performed poorly on both tests [17]. In our study, strain-dependent differences in the level of AHN also suggest that there is an effect of genetic background, which may explain strain-dependent differences in memory function. Furthermore, the population differences of newborn and integrated neurons between 9 mouse strains may explain differences in the learning and memory functions of the hippocampus.

In the present study, we could not elucidate the factors that induce differences in neurogenesis among mouse strains. There has been a report, however, that pregnenolone sulfate (PREGS) level is an important factor in differences in neurogenesis that are observed among the strains. In the DBA/2 strain, PREGS levels are significantly lower than in the C57BL/6, BALB/c, ddY, and ICR strains, while dehydroepiandrosterone sulfate (DHEAS) concentrations in the DBA/2 strain were significantly higher than those in other strains [37]. PREGS is known to promote neurogenesis [38] and increase the survival of newly generated cells [39]. In addition, PREGS improves spatial cognitive performance, as well as ameliorates the reduction in the survival and maturation of newborn neuronal cells in a mouse model of Alzheimer's disease [40]. In contrast, DHEAS decreases activated Akt levels and increases apoptosis [41].

Neurogenesis in the hippocampus is regulated at each level of cell proliferation, neuroblast differentiation, and survival. Regulation of neurogenesis has been controlled in many paradigms, including physical exercise [8, 42]. Physical exercise enhances AHN and improves learning and memory and long-term potentiation [43]. In the present study, we observed that physical exercise significantly increased cell proliferation, neuroblast differentiation, and integration into mature neurons in 8 mouse strains, but not in the DBA/2 strain. This result is consistent with our previous studies in which we showed that physical exercise increases neurogenesis and the number of dendrites of DCX-immunoreactive neuroblasts in the dentate gyrus [44–46]. The responsiveness to physical exercise was most prominent in the BALB/c strain and least prominent in the C57BL/6 strain. This result is consistent with a previous study that showed that running for 43 days increases neurogenesis to the greatest extent in BALB/cByJ mice and to the least extent in C57BL/6 mice [28].

The mechanism by which exercise increases AHN may be explained by systemic improvement and changes in neurotrophins, signaling pathway-related ligands, and receptors. Exercise increases the growth of blood vessels in the hippocampus and blood flow in the dentate gyrus of the hippocampus [8, 47]. In addition, exercise training increases the size of the hippocampus and improves memory function and also reduces normal shrinking of the hippocampal region in aging humans [9]. Some investigations provide clues about androgenic mediation of neurogenesis; mild exercise increases neurogenesis through an increase in androgenic enzyme and androgenic receptor in the hippocampus [48]. Exercise increases the production and secretion of brain-derived neurotrophic factor (BDNF) and mRNA expression of its receptor, tyrosine kinase (TrkB), in the hippocampus [49–52]. Inhibiting the action of BDNF with TrkB-IgG blocks the effect of exercise on downstream pathways regulated by BDNF that are important for synaptic plasticity, including cAMP response elements binding protein (CREB) and synapsin I [50]. Other studies have also shown that physical exercise increases neurogenesis by the induction of insulin-like growth factor-1 and vascular endothelial growth factor [53, 54] and also has beneficial effects on LTP by altering N-methyl-D-aspartate subunit contribution [55].

In conclusion, we showed that there are basal strain-dependent differences in AHN, as well as differences in the effectiveness of physical exercise on AHN in 9 mouse strains. In normal mice, AHN was the most abundant in C57BL/6 mice and was the least abundant in DBA/2 mice. However, integration into mature neurons was most effective in ICR mice. The responsiveness to physical exercise was most prominent in the BALB/c strain, and least prominent in the C57BL/6 strain. Choosing the correct inbred mouse strain for transgenic or knockout mouse models for common neurological studies requires significant knowledge of the origin of phenotype for each inbred mouse strain. Furthermore, knowledge about the differences in phenotype between inbred mouse strains may contribute to our understanding of strain-dependent genetic influences on AHN and may therefore aid in choosing the correct approach for generating a suitable animal disease model. Our data showed varying degrees of basal AHN level in 9 mouse strains. Therefore, in the design of AHN studies, it is necessary to take into account the genetic differences related to AHN in each mouse strain. Our study also indicates that the level of physical activity in the study, such as treadmill exercise, should be taken into consideration. Current approaches to reveal the mechanism of AHN use reverse genetics, but the elucidation of clear mechanisms for differences in AHN requires a forward genetics approach with different mouse strains. These results provide information for the selection of appropriate mouse strains and the ideal conditions for AHN experiments in the field of neuroscience.

Conflicts of Interest

The authors declare that they have no conflict of interests.

Acknowledgments

This work was supported by the Basic Science Research Program through the National Research Foundation of Korea (NRF) funded by the Ministry of Education (NRF-2015R1D1A1A01059314) and by the Korea Mouse Phenotyping Project (NRF-2015M3A9D5A01076747) of the Ministry of Science, ICT, and Future Planning through the National Research Foundation (NRF), Korea. This study was partially supported by the Research Institute for Veterinary Science, Seoul National University.

Supplementary Materials

Table 1: statistical data of proliferative NCSs in 9 mouse strains and the effects of exercise. A red box indicates a significant increase and a blue box indicates a significant reduction as compared to the cross-matched group. p value in the table shown compared to the cross-matched group obtained from LSD post hoc analysis. Between-subject effects F value and p value of mouse strain, exercise, and mouse strain and exercise ($n = 5$ per group). Table 2: statistical data of differentiating neuroblasts in 9 mouse strains and the effects of exercise. A red box indicates a significant increase and a blue box indicates a significant reduction as compared to the cross-matched group. p value in the table shown compared to the cross-matched group obtained from LSD post hoc analysis. Between-subject effects F value and p value of mouse strain, exercise, and mouse strain and exercise ($n = 5$ per group). Table 3: statistical data of integrated neurons in 9 mouse strains and the effects of exercise. A red box indicates a significant increase and a blue box indicates a significant reduction as compared to the cross-matched group. p value in the table shown compared to the cross-matched group obtained from LSD post hoc analysis. Between-subject effects F value and p value of mouse strain, exercise, and mouse strain and exercise ($n = 5$ per group). (Supplementary Materials)

References

[1] F. H. Gage, "Mammalian neural stem cells," *Science*, vol. 287, no. 5457, pp. 1433–1438, 2000.

[2] F. H. Gage, "Neurogenesis in the adult brain," *The Journal of Neuroscience: The Official Journal of the Society for Neuroscience*, vol. 22, no. 3, pp. 612–613, 2002.

[3] G. Kempermann, H. G. Kuhn, and F. H. Gage, "Genetic influence on neurogenesis in the dentate gyrus of adult mice," *Proceedings of the National Academy of Sciences of the United States of America*, vol. 94, no. 19, pp. 10409–10414, 1997.

[4] T. D. Palmer, J. Takahashi, and F. H. Gage, "The adult rat hippocampus contains primordial neural stem cells,"

Molecular and Cellular Neurosciences, vol. 8, no. 6, pp. 389–404, 1997.

[5] G. Kempermann, H. G. Kuhn, and F. H. Gage, "More hippocampal neurons in adult mice living in an enriched environment," *Nature*, vol. 386, no. 6624, pp. 493–495, 1997.

[6] H. van Praag, G. Kempermann, and F. H. Gage, "Running increases cell proliferation and neurogenesis in the adult mouse dentate gyrus," *Nature Neuroscience*, vol. 2, no. 3, pp. 266–270, 1999.

[7] R. M. O'Callaghan, R. Ohle, and A. M. Kelly, "The effects of forced exercise on hippocampal plasticity in the rat: a comparison of LTP, spatial- and non-spatial learning," *Behavioural Brain Research*, vol. 176, no. 2, pp. 362–366, 2007.

[8] H. van Praag, T. Shubert, C. Zhao, and F. H. Gage, "Exercise enhances learning and hippocampal neurogenesis in aged mice," *The Journal of Neuroscience: The Official Journal of the Society for Neuroscience*, vol. 25, no. 38, pp. 8680–8685, 2005.

[9] K. I. Erickson, M. W. Voss, R. S. Prakash et al., "Exercise training increases size of hippocampus and improves memory," *Proceedings of the National Academy of Sciences of the United States of America*, vol. 108, no. 7, pp. 3017–3022, 2011.

[10] J. L. Bergen, T. Toole, R. G. Elliott 3rd, B. Wallace, K. Robinson, and C. G. Maitland, "Aerobic exercise intervention improves aerobic capacity and movement initiation in Parkinson's disease patients," *NeuroRehabilitation*, vol. 17, no. 2, pp. 161–168, 2002.

[11] A. M. Crizzle and I. J. Newhouse, "Is physical exercise beneficial for persons with Parkinson's disease?" *Clinical Journal of Sport Medicine*, vol. 16, no. 5, pp. 422–425, 2006.

[12] T. Y. Pang, N. C. Stam, J. Nithianantharajah, M. L. Howard, and A. J. Hannan, "Differential effects of voluntary physical exercise on behavioral and brain-derived neurotrophic factor expression deficits in Huntington's disease transgenic mice," *Neuroscience*, vol. 141, no. 2, pp. 569–584, 2006.

[13] P. A. Adlard, V. M. Perreau, V. Pop, and C. W. Cotman, "Voluntary exercise decreases amyloid load in a transgenic model of Alzheimer's disease," *The Journal of Neuroscience: The Official Journal of the Society for Neuroscience*, vol. 25, no. 17, pp. 4217–4221, 2005.

[14] T. M. Keane, L. Goodstadt, P. Danecek et al., "Mouse genomic variation and its effect on phenotypes and gene regulation," *Nature*, vol. 477, no. 7364, pp. 289–294, 2011.

[15] G. Kempermann and F. H. Gage, "Genetic influence on phenotypic differentiation in adult hippocampal neurogenesis," *Brain Research Developmental Brain Research*, vol. 134, no. 1-2, pp. 1–12, 2002.

[16] G. M. McKhann 2nd, H. J. Wenzel, C. A. Robbins, A. A. Sosunov, and P. A. Schwartzkroin, "Mouse strain differences in kainic acid sensitivity, seizure behavior, mortality, and hippocampal pathology," *Neuroscience*, vol. 122, no. 2, pp. 551–561, 2003.

[17] L. A. Schimanski and P. V. Nguyen, "Multidisciplinary approaches for investigating the mechanisms of hippocampus-dependent memory: a focus on inbred mouse strains," *Neuroscience and Biobehavioral Reviews*, vol. 28, no. 5, pp. 463–483, 2004.

[18] J. N. Crawley, J. K. Belknap, A. Collins et al., "Behavioral phenotypes of inbred mouse strains: implications and recommendations for molecular studies," *Psychopharmacology*, vol. 132, no. 2, pp. 107–124, 1997.

[19] G. W. Bothe, V. J. Bolivar, M. J. Vedder, and J. G. Geistfeld, "Genetic and behavioral differences among five inbred mouse strains commonly used in the production of transgenic and knockout mice," *Genes, Brain, and Behavior*, vol. 3, no. 3, pp. 149–157, 2004.

[20] J. S. Kim, J. Jung, H. J. Lee et al., "Differences in immunoreactivities of Ki-67 and doublecortin in the adult hippocampus in three strains of mice," *Acta Histochemica*, vol. 111, no. 2, pp. 150–156, 2009.

[21] I. K. Hwang, I. Y. Kim, D. W. Kim et al., "Strain-specific differences in cell proliferation and differentiation in the dentate gyrus of C57BL/6N and C3H/HeN mice fed a high fat diet," *Brain Research*, vol. 1241, pp. 1–6, 2008.

[22] C. W. Wu, Y. T. Chang, L. Yu et al., "Exercise enhances the proliferation of neural stem cells and neurite growth and survival of neuronal progenitor cells in dentate gyrus of middle-aged mice," *Journal of Applied Physiology*, vol. 105, no. 5, pp. 1585–1594, 2008.

[23] R. W. Overall, T. L. Walker, O. Leiter, S. Lenke, S. Ruhwald, and G. Kempermann, "Delayed and transient increase of adult hippocampal neurogenesis by physical exercise in DBA/2 mice," *PloS One*, vol. 8, no. 12, article e83797, 2013.

[24] K. B. J. Franklin and G. Paxinos, *Paxinos and Franklin's the Mouse Brain in Stereotaxic Coordinates*, Academic Press, an imprint of Elsevier, Amsterdam, 2013.

[25] P. M. Petkov, Y. Ding, M. A. Cassell et al., "An efficient SNP system for mouse genome scanning and elucidating strain relationships," *Genome Research*, vol. 14, no. 9, pp. 1806–1811, 2004.

[26] G. Kempermann and F. H. Gage, "Genetic determinants of adult hippocampal neurogenesis correlate with acquisition, but not probe trial performance, in the water maze task," *The European Journal of Neuroscience*, vol. 16, no. 1, pp. 129–136, 2002.

[27] G. Kempermann, E. J. Chesler, L. Lu, R. W. Williams, and F. H. Gage, "Natural variation and genetic covariance in adult hippocampal neurogenesis," *Proceedings of the National Academy of Sciences of the United States of America*, vol. 103, no. 3, pp. 780–785, 2006.

[28] P. J. Clark, R. A. Kohman, D. S. Miller, T. K. Bhattacharya, W. J. Brzezinska, and J. S. Rhodes, "Genetic influences on exercise-induced adult hippocampal neurogenesis across 12 divergent mouse strains," *Genes, Brain, and Behavior*, vol. 10, no. 3, pp. 345–353, 2011.

[29] P. E. Schauwecker, "Genetic influence on neurogenesis in the dentate gyrus of two strains of adult mice," *Brain Research*, vol. 1120, no. 1, pp. 83–92, 2006.

[30] P. V. Nguyen, T. Abel, E. R. Kandel, and R. Bourtchouladze, "Strain-dependent differences in LTP and hippocampus-dependent memory in inbred mice," *Learning & Memory (Cold Spring Harbor, New York)*, vol. 7, no. 3, pp. 170–179, 2000.

[31] N. Toni, D. A. Laplagne, C. Zhao et al., "Neurons born in the adult dentate gyrus form functional synapses with target cells," *Nature Neuroscience*, vol. 11, no. 8, pp. 901–907, 2008.

[32] N. Toni, E. M. Teng, E. A. Bushong et al., "Synapse formation on neurons born in the adult hippocampus," *Nature Neuroscience*, vol. 10, no. 6, pp. 727–734, 2007.

[33] C. Zhao, E. M. Teng, R. G. Summers Jr., G. L. Ming, and F. H. Gage, "Distinct morphological stages of dentate granule neuron maturation in the adult mouse hippocampus," *The Journal of Neuroscience*, vol. 26, no. 1, pp. 3–11, 2006.

[34] W. Deng, J. B. Aimone, and F. H. Gage, "New neurons and new memories: how does adult hippocampal neurogenesis affect learning and memory?" *Nature Reviews Neuroscience*, vol. 11, no. 5, pp. 339–350, 2010.

[35] Y. S-y, A. Li, and K.-F. So, "Involvement of adult hippocampal neurogenesis in learning and forgetting," *Neural Plasticity*, vol. 2015, Article ID 717958, 13 pages, 2015.

[36] K. McAvoy, A. Besnard, and A. Sahay, "Adult hippocampal neurogenesis and pattern separation in DG: a role for feedback inhibition in modulating sparseness to govern population-based coding," *Frontiers in Systems Neuroscience*, vol. 9, p. 120, 2015.

[37] N. Tagawa, Y. Sugimoto, J. Yamada, and Y. Kobayashi, "Strain differences of neurosteroid levels in mouse brain," *Steroids*, vol. 71, no. 9, pp. 776–784, 2006.

[38] W. Mayo, V. Lemaire, J. Malaterre et al., "Pregnenolone sulfate enhances neurogenesis and PSA-NCAM in young and aged hippocampus," *Neurobiology of Aging*, vol. 26, no. 1, pp. 103–114, 2005.

[39] R. Yang, R. Zhou, L. Chen et al., "Pregnenolone sulfate enhances survival of adult-generated hippocampal granule cells via sustained presynaptic potentiation," *Neuropharmacology*, vol. 60, no. 2-3, pp. 529–541, 2011.

[40] B. Xu, R. Yang, F. Chang et al., "Neurosteroid PREGS protects neurite growth and survival of newborn neurons in the hippocampal dentate gyrus of APPswe/PS1dE9 mice," *Current Alzheimer Research*, vol. 9, no. 3, pp. 361–372, 2012.

[41] L. Zhang, B. Li, W. Ma et al., "Dehydroepiandrosterone (DHEA) and its sulfated derivative (DHEAS) regulate apoptosis during neurogenesis by triggering the Akt signaling pathway in opposing ways," *Brain Research. Molecular Brain Research*, vol. 98, no. 1-2, pp. 58–66, 2002.

[42] S. Lugert, O. Basak, P. Knuckles et al., "Quiescent and active hippocampal neural stem cells with distinct morphologies respond selectively to physiological and pathological stimuli and aging," *Cell Stem Cell*, vol. 6, no. 5, pp. 445–456, 2010.

[43] H. van Praag, B. R. Christie, T. J. Sejnowski, and F. H. Gage, "Running enhances neurogenesis, learning, and long-term potentiation in mice," *Proceedings of the National Academy of Sciences of the United States of America*, vol. 96, no. 23, pp. 13427–13431, 1999.

[44] I. K. Hwang, S. S. Yi, W. Song, M. H. Won, Y. S. Yoon, and J. K. Seong, "Effects of age and treadmill exercise in chronic diabetic stages on neuroblast differentiation in a rat model of type 2 diabetes," *Brain Research*, vol. 1341, pp. 63–71, 2010.

[45] S. M. Nam, J. W. Kim, D. Y. Yoo et al., "Physical exercise ameliorates the reduction of neural stem cell, cell proliferation and neuroblast differentiation in senescent mice induced by D-galactose," *BMC Neuroscience*, vol. 15, p. 116, 2014.

[46] S. S. Yi, I. K. Hwang, K. Y. Yoo et al., "Effects of treadmill exercise on cell proliferation and differentiation in the subgranular zone of the dentate gyrus in a rat model of type II diabetes," *Neurochemical Research*, vol. 34, no. 6, pp. 1039–1046, 2009.

[47] A. C. Pereira, D. E. Huddleston, A. M. Brickman et al., "An in vivo correlate of exercise-induced neurogenesis in the adult dentate gyrus," *Proceedings of the National Academy of Sciences of the United States of America*, vol. 104, no. 13, pp. 5638–5643, 2007.

[48] M. Okamoto, Y. Hojo, K. Inoue et al., "Mild exercise increases dihydrotestosterone in hippocampus providing evidence for androgenic mediation of neurogenesis," *Proceedings of the National Academy of Sciences of the United States of America*, vol. 109, no. 32, pp. 13100–13105, 2012.

[49] A. Russo-Neustadt, R. C. Beard, and C. W. Cotman, "Exercise, antidepressant medications, and enhanced brain derived neurotrophic factor expression," *Neuropsychopharmacology*, vol. 21, no. 5, pp. 679–682, 1999.

[50] S. Vaynman, Z. Ying, and F. Gomez-Pinilla, "Hippocampal BDNF mediates the efficacy of exercise on synaptic plasticity and cognition," *The European Journal of Neuroscience*, vol. 20, no. 10, pp. 2580–2590, 2004.

[51] S. A. Neeper, F. Gomez-Pinilla, J. Choi, and C. W. Cotman, "Physical activity increases mRNA for brain-derived neurotrophic factor and nerve growth factor in rat brain," *Brain Research*, vol. 726, no. 1-2, pp. 49–56, 1996.

[52] Y. Li, B. W. Luikart, S. Birnbaum et al., "TrkB regulates hippocampal neurogenesis and governs sensitivity to antidepressive treatment," *Neuron*, vol. 59, no. 3, pp. 399–412, 2008.

[53] J. L. Trejo, E. Carro, and I. Torres-Aleman, "Circulating insulin-like growth factor I mediates exercise-induced increases in the number of new neurons in the adult hippocampus," *The Journal of Neuroscience*, vol. 21, no. 5, pp. 1628–1634, 2001.

[54] K. Fabel, K. Fabel, B. Tam et al., "VEGF is necessary for exercise-induced adult hippocampal neurogenesis," *The European Journal of Neuroscience*, vol. 18, no. 10, pp. 2803–2812, 2003.

[55] C. Vasuta, C. Caunt, R. James et al., "Effects of exercise on NMDA receptor subunit contributions to bidirectional synaptic plasticity in the mouse dentate gyrus," *Hippocampus*, vol. 17, no. 12, pp. 1201–1208, 2007.

9

Effects of Various Extents of High-Frequency Hearing Loss on Speech Recognition and Gap Detection at Low Frequencies in Patients with Sensorineural Hearing Loss

Bei Li, Yang Guo, Guang Yang, Yanmei Feng, and Shankai Yin

Department of Otolaryngology Head and Neck Surgery, Shanghai Jiao Tong University Affiliated Sixth People's Hospital, No. 600, Yishan Road, Xuhui District, Shanghai 200233, China

Correspondence should be addressed to Yanmei Feng; feng.yanmei@126.com and Shankai Yin; yinshankai@china.com

Academic Editor: Hai Huang

This study explored whether the time-compressed speech perception varied with the degree of hearing loss in high-frequency sensorineural hearing loss (HF SNHL) individuals. 65 HF SNHL individuals with different cutoff frequencies were recruited and further divided into mildly, moderately, and/or severely affected subgroups in terms of the averaged thresholds of all frequencies exhibiting hearing loss. Time-compressed speech recognition scores under both quiet and noisy conditions and gap detection thresholds within low frequencies that had normal thresholds were obtained from all patients and compared with data from 11 age-matched individuals with normal hearing threshold at all frequencies. Correlations of the time-compressed speech recognition scores with the extents of HF SNHL and with the 1 kHz gap detection thresholds were studied across all participants. We found that the time-compressed speech recognition scores were significantly affected by and correlated with the extents of HF SNHL. The time-compressed speech recognition scores also correlated with the 1 kHz gap detection thresholds except when the compression ratio of speech was 0.8 under quiet condition. Above all, the extents of HF SNHL were significantly correlated with the 1 kHz gap thresholds.

1. Introduction

In ENT clinical, patients with high-frequency sensorineural hearing loss (HF SNHL) always complain about the intelligibility of the fast speech. Sensorineural hearing loss (SNHL) is very commonly encountered in the clinic. Researches showed that compared to the normal-hearing (NH) individuals, the ability to comprehend speech in noise decreased in the SNHL individuals [1–3]. Low-intensity signals masked in speech cannot be perceived by those with SNHL, rendering poor speech recognition. Although speech contains a wide range of frequencies [4], according to Ardoint and Lorenzi [5], the most important frequency range in terms of speech perception is 1-2 kHz. Usually, the SNHL begins at high frequencies and slowly spreads to lower frequencies. Once SNHL extends into the low-frequency region (1-2 kHz), the

speech recognition ability of SNHL individuals becomes even worse.

Of all those with SNHL, even individuals with only HF SNHL usually complain about the intelligibility of fast speech, especially in noise. Accumulated evidence shows that the speech recognition scores of HF SNHL patients with normal low-frequency hearing are poorer than those of NH individuals, even when speech stimuli are limited to low frequencies [6–10]. Age also played an important role in speech perception [11]. Leigh-Paffenroth and Elangovan [12] found significant poorer temporal processing in the low-frequency regions (with normal thresholds) in middle-aged individuals even without HF SNHL, compared to the younger individuals. Fullgrabe et al. [13] found declines in speech perception in older persons compared to the youth persons, even the audiometric sensitivities of both were within normal ranges. It is necessary to exclude the influence of age and hearing differences in low-frequency region to study the impact of HF SNHL in speech perception in low frequencies. After auditory sensitivity and age were controlled, research suggested that suprathreshold temporal processing deficits did exist [6, 14]. Others showed that noise-induced HF SNHL affected low-frequency temporal resolution in guinea pigs, even though the thresholds in the low-frequency region were within normal ranges [15, 16]. In this point of view, the speech perception difficulties that many SNHL individuals experienced probably consist of not only SNHL of the high-frequency region but also the temporal processing disability in the low-frequency region.

Previous studies found that speech recognition ability varied among individuals with different extents of SNHL [12, 17–20]. Andrade et al. [18] reported that the speech recognition thresholds correlated with the extents of SNHL in individuals with nonflat audiograms. Also, self-assessed scores of hearing disability were associated with the pure-tone thresholds [17, 19, 20]. Notably, Dobie [19] explored the relationships between pure-tone averages (at 0.5, 1, 2, and 3 kHz) and self-assessed hearing disability scores of 1001 patients and found no correlation between self-assessed scores and pure-tone averages in patients whose pure-tone averages were below 25 dB HL. However, a linear correlation was evident between the self-assessed hearing disability scores and pure-tone averages in patients whose pure-tone averages were above 25 dB HL [19].

However, whether and how HF SNHL affects low-frequency speech perception and temporal resolution remains largely unknown. In the present work, we grouped patients by cutoff frequency (1, 2, and 4 kHz) of HF SNHL. Thus, the thresholds at and below each cutoff frequency were within normal ranges, and the thresholds beyond the cutoff frequencies were higher than 25 dB HL. And gap detection tasks were used to evaluate the temporal resolution of low-frequency region. Speech recognition scores upon delivery of time-compressed sentences under both quiet and noisy conditions and gap detection thresholds were measured and compared between HF SNHL groups with the same cutoff frequency but various degrees of HF SNHL and age-matched NH group.

2. Materials and Methods

2.1. Participants. A total of 76 individuals were recruited, including 65 HF SNHL patients and 11 NH individuals. All HF SNHL participants were recruited from the Department of Otolaryngology Head and Neck Surgery at Shanghai Jiao Tong University Affiliated Sixth People's Hospital, and NH individuals from the staff of the same hospital. No neurological, psychiatric, or other disorders that would undermine speech recognition ability were identified in all participants including the HF SNHL participants. The program was approved by the Ethics Committee of Shanghai Jiao Tong University Affiliated Sixth People's Hospital. All participants gave written informed consent prior to study commencement.

All participants were native Mandarin-speaking Chinese. All NH individuals had pure-tone thresholds 25 dB HL or less at all octave frequencies between 250 and 8000 Hz, in both ears. HF SNHL patients were rigorously selected according to the following criteria: (1) symmetrical SNHL, with threshold differences of 15 dB or less (at all frequencies) between both ears for more than 6 months; (2) pure-tone thresholds of 25 dB HL or less, both at and below the cutoff frequencies; (3) pure-tone thresholds > 25 dB HL above the cutoff frequencies; and (4) type A or Ad type tympanograms.

HF SNHL patients were grouped by the HF SNHL cutoff frequencies evident on audiograms (e.g., 1, 2, and 4 kHz). In each of these three groups, patients were further subdivided into those with mild (25–40 dB HL), moderate (41–60 dB HL), and severe (>60 dB HL) HF SNHL subgroups, defined by the means of averaged pure-tone threshold across frequencies higher than the cutoff frequency. Thus, finally, we formed eight HF SNHL groups, including mild, moderate, and severe groups with cutoff frequencies at 1 and 2 kHz and mild and moderate groups with cutoff frequency at 4 kHz, and one NH group. The means and standard deviations of the auditory thresholds of the tested ears for all groups are shown in Figure 1. Demographic data of all groups are shown in Table 1.

2.2. Stimuli and Procedure. The gap detection task was measured in a three-interval forced-choice procedure. For the gap marker, white noise was low-pass filtered at cutoff frequencies of 1, 2, and 4 kHz, respectively, via 3000th-order finite impulse response filter with an approximately −116 dB/octave filter slope.

In brief, a three-interval forced-choice program had been run on MATLAB software (version 7.0). Three buttons were presented on a monitor to the participant who was asked to indicate which one of the three stimuli was different (i.e., which of the three stimuli was inserted with a gap). As each of the three stimuli playing, the corresponding button was highlighted in red (from left to right). Participant was instructed to click one of the three buttons with the mouse as a response after each presentation of three signals. The next trial was initiated after an answer was given. All subjects were trained to be familiar with the procedure before formal test. The training would last until their performances reached platforms, respectively. No feedback was given to the subject throughout the test. The gap varying in size from 20 to 1 ms was embedded in the middle of one of the three noise bursts (total duration: 1000 ms for each). The gap was shaped using a 1 ms, raised cosine envelope. Each test, commenced with a gap of 20 ms, was followed by a down sequence (in 2 ms steps) until the first erroneous answer was recorded. The two-down, one-up procedure was then adopted (with a gap step size of 1 ms) until the appointed reversals were reached. In gap detection tests, the frequency spectra of the gap markers tested in the HF SNHL groups differed. For example, 4 kHz group members were tested separately with 1, 2, and 4 kHz gap markers. Those of the 2 kHz groups were tested using 1 and 2 kHz gap markers. For those of the 1 kHz groups, only the 1 kHz gap marker test was tested.

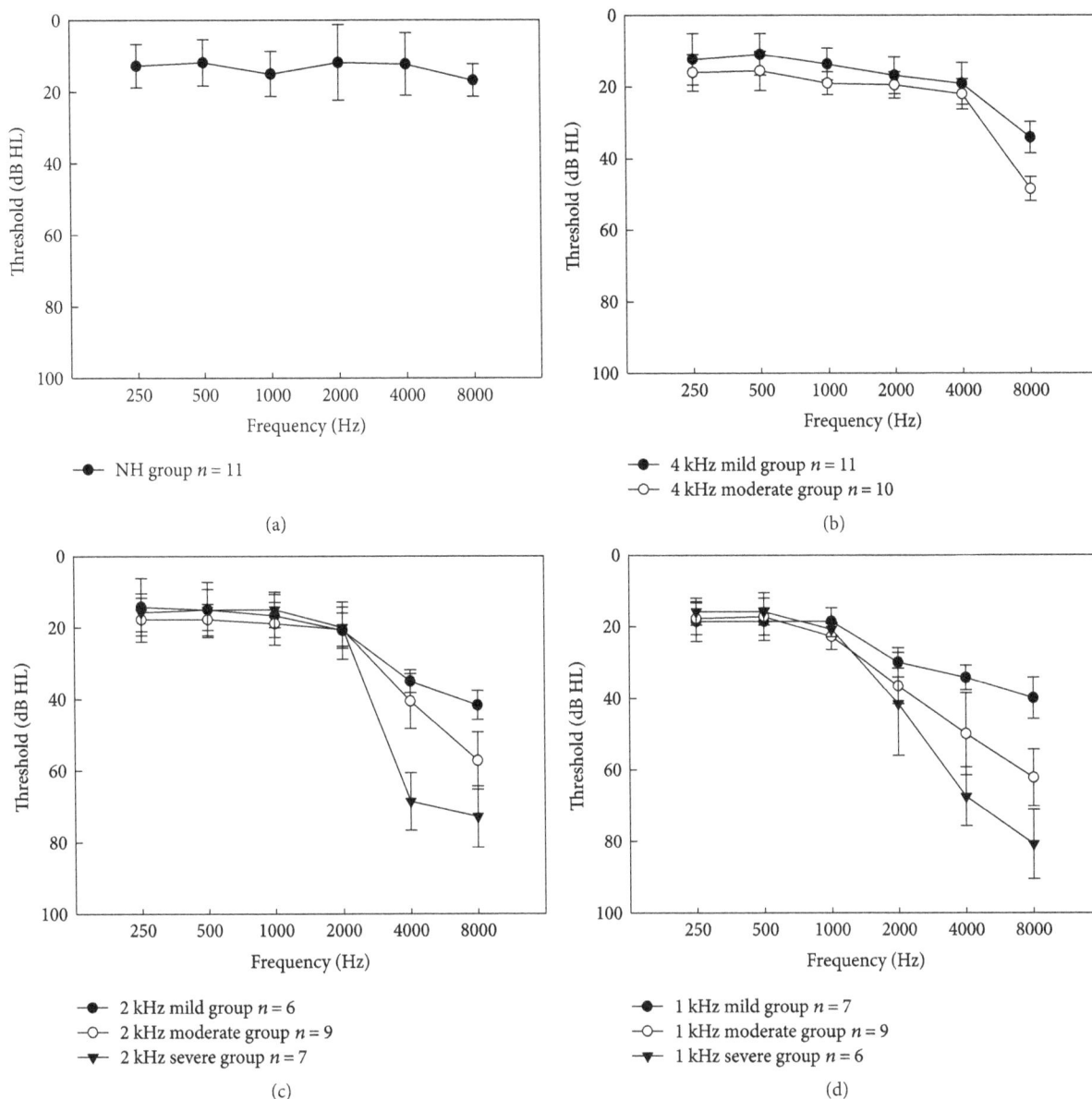

FIGURE 1: Mean audiometric thresholds (dB HL), with standard deviations, for each group. The audiometric thresholds of the tested ears for the normal hearing (NH) and 4, 2, and 1 kHz HF SNHL groups are shown in (a), (b), (c) and (d), respectively.

TABLE 1: Demographic data for the NH group and HF SNHL subgroups.

Group	Male	Female	Age mean ± SD (yrs)
NH	2	9	45.6 ± 13.5
4 kHz mild	5	6	51.2 ± 8.5
4 kHz moderate	5	5	48.3 ± 5.3
2 kHz mild	3	3	52.0 ± 5.4
2 kHz moderate	3	6	46.4 ± 7.9
2 kHz severe	3	4	52.9 ± 11.3
1 kHz mild	3	4	42.6 ± 8.2
1 kHz moderate	4	5	52.7 ± 13.4
1 kHz severe	3	3	51.0 ± 8.6

NH: normal hearing; SD: standard deviation.

Speech perception was assessed using the Mandarin version of the Hearing in Noise Test (MHINT) of the House Ear Institute [21], representing a daily and communicative style of speech, which could be easily understood by native Mandarin-speaking listeners with various degrees of education. Speech was time-compressed using Praat software (version 5.3), without any significant change in the power spectrum [22]. We used three compression ratios: 0.6, 0.8, and 1.0 that of the normal speech rate (the compression ratio of 1.0, namely, was normal speech rate). Speech recognition tests were run under both quiet and noisy [signal-to-noise ratio (SNR): −5 dB] conditions.

All test signals were presented at 75 dB SPL under both quiet and noisy conditions and were delivered monaurally through Sennheiser HD580 headphones. Only right ears were tested, and a 40 dB SPL speech-shaped noise was conducted to the left ears as masker all along the tests. To create noisy conditions, a speech-shaped noise of the same spectrum as that of the MHINT sentence was presented with SNR at −5 dB. The noise began 500 ms before the sentence and continued for 500 ms after the sentence had concluded. A complete set of tests required approximately 30 min. Practice was conducted before each test, and feedback was provided. After practice, each participant achieved stable recognition scores. During a speech recognition test, each sentence was played only once, and no feedback was given. The same methods were also applied by Feng et al. [14].

3. Results

3.1. Age Matching and Pure-Tone Thresholds of the NH and HF SNHL Groups. One-way analysis of variance (ANOVA) showed that the mean ages of all nine groups did not differ significantly ($F_{(8,75)} = 1.097$, $p = 0.376$).

Comparisons of the averaged thresholds across the frequencies with normal thresholds in all groups showed that the thresholds of frequencies exhibiting normal hearing did not differ significantly among the groups ($F_{(8,75)} = 1.899$, $p = 0.075$).

3.2. Gap Detection Task. The gap thresholds of groups varying in terms of gap marker cutoff frequency are shown in Figure 2. The gap thresholds of the gap markers with different cutoff frequencies for the same listener group were compared firstly. Paired *t*-tests showed that the gap thresholds of 1 kHz gap marker were significantly higher than those of 2 kHz gap marker for 2 kHz mild HF SNHL group ($t = 5.349$, $p = 0.003$), 2 kHz moderate HF SNHL group ($t = 10.639$, $p < 0.001$), and 2 kHz severe HF SNHL group ($t = 7.22$, $p < 0.001$). One-way repeated ANOVA showed significant main effects of cutoff frequencies of gap marker on gap thresholds of 4 kHz mild HF SNHL group ($F_{(2,20)} = 19.334$, $p < 0.001$), 4 kHz moderate HF SNHL group ($F_{(2,18)} = 21.063$, $p < 0.001$), and NH group ($F_{(2,20)} = 57.133$, $p < 0.001$); the post hoc analyses (LSD tests) revealed that gap thresholds of 1 kHz gap marker, 2 kHz gap marker, and 4 kHz gap marker differed from each other significantly for the three groups, respectively. Generally, the gap thresholds of all groups gradually decrease as cutoff frequencies of the gap marker increase gradually.

Then, data derived from different groups with the same gap marker frequency were analyzed by one-way ANOVA. There was a significant difference when the cutoff frequency of gap marker is 1 kHz ($F_{(8,75)} = 2.189$, $p = 0.039$); the post hoc analysis (LSD test) revealed that the gap thresholds of the NH group and 4 kHz mild HF SNHL group were significantly lower than those of the 1 kHz mild HF SNHL group, 1 kHz moderate HF SNHL group, and 1 kHz severe HF SNHL group. And there was also a significant difference when the cutoff frequency of gap marker is 4 kHz ($F_{(2,31)} = 3.515$, $p = 0.043$); the post hoc analysis (LSD test) revealed that the gap thresholds of the NH group were significantly lower than those of the 4 kHz moderate HF SNHL group with 4 kHz gap marker. However, no difference was evident with 2 kHz gap marker ($F_{(5,53)} = 0.231$, $p = 0.947$).

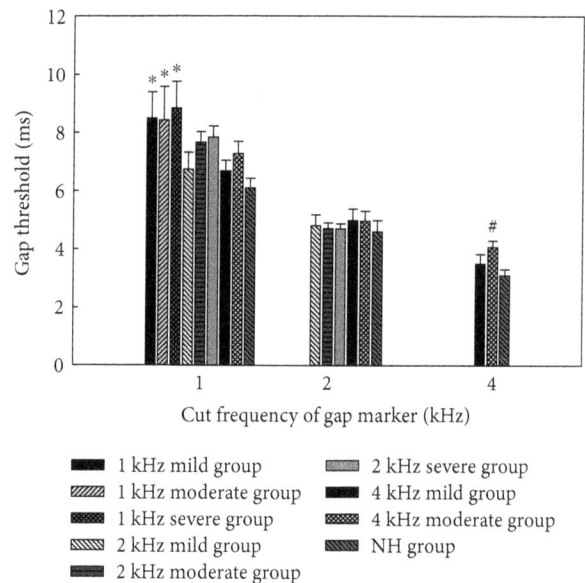

FIGURE 2: The mean gap thresholds in the high-frequency sensorineural hearing loss (HF SNHL) groups and normal-hearing (NH) group. The error bars indicate standard errors. ∗ indicates gap thresholds of the 1 kHz mild, moderate, and severe HF SNHL groups with 1 kHz gap marker which were significantly higher than those of the NH group and the 4 kHz mild HF SNHL group; # indicates gap thresholds of the 4 kHz moderate HF SNHL group which were significantly higher than those of the NH group for 4 kHz gap marker.

When presented with gap marker of the same cutoff frequency, in general, the gap thresholds of various groups tended to be higher if the range of HF SNHL was wider or the degrees of hearing impairment were higher.

3.3. Time-Compressed Speech Recognition. The original scores under quiet and noisy conditions are shown in Figures 3 and 4, respectively. Overall, the speech recognition scores of all groups decreased as the time compression ratio fell from 1.0 (normal speech rate) to 0.6 and the scores were lower under noisy conditions than those under quiet conditions at the same time compression ratio.

Before analysis, all speech recognition scores were arcsine-transformed to avoid ceiling or floor effects. Data from the NH and eight HF SNHL groups in quiet were subjected to two-way repeated-measures ANOVA to test the effects of group and time compression ratio on speech recognition. The effects of group and compression ratio were both significant: $F_{group(8,67)} = 5.368$, $p < 0.001$ and $F_{compression(2,134)} = 114.028$, $p < 0.001$. There was a statistically significant two-way interaction between group and time compression ratio ($F_{(16,134)} = 2.130$, $p = 0.010$). The LSD method was applied in post hoc comparisons, to explore the effect of the extent of HF SNHL on speech recognition scores in quiet. When speech compression ratio was 0.6, all HF SNHL groups scored significantly lower than the NH group except the 2 kHz mild and severe HF SNHL groups and 4 kHz mild HF SNHL group; when speech compression ratio was 0.8, the NH group scored significantly higher than the 1 kHz moderate and severe HF SNHL groups and 4 kHz

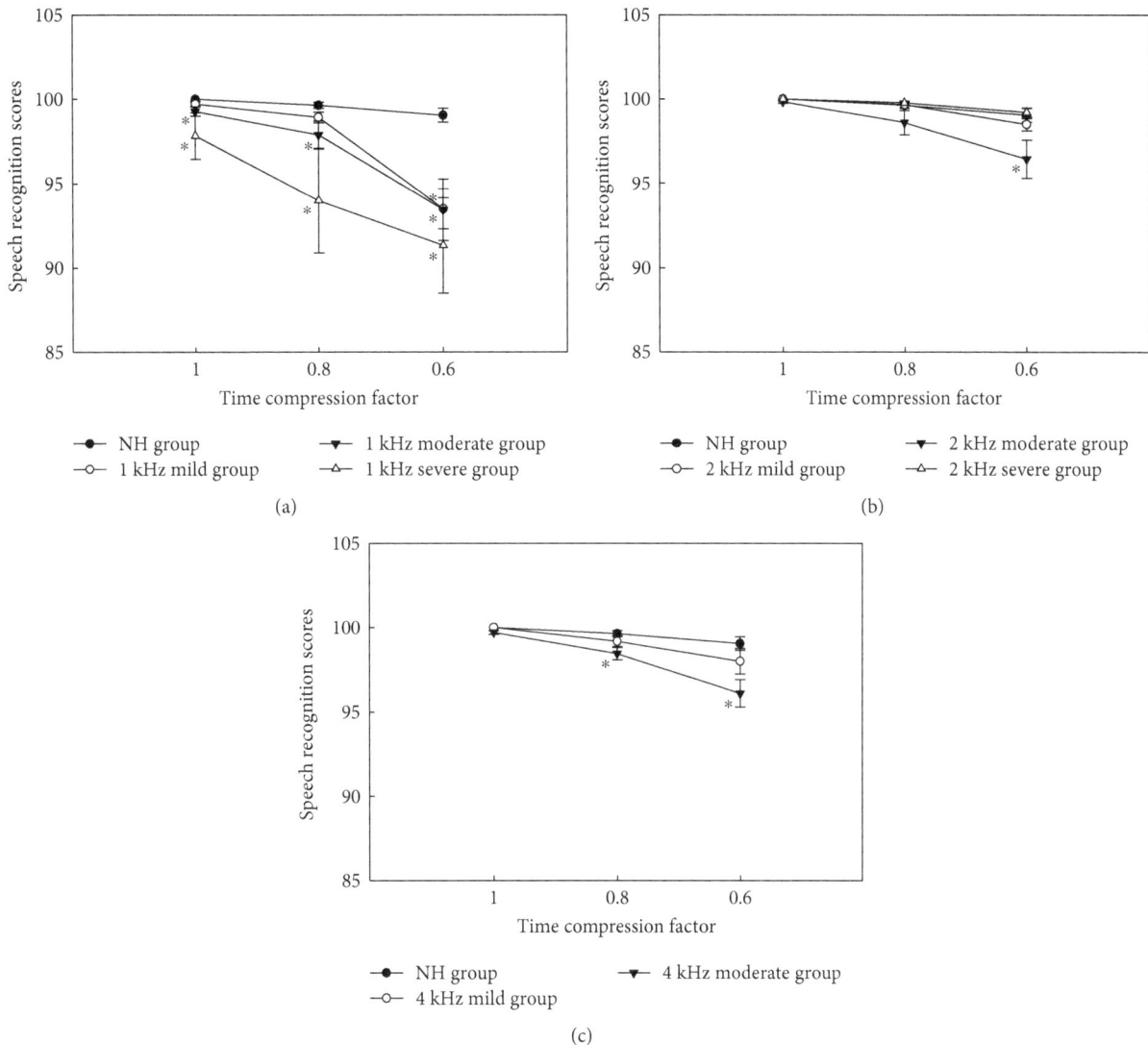

FIGURE 3: Speech recognition scores under quiet conditions for the normal-hearing (NH) and high-frequency sensorineural hearing loss (HF SNHL) groups, as a function of the time compression ratio. The scores for the 1, 2, and 4 kHz HF SNHL groups are shown in (a), (b), and (c), respectively. The error bars indicate standard errors. * indicates significant difference of speech recognition scores when compared with that of the NH group at the same time compression factor.

moderate HF SNHL group, while the NH group scored significantly higher than the 1 kHz moderate and severe HF SNHL groups when speech compression ratio was 1.0. The differences among the 1 kHz mild, moderate, and severe HF SNHL groups were not statistically significant when speech compression ratio was 0.6 or 1.0, but the scores of the 1 kHz mild HF SNHL groups were significantly higher than the 1 kHz severe HF SNHL groups when speech compression ratio was 0.8; the differences among the 2 kHz mild, moderate, and severe HF SNHL groups and the differences between the 4 kHz mild and moderate HF SNHL groups were not statistically significant for all three speech compression ratios.

A two-way repeated-measures ANOVA was used to evaluate the effects of group and time compression ratio on speech recognition in noise. The effects of group and compression ratio were both significant: $F_{group(8,67)} = 11.541$,

$p < 0.001$ and $F_{compression(2,134)} = 144.785$, $p < 0.001$. There was a statistically significant two-way interaction between group and time compression ratio ($F_{(16,134)} = 4.434$, $p \leq 0.001$). The LSD method was used in post hoc comparisons to explore the effect of the extent of HF SNHL on speech recognition scores in noise. When speech compression ratio was 0.8 and 1.0, the differences between scores of the NH group and all HF SNHL groups were significant; when speech compression ratio was 0.6, the NH group scored significantly higher than all HF SNHL groups except the 2 kHz mild HF SNHL group. The differences among the 1 kHz mild, moderate, and severe HF SNHL groups were not statistically significant when speech compression ratio was 0.6 or 0.8, but the scores of the 1 kHz mild HF SNHL groups were significantly higher than those of 1 kHz severe HF SNHL groups when speech compression ratio was 1.0; the 2 kHz mild HF SNHL group scored significantly higher

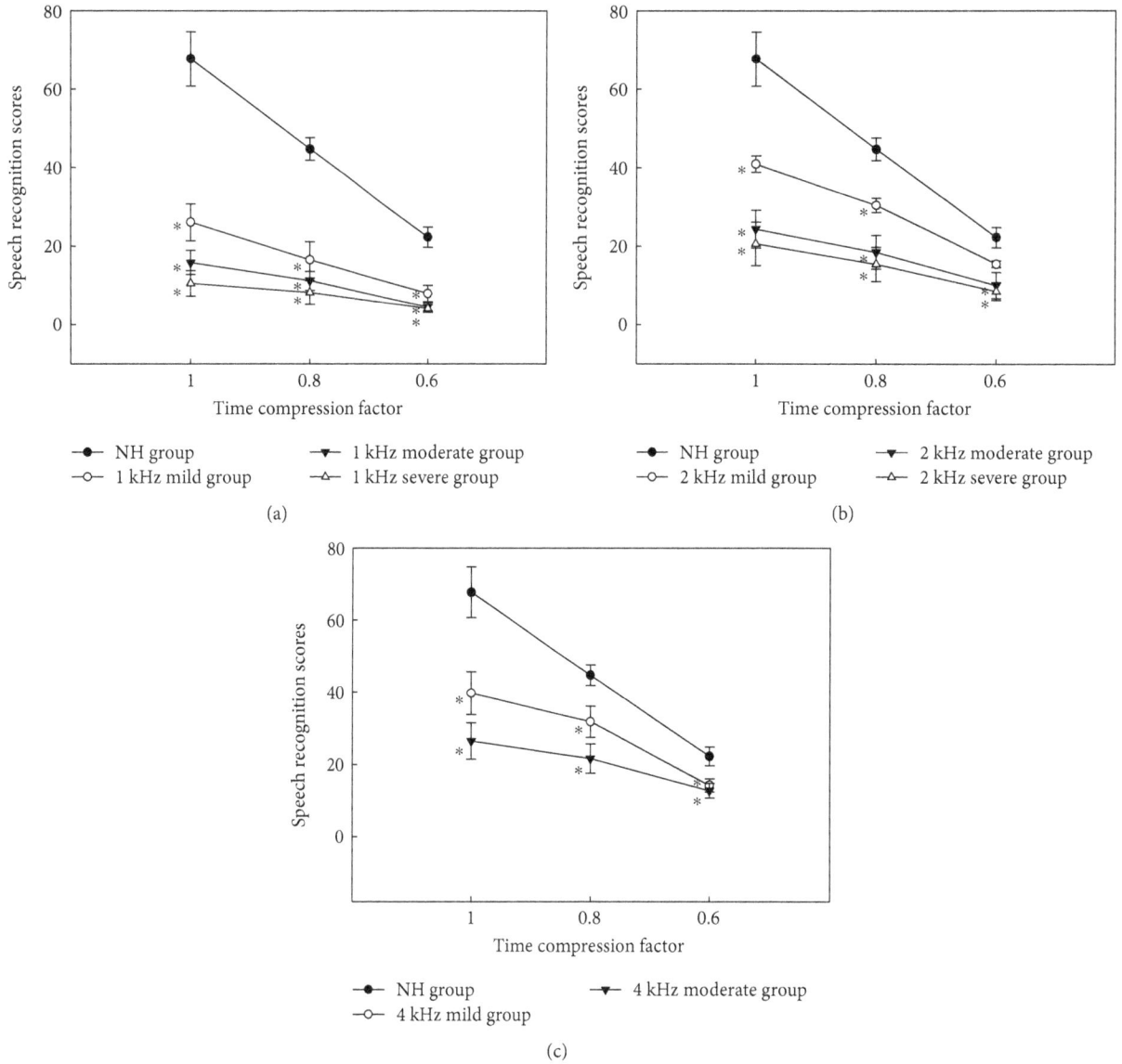

FIGURE 4: Speech recognition scores under noisy conditions (SNR = −5 dB) for the normal-hearing (NH) and high-frequency sensorineural hearing loss (HF SNHL) groups, as a function of the time compression ratio. The scores for the 1, 2, and 4 kHz HF SNHL groups are shown in (a), (b), and (c), respectively. The error bars indicate standard errors. ∗ indicates significant difference of speech recognition scores when compared with that of the NH group at the same time compression factor.

than the 2 kHz moderate and severe HF SNHL groups when speech compression ratio was 0.6 and 0.8, and the 2 kHz mild HF SNHL group scored significantly higher than the 2 kHz severe HF SNHL group when speech compression ratio was 1.0. The differences between the 4 kHz mild and moderate HF SNHL groups were not statistically significant for all three speech compression ratios.

As a whole, at the same time compression ratio, the scores of the NH group were better than those of any HF SNHL group, and the scores of those with HF SNHL decreased as the degree of HF SNHL increased, which was more obvious under noisy conditions.

3.4. Correlation Analysis. We explored relationships between time-compressed speech recognition scores, pure-tone HF

averages, and gap detection thresholds, by calculating *Pearson* correlations as follows: (1) between pure-tone HF averages (for NH groups, the average was calculated across 2, 4, and 8 kHz; for HF SNHL groups, the average was calculated across frequencies where exhibited hearing loss) and time-compressed speech recognition scores; (2) between pure-tone HF averages and the 1 kHz gap detection thresholds; and, (3) between the time-compressed speech recognition scores and the 1 kHz gap detection thresholds (all participants underwent 1 kHz gap detection testing). As shown in Table 2, the pure-tone HF averages were significantly correlated with time-compressed speech recognition scores at compression ratios of both 0.6 and 0.8, and normal speech recognition scores (all p values < 0.05), under both quiet and noisy conditions. What is noteworthy is that pure-tone

TABLE 2: Correlation analysis between pure-tone averages of high-frequency hearing loss and speech recognition scores with different compression and different test backgrounds.

	Compression ratio of speech in quiet			Compression ratio of speech in noise		
	1	0.8	0.6	1	0.8	0.6
Pearson correlation	−0.279	−0.269	−0.329	−0.694	−0.627	−0.536
p value	0.015*	0.019*	0.004*	<0.001*	<0.001*	<0.001*

For NH groups, the average was calculated across 2, 4, and 8 kHz; for HF SNHL groups, the average was calculated across frequencies where exhibited hearing loss. * indicates *p* values smaller than 0.05.

TABLE 3: Correlation analysis between 1 kHz gap thresholds and speech recognition scores with different compression ratios under different test backgrounds.

	Compression ratio of speech in quiet			Compression ratio of speech in noise		
	1	0.8	0.6	1	0.8	0.6
Pearson correlation	−0.231	−0.185	−0.427	−0.388	−0.394	−0.381
p value	0.045*	0.109	<0.001*	0.001*	<0.001*	0.001*

* indicates *p* values smaller than 0.05.

HF averages were significantly correlated with the 1 kHz gap detection thresholds (*Pearson* correlation = 0.367, $p = 0.001$). In Table 3, the results showed that 1 kHz gap thresholds were significantly correlated with the speech recognition scores at all compression ratios under noisy conditions (all p values ≤ 0.001). This was also true under quiet conditions for both normal speech and that at a 0.6 compression ratio ($p_{0.6\text{compression}} \leq 0.001$, $p_{\text{normal speed}} = 0.045$).

4. Discussion

Our primary purpose in the present study was to explore whether and how HF SNHL affected time-compressed speech perception and gap detection in low-frequency region with normal auditory threshold. We found that the time-compressed speech recognition scores of the HF SNHL group were poorer than those of the NH group and decreased as the extent of HF SNHL increased in patients with the same cutoff frequency. Generally, the recognition scores of patients with severe HF SNHL were poorer than the scores of those with moderate HF SNHL, which in turn were poorer than those of patients with mild HF SNHL at the same cutoff frequencies, under both quiet and noisy conditions (Figures 3 and 4).

As shown in Table 2, pure-tone averages of HF SNHL were significantly correlated with the time-compressed speech recognition scores. These results suggested that the ability to recognize time-compressed speech was affected by HF SNHL and correlated with the extent of HF SNHL. These results are similar to those of our previous study and indeed extend our earlier work [14]. We previously showed that the time-compressed speech recognition scores of the HF SNHL subjects were poorer than those of NH individuals [14]. However, the effect of the extent of HF SNHL on speech recognition was not explored in detail. Therefore, in the present study, we focused on the effect of varying levels of HF SNHL on time-compressed speech recognition abilities.

Indeed, the extent of HF SNHL affects the ability of speech recognition. Moore [23] found that, in individuals with cochlear hearing loss of up to approximately 45 dB, a change in audibility was the single most important contributor to speech perception problems. However, when the extent of hearing loss was greater, poor discrimination of suprathreshold stimuli also became of major importance. Nimitbunnasarn et al. [24] examined tonal identification in Thai speakers with normal hearing and different extents of SNHL. Identification ability was affected by SNHL per se and the extent thereof [24]. Jerger et al. [25] explored correlations among speech recognition performance, the pure-tone hearing level, and the age of individuals with SNHL. The relationship between the extent of hearing loss and speech recognition score was strongest in older individuals with SNHL. Other studies sought correlations between self-assessed hearing inventories and individual pure-tone thresholds [12, 17, 19] or between speech reception and pure-tone thresholds [20]. All data suggested that the extents of SNHL correlated with the speech recognition scores. Our results are consistent with such findings and suggest that the extents of HF SNHL are also correlated with the time-compressed speech recognition scores. Similar hearing configurations that vary in the extent of hearing loss may impact speech recognition differently, especially when speech is fast. More severe speech disruption is evident as the severity of hearing loss rises.

It is worth noting that the pure-tone averages of HF SNHL correlated with the 1 kHz gap thresholds significantly, which indicates that the HF SNHL could impair the temporal resolution of the low-frequency region. This is in line with our previous research results, which suggests that HF SNHL exerted an off-channel effect on temporal processing ability in the low-frequency region of the auditory system, whether in guinea pigs or humans [14, 15]. This off-channel effect may contribute to the difficulty, which is experienced by patients with normal hearing in low frequencies but suffered from HF SNHL, of perceiving the time-compressed speech [14] and temporal fine structure speech [6].

The relationship between speech recognition and temporal resolution, another focus of the present study, remains unclear. Previous studies suggested that temporal resolution played an important role in speech recognition [26–29]. However, no influence of any temporal processing ability, such as gap detection, on speech perception, has been conclusively shown [11].

To determine whether the gap detection threshold correlated with time-compressed speech recognition ability, we carefully controlled for age and the extent of HF SNHL. As shown in Table 3, the gap thresholds with 1 kHz-low-pass-filtered noise were negatively correlated with the time-compressed speech recognition scores, suggesting that speech recognition ability was also affected by temporal resolution of the low-frequency region, even whose auditory sensitivity was normal.

5. Conclusions

Even when age was controlled, the extent of HF SNHL impacted the ability to recognize compressed speech. The greater the extent of HF SNHL was, the poorer the speech recognition ability was. The significant correlation between the extents of HF SNHL and gap detection thresholds implied that there was probable off-channel mechanism underlying. The decrease of time-compressed speech recognition ability may be partly attributable to the increased thresholds in gap detection task, which signified the deterioration of suprathresholdly temporal resolution.

Conflicts of Interest

The authors declare that there is no competing interest relevant to the publication of this paper.

Authors' Contributions

Bei Li and Yang Guo contributed equally to this paper.

Acknowledgments

The study was supported by a grant from the National Natural Science Foundation of China (81771015), Shanghai Municipal Education Commission—Gaofeng Clinical Medicine Grant Support (20152526), and Three-Year Action Program on Promotion of Clinical Skills and Clinical Innovation for Municipal Hospitals (16CR4027A) to Yanmei Feng and a grant from the National Natural Science Foundation of China (81530029) to Shankai Yin.

References

[1] J. R. Dubno, D. D. Dirks, and D. E. Morgan, "Effects of age and mild hearing loss on speech recognition in noise," *The Journal of the Acoustical Society of America*, vol. 76, no. 1, pp. 87–96, 1984.

[2] A. R. Needleman and C. C. Crandell, "Speech recognition in noise by hearing-impaired and noise-masked normal-hearing listeners," *Journal of the American Academy of Audiology*, vol. 6, no. 6, pp. 414–424, 1995.

[3] A. J. Klein, J. H. Mills, and W. Y. Adkins, "Upward spread of masking, hearing loss, and speech recognition in young and elderly listeners," *The Journal of the Acoustical Society of America*, vol. 87, no. 3, pp. 1266–1271, 1990.

[4] B. C. J. Moore, "The role of temporal fine structure processing in pitch perception, masking, and speech perception for normal-hearing and hearing-impaired people," *Journal of the Association for Research in Otolaryngology*, vol. 9, no. 4, pp. 399–406, 2008.

[5] M. Ardoint and C. Lorenzi, "Effects of lowpass and highpass filtering on the intelligibility of speech based on temporal fine structure or envelope cues," *Hearing Research*, vol. 260, no. 1-2, pp. 89–95, 2010.

[6] B. Li, L. Hou, L. Xu et al., "Effects of steep high-frequency hearing loss on speech recognition using temporal fine structure in low-frequency region," *Hearing Research*, vol. 326, pp. 66–74, 2015.

[7] A. C. Leger, D. T. Ives, and C. Lorenzi, "Abnormal intelligibility of speech in competing speech and in noise in a frequency region where audiometric thresholds are near-normal for hearing-impaired listeners," *Hearing Research*, vol. 316, pp. 102–109, 2014.

[8] A. C. Léger, B. C. J. Moore, and C. Lorenzi, "Abnormal speech processing in frequency regions where absolute thresholds are normal for listeners with high-frequency hearing loss," *Hearing Research*, vol. 294, no. 1-2, pp. 95–103, 2012.

[9] C. Lorenzi, L. Debruille, S. Garnier, P. Fleuriot, and B. C. J. Moore, "Abnormal processing of temporal fine structure in speech for frequencies where absolute thresholds are normal," *The Journal of the Acoustical Society of America*, vol. 125, no. 1, pp. 27–30, 2009.

[10] V. Summers, M. J. Makashay, S. M. Theodoroff, and M. R. Leek, "Suprathreshold auditory processing and speech perception in noise: hearing-impaired and normal-hearing listeners," *Journal of the American Academy of Audiology*, vol. 24, no. 4, pp. 274–292, 2013.

[11] A. Strouse, D. H. Ashmead, R. N. Ohde, and D. W. Grantham, "Temporal processing in the aging auditory system," *The Journal of the Acoustical Society of America*, vol. 104, no. 4, pp. 2385–2399, 1998.

[12] E. D. Leigh-Paffenroth and S. Elangovan, "Temporal processing in low-frequency channels: effects of age and hearing loss in middle-aged listeners," *Journal of the American Academy of Audiology*, vol. 22, no. 7, pp. 393–404, 2011.

[13] C. Fullgrabe, B. C. Moore, and M. A. Stone, "Age-group differences in speech identification despite matched audiometrically normal hearing: contributions from auditory temporal processing and cognition," *Frontiers in Aging Neuroscience*, vol. 6, p. 347, 2014.

[14] Y. Feng, S. Yin, M. Kiefte, and J. Wang, "Temporal resolution in regions of normal hearing and speech perception in noise for adults with sloping high-frequency hearing loss," *Ear and Hearing*, vol. 31, no. 1, pp. 115–125, 2010.

[15] Y. Feng, S. Yin, and J. Wang, "Deterioration of cortical responses to amplitude modulations of low-frequency carriers after high-frequency cochlear lesion in guinea pigs," *International Journal of Audiology*, vol. 49, no. 3, pp. 228–237, 2010.

[16] S. K. Yin, Y. M. Feng, Z. N. Chen, and J. Wang, "The effect of noise-induced sloping high-frequency hearing loss on the gap-response in the inferior colliculus and auditory cortex of guinea pigs," *Hearing Research*, vol. 239, no. 1-2, pp. 126–140, 2008.

[17] C. H. Chien, T. Y. Tu, A. S. Shiao et al., "Prediction of the pure-tone average from the speech reception and auditory brainstem response thresholds in a geriatric population," *ORL*, vol. 70, no. 6, pp. 366–372, 2008.

[18] K. C. Andrade, P. L. Menezes, A. T. Carnauba, R. G. Rodrigues, M. C. Leal, and L. D. Pereira, "Non-flat audiograms in sensorineural hearing loss and speech perception," *Clinics*, vol. 68, no. 6, pp. 815–819, 2013.

[19] R. A. Dobie, "The AMA method of estimation of hearing disability: a validation study," *Ear and Hearing*, vol. 32, no. 6, pp. 732–740, 2011.

[20] S. Coren and A. R. Hakstian, "The development and cross-validation of a self-report inventory to assess pure-tone threshold hearing sensitivity," *Journal of Speech and Hearing Research*, vol. 35, no. 4, pp. 921–928, 1992.

[21] L. L. Wong, S. D. Soli, S. Liu, N. Han, and M. W. Huang, "Development of the Mandarin hearing in noise test (MHINT)," *Ear and Hearing*, vol. 28, 2 Supplement, pp. 70S–74S, 2007.

[22] P. Boersma and D. Weenink, "Praat: Doing phoenetics by computer [computer program]," in *Version 4.3.14 Amsterdam*, Institute of Phonetic Sciences, University of Amsterdam; 2005, Netherlands, 2008.

[23] B. C. Moore, "Perceptual consequences of cochlear hearing loss and their implications for the design of hearing aids," *Ear and Hearing*, vol. 17, no. 2, pp. 133–161, 1996.

[24] C. Nimitbunnasarn, P. Amatyakul, J. Gandour, A. Carney, C. Nimitbunnasarn, and P. Amatyakul, "Tonal confusions in Thai patients with sensorineural hearing loss," *Journal of Speech and Hearing Research*, vol. 27, no. 1, pp. 89–97, 1984.

[25] J. Jerger, S. Jerger, and F. Pirozzolo, "Correlational analysis of speech audiometric scores, hearing loss, age, and cognitive abilities in the elderly," *Ear and Hearing*, vol. 12, no. 2, pp. 103–109, 1991.

[26] R. Drullman, J. M. Festen, and R. Plomp, "Effect of temporal envelope smearing on speech reception," *The Journal of the Acoustical Society of America*, vol. 95, no. 2, pp. 1053–1064, 1994.

[27] K. W. Grant and T. C. Walden, "Understanding excessive SNR loss in hearing-impaired listeners," *Journal of the American Academy of Audiology*, vol. 24, no. 4, pp. 258–273, 2013.

[28] B. R. Glasberg, B. C. Moore, and S. P. Bacon, "Gap detection and masking in hearing-impaired and normal-hearing subjects," *The Journal of the Acoustical Society of America*, vol. 81, no. 5, pp. 1546–1556, 1987.

[29] R. S. Tyler, Q. Summerfield, E. J. Wood, and M. A. Fernandes, "Psychoacoustic and phonetic temporal processing in normal and hearing-impaired listeners," *The Journal of the Acoustical Society of America*, vol. 72, no. 3, pp. 740–752, 1982.

10

Action Observation Treatment Improves Upper Limb Motor Functions in Children with Cerebral Palsy: A Combined Clinical and Brain Imaging Study

Giovanni Buccino ⓘ,[1] **Anna Molinaro,**[2,3] **Claudia Ambrosi,**[4] **Daniele Arisi,**[5] **Lorella Mascaro,**[6] **Chiara Pinardi,**[7] **Andrea Rossi,**[8] **Roberto Gasparotti,**[4] **Elisa Fazzi,**[2,3] **and Jessica Galli**[2,3]

[1]*Department of Medical and Surgical Sciences, University of Magna Graecia, Catanzaro, Italy*
[2]*Unit of Child Neurology and Psychiatry, ASST Spedali Civili, Brescia, Italy*
[3]*Department of Clinical and Experimental Sciences, University of Brescia, Brescia, Italy*
[4]*Department of Diagnostic Imaging, Neuroradiology Unit, University of Brescia, Brescia, Italy*
[5]*Department of Paediatrics, Ospedale di Cremona, Cremona, Italy*
[6]*Department of Diagnostic Imaging, Medical Physics Unit, ASST Spedali Civili, Brescia, Italy*
[7]*Neuroscience Unit, Department of Medicine and Surgery, University of Parma, Parma, Italy*
[8]*Unit of Child Neurology and Psychiatry, ASST Spedali Civili, Brescia, Italy*

Correspondence should be addressed to Giovanni Buccino; buccino@unicz.it

Academic Editor: Michela Bassolino

The aim of the present study was to assess the role of action observation treatment (AOT) in the rehabilitation of upper limb motor functions in children with cerebral palsy. We carried out a two-group, parallel randomized controlled trial. Eighteen children (aged 5–11 yr) entered the study: 11 were treated children, and 7 served as controls. Outcome measures were scores on two functional scales: Melbourne Assessment of Unilateral Upper Limb Function Scale (MUUL) and the Assisting Hand Assessment (AHA). We collected functional scores before treatment (T1), at the end of treatment (T2), and at two months of follow-up (T3). As compared to controls, treated children improved significantly in both scales at T2 and this improvement persisted at T3. AOT has therefore the potential to become a routine rehabilitation practice in children with CP. Twelve out of 18 enrolled children also underwent a functional magnetic resonance study at T1 and T2. As compared to controls, at T2, treated children showed stronger activation in a parieto-premotor circuit for hand-object interactions. These findings support the notion that AOT contributes to reorganize brain circuits subserving the impaired function rather than activating supplementary or vicariating ones.

1. Introduction

There is an urgent need in neurorehabilitation of both adults and children of approaches that take into account the progresses of our knowledge in basic neuroscience. These approaches should aim at transferring ideas and facts from basic neuroscience to clinical practice with the final goal to build up tools well-grounded in neurophysiology and to provide a cure for several neurological (and nonneurological) diseases [1, 2]. Such a rehabilitation approach,

grounded in basic neuroscience, would also be a model of translational medicine.

The use of such approaches may help to overwhelm a general attitude in neurorehabilitation to focus on ways to circumvent functional deficits, thus leading to a compensation or a reeducation of functions rather than a cure for them through remediation (for a more general discussion on the notion of compensation and remediation, see [3–5]). Although compensation sometimes works and helps patients to recover in daily activities, it does not aim at repairing the neural circuits underlying specific functions through a direct or indirect restoration. Moving to a translational model in neurorehabilitation would imply to plan specific rehabilitative tools aiming at restoring the neural structures whose damage caused the impaired functions or activating supplementary or related pathways, which may perform the original functions. Last, but not least, rehabilitation tools well-grounded in basic neuroscience allow researchers to plan well-designed randomized controlled trials. This in turn allows clinicians and therapists to measure outcomes not only in terms of functional and/or behavioural gains (as it currently happens by means of functional scales) but also in terms of changes in biological parameters, which researchers can test using neurophysiological and brain imaging techniques. There are indeed some approaches in the neurorehabilitation of children that fit these criteria. For example, constraint-induced movement therapy (CIMT) has a well-established neurophysiological basis grounded on the experimental evidence that monkeys can be induced to use a deafferented limb by restricting movements of the unaffected limb over a period of days [6]. CIMT has been widely applied in patients with acute and chronic stroke and in children with cerebral palsy [7]; similarly, HABIT (hand-arm bimanual intensive training) is a highly structured form of bimanual training, whose goal is to improve the quality and quantity of hand use in bimanual tasks in children with hemiplegic CP [7]. Another example is the mirror therapy [8]. In this treatment, a mirror is placed in the patient's mid-sagittal plane so that he/she can see her unaffected arm/hand as if it were the affected one. This strategy has been proven to be effective to relieve phantom pain in arm amputees as well as in the recovery of upper limb in chronic stroke patients and in children with cerebral palsy [9, 10]. This approach grounds on a neurophysiological mechanism known as mirror mechanism. Based on this mechanism, the observation of actions performed by other individuals recruits in the observer the same areas involved in the actual execution of those same actions [11]. In the case of mirror therapy, patients have the opportunity to look at their own actions performed with the unaffected arm/hand. More recently, we proposed a novel approach in neurorehabilitation known as action observation treatment (for a review, see Buccino [12]). AOT exploits the mirror mechanism in an even more straightforward manner than mirror therapy, because patients observe daily actions performed by other healthy individuals. During one typical session, patients observe a daily action and afterwards execute it in context. So far, this approach has been successfully applied in the rehabilitation of upper limb motor functions in chronic stroke patients, in motor recovery of Parkinson's disease patients, including those presenting with freezing of gait; interestingly, this approach also improved lower limb motor functions in post-surgical orthopaedic patients [13–16]. Pivotal studies were conducted also in children with cerebral palsy [17–19]. AOT is well-grounded in basic neuroscience, thus representing a valid model of translational medicine in the field of neurorehabilitation. Moreover, the results concerning its effectiveness have been collected in randomized controlled studies, thus being an example of evidence-based clinical

practice. The present study aimed at assessing whether this novel rehabilitation approach has the potential to improve the functional recovery of children with CP aged 5–11 (primary school cycle in Italy), within a comprehensive rehabilitation program. The focus was on the recovery of upper limb motor functions. We used the same protocol of an earlier pilot study from our group [17]. We also tested whether this approach may lead to neural changes in the brain by means of a functional magnetic resonance study, in which we asked some of the children that entered the study to manipulate complex objects in the scanner. Control condition was the manipulation of a small sphere.

2. Methods

2.1. Study Design. We used a two-group, parallel randomized controlled trial. Recruitment criteria and methodological procedures were approved by the Ethical Committee of the Hospital of Brescia.

2.2. Participants. All children referred to the Centre of Child Neurology and Psychiatry at the Hospital of Brescia with a diagnosis of cerebral palsy (CP) were eligible. Inclusion criteria were the presence of CP confirmed by neuroimaging techniques (MRI), Manual Ability Classification System (MACS) ≤ 4 [20], verbal IQ > 70, age between 5 and 11 (primary school cycle in Italy), absence of major visual and/or auditory deficits, and no antiepileptic treatment. We enrolled a group of 18 children that met the inclusion/exclusion criteria. Before entering the study, the parents of each child gave written informed consent.

2.3. Allocation and Assessment. Patients were enrolled by one of the authors (Elisa Fazzi); enrolled children were randomly allocated to the treatment ($n = 11$) or the control group ($n = 7$) by means of a dedicated software. Both children and their parents were blind to group allocation. After randomization, children were evaluated clinically with a neurological examination carried out by two expert child neurologists (Elisa Fazzi, Anna Molinaro), while functional assessment was carried out by a physician blind to treatment allocation, using the Melbourne Assessment of Unilateral Upper Limb Function Scale (MUUL) and the Assisting Hand Assessment (AHA). MUUL consists of 16 items involving reaching, grasping, releasing, and manipulation, specifically developed to measure quality of upper limb motor functions in children with CP aged 5 to 16 [21]. It has been shown to have a good reliability on a sample of 20 children with different severity degrees of CP. AHA is a hand function evaluation instrument that measures and describes how children with an upper limb disability in one hand use his/her affected hand collaboratively with the nonaffected hand in bimanual actions [22]. In the present study, children underwent functional evaluation with MUUL and AHA at three different time points: at baseline (T1), at the end of the treatment (T2), and at two months of follow-up (T3).

2.4. Stimuli. We prepared fifteen video clips to be used during AOT in the treatment group, each showing a specific daily action implying the use of the arms/hands, (i.e., grasping an object, using a pencil, and playing with Lego). All recorded actions were chosen among those which are familiar to children in primary school age. We used the same videos as in a previous study from our group [17]. In that study, we report also a complete list of all seen actions. In the videos, these everyday actions, performed both by normal children and adults, were recorded from different perspectives, to make the video clips more interesting and to sustain the attention of children during the rehabilitation sessions. Each action was subdivided into 3 or 4 constituent motor segments. For instance, eating a candy, one of the shown actions, was subdivided into taking the candy from the table, approaching it to the mouth, and giving back to the therapist. Each motor act was presented for 3 minutes so that the total duration of each video clip was 9–12 minutes. We also prepared the same number of video clips addressing various topics (geography, history, and science adapted for children) but with no motor content, for the control group. Video clips for the control group were also divided into three-four parts, each lasting 3 minutes.

2.5. Treatment Procedure. For 3 weeks, children in the treatment group attended daily rehabilitation sessions from Monday to Friday, during which they were asked to observe one movie showing an actor/an actress performing one specific daily action with the hand. Actions were presented in a fixed order according to their complexity, as judged by the experimenter.

After observation of each motor segment (3-4 per each video clip), children were required to execute for 2 minutes what observed to the best of their ability. They were advised that the quality of their imitation was not the goal of the rehabilitation treatment. Children in the control group viewed short video clips (for the same time as treated participants) showing scenes with no motor content (e.g., geographical documentaries). After observing each part of a video clip (3-4 parts per each video clip), controls were also asked to execute the same actions as treated participants for the same duration. In this way, the total amount of visual stimulation and motor activity following observation was similar in the two groups. The only difference concerned the content of videos: treated participants observed videos with motor content (everyday arm/hand actions), while controls observed videos with no specific motor content. As a whole, each rehabilitation session lasted about half an hour. The physiotherapist devoted up to 10 minutes to explain the task and encourage children to observe carefully the videos and perform the seen actions at their best. Twelve minutes was devoted to observation (motor acts for cases, documentaries for controls) and 8 minutes to the execution of the observed actions (cases) or just execution of the same actions, but without a model (controls).

Both treated participants and controls received written instructions. The physiotherapist read them aloud twice. This was in order to avoid any influence of the physiotherapist in giving instructions.

During the treatment, children continued to follow their routine conventional rehabilitation program that was the same for cases and controls. All children (treated participants and controls) completed the study.

2.6. Outcome Measures. Primary outcome measures were score changes on the MUUL and AHA.

2.7. Statistical Analysis. A mixed linear model, with fixed effects: time (T1, T2, and T3) and group (treatment, control), was carried out on MUUL and AHA scores. The best model was identified using the Akaike information criterion (AIC). The significance level was set at 0.05. Statistical analyses were carried out using SPSS version 23.

2.8. fMRI Study. Twelve children (six treated participants) out of 18 enrolled children also entered an fMRI study to assess a reorganization of brain neural structures following treatment. While being scanned, children with CP from both groups manipulated complex objects with both hands, in order to explore all the motor properties of the manipulated object. As a control condition, children manipulated a simple object, a sphere. All objects used in the scanner were different from those used during the treatment. Figure 1(a) shows the experimental paradigm. fMRI data were collected on a 1.5T Siemens Avanto scanner. The protocol included four EPI sequences (TR/TE 2500/50 ms, $3.3 \times 3.3 \times 3.3$ mm isotropic voxel) and a high resolution T1W 3D MP-RAGE sequence for anatomical reference (TR/TE 2050/2.56 ms, $1 \times 1 \times 1$ mm isotropic voxel). Imaging data were collected before starting treatment (T1) and at the end of treatment (T2). The fMRI paradigm consisted of 14 alternating task-rest blocks (8 volumes/block were acquired) repeated 4 times to increase statistics. fMRI data underwent the following preprocessing. The mean EPI was first computed for each participant and visually inspected to ensure that none showed artifacts. The first 2 EPI volumes of each functional run were discarded to allow for T1 equilibration effects. For each subject, all volumes were spatially realigned to the mean volume of the four runs. Next, the 3D structural data of each subject were normalized to the ANTS standard space, a T1 pediatric template in a standardized MNI space [23]. The normalization matrix was subsequently transferred to the fMRI images, resampled in $1 mm \times 1 mm \times 1 mm$ voxels using trilinear interpolation in space and then the images were spatially smoothed with a 6 mm full width at half maximum isotropic Gaussian kernel for the group analysis. No participant showed head movements greater than 3 mm; thus, none was excluded from further analyses.

Data were analyzed using a random effects model [24], implemented in a two-level procedure. In the first level, single-subject fMRI data entered an independent general linear model (GLM) by design matrixes modelling the onsets and durations of two experimental factors, one related to the experimental task and one related to its corresponding baseline. For each participant, we generated contrast images displaying the effect of the experimental task (manipulating complex objects) contrasted with the respective baseline (manipulating a sphere). Next, each contrast entered a second level GLM to obtain (i) SPM{T} maps (one sample *t*-test) related to each task at group level and (ii) to test for the

(a)

(b)

(c)

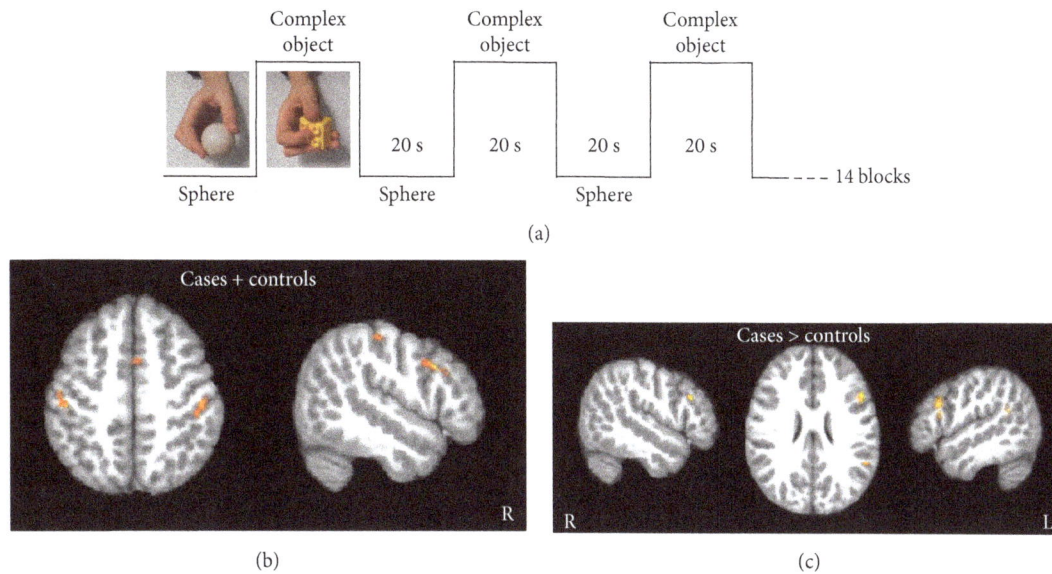

FIGURE 1: (a) Graphic representation of the fMRI experimental paradigm, alternating manipulation of a simple object (a sphere), and manipulation of complex objects. (b) Clusters of activations transposed on sections from standard pediatric brain (ANTS) before treatment (T1), when comparing manipulation of complex objects versus manipulation of a sphere. Cases and controls are taken as a whole group, $p < 0.001$. Note that at T1, no activation was present when directly comparing cases versus controls. (c) After treatment (T2), direct comparison between cases and controls shows increased activations in frontal and parietal areas known to be involved in hand-object interactions, $p < 0.001$. Clusters of activations transposed on sections from standard pediatric brain (ANTS), as in (b).

existence of brain areas specifically involved in manipulating complex objects. Moreover, we were interested in assessing differences in brain area recruitment between treated children and controls. For all analyses, location of the activation foci was determined in the stereotaxic space of the MNI coordinates system. A significance level of $p < 0.001$ uncorrected and an extended threshold on cluster dimension of 10 voxels was applied.

3. Results

Demographic data, clinical features, and brain imaging findings of children in the two groups are shown in Table 1. Mean scores and SD of AHA and MUUL in treated participants and controls at T1, T2, and T3 are shown in Table 2.

Mixed linear model showed that for MUUL, the best model included the random effects of intercept and the fixed effect of group, time, and interaction. For the AHA, the best model included the random effects of intercept and time and the fixed effects of group and interaction. The mixed linear model analysis disclosed a significant interaction between time and treatment, both for MUUL (b_1 interaction = 2.71, $t_{36} = 3.99$, and $p = 0.000$) and for AHA (b_1 interaction = 2.36, $t_{18} = 3.61$, $p = 0.002$). Score improvements, in both scales, were higher in the treated participants than in the controls; furthermore, in the treatment group, those improvements were not only maintained but became even stronger at T3.

Post hoc analysis showed that for MUUL, results at T2 were significantly different from results at T1 only in cases ($p < 0.001$), but not in controls. As for AHA, results at T2 were significantly different from results at T1 ($p < 0.001$). Even more interestingly, results at T3 were different from

results at T2 ($p < 0.001$) for both scales, but again only in cases, but not in controls. Figure 2 shows the results.

4. fMRI Results

For the aim of the present study, we will present results concerning the differences between treated children and controls. It is worth stressing that at baseline (T1), there were no differential activations when comparing cases versus controls. In contrast, after treatment (T2), differential activations were located in the left premotor cortex extending to the inferior frontal gyrus (−49; 19; 26), in the right premotor cortex (53; 14; 31), in the left supramarginal gyrus (−47; −51; 37), and finally a weaker activation in the left superior temporal gyrus (−52; −47; 23). Figures 1(a) and 1(b) shows fMRI findings.

5. Discussion

The results of the present study are relevant within the literature devoted to rehabilitation of children with cerebral palsy. Treated children improved significantly as compared to controls in both MUUL and AHA. These results are in keeping with earlier, pilot studies using AOT as a rehabilitation tool [17, 18]. It is worth stressing that our sample consisted of hemiplegic (both right and left) and tetraplegic children, thus suggesting that AOT may be useful for different clinical presentations of CP. As reported above, AOT exploits a neurophysiological mechanism known as mirror mechanism. The observation of actions performed by other individuals recruits in the observer the same areas involved in the actual execution of those same actions [11], this whatever the biological effector involved in the observed

TABLE 1: Demographic data, clinical features, and radiological findings in treated participants and controls.

Pt. number	Case/control	Sex (M, F)	GA (wk)	Age (yr, m)	CP type Hagberg	Motor abnormalities	GMFCS	MACS	CFCS	Associated impairments	Total IQ	Verbal IQ	Performance IQ	Radiological findings (brain MRI)
1	Case	M	33	9 yr, 5 m	Right hemiplegia	Unilateral spastic hypertonia	2	2	1	V: CVI; H: no; M/A: no; LD: no; E: no	85	92	82	Right temporooccipital, left occipitoparietal, bilateral periventricular, and left frontotemporal subdural hematomas
2	Case	F	27	8 yr, 2 m	Right hemiplegia	Unilateral spastic hypertonia	1	2	1	V: ROP; H: no; M/A: no; LD: no; E: no	100	106	107	Mild bilateral periventricular leukomalacia, mild ventricular dilatation
3	Control	M	40	7 yr, 10 m	Right hemiplegia	Unilateral spastic hypertonia	2	2	1	V: no; H: no; M/A: no; LD: no; E: no	99	101	97	Left subdural occipitotemporal hematoma and epidural parietotemporal hematoma; hypoxic ischemic encephalopathy characterized by signal alterations in both putamen tail and anterior thalamus
4	Control	M	34	8 yr, 3 m	Tetraplegia	Bilateral spastic hypertonia, left side more affected	4	3	2	V: CVI; H: no; M/A: yes; LD: no; E: no	73	97	50	Hypoxic ischemic injury with thinning of the corpus callosum, enlargement of CSF spaces, widespread hyperintensity of centrum semiovale, corona radiata, and periventricular white matter, dilation of the ventricles
5	Control	F	40	6 yr, 8 m	Tetraplegia	Bilateral spastic hypertonia, left side more affected	4	2	3	V: CVI; H: no; M/A: yes; LD: no; E: no	114	139	77	Diffuse periventricular hyperintensity with parietal bilateral white matter involvement; mild dilatation of bilateral ventricular trigone
6	Case	F	30	11 yr, 9 m	Tetraplegia	Bilateral spastic hypertonia, left side more affected	4	3	2	V: CVI; H: no; M/A: yes; LD: yes; E: yes	56	89	50	Periventricular leukomalacia, fronto-parieto-occipital white matter reduction, ex vacuo enlargement of bilateral ventricles

Table 1: Continued.

Pt. number	Case/control	Sex (M, F)	GA (wk)	Age (yr, m)	CP type Hagberg	Motor abnormalities	GMFCS	MACS	CFCS	Associated impairments	Total IQ	Verbal IQ	Performance IQ	Radiological findings (brain MRI)
7	Control	F	37	9 yr, 1 m	Right hemiplegia	Unilateral spastic hypertonia	1	2	1	V: CVI; H: no; M/A: yes; LD: no; E: no	87	84	100	Left periventricular malacic area with gliosis, extended into the corona radiata; left corticospinal projection hyperintensisty with mild cerebellar peduncle hypotrophy (Wallerian degeneration)
8	Control	F	31	8 yr, 9 m	Right hemiplegia	Unilateral spastic hypertonia	2	1	1	V: CVI; H: no; M/A: no; LD: no; E: no	87	99	77	Bilateral parietal cystic periventricular leukomalacia, with centrum semiovale white matter involvement, short distance between cortex and ventricular walls in temporoparietal areas, thinning of the corpus callosum
9	Case	F	Not known	11 yr, 9 m	Left hemiplegia	Unilateral spastic hypertonia	2	2	1	V: no; H: no; M/A: no; LD: no; E: yes	Leiter -R 82			Right fronto-parieto-temporal malacic area, ex vacuo enlargement of the ventricle and Wallerian degeneration of the corticospinal tract
10	Case	M	32	6 yr, 10 m	Tetraplegia	Bilateral spastic hypertonia, right side more affected	3	2	2	V: CVI; H: no; M/A: yes; LD: no; E: no	89	120	70	Periventricular leukomalacia, corpus callosum hypoplasia, hippocampal commissure agenesis
11	Control	M	38	5 yr, 2 m	Right hemiplegia	Unilateral spastic hypertonia	2	3	2	V: CVI; H: no; M/A: no; LD: no; E: no	98	118	87	Cortical laminar necrosis (left insular cortex, left frontoparietal areas, and left temporal lobe). Signal T2 and FLAIR hyperintensity in the left caudate nucleus and in the left corona radiata (ischemic event)

TABLE 1: Continued.

Pt. number	Case/control	Sex (M, F)	GA (wk)	Age (yr, m)	CP type Hagberg	Motor abnormalities	GMFCS	MACS	CFCS	Associated impairments	Total IQ	Verbal IQ	Performance IQ	Radiological findings (brain MRI)
12	Case	F	31	10 yr, 1 m	Tetraplegia	Bilateral spastic hypertonia, left side more affected	4	3	3	V: CVI; H: no; M/A: yes; LD: no; E: no	85	92	82	Severe periventricular leukomalacia with major involvement of the posterior area, associated with supra- and subtentorial ventricular dilatation and subarachnoid spaces enlargement, thinning of the corpus callosum
13	Case	F	41	8 yr, 2 m	Right hemiplegia	Unilateral spastic hypertonia	3	2	1	V: CVI; H: no; M/A: no; LD: no; E: yes	87	99	77	Left hemispheric atrophy (previous extensive left frontoparietal intraparenchymal hemorrhage, wide left parietal subdural hematoma), ex vacuo dilatation of the ipsilateral ventricles and midline brain right to left shift, Wallerian degeneration of the corticospinal tract and ipsilateral cerebellar peduncle atrophy
14	Case	M	33	5 yr, 10 m	Right hemiplegia	Unilateral spastic hypertonia	2	3	2	V: strabismus; H: no; M/A: no; LD: no; E: no	85	92	82	Left fronto-parieto-temporo-insular polymicrogyria (perisylvian and perirolandic with cortical infolding), mild left temporal atrophy with subarachnoid spaces enlargement
15	Case	F		6 yr, 8 m	Left hemiplegia	Unilateral spastic hypertonia	4	3	1	V: no; H: no; M/A: yes; LD: no; E: yes	100	106	107	Ischemic right frontoparietal malacic area with focal cortical atrophy, gliosis, subarachnoid space enlargement, and mid ipsilateral ventricular dilatation. Mild controlateral periventricular white matter hyperintensity

TABLE 1: Continued.

Pt. number	Case/ control	Sex (M, F)	GA (wk)	Age (yr, m)	CP type Hagberg	Motor abnormalities	GMFCS	MACS	CFCS	Associated impairments	Total IQ	Verbal IQ	Performance IQ	Radiological findings (brain MRI)
16	Case	M	38	6yr, 3 m	Left hemiplegia	Unilateral spastic hypertonia	2	3	2	V: no; H: no; M/A: no; LD: no; E: no	99	101	97	Malacic areas affecting the right middle cerebral artery territory with Wallerian degeneration of the corticospinal tract and of the thalamus, left hemisphere hypotrophy
18	Case	M	40	5yr, 3 m	Left hemiplegia	Unilateral spastic hypertonia	2	3	1	V: strabismus; H: no; M/A: no; LD: no; E: yes	101	106	100	Right periventricular porencephalic lesion (hemorrhagic venous infarct) with hemosiderin deposition and Wallerian degeneration of the ipsilateral corticospinal tract
18	Control	M	36	6yr, 4 m	Left hemiplegia	Unilateral spastic hypertonia	1	2	1	V: no; H: no; M/A: no; LD: no; E: no	90	94	93	Supratentorial right malacic areas with right lateral ventricular dilatation; hemosiderin deposition secondary to germinal matrix hemorrhage

M: male; F: female; GA: gestational age; CP: cerebral palsy; GMFCS: Gross Motor Function Classification System; MACS: Manual Ability Classification System; CFCS: Communication Function Classification System; V: vision; CVI: cerebral visual impairment; H: hearing; M/A: memory and attention; LD: learning disabilities (North American usage; mental retardation); E: epilepsy; MRI: magnetic resonance imaging.

TABLE 2: Mean scores (and SD) of AHA and MUUL in controls and treated participants at different time points.

Group	Score	Time point		
		T1	T2	T3
Control	AHA	65.71 (7.23)	66.86 (7.31)	66.71 (7.52)
	MUUL	96.00 (16.73)	98.00 (16.69)	98.14 (16.52)
Treatment	AHA	57.45 (12.18)	61.09 (10.79)	63.18 (11.06)
	MUUL	81.73 (22.38)	87.27 (22.36)	89.27 (22.41)

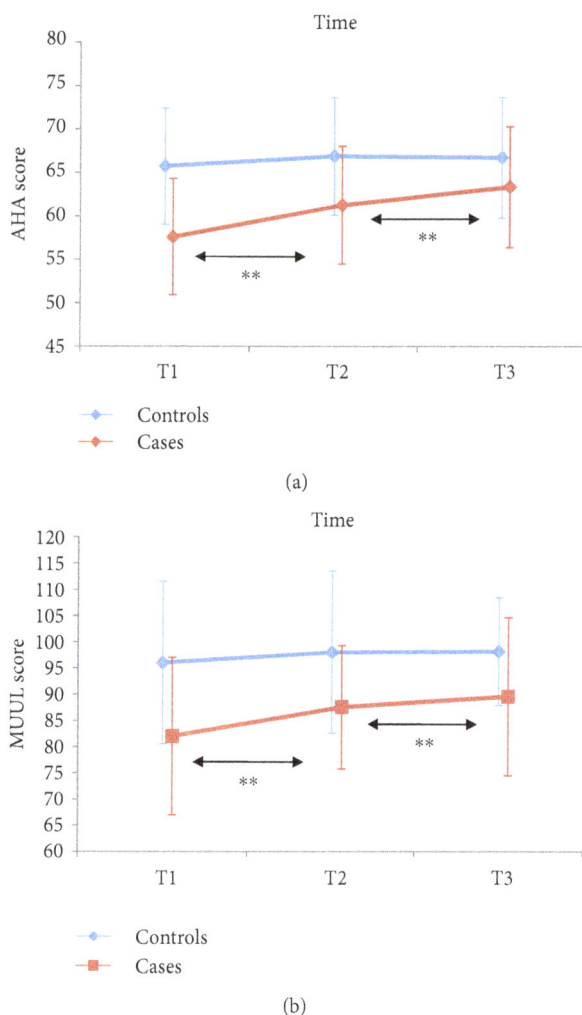

(a)

(b)

FIGURE 2: Scores obtained by cases (red line) and controls (blue line) at T1, T2, and T3 in two different functional scales (AHA, MUUL). Statistical analysis (see text for details) showed that only in case scores obtained at T2 differed significantly from scores at T1 in both scales. This was true also when comparing T3 with T2 in both scales (error bars: 95% CI). ** refers to statistical significant effects.

action. This mechanism may underlie the capacity to understand and imitate others' actions even at an early stage of life [25, 26] and contribute to interact with other people in an empathic manner (for review see, Hari and Kujala) [27]. This same mechanism may be helpful during learning motor tasks or relearning daily actions following brain lesions and therefore during rehabilitation [28–30]. AOT has the potential to become a routine approach in the rehabilitation of children with CP and could be easily applied by physiotherapists working with children. During the rehabilitation session, physiotherapists have the role to motivate little patients to observe carefully every detail of the observed actions and to push children to use the objects provided at hand, as in the videos, but also to reassure if children fail in performing the observed actions. Patients, even children as in the present study, may follow the rehabilitation program without difficulties. It is worth stressing that AOT may be applied in a very flexible manner: in fact, the trained actions, presented through videos, may vary depending on the real need of patients. For example, children that have more difficulties in performing distal hand/arm actions (i.e., grasping, manipulating) should focus their training on these motor tasks, while children that present with impairment of proximal arm actions (i.e., reaching objects, coding objects in space) should train this kind of motor tasks. Last, but not least, AOT may be used also at home where children may get their rehabilitation session with the help of their parents or even in telerehabilitation with a physiotherapist monitoring from a dedicated position what children perform at home.

In the present study, we collected functional scores on MUUL and AHA also at two months of follow-up. Interestingly, treated children, as compared to controls, maintained and even improved their functional gain at follow-up. In our opinion, these findings may be explained by the fact that during AOT, children learn novel strategies to interact with other people and common objects. They learn to look very carefully at all details present in the scene, they pay attention at the different motor segments of an action, and they spontaneously prepare themselves to imitate a seen action or to interact upon objects available in the environment. Eventually, they transfer these strategies in everyday life situations; thus at the very end, they accomplish the goal of gaining better motor performances.

A main point of interest in the present study is that some of the treated children also underwent an fMRI study aimed at assessing whether AOT may recruit areas within the motor system and eventually contribute to their reorganization. It is worth noting that, while being scanned, children performed an independent task, namely, manipulation of complex objects that were not included in the set of actions trained during the treatment. When comparing treated participants and controls, differential activation was present in a sector of the premotor cortex and parietal cortex also involved in object manipulation in both healthy adults and children [31, 32] and known to be endowed with a motor representation of distal upper limb movements. This premotor sector is strictly connected with a parietal area with which it builds up a sensorimotor circuit allowing individuals to code for the motor properties of objects and the implementation of the most appropriate actions to act upon objects [33]. These findings suggest that the brain target of AOT is exactly a hand motor area possibly involved in executing actions as well as in their processing. It therefore appears that there are not vicariating areas emerging from AOT treatment, but rather a recovery of areas normally involved in a specific hand motor task. Further studies should assess to what extent this concerns also other biological effectors (e.g., the foot) and contributes to rebuild physiological sensorimotor circuits. Another issue that future studies should help to ascertain is whether there are specific subgroups of children with cerebral palsy that may mostly benefit from AOT, or rather this approach may help clinical conditions in all children affected.

Conflicts of Interest

The authors declare that they have no conflicts of interest.

Acknowledgments

The authors are grateful to Anna Alessandrini, Nicole D'Adda, Maria Fezzardi, and Federica Tansini for their valuable help in performing the treatment of the children included in this study and to Federica Pagani for her help in collecting data. The authors are also grateful to Serena Micheletti for her precious assistance in evaluating cognitive profile of all the children and to Annalisa Pelosi for her great support on statistical analysis.

References

[1] S. L. Small, G. Buccino, and A. Solodkin, "Brain repair after stroke-a novel neurological model," *Nature Reviews Neurology*, vol. 9, no. 12, pp. 698–707, 2013.

[2] E. Taub, G. Uswatte, and T. Elbert, "New treatments in neurorehabilitation founded on basic research," *Nature Reviews Neuroscience*, vol. 3, no. 3, pp. 228–236, 2002.

[3] A. Roby-Brami, A. Feydy, M. Combeaud, E. V. Biryukova, B. Bussel, and M. F. Levin, "Motor compensation and recovery for reaching in stroke patients," *Acta Neurologica Scandinavica*, vol. 107, no. 5, pp. 369–381, 2003.

[4] M. F. Levin, J. A. Kleim, and S. L. Wolf, "What do motor "recovery" and "compensation" mean in patients following stroke?," *Neurorehabilitation and Neural Repair*, vol. 23, no. 4, pp. 313–319, 2009.

[5] P. S. Lum, S. Mulroy, R. L. Amdur, P. Requejo, B. I. Prilutsky, and A. W. Dromerick, "Gains in upper extremity function after stroke via recovery or compensation: potential differential effects on amount of real-world limb use," *Topics in Stroke Rehabilitation*, vol. 16, no. 4, pp. 237–253, 2009.

[6] R. J. Nudo, "Mechanisms for recovery of motor function following cortical damage," *Current Opinion in Neurobiology*, vol. 16, no. 6, pp. 638–644, 2006.

[7] L. Sakzewski, A. Gordon, and A. C. Eliasson, "The state of the evidence for intensive upper limb therapy approaches for children with unilateral cerebral palsy," *Journal of Child Neurology*, vol. 29, no. 8, pp. 1077–1090, 2014.

[8] V. S. Ramachandran and E. L. Altschuler, "The use of visual feedback, in particular mirror visual feedback, in restoring brain function," *Brain*, vol. 132, no. 7, pp. 1693–1710, 2009.

[9] H. Thieme, J. Mehrholz, M. Pohl, J. Behrens, and C. Dohle, "Mirror therapy for improving motor function after stroke," *Stroke*, vol. 44, no. 1, pp. e1–e2, 2013.

[10] R. Bruchez, M. Jequier Gygax, S. Roches et al., "Mirror therapy in children with hemiparesis: a randomized observer-blinded trial," *Developmental Medicine & Child Neurology*, vol. 58, no. 9, pp. 970–978, 2016.

[11] G. Rizzolatti and L. Craighero, "The mirror-neuron system," *Annual Review of Neuroscience*, vol. 27, no. 1, pp. 169–192, 2004.

[12] G. Buccino, "Action observation treatment: a novel tool in neurorehabilitation," *Philosophical Transactions of the Royal Society B: Biological Sciences*, vol. 369, no. 1644, article 20130185, 2014.

[13] G. Bellelli, G. Buccino, B. Bernardini, A. Padovani, and M. Trabucchi, "Action observation treatment improves recovery of postsurgical orthopedic patients: evidence for a topdown effect?," *Archives of Physical Medicine and Rehabilitation*, vol. 91, no. 10, pp. 1489–1494, 2010.

[14] D. Ertelt, S. Small, A. Solodkin et al., "Action observation has a positive impact on rehabilitation of motor deficits after stroke," *NeuroImage*, vol. 36, Supplement 2, pp. T164–T173, 2007.

[15] E. Pelosin, L. Avanzino, M. Bove, P. Stramesi, A. Nieuwboer, and G. Abbruzzese, "Action observation improves freezing of gait in patients with Parkinson's disease," *Neurorehabilitation and Neural Repair*, vol. 24, no. 8, pp. 746–752, 2010.

[16] G. Buccino, R. Gatti, M. C. Giusti et al., "Action observation treatment improves autonomy in daily activities in Parkinson's disease patients: results from a pilot study," *Movement Disorders*, vol. 26, no. 10, pp. 1963-1964, 2011.

[17] G. Buccino, D. Arisi, P. Gough et al., "Improving upper limb motor functions through action observation treatment: a pilot study in children with cerebral palsy," *Developmental Medicine & Child Neurology*, vol. 54, no. 9, pp. 822–828, 2012.

[18] G. Sgandurra, A. Ferrari, G. Cossu, A. Guzzetta, L. Fogassi, and G. Cioni, "Randomized trial of observation and execution of upper extremity actions versus action alone in children with unilateral cerebral palsy," *Neurorehabilitation and Neural Repair*, vol. 27, no. 9, pp. 808–815, 2013.

[19] J. Y. Kim, J. M. Kim, and E. Y. Ko, "The effect of the action observation physical training on the upper extremity function in children with cerebral palsy," *Journal of Exercise Rehabilitation*, vol. 10, no. 3, pp. 176–183, 2014.

[20] A. C. Eliasson, L. Krumlinde-Sundholm, B. Rösblad et al., "The Manual Ability Classification System (MACS) for children with cerebral palsy: scale development and evidence of validity and reliability," *Developmental Medicine & Child Neurology*, vol. 48, no. 7, pp. 549–554, 2006.

[21] M. Randall, J. B. Carlin, P. Chondros, and D. Reddihough, "Reliability of the Melbourne Assessment of Unilateral Upper Limb Function," *Developmental Medicine & Child Neurology*, vol. 43, no. 11, pp. 761–767, 2001.

[22] L. Krumlinde-Sundholm, M. Holmefur, A. Kottorp, and A. C. Eliasson, "The Assisting Hand Assessment: current evidence of validity, reliability, and responsiveness to change," *Developmental Medicine & Child Neurology*, vol. 49, no. 4, pp. 259–264, 2007.

[23] S. S. Ghosh, S. Kakunoori, J. Augustinack et al., "Evaluating the validity of volume-based and surface-based brain image registration for developmental cognitive neuroscience studies in children 4 to 11 years of age," *NeuroImage*, vol. 53, no. 1, pp. 85–93, 2010.

[24] K. J. Friston, A. P. Holmes, C. J. Price, C. Buchel, and K. J. Worsley, "Multisubject fMRI studies and conjunction analyses," *NeuroImage*, vol. 10, no. 4, pp. 385–396, 1999.

[25] A. N. Meltzoff and M. K. Moore, "Imitation of facial and manual gestures by human neonates," *Science*, vol. 198, no. 4312, pp. 75–78, 1977.

[26] T. Falck-Ytter, G. Gredebäck, and C. von Hofsten, "Infants predict other people's action goals," *Nature Neuroscience*, vol. 9, no. 7, pp. 878-879, 2006.

[27] R. Hari and M. V. Kujala, "Brain basis of human social interaction: from concepts to brain imaging," *Physiological Reviews*, vol. 89, no. 2, pp. 453–479, 2009.

[28] P. Celnik, B. Webster, D. M. Glasser, and L. G. Cohen, "Effects of action observation on physical training after stroke," *Stroke*, vol. 39, no. 6, pp. 1814–1820, 2008.

[29] K. Stefan, L. G. Cohen, J. Duque et al., "Formation of a motor memory by action observation," *The Journal of Neuroscience*, vol. 25, no. 41, pp. 9339–9346, 2005.

[30] R. Gatti, A. Tettamanti, P. M. Gough, E. Riboldi, L. Marinoni, and G. Buccino, "Action observation versus motor imagery in learning a complex motor task: a short review of literature and a kinematics study," *Neuroscience Letters*, vol. 540, pp. 37–42, 2013.

[31] F. Binkofski, G. Buccino, S. Posse, R. J. Seitz, G. Rizzolatti, and H. J. Freund, "A fronto-parietal circuit for object manipulation in man: evidence from an fMRI-study," *The European Journal of Neuroscience*, vol. 11, no. 9, pp. 3276–3286, 1999.

[32] L. Biagi, G. Cioni, L. Fogassi, A. Guzzetta, G. Sgandurra, and M. Tosetti, "Action observation network in childhood: a comparative fMRI study with adults," *Developmental Science*, vol. 19, no. 6, pp. 1075–1086, 2016.

[33] M. Jeannerod, M. A. Arbib, G. Rizzolatti, and H. Sakata, "Grasping objects: the cortical mechanisms of visuomotor transformation," *Trends in Neurosciences*, vol. 18, no. 7, pp. 314–320, 1995.

11

The Neural Basis of Fear Promotes Anger and Sadness Counteracts Anger

Jun Zhan ⓘ,[1,2] Jingyuan Ren,[1] Pei Sun,[3] Jin Fan,[4] Chang Liu ⓘ,[5] and Jing Luo ⓘ[1]

[1]School of Psychology, Capital Normal University, Beijing, China
[2]School of Marxism, Fujian Agriculture and Forestry University, Fuzhou, China
[3]Department of Psychology, Tsinghua University, Beijing, China
[4]Department of Psychology, The City University of New York, New York City, NY, USA
[5]School of Psychology, Nanjing Normal University, Nanjing, China

Correspondence should be addressed to Chang Liu; cglew@163.com and Jing Luo; luoj@psych.ac.cn

Academic Editor: Fushun Wang

In contrast to cognitive emotion regulation theories that emphasize top-down control of prefrontal-mediated regulation of emotion, in traditional Chinese philosophy and medicine, different emotions are considered to have mutual promotion and counteraction relationships. Our previous studies have provided behavioral evidence supporting the hypotheses that "fear promotes anger" and "sadness counteracts anger"; this study further investigated the corresponding neural correlates. A basic hypothesis we made is the "internal versus external orientation" assumption proposing that fear could promote anger as its external orientation associated with motivated action, whereas sadness could counteract anger as its internal or homeostatic orientation to somatic or visceral experience. A way to test this assumption is to examine the selective involvement of the posterior insula (PI) and the anterior insula (AI) in sadness and fear because the posterior-to-anterior progression theory of insular function suggests that the role of the PI is to encode primary body feeling and that of the AI is to represent the integrative feeling that incorporates the internal and external input together. The results showed increased activation in the AI, parahippocampal gyrus (PHG), posterior cingulate (PCC), and precuneus during the fear induction phase, and the activation level in these areas could positively predict subsequent aggressive behavior; meanwhile, the PI, superior temporal gyrus (STG), superior frontal gyrus (SFG), and medial prefrontal cortex (mPFC) were more significantly activated during the sadness induction phase, and the activation level in these areas could negatively predict subsequent feelings of subjective anger in a provocation situation. These results revealed a possible cognitive brain mechanism underlying "fear promotes anger" and "sadness counteracts anger." In particular, the finding that the AI and PI selectively participated in fear and sadness emotions was consistent with our "internal versus external orientation" assumption about the different regulatory effects of fear and sadness on anger and aggressive behavior.

1. Introduction

Western psychology generally advocates the use of cognitive methods, such as rational or cognitive reappraisal, to downregulate negative emotions. However, hormones released in response to stress can impair the advanced function of the prefrontal cortex (PFC), leading to a failure of cognitive reappraisal in regulating conditioned fear under stress [1, 2]; thus, emotion regulation strategies that are less reliant on the PFC could be more suitable for changing negative responses to emotional arousal under stress than normal downregulating strategies [3]. In contrast to cognitive emotion regulation theories, traditional Chinese philosophy and medicine consider different types of emotions to have mutual promotion and mutual counteraction (MPMC) relationships (Figure 1) involving a down-up process that depends less on the PFC

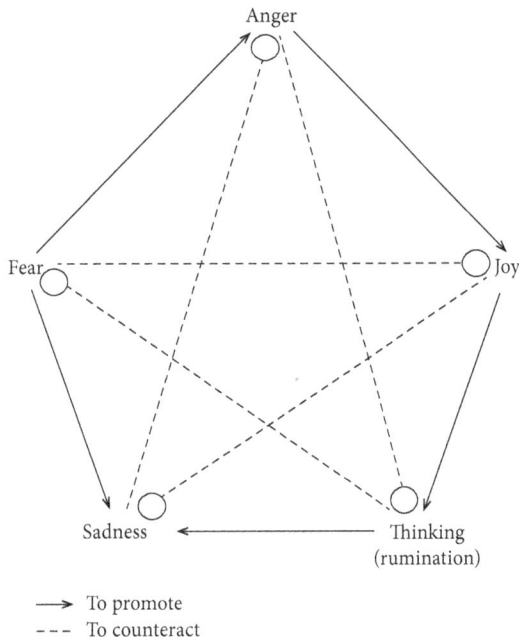

FIGURE 1: Relationships of mutual promotion and mutual restraint and the emotions of joy, thinking/anxiety (The original word for "thinking" in the Chinese literature is 思 [read as si]; 思 may indicate either the pure cognitive thinking and reasoning process that is nonpathogenic or the maladaptive repetitive thinking or ruminative thinking that is typically associated with negative emotion and has pathogenic potential. Thus, 思 may have different meanings in different contexts of the MPMC theory. The implication of maladaptive "thinking" in the MPMC theory of emotionality includes not only ruminative thought per se but also the negative, depression-like emotion associated with it. Therefore, in specific contexts, particularly the context discussed in this study, 思 indicates the ruminative or repetitive thinking that is closely related to rumination in modern psychology, which is defined as a pattern of repetitive self-focus and recursive thinking focused on negative cases or problems (e.g., unfulfilled goals or unemployment) that is always associated with the aggravation of negative mood states (e.g., sadness, tension, and self-focus) and has been shown to increase one's vulnerability to developing or exacerbating depression [4].), sadness, fear, and anger. The promotion relationships include the following: joy promotes thinking/anxiety, thinking/anxiety promotes sadness, sadness promotes fear, fear promotes anger, and anger promotes joy. The restraint relationships include the following: joy counteracts sadness, sadness counteracts anger, anger counteracts thinking/anxiety, thinking/anxiety counteracts fear, and fear counteracts joy.

[4], thereby suggesting a novel approach for emotion regulation that may overcome the shortcomings of traditional cognitive regulation strategies.

In our recent study, aggressive behavior associated with anger was found to be effectively reduced by inducing sadness, while the induction of fear significantly increased self-reported anger; these findings provided behavioral evidence supporting the hypotheses proposed by the MPMC theory of emotionality that suggest "sadness counteracts anger" and "fear promotes anger" [3, 4]. In that experiment, anger was first induced by asking the participants to read an extremely negative comment regarding their viewpoints (the

mutual article evaluation paradigm) or watch standardized anger-inducing movie clips; then, fear, sadness, or a neutral mood was induced. The participants who were provoked exhibited less aggressive behavior if sadness was subsequently induced; however, the participants became increasingly angry if fear was subsequently induced.

More importantly, the principle of "sadness counteracts anger" may have application value because the induction of sadness (e.g., passively watching a clip from a sad movie or listening to sad music) requires obviously fewer cognitive control resources mediated by the PFC and may regulate negative emotion; therefore, this principle could have some advantages in regulating emotion relative to cognitive-regulation strategies that may fail to work under stress. To test this hypothesis, in our recent study, we directly compared the effects of cognitive reappraisal and sadness induction on reducing anger or anger-related aggression in nonstressful and stressful situations [3]. Expectedly, cognitive reappraisal was unable to effectively relieve the subjective feeling of anger under the stress condition; however, the stressful condition did not influence the efficiency of sadness induction in reducing aggressive behavior. First, all the participants were assigned to a nonstressful or stressful condition and were provoked using the mutual article evaluation paradigm; then, the participants were asked to make a cognitive reappraisal or watch sad movie clips. The cognitive reappraisal effectively reduced self-reported anger under the nonstress condition but failed to have such an effect under the stress condition; meanwhile, high cortisol levels were found to be maintained in and after the reappraisal. It is possible that cortisol activation triggered by the arousal of the hypothalamic-pituitary-adrenal (HPA) axis disrupted the PFC function and further impaired the efficiency of cognitive regulation, while stress did not influence the effects of sadness induction on aggressive behavior and related skin conductance, suggesting that the emotion regulation strategy is relatively immune to stress.

However, the cognitive brain processes underlying the phenomenon of "sadness counteracts anger" and "fear promotes anger" are still unknown. A general perspective for understanding these mechanisms is to consider the ways in which different types of emotions interact, that is, how an antecedent or subsequent emotion (such as sadness or fear) could interact with the targeted emotion (such as anger). This investigation of the process and neural mechanism of the interactions among different emotions could increase our understanding of the effective principle of the "sadness counteracts anger" strategy. For example, if an individual is aroused by sadness or fear before or after being provoked, a certain pattern of neuropsychological components activated by the sadness or fear could affect the expression of anger or aggressive behavior.

More specifically, according to a meta-analysis of the neural activation patterns associated with different types of basic emotions, the anger and fear categories both prioritized cortical processes that support an "external orientation/object-focused" schema, which is characterized by goal-driven responses in which objects and events in the world are in the foreground [5]. In contrast, the cortical patterns associated with sadness support an internal orientation/homeostatic-focused schema characterized by an orientation toward immediate somatic or visceral experiences, which prioritizes the processing of interoceptive and homeostatic events [5]. Thus, the neural circuits mediating anger and related aggression may be more easily triggered by the neural activity underlying fear but more efficiently eliminated by the neural activity underlying sadness [4].

To test this hypothesis, this study investigated the regulatory effects of antecedently induced sadness or fear on the subsequent anger and related aggressive behavior in a provoking situation and analyzed the accompanying brain mechanisms using functional magnetic resonance imaging (fMRI). Specifically, we explored and verified the possibility that following antecedent-induced sadness, individuals are less likely to become angry or aggressive ("sadness counteracts anger") in a provoking situation, while following antecedent-induced fear, individuals are more likely to become angry or display more aggression ("fear promotes anger") in a provoking situation. We identified the key brain regions activated by sadness or fear inducing and further analyzed the correlation between the activations of these regions and the subsequent anger-related responses in subsequent provocation.

In particular, we made an "internal versus external orientation" assumption proposing that fear could promote anger because of its external orientation associated with motivated action, whereas sadness could counteract anger because of its internal or homeostatic orientation to somatic or visceral experience. This assumption could be examined by detecting the selective involvement of the posterior insula (PI) and the anterior insula (AI) in sadness and fear. According to the theory of the posterior-to-anterior progression of insular function in re-representing human feeling and emotion, the PI represents more primary quantities, whereas the AI integrates more contextual information in its representation of emotion [6, 7]. Therefore, we propose that fear could be more intensively represented in the AI by its external encoding or contextual integrating orientation and that this orientation, because of its similarities with anger, will promote anger-related feeling and behavior, whereas sadness could be more intensively represented in the PI by its internal orientation or homeostatic-focused schema and that this orientation, because of its dissimilarities with anger, will counteract with anger-related feeling and behavior.

2. Materials and Methods

2.1. Participants. The sample size was 24, which was calculated with the G*Power software 3.1.9.2 (input parameter: α: 0.05; power $(1 - \beta)$: 0.8). In addition, to minimize the potential impact of age differences, twenty-six college students (17 females and 9 males, aged 19–25 years, mean age = 22 years, all native Chinese speakers) at universities in Beijing were recruited to participate in this study as paid volunteers. All the participants were right-handed, had normal or corrected-to-normal vision, and had no history of neurological or psychiatric problems. Prior to the scanning session, the participants signed informed consent forms, and the study was approved by the Institutional Review Board of

the Center for Biomedical Imaging Research of Tsinghua University. After the experiment, each participant was compensated with 120 RMB for participating in the study. Two participants (1 male and 1 female) were excluded from the analysis due to excessive head motion during the scanning.

2.2. Experimental Design and Procedures

2.2.1. Overview of the Experimental Procedure. In contrast to the experimental procedure used in our previous study, which examined the regulatory effects of subsequently evoked sadness or fear on the anger emotion that had already been evoked [3, 4], in this study, we adopted a modified experimental procedure to examine the interaction between anger and sadness or fear, which could be more suitable for within-subject design. We examined the inhibitory or facilitatory effects of the antecedently evoked sadness or fear on anger or aggressive behavior in an offensive situation subsequently experienced by the participants. A single-factor (mood induction: fear versus sadness versus neutral mood) within-subject design was adopted in this study in which the participants experienced three episodes of fear, sadness, or neutral emotion induction, and each emotion induction was followed by a modified competitive reaction time task to provoke the participants; the level of subjective anger was measured at baseline and after the competitive reaction time task. Using this paradigm, a within-subject design that is more suitable for an fMRI investigation could be applied.

2.2.2. Evaluation of Subjective Anger. The subjective feeling of anger was measured using the hostility subscale of the revised Multiple Affect Adjective Checklist (MAACL) [8, 9]. In the Chinese version of the MAACL [10], the hostility subscale contains 22 adjectives, including 11 words that are positively associated with anger (i.e., irritable, cruel, jealous, disgruntled, indignant, impatient, hostile, irritated, violent, furious, and exasperated) and 11 words that are negatively associated with anger (i.e., gracious, easy-going, good-natured, helpful, friendly, courteous, gentle, pleasantly agreeable, kind, affable, and cooperative). All the participants were required to assess these 22 adjectives according to their current feelings and to select each positive anger word (press the "1" button) or to unselect each negative anger word (press the "2" button). Each selection accumulated one point, and the final scores were the sum of the total points of the selected positive anger words and unselected negative anger words. A high total score indicated a high level of anger.

2.2.3. Fear/Sadness/Neutral Mood Induction. In this study, 3 video clips were used to induce fear (duration, 2 min 20 sec; from the movie "Help"; intensity, M = 3.33, SD = 2.1), sadness (duration, 2 min 20 sec; from the movie "Mom Love Me Once Again"; intensity, M = 3.17, SD = 1.56), and a neutral emotion (duration, 2 min 20 sec; from the movie "Computer Repair"; intensity, M = 1.0625, SD = 0.25). The movie clips were extracted from the Chinese Emotional Visual Stimulus (CEVS) database [11]. While watching the clips, the participants were asked to be as attentive to the clips as possible, to express their natural feelings, and to avoid suppressing any emotion.

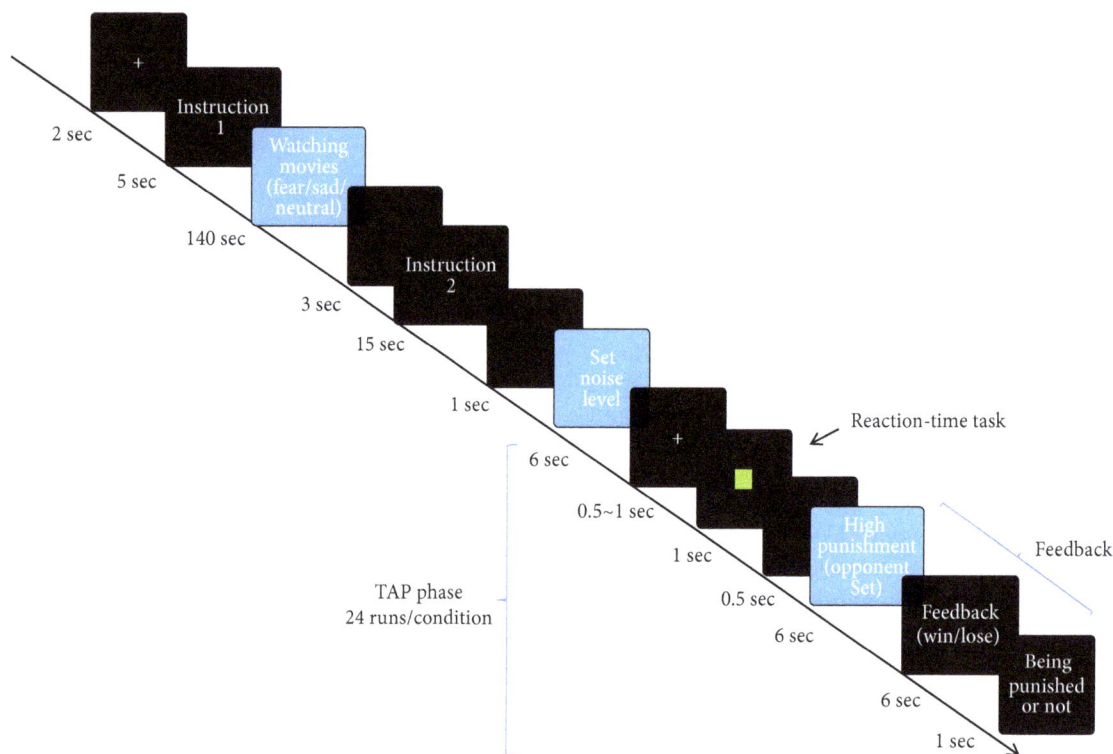

FIGURE 2: Overview of the presentations experienced by each subject over the course of the experiment. The entire experiment consisted of three runs (i.e., fear/sadness/neutral mood conditions) of the procedure.

2.2.4. Anger Induction and Aggressive Behavior Measure. The Taylor Aggression Paradigm (TAP) was used to induce anger and measure aggressive behaviors [12–15]. The modified version of the TAP was used in this study, and the task paradigm was adopted from a previous study [16]. In this task, the participants were informed that they would be playing 24 successive competitive reaction-time trials against an opponent. However, there was no opponent, and the entire program was established in advance. At the beginning of each trial, the participant was shown the opponent number for the upcoming competition (each of the three runs was supposedly played against a different opponent to avoid the possible influence of the competition experience with the opponent against whom they had competed in the previous run). Each participant was allowed to determine the intensity of the noise, that is, between 65 decibels (1—very weak) and 95 decibels (4—very strong), his/her opponent would hear if the opponent lost; each noise had a 2-second duration. Participants were instructed to select the noise intensity from 1 to 4 before each competition trial, and the average noise intensity selected by the participants over 24 rounds was used to indicate participants' aggression levels. After the participants selected the noise intensity, they were provoked by being shown the high-punishment selection (level 3 or 4, each 50%) of their opponents. Finally, feedback was provided regarding whether the participant won or lost. In the losing trials, the participants were exposed to aversive noise; in the winning trials, the participants did not receive a punishment. However, all win and fail trials were secretly controlled by the

experimenter, and the participants won 12 of the 24 trials of the competition game.

2.3. Imaging Procedure. The scanning was divided into three runs according to the mood induction (fear, sadness, or neutral mood), and the run sequence was balanced across all participants. The interval between two runs was 3 min to allow the participants' mood to return to the baseline level and minimize any carryover effect [17]. The duration of each run was 12 min and 54 sec, and the total time of the functional imaging was 38 min and 42 sec. Each run consisted of two sessions (Figure 2). The first session included the phases of "introduction 1" and "watching movies." During "introduction 1," the participant was required to pay attention to watching movies, and in the phase of "watching movies," the participant was assigned to watch one of three different emotional movie clips to induce sadness, fear, or neutral emotions, with a clip duration of 140 sec. During the second session, "instruction 2" was used to introduce the rules of the TAP, which consisted of 24 trials and was used to elicit and assess aggression [16]. Each trial included the phase of "set noise level" (duration: 6 sec), in which the participant set the noise intensity for the opponent; the phase of "reaction-time task" (duration: 1 sec), in which the participant played against an opponent; and the phase of "feedback" (duration: 13 sec), in which the participant was provoked by being shown the opponent's high-punishment selection.

2.4. Image Acquisition. The data were acquired from the Center for Biomedical Imaging Research of Tsinghua University.

TABLE 1: Illustration of the eighteen events defined in the image analysis.

Number	Run—condition	Session	Event	Onset time (sec)	Duration (sec)
1			Instruction 1	20	5
2		Fear induction	Watching fear movie clip	25	140
3	Run 1—fear		Instruction 2	168	15
4			Determining noise level	186	6
5		TAP (first trial)	Reaction time task	192	1
6			Provocation	193	13
7			Instruction 1	20	5
8		Sadness induction	Watching sad movie clip	25	140
9	Run 2—sadness		Instruction 2	168	15
10			Determining noise level	186	6
11		TAP (first trial)	Reaction time task	192	1
12			Provocation	193	13
13			Instruction 1	20	5
14		Neutral induction	Watching neutral movie clip	25	140
15	Run 3—neutral		Instruction 2	168	15
16			Determining noise level	186	6
17		TAP (first trial)	Reaction time task	192	1
18			Provocation	193	13

The fMRI scanning was performed using a 3 T magnetic resonance scanner (Philips, Netherlands) with a 32-channel frequency head coil. To restrict head movements, the participants' heads were fixed with plastic braces and foam pads during the entire experiment. To perform the functional imaging, we used an echo-planar sequence based on blood oxygenation level-dependent (BOLD) contrast with the following parameters: time (TR) = 2000 ms, echo time (TE) = 35 ms, flip angle (FA) = 90°, field of view (FOV) = 200 mm × 200 mm, 64 × 64 matrix, voxel size = $2.5 \times 2.5 \times 4$ mm^3, 30 slices, and 4 mm thickness. T2*-weighted function images parallel to the anterior commissure-posterior commissure (AC-PC) were obtained. To obtain structural images, high-resolution structural T1*-weighted anatomical scanning was performed using a 3D gradient-echo pulse sequence (TR = 7.65, TE = 3.73, flip = 90°, FOV = 230 mm × 230 mm, and voxel size = 0.96 mm × 0.96 mm × 1 mm).

2.5. Image Analysis. The imaging data were analyzed using SPM 8 (Statistical Parametric Mapping, Wellcome Department of Cognitive Neurology, London, UK). During preprocessing, the images of each participant were corrected with slice-timing, realigned to correct for head motion, spatially normalized into a standard echo planar imaging (EPI) template in the Montreal Neurological Institute (MNI) space, and smoothed using an 8 mm Gaussian kernel full width at half maximum (FWHM).

For each participant, a general linear model with eighteen events was defined. Specifically, each run consisted of six events, including "instruction 1," "watching movies," "instruction 2," "set noise level," "reaction-time task," and "feedback" (merged with "the presentation of a high punishment by the opponent," "feedback regarding winning or losing," and "being punished or not punished"). Because

each run included one experimental condition (fearful, sad, or neutral), the three runs had eighteen (3 runs × 6 events/run) events (Figure 2 and Table 1). All the events were modeled with a canonical hemodynamic response function using the standard SPM8 settings. Six covariates (i.e., three rigid-body translations and three rotations resulting from the realignment) were also included to account for movement-related variability. Regionally specific condition effects were tested with performing linear contrasts for each key event relative to the baseline and each participant.

During the mood-induction phase, we were primarily interested in the differences in the cognitive brain responses among the different mood inductions (i.e., fear versus neutral mood induction, fear versus sadness induction, sadness versus neutral mood induction, and sadness versus fear induction). We additionally performed conjunction analyses of "fear induction > neutral mood induction," "fear induction > sadness induction," "sadness induction > neutral mood induction," and "sadness induction > fear induction" to identify the selective effects of the fear and sadness inductions.

The threshold of the whole-brain analyses was generally set at the threshold of $p < 0.001$ (uncorrected for multiple comparisons). All ROIs were created by superimposing the activated clusters obtained from the given contrast (e.g., the parahippocampal activation obtained in the conjunction analysis of "fear induction > neutral mood induction" and "fear induction > sadness induction") on the mask defined in the WFU PickAtlas (Version 3.0, http://fmri.wfubmc.edu/software/PickAtlas), and the percentage signal changes were extracted from MarsBar (http://marsbar.sourceforge.net). The percentage signal changes within each ROI were extracted separately for each participant under each condition.

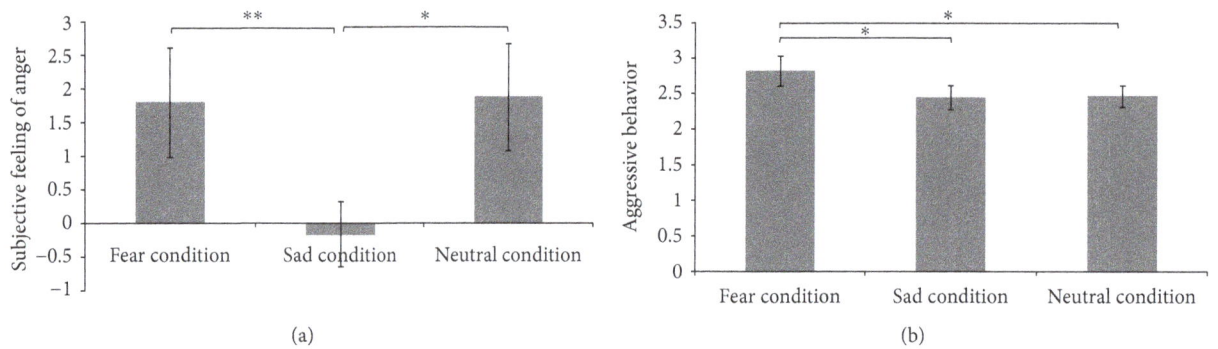

(a)   (b)

FIGURE 3: Comparison of the subjective feeling of anger and aggressive behavior under the fear, sad, and neutral conditions. The difference between the subjective anger feeling in each condition and that at baseline is shown in (a). The aggressive behavior under the three conditions is shown in (b). The error bars (capped vertical bars) represent $(-1)/(+1)$SE. ** indicates a significant difference at $p < 0.01$; * indicates a significant difference at $p < 0.05$.

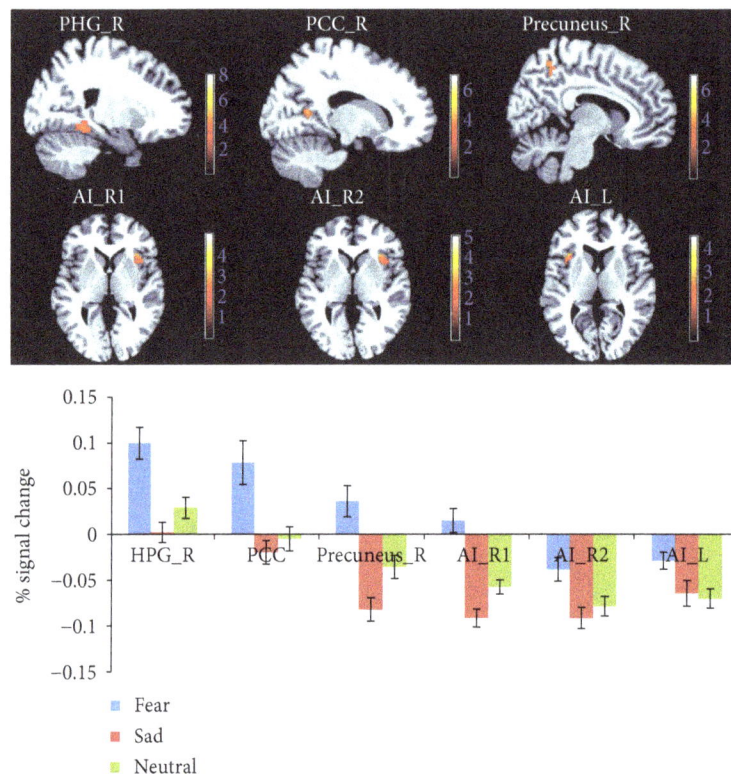

FIGURE 4: Neuroimaging results showing brain activation associated with fear induction (i.e., watching movies). The activation of the PHG_R, PCC_R, and precuneus_R result was taken from the conjunction analysis of "fear > neutral" and "fear > sadness" (depicted at threshold of $p < 0.001$), the activation of AI_R1 was taken from the contrast of "fear > sadness" (depicted at threshold of $p < 0.05$), and the activation of AI_R2 and AI_L was taken from the contrast of "fear > neutral" (depicted at $p < 0.05$). The graphs show the mean percent signal changes for the PHG_R, PCC_R, precuneus_R, AI_R1, AI_R2, and AI_L across the three experimental conditions.

3. Results

3.1. Behavioral Results. The change in subjective anger (the difference between subjective anger after the TAP session and at baseline) was significantly lower under the sadness condition than under the fear $[t(23) = -2.964,$ $p < 0.05,$ $d = 0.526]$ and neutral mood $[t(23) = -2.553,$

$p < 0.05,$ $d = 0.470]$ conditions, and no significant differences were observed between the fear and neutral mood conditions (Figure 3(a)). In addition, aggressive behavior, as determined with the average noise intensity set by the participant to punish his/her opponent over 24 rounds of the competition, under the fear condition was significantly higher than under the sadness $[t(23) = 2.382, p < 0.05, d = 0.445]$

TABLE 2: Brain regions associated with the effects of fear induction.

Brain regions	Hemisphere	Brodmann's area	MNI coordinates			$t(24)$	k
			x	y	z		
(fear > neutral) ∩ *(fear > sadness) (conjunction)*							
Parahippocampal gyrus	Right	19	24	−46	−5	4.46	48
Culmen	Left		−18	−46	−8	4.42	58
Posterior cingulate	Right	30	18	−55	13	4.02	19
Precuneus	Right	7	9	−49	55	3.96	27
Precuneus	Right	7	9	−52	46	3.37	
Cingulate gyrus	Left	31	−15	−37	43	3.82	7
Uvula	Left		0	−70	−29	3.77	6
Claustrum	Right		30	29	1	3.69	9
fear > sadness							
Parahippocampal gyrus	Right	36	30	−46	−11	7.35	214
Parahippocampal gyrus	Left	36	−30	−40	−11	7.14	290
Fusiform gyrus	Left	37	−30	−52	−11	6.95	
Declive	Left		−30	−67	−14	3.33	
Cingulate gyrus	Left	31	−15	−37	43	6.8	1270
Middle occipital gyrus	Right	19	42	−79	19	5.8	
Precuneus	Right	7	9	−52	55	5.78	
Middle temporal gyrus	Left	19	−36	−82	28	5.06	89
Middle occipital gyrus	Left	19	−48	−79	13	4.48	
Middle occipital gyrus	Left	19	−36	−85	19	4.4	
Superior frontal gyrus	Right	8	30	41	43	4.51	9
Middle frontal gyrus	Right	8	42	35	37	3.61	
Middle frontal gyrus	Right	6	30	8	64	4.4	11
Pyramis	Right		6	−76	−26	4.31	88
Pyramis	Left		−6	−73	−26	4.16	
Posterior cingulate	Right	30	18	−55	13	4.16	26
Posterior cingulate	Right	30	24	−58	22	3.6	
Inferior parietal lobule	Right	40	57	−40	40	4.04	40
Insula	Right	13	33	29	4	3.8	19
Middle frontal gyrus	Right	9	39	47	25	3.7	11
Inferior frontal gyrus	Left	46	−45	44	7	3.64	5
fear > neutral							
Parahippocampal gyrus	Right	30	21	−43	−5	4.68	95
Insula	Right	13	36	14	−14	4.52	104
Inferior frontal gyrus	Right	45	48	23	−2	4.29	
Insula	Right	13	33	29	−2	3.82	
Culmen	Left		−18	−46	−8	4.42	90
Culmen	Right		3	−40	−2	3.84	
Culmen	Left		−18	−37	−17	3.54	
Uvula	Right		0	−67	−29	4.11	17
Thalamus (medial dorsal nucleus)	Right		6	−10	13	4.1	36
Posterior cingulate	Right	30	18	−55	13	4.02	28
Posterior cingulate	Right	31	24	−61	22	3.38	
Precuneus	Right	7	9	−49	55	3.96	27
Precuneus	Right	7	9	−52	46	3.37	
Thalamus	Left		0	−31	7	3.92	30

TABLE 2: Continued.

Brain regions	Hemisphere	Brodmann's area	MNI coordinates			$t(24)$	k
			x	y	z		
Cingulate gyrus	Left	31	−15	−37	43	3.82	7
Precuneus	Left	7	−9	−52	58	3.54	9
Insula	Left	13	−39	23	1	3.54	11
Supramarginal gyrus	Right	40	63	−49	31	3.53	9

Note: threshold was set at $p < 0.001$ (uncorrected). Cluster size is represented by k. MNI = Montreal Neurological Institute.

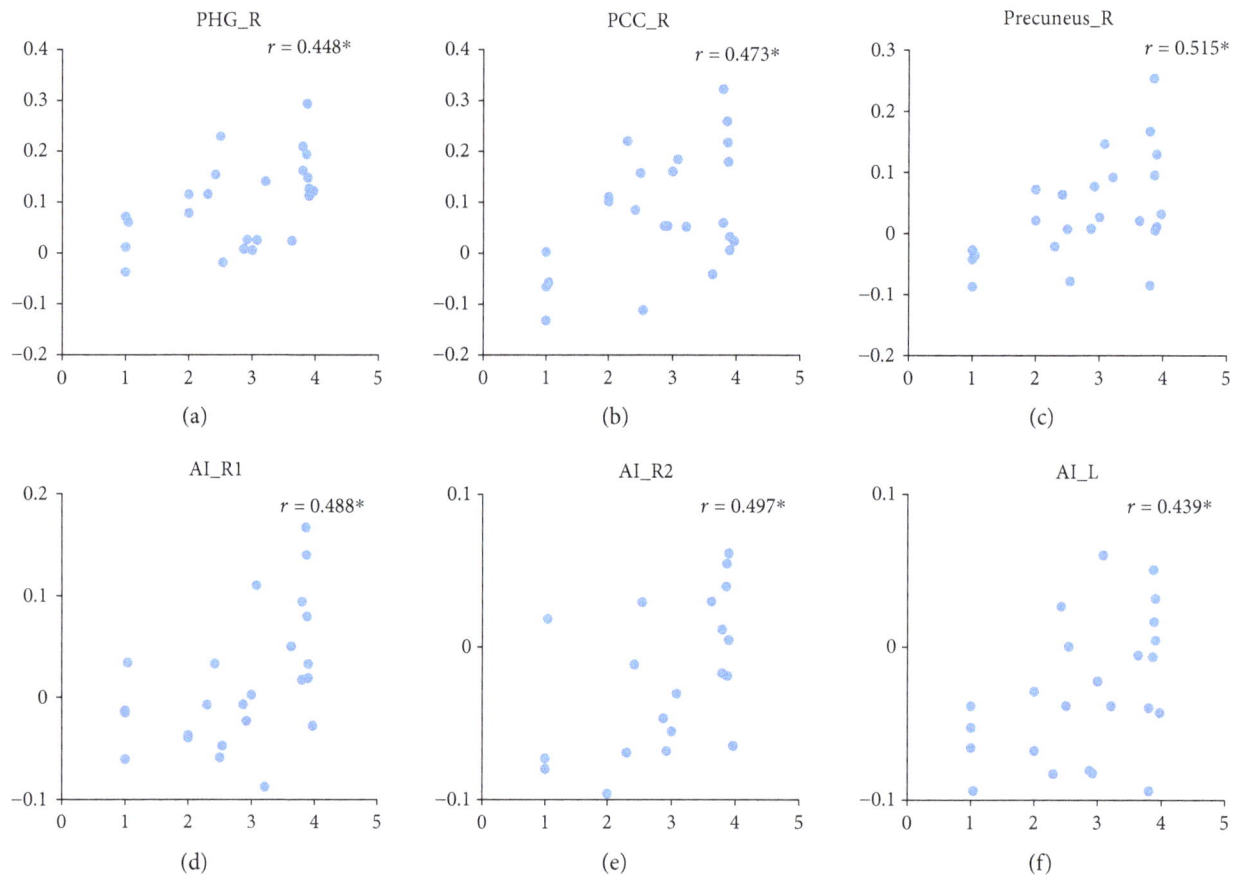

FIGURE 5: Relationships between brain activation associated with fear induction and aggressive behavior under the fear condition. r represents the correlation coefficient. * indicates a significant difference at $p < 0.05$.

and neutral mood [$t(23) = 2.384$, $p < 0.05$, $d = 0.445$] conditions, and no significant differences were observed between the sadness and neutral mood conditions (Figure 3(b)).

3.2. Imaging Results. The effect of fear induction was examined using the contrasts of "fear induction > sadness induction" and "fear induction > neutral mood induction" (both sampled during the emotional movie-clip-viewing) and with the conjunction analyses of these two contrasts. Increased neural activity selectively associated with fear was identified in the right parahippocampal gyrus (PHG_R, BA19), right posterior cingulate cortex (PCC_R, BA30), and right precuneus (precuneus_R, BA7) by the conjunction analyses of "fear induction > sadness induction" and "fear induction > -neutral mood induction." Right anterior insula (AI_R,

BA13) and left anterior insula (AI_L, BA13) activation was detected in both contrasts of "fear induction > sadness induction" and "fear induction > neutral mood induction" but was located in different AI regions in these two contrasts. Thus, the conjunction analysis did not identify AI activation (Figure 4 and Table 2). In addition, under the fear condition, the BOLD responses in the ROIs of the PHG, PCC, precuneus, and AI positively predicted the subsequent aggressive behavior levels (i.e., noise intensity determined by the participants to punish their opponents) [$r_{PHG\_R} = 0.488$, $p < 0.05$; $r_{PCC\_R} = 0.473$, $p < 0.05$; $r_{precuneus\_R} = 0.515$, $p < 0.05$; $r_{AI\_R(fear>sadness)} = 0.488$, $p < 0.05$; $r_{AI\_R(fear>neutral)} = 0.497$, $p < 0.05$; and $r_{AI\_L(fear>neutral)} = 0.439$, $p < 0.05$] (Figure 5).

The effects of the sadness induction were examined by the contrasts of "sadness induction > fear induction" and

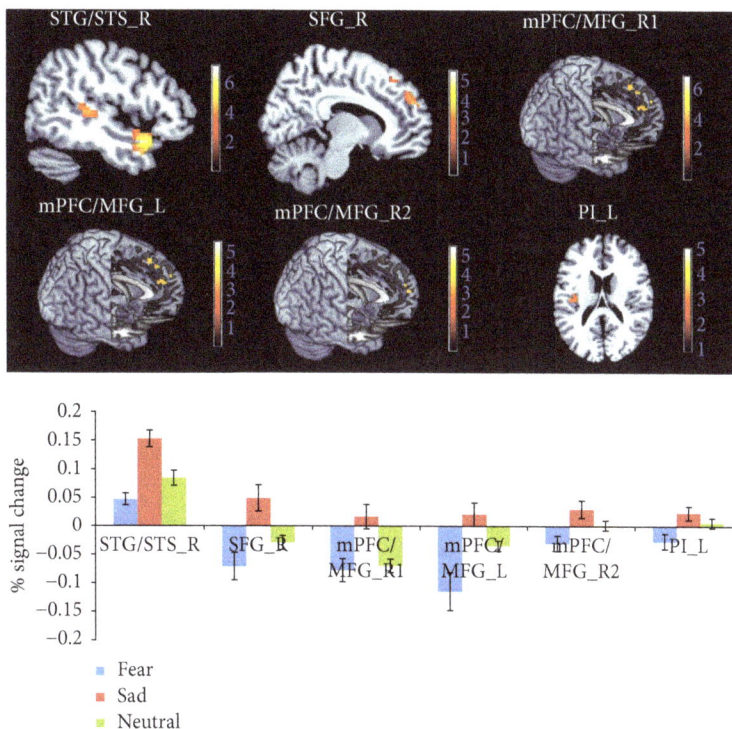

FIGURE 6: Neuroimaging results showing brain activation associated with sadness induction (i.e., watching movies). The activation of the STG/STS_R and SFG_R was taken from the conjunction analysis of "sadness > neutral" and "sadness > fear" (depicted at $p < 0.001$), the activation of the mPFC/MFG_R1 and mPFC/MFG_L was taken from the contrast of "sadness > fear", the activation of the mPFC/MFG_R2 was taken from the contrast of "sadness > neutral" (depicted at $p < 0.05$), and the activation of PI was taken from the contrast of "sadness > fear" (depicted at $p < 0.005$). The graphs show the mean percent signal changes separately for the STG/STS_R, SFG_R, mPFC/MFG_L, mPFC/MFG_R2, and PI_L across the three experimental conditions.

"sadness induction > neutral mood induction" (both sampled during the emotional movie-clip-viewing) and by the conjunction analyses of these two contrasts. Increased neural activity selectively associated with sadness induction was identified in the right superior temporal gyrus/sulcus (STG/STS_R, BA 22/38/41) and right superior frontal gyrus (SFG_R, BA9) by the conjunction analysis. Left and right medial prefrontal cortex/medial frontal gyrus (mPFC/MFG_L, mPFC/MFG_R) activation was detected in both contrasts of "sadness induction > fear induction" and "sadness induction > neutral mood induction," but the exact location in the mPFC/MFG differed between these two contrasts (Figure 6 and Table 3), and left posterior insula (PI_L) activation was only detected in the contrast of "sadness induction > fear induction." Under the sadness condition, the BOLD responses in the ROIs of the STG/STS, SFG, mPFC/MFG, and PI were negatively correlated with the subjective anger feeling [$r_{STG/STS\_R} = -0.661$, $p < 0.001$; $r_{SFG\_R} = -0.519$, $p < 0.01$; $r_{mPFC/MFG\_R (sadness > fear)} = -0.471$, $p < 0.05$; $r_{mPFC/MFG\_L (sadness > fear)} = -0.560$, $p < 0.01$; $r_{mPFC/MFG\_R (sadness > neutral)} = -0.517$, $p < 0.01$; and $r_{PI\_L (sadness > fear)} = -0.564$, $p < 0.01$] (Figure 7).

4. Discussion

In the current study, the participants showed more aggressive behavior after they were induced with fear and a lower level of anger after they were induced with sadness, thus supporting the hypotheses of the MPMC theory of emotionality that "sadness counteracts anger" and "fear promotes anger" from a "proactive interference perspective" that is different from the "retroactive interference perspective" in our previous studies [3, 4]. In our previous study, participants were first provoked, and we found that afterward-induced sadness could reduce the subsequent aggressiveness level, whereas afterward-induced fear promoted angry feelings [3, 4]. Therefore, the MPMC theory principle of "sadness counteracts anger" may refer to the following two different situations: the subsequently induced sadness could help to control anger-related aggressive behavior (the retroactive regulatory effects) and the antecedently induced sadness could help to reduce angry feelings (the proactive regulatory effects). Similarly, the principle of "fear promotes anger" also involves the following two situations: feelings of anger could increase if fear is subsequently experienced, indicating that fear promotes existing anger (the retroactive regulatory effects), and an individual may express more aggressive behavior during an aggravating situation if he/she is antecedently evoked by fear, indicating that existing fear could foster aggressive behavior (the proactive regulatory effects). Interestingly, the principles of "sadness counteracts anger" and "fear promotes anger" have different effects on subjectively reported anger and aggressive behavior in their retroactive or proactive regulation form. In the retroactive regulation form, "sadness

TABLE 3: Brain regions associated with the effects of the sadness induction.

Brain regions	Hemisphere	Brodmann's area	MNI coordinates			$t(24)$	k
			x	y	z		
(sadness > neutral) ∩ (sadness > fear) (conjunction)							
Superior temporal gyrus/superior temporal sulcus	Right	38	51	11	−20	7.11	127
Superior temporal gyrus/superior temporal sulcus	Right	41	51	−31	4	4.41	57
Superior temporal gyrus/superior temporal sulcus	Right	22	60	−37	10	3.41	
Superior temporal gyrus/superior temporal sulcus	Left	38	−48	11	−17	4.12	36
Superior temporal gyrus/superior temporal sulcus	Left	38	−48	8	−26	4.02	
Superior frontal gyrus	Right	9	12	53	28	3.53	17
sadness > fear							
Superior temporal gyrus/superior temporal sulcus	Right	38	54	11	−17	7.74	449
Superior temporal gyrus/superior temporal sulcus	Right	22	66	−10	−2	6.27	
Superior temporal gyrus/superior temporal sulcus	Right	41	54	−31	7	6.26	
Superior temporal gyrus/superior temporal sulcus	Left	22	−60	−4	1	5.3	287
Superior temporal gyrus/superior temporal sulcus	Left	38	−48	11	−17	5.02	
Middle temporal gyrus	Left	22	−51	−37	1	4.92	
Superior frontal gyrus	Right	9	15	53	25	4.66	279
Superior frontal gyrus	Right	6	15	23	52	3.72	
Medial prefrontal cortex/medial frontal gyrus	Right	32	21	20	43	3.66	
Parahippocampal gyrus	Left	27	−27	−28	−5	4.27	30
Superior frontal gyrus	Left	9	−15	50	25	4.14	143
Medial prefrontal cortex/medial frontal gyrus	Left	8	−15	38	37	3.59	
Medial prefrontal cortex/medial frontal gyrus	Left	9	−24	50	7	3.56	
Postcentral gyrus	Left	3	−51	−16	55	4.05	11
Insula	Left	13	−48	−16	22	3.77	46
Insula	Left	13	−39	−16	25	3.72	
sadness > neutral							
Superior temporal gyrus/superior temporal sulcus	Right	38	51	11	−20	7.11	209
Parahippocampal gyrus (amygdala)	Left		−18	−7	−14	4.84	29
Insula	Right	13	39	14	−14	4.7	
Superior temporal gyrus/superior temporal sulcus	Right	41	51	−31	4	4.41	58
Superior temporal gyrus/superior temporal sulcus	Right	22	63	−37	10	3.42	
Superior temporal gyrus/Superior temporal sulcus	Left	38	−48	11	−17	4.12	36
Superior temporal gyrus/superior temporal sulcus	Left	38	−48	8	−26	4.02	
Inferior frontal gyrus	Right	47	48	32	−8	3.73	15
Inferior frontal gyrus	Right	45	51	23	−2	3.42	
Medial prefrontal cortex/medial frontal gyrus	Right	6	9	53	31	3.63	28
Medial prefrontal cortex/medial frontal gyrus	Right	9	6	59	16	3.48	

Note: threshold was set at $p < 0.001$ (uncorrected). Cluster size is represented by k. MNI = Montreal Neurological Institute.

counteracts anger" significantly reduces aggressive behavior, whereas in the proactive regulation form, "sadness counteracts anger" significantly reduces anger. Similarly, in the retroactive regulation form, "fear promotes anger" significantly promotes anger, whereas in the proactive regulation form, "fear promotes anger" significantly promotes aggressive behavior. Thus, aggressive behavior, despite its close relationship with anger [12, 18], may be selectively regulated in different ways depending on the context. Further studies should investigate the difference between anger and aggressive behavior in terms of their regulatory approaches and context.

The main goal of this study was to explore the cognitive brain mechanism underlying the principles of "fear promotes anger" and "sadness counteracts anger." Compared with the sadness and neutral mood induction, the fear mood induction was associated with more activation in the AI, PHG, PCC, and precuneus, and activation in these regions could positively predict the individuals' anger feelings in a subsequent provocation situation. However, compared with the fear and neutral mood inductions, the sadness mood induction was associated with more activation in the PI, STG/STS, and SFG, and the activation in these regions

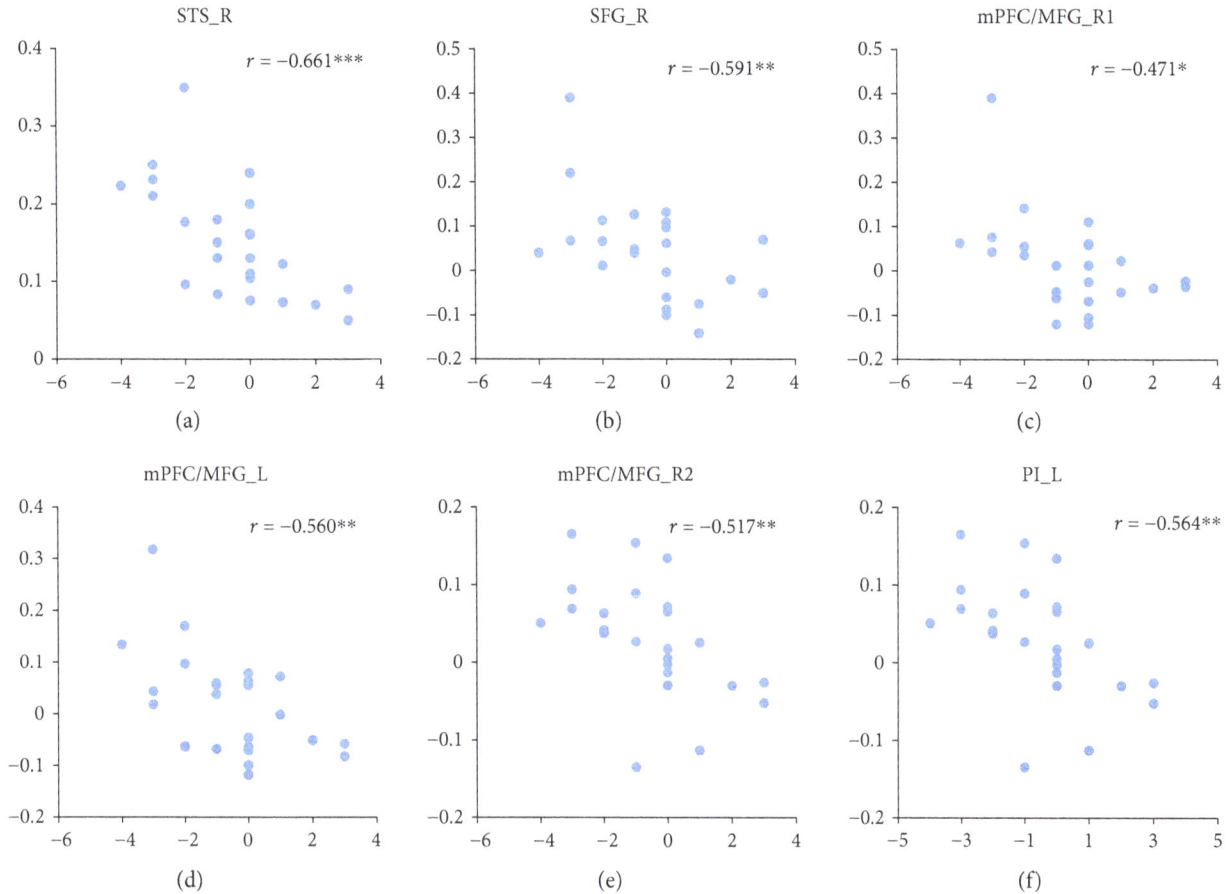

FIGURE 7: Relationships between brain activation associated with sadness induction and subjective anger feelings under the sadness condition. r represents the correlation coefficient. *** indicates a significant difference at $p < 0.001$, ** indicates a significant difference at $p < 0.01$, * indicates a significant difference at $p < 0.05$.

could negatively predict the individuals' aggressive behavior in subsequent provocation situations.

First, the AI, PHG, PCC, and precuneus activation was associated with the processing of the fear-inducing movie clip, which is consistent with previous neuroscience studies showing that fearful or threatening stimuli elicit activity in the AI, hippocampus, PCC, and precuneus, and this activation is mainly characterized by wakefulness and goal-driven responses [5, 19]. Second, areas in the PI, frontal lobe (e.g., superior frontal gyrus and medial frontal gyrus) and superior temporal gyrus were selectively activated during the processing of the sadness-inducing movie clip, which is also consistent with previous studies investigating the neural correlates of sadness [20–23]. These findings, together with the significant correlation between the brain activation and subsequent anger or aggressive behavior, may imply the possible neural mechanism of "fear promotes anger" and "sadness counteracts anger."

Most importantly, our results demonstrate a clear functional dissociation between the AI and PI in which the AI is more involved in fear induction, and this AI activation positively predicted later anger, whereas the PI was more involved in sadness induction, and this PI activation negatively predicted later aggressive behavior. This result not only proved that sadness and fear could be different in their

representation location in the posterior-to-anterior progression of insular structure but also implied that the mechanism mediating the different inducing effects of sadness and fear on anger and aggressive behavior could be related to this difference. The AI is generally considered a part of the neural loop that notices, evaluates, and adapts to threat signals [7, 24]; the AI also reflects negative emotions, such as anxiety, aversion and alertness, arising from individual conflicts in the face of unfair events [25]. The AI activation in fear, together with the activation in the PHG, PCC, and precuneus, which could be related to conscious information processing such as attentive focusing and awakening [26–29], implied that the reason fear enhanced aggressive behavior could be attributed to an externally oriented threat-driven arousal state. Different from fear, sadness tended to be selectively represented in the PI and was associated with the representation of feeling oriented toward one's internal feeling and experience. The PI has been shown to connect reciprocally with the secondary somatosensory cortex and is highly specialized to convey homeostatic information such as pain, temperature, itch, and sensual touch [6, 30, 31], and a number of studies indicate that a subsection of the PI both anatomically and functionally serves a primary and fundamental role in pain processing [30, 32–34]. In addition, the induction of sadness was also accompanied by the empathy-

or sympathy-related neural processing process embodied by the activation of STG/STS and mPFC [35, 36]. Previous studies suggested that STS was engaged in tasks that required one to infer and share in another individual's mental [37, 38] and emotional state [39, 40]. For example, Zelinková and colleagues found that videos depicting dangerous behavior in a traffic campaign ending with tragic consequences activated the STS and that this activation was directly related to the participants' empathy and sympathy [41]. Thus, the possible neurological basis of "sadness counteracts anger" is that sadness induced internally oriented feeling represented in the PI, while eliciting empathy and sympathy processes mediated by STS/STG and mPFC, and finally producing less of a tendency to feel anger when provoked by others.

The current findings and conclusions must be considered in light of our study's limitations. First, as discussed above, the self-reported anger and aggressive behavior were inconsistent because the sadness induction successfully decreased the self-reported anger but not aggressive behavior; thus, whether the target of "fear promotes anger" or "sadness counteracts anger" occurs at the cognition or behavior level or both requires further confirmation in future studies. Second, we only examined 24 healthy, young Chinese college students. Thus, our findings cannot be generalized to larger populations, a nationality-unspecific context, or any clinical population. Finally, the mood (fear, sadness, or anger) inductions in this study were almost controlled in a moderate intensity. Regulating different intensities of emotional stimuli, however, may involve different neural mechanisms [42]; thus, studies should investigate the influence of the inducing mood intensity on the neural responses of "fear promotes anger" and "sadness counteracts anger."

5. Conclusions

In summary, our findings suggest a clear functional dissociation between the anterior and posterior parts of insula in which the AI is more involved in the processing of "fear promotes anger" than the PI and the PI is more involved in the processing of "sadness counteracts anger" than the AI. Specifically, fear-induced AI activity is associated with negative feelings (e.g., disgust and cognitive conflict) and neural responses are related to arousal (PHG, PCC, and precuneus), further promoting more aggression to external irritation. In contrast, sadness elicited the activation of the PI, which is involved in the processing of primary feeling and neural regions that may be related to empathy/sympathy (STG/STS, SFG, and mPFC), further producing less of a tendency to feel anger when provoked by others. These findings provide compelling neurological evidence supporting the "fear promotes anger" and "sadness counteracts anger" hypotheses of the MPMC theory of emotionality, which is based on traditional Chinese medicine.

Conflicts of Interest

The authors declare that this study was conducted in the absence of any commercial or financial relationships that could be construed as potential conflicts of interest.

Acknowledgments

This work was supported by the Fundamental Research Funds from CNU's special construction project on supporting capacity for scientific and technological innovation (025-185305000), the National Natural Science Foundation of China (31671124 and 31471000), and the Beijing Municipal Commission of Education (TJSH20161002801).

References

[1] C. M. Raio, T. A. Orederu, L. Palazzolo, A. A. Shurick, and E. A. Phelps, "Cognitive emotion regulation fails the stress test," *Proceedings of the National Academy of Sciences of the United States of America*, vol. 110, no. 37, pp. 15139–15144, 2013.

[2] C. M. Raio and E. A. Phelps, "The influence of acute stress on the regulation of conditioned fear," *Neurobiology of Stress*, vol. 1, pp. 134–146, 2015.

[3] J. Zhan, X. Wu, J. Fan et al., "Regulating anger under stress via cognitive reappraisal and sadness," *Frontiers in Psychology*, vol. 8, p. 1372, 2017.

[4] J. Zhan, J. Ren, J. Fan, and J. Luo, "Distinctive effects of fear and sadness induction on anger and aggressive behavior," *Frontiers in Psychology*, vol. 6, p. 725, 2015.

[5] T. D. Wager, J. Kang, T. D. Johnson, T. E. Nichols, A. B. Satpute, and L. F. Barrett, "A Bayesian model of category-specific emotional brain responses," *PLoS Computational Biology*, vol. 11, no. 4, article e1004066, 2015.

[6] A. D. Craig, "How do you feel? Interoception: the sense of the physiological condition of the body," *Nature Reviews Neuroscience*, vol. 3, no. 8, pp. 655–666, 2002.

[7] A. D. Craig, "How do you feel — now? The anterior insula and human awareness," *Nature Reviews Neuroscience*, vol. 10, no. 1, pp. 59–70, 2009.

[8] B. J. Bushman, R. F. Baumeister, and C. M. Phillips, "Do people aggress to improve their mood? Catharsis beliefs, affect regulation opportunity, and aggressive responding," *Journal of Personality and Social Psychology*, vol. 81, no. 1, pp. 17–32, 2001.

[9] M. Zuckerman and B. Lubin, *Manual for the MAACL-R: The Multiple Affect Adjetive Check List Revised*, Educational and Industrial Testing Service, 1985.

[10] Y. Zhang, "The measurement of experimentally induced affects," *Acta Psychologica Sinica*, vol. 23, no. 1, pp. 101–108, 1991.

[11] P. Xu, Y. Huang, and Y. Luo, "Establishment and assessment of native Chinese affective video system," *Chinese Mental Health Journal*, vol. 24, no. 7, pp. 551–554, 2010.

[12] B. J. Bushman, R. F. Baumeister, and A. D. Stack, "Catharsis, aggression, and persuasive influence: self-fulfilling or self-defeating prophecies?," *Journal of Personality and Social Psychology*, vol. 76, no. 3, pp. 367–376, 1999.

[13] F. Dambacher, A. T. Sack, J. Lobbestael, A. Arntz, S. Brugman, and T. Schuhmann, "Out of control: evidence for anterior insula involvement in motor impulsivity and reactive aggression," *Social Cognitive and Affective Neuroscience*, vol. 10, no. 4, pp. 508–516, 2015.

[14] P. R. Giancola and D. J. Parrott, "Further evidence for the validity of the Taylor aggression paradigm," *Aggressive Behavior*, vol. 34, no. 2, pp. 214–229, 2008.

[15] S. P. Taylor, "Aggressive behavior and physiological arousal as a function of provocation and the tendency to inhibit aggression," *Journal of Personality*, vol. 35, no. 2, pp. 297–310, 1967.

[16] U. M. Krämer, H. Jansma, C. Tempelmann, and T. F. Münte, "Tit-for-tat: the neural basis of reactive aggression," *NeuroImage*, vol. 38, no. 1, pp. 203–211, 2007.

[17] C. Fernández, J. C. Pascual, J. Soler, M. Elices, M. J. Portella, and E. Fernández-Abascal, "Physiological responses induced by emotion-eliciting films," *Applied Psychophysiology and Biofeedback*, vol. 37, no. 2, pp. 73–79, 2012.

[18] D. J. Parrott and P. R. Giancola, "Addressing "the criterion problem" in the assessment of aggressive behavior: development of a new taxonomic system," *Aggression and Violent Behavior*, vol. 12, no. 3, pp. 280–299, 2007.

[19] N. Kirlic, R. Aupperle, J. Rhudy, and R. Alvarez, "122. pain-related negative affect relates to anxious reactivity and anterior insula activity during unpredictable threat of shock," *Biological Psychiatry*, vol. 81, no. 10, article S51, 2017.

[20] M. E. Sachs, A. Damasio, and A. Habibi, "The pleasures of sad music: a systematic review," *Frontiers in Human Neuroscience*, vol. 9, p. 404, 2015.

[21] E. Brattico, B. Bogert, V. Alluri, M. Tervaniemi, T. Eerola, and T. Jacobsen, "It's sad but I like it: the neural dissociation between musical emotions and liking in experts and laypersons," *Frontiers in Human Neuroscience*, vol. 9, p. 676, 2016.

[22] H. S. Mayberg, M. Liotti, S. K. Brannan et al., "Reciprocal limbic-cortical function and negative mood: converging PET findings in depression and normal sadness," *The American Journal of Psychiatry*, vol. 156, no. 5, pp. 675–682, 1999.

[23] K. Vytal and S. Hamann, "Neuroimaging support for discrete neural correlates of basic emotions: a voxel-based meta-analysis," *Journal of Cognitive Neuroscience*, vol. 22, no. 12, pp. 2864–2885, 2010.

[24] R. Kalisch and A. M. V. Gerlicher, "Making a mountain out of a molehill: on the role of the rostral dorsal anterior cingulate and dorsomedial prefrontal cortex in conscious threat appraisal, catastrophizing, and worrying," *Neuroscience & Biobehavioral Reviews*, vol. 42, pp. 1–8, 2014.

[25] C. Corradi-Dell'Acqua, C. Civai, R. I. Rumiati, and G. R. Fink, "Disentangling self- and fairness-related neural mechanisms involved in the ultimatum game: an fMRI study," *Social Cognitive and Affective Neuroscience*, vol. 8, no. 4, pp. 424–431, 2013.

[26] R. Leech and D. J. Sharp, "The role of the posterior cingulate cortex in cognition and disease," *Brain*, vol. 137, no. 1, pp. 12–32, 2014.

[27] P. Qin, Y. Liu, J. Shi et al., "Dissociation between anterior and posterior cortical regions during self-specificity and familiarity: a combined fMRI–meta-analytic study," *Human Brain Mapping*, vol. 33, no. 1, pp. 154–164, 2012.

[28] X. Xu, H. Yuan, and X. Lei, "Activation and connectivity within the default mode network contribute independently to future-oriented thought," *Scientific Reports*, vol. 6, no. 1, article 21001, 2016.

[29] B. A. Vogt and S. Laureys, "Posterior cingulate, precuneal and retrosplenial cortices: cytology and components of the neural network correlates of consciousness," *Progress in Brain Research*, vol. 150, pp. 205–217, 2005.

[30] A. R. Segerdahl, M. Mezue, T. W. Okell, J. T. Farrar, and I. Tracey, "The dorsal posterior insula subserves a fundamental role in human pain," *Nature Neuroscience*, vol. 18, no. 4, pp. 499–500, 2015.

[31] A. D. Craig, K. Chen, D. Bandy, and E. M. Reiman, "Thermosensory activation of insular cortex," *Nature Neuroscience*, vol. 3, no. 2, pp. 184–190, 2000.

[32] L. Mazzola, J. Isnard, R. Peyron, M. Guénot, and F. Mauguière, "Somatotopic organization of pain responses to direct electrical stimulation of the human insular cortex," *Pain*, vol. 146, no. 1, pp. 99–104, 2009.

[33] J. D. Greenspan, R. R. Lee, and F. A. Lenz, "Pain sensitivity alterations as a function of lesion location in the parasylvian cortex," *Pain*, vol. 81, no. 3, pp. 273–282, 1999.

[34] L. Garcia-Larrea and R. Peyron, "Pain matrices and neuropathic pain matrices: a review," *Pain*, vol. 154, pp. S29–S43, 2013.

[35] J. Decety and T. Chaminade, "Neural correlates of feeling sympathy," *Neuropsychologia*, vol. 41, no. 2, pp. 127–138, 2003.

[36] S. Nichols, "Mindreading and the cognitive architecture underlying altruistic motivation," *Mind & Language*, vol. 16, no. 4, pp. 425–455, 2001.

[37] H. L. Gallagher and C. D. Frith, "Functional imaging of 'theory of mind'," *Trends in Cognitive Sciences*, vol. 7, no. 2, pp. 77–83, 2003.

[38] U. M. Krämer, B. Mohammadi, N. Doñamayor, A. Samii, and T. F. Münte, "Emotional and cognitive aspects of empathy and their relation to social cognition—an fMRI-study," *Brain Research*, vol. 1311, pp. 110–120, 2010.

[39] C. Lamm, J. Decety, and T. Singer, "Meta-analytic evidence for common and distinct neural networks associated with directly experienced pain and empathy for pain," *NeuroImage*, vol. 54, no. 3, pp. 2492–2502, 2011.

[40] I. Dziobek, S. Preißler, Z. Grozdanovic, I. Heuser, H. R. Heekeren, and S. Roepke, "Neuronal correlates of altered empathy and social cognition in borderline personality disorder," *NeuroImage*, vol. 57, no. 2, pp. 539–548, 2011.

[41] J. Zelinková, D. J. Shaw, R. Mareček et al., "An evaluation of traffic-awareness campaign videos: empathy induction is associated with brain function within superior temporal sulcus," *Behavioral and Brain Functions*, vol. 10, no. 1, p. 27, 2014.

[42] J. A. Silvers, J. Weber, T. D. Wager, and K. N. Ochsner, "Bad and worse: neural systems underlying reappraisal of high- and low-intensity negative emotions," *Social Cognitive and Affective Neuroscience*, vol. 10, no. 2, pp. 172–179, 2015.

12

Anatomical and Functional MRI Changes after One Year of Auditory Rehabilitation with Hearing Aids

M. R. Pereira-Jorge,[1] K. C. Andrade,[2] F. X. Palhano-Fontes,[2] P. R. B. Diniz,[3] M. Sturzbecher,[1] A. C. Santos,[1,4] and D. B. Araujo [2]

[1]Department of Neuroscience and Behavior, University of São Paulo, Ribeirao Preto, SP, Brazil
[2]Brain Institute/Onofre Lopes University Hospital, Federal University of Rio Grande do Norte (UFRN), Natal, RN, Brazil
[3]Department of Internal Medicine, Federal University of Pernambuco, Recife, PE, Brazil
[4]Department of Internal Medicine, University of São Paulo, Ribeirao Preto, SP, Brazil

Correspondence should be addressed to D. B. Araujo; draulio@neuro.ufrn.br

Academic Editor: Surjo R. Soekadar

Hearing aids (HAs) are an effective strategy for auditory rehabilitation in patients with peripheral hearing deficits. Yet, the neurophysiological mechanisms behind HA use are still unclear. Thus far, most studies have focused on changes in the auditory system, although it is expected that hearing deficits affect a number of cognitive systems, notably speech. In the present study, we used audiometric evaluations in 14 patients with bilateral hearing loss before and after one year of continuous HA use and functional magnetic resonance imaging (fMRI) and cortical thickness analysis in 12 and 10 of them compared with a normal hearing control group. Prior to HA fitting, fMRI activity was found reduced in the auditory and language systems and increased in visual and frontal areas, expanding to multimodal integration cortices, such as the superior temporal gyrus, intraparietal sulcus, and insula. One year after rehabilitation with HA, significant audiometric improvement was observed, especially in free-field Speech Reception Threshold (SRT) test and functional gain, a measure of HA efficiency. HA use increased fMRI activity in the auditory and language cortices and multimodal integration areas. Individual fMRI signal changes from all these areas were positively correlated with individual SRT changes. Before rehabilitation, cortical thickness was increased in parts of the prefrontal cortex, precuneus, fusiform gyrus, and middle temporal gyrus. It was reduced in the insula, supramarginal gyrus, medial temporal gyrus, occipital cortex, posterior cingulate cortex, and claustrum. After HA use, increased cortical thickness was observed in multimodal integration regions, particularly the very caudal end of the superior temporal sulcus, the angular gyrus, and the inferior parietal gyrus/superior temporal gyrus/insula. Our data provide the first evidence that one year of HA use is related to functional and anatomical brain changes, notably in auditory and language systems, extending to multimodal cortices.

1. Introduction

Peripheral hearing deficits have a profound impact on the central auditory system, hampering individual communication and social interaction [1]. Individuals with hearing impairment can benefit from rehabilitation with cochlear implant (CI) and acoustic hearing aid (HA) devices. In both cases, patients experience significant improvement in their general condition, including cognitive abilities such as memory and language comprehension [2, 3].

Little is known, however, about neurophysiological mechanisms underlying these beneficial changes, and most knowledge on the topic is still based on animal models. Lesions to different segments of the auditory system are associated with specific changes in the neuronal representation of sound stimuli in cats [4], monkeys [5], mice [6], birds [7], and rabbits [8]. Furthermore, molecular and electrophysiological evidences show that rehabilitation with CI, for instance, leads to changes in the auditory system [8, 9].

In humans, advances in neuroimaging have expanded considerably the exploration of the auditory system, both in normal hearing subjects [10] and in patients with hearing impairment [11, 12]. Positron emission tomography (PET) and functional MRI (fMRI) have already found consistent reduced activity of the auditory cortex in patients with hearing deficits [13, 14], which is at least partially recovered with CI and HA [12, 14, 15].

Only very few studies used neuroimaging to probe the impact of auditory rehabilitation over higher cognitive functions, and most of them have focused on language cortices, particularly Wernicke's area (Brodmann area—BA22) [12, 16]. In general, auditory deprivation leads to decreased activation of this area, which is recovered at least partially by rehabilitation, for instance, with CI [17]. It has been regarded as a fact that the use of hearing devices allows access to the auditory information to language centers, therefore leading to increased activity of this area. However, to our knowledge, these are still no solid evidence suggesting that this is the case or if there are other mechanisms involved. Thus, the first aim of this longitudinal study is to investigate the impact of HA use over audiometric scales, anatomical and functional MRI, and their correlations.

Furthermore, it is well known that the integration of auditory and visual information greatly improves the ability of language comprehension [18]. In fact, patients with hearing deficits often exhibit increased activity in areas related to visual functions, during auditory stimulation [19, 20]. Therefore, we also aimed to deeply explore brain areas involved in multimodal integration, such as the superior temporal sulcus (STS), the middle intraparietal sulcus (IT, BA40), the inferior frontal gyrus (IFG, BA44, BA45, and BA47), and the insula (BA13). The second objective of this study was to explore effects of auditory deprivation and recovery in sensory integration systems, for aurally delivered stimuli.

2. Material and Methods

This work was approved by the Ethics and Research Committee of the University of São Paulo, Ribeirao Preto School of Medicine (no. 2413/2007). Written informed consent was obtained from all participants. The data that support the findings of this study are available from the corresponding author upon request.

2.1. Subjects. Two groups participated in the current study: 14 postlingual deaf patients (P) with sensorineural hearing loss (5 women, age = 51.29 ± 18.8 years) and 11 normal hearing control group (CG) (5 women, age = 46.54 ± 19.88 years). At the time of recruitment, all patients had mild to severe bilateral sensorineural hearing loss and were referred to us by an otorhinolaryngologist for HA use (see Suppl. Table 1 for clinical details).

2.2. Audiometric Evaluation and Hearing Aid. The HAs used were manufactured by Widex (Lynge, Denmark). Four patients were fitted with completely in the canal (CIC) HA, and ten patients were fitted with intracanal (ITC) HA, with digital processing and compression (Suppl. Table 1). During the first two months of HA fitting, patients were evaluated weekly. After acclimatization, all patients were asked to use the HA for at least 10 hours a day.

Audiological evaluation followed the Brazilian protocol and occurred twice: right before HA fitting and right after

one year of continuous HA use. All patients underwent pure tone audiometry tests by air and bone in an acoustic cabin, with headphones, for the following frequencies: 250 Hz, 500 Hz, 1000 Hz, 2000 Hz, 3000 Hz, 4000 Hz, 6000 Hz, and 8000 Hz. The pure tone auditory threshold was defined as the minimum level of sound intensity necessary for the pure tone, at each frequency, to be perceived. Patients were instructed to press a button every time they heard a sound (whistle) in the ear being tested. The tones began at higher sound levels that were gradually lowered from 120 dB to 15 dB. In patients with asymmetric loss, we started with the better ear. The test was performed for all frequencies on one ear first and then the other ear. Pure tone averages (PTA) were computed as the average of the thresholds obtained for the frequencies of 500, 1000, and 2000, according to Davis and Silverman [21].

Also, in an acoustic cabin, we evaluated the patient's ability to recognize speech sounds and measured the Speech Reception Threshold (SRT) for disyllables [22]. SRT is defined as the lowest sound level in which the patient is able to perceive and to repeat out loud correctly 50% of the words presented.

Subjects were also submitted to bone pure tone audiometry in which a pure tone signal is delivered by a bone vibrator (coupled to the arc) placed onto the individuals' mastoid. Hearing thresholds were obtained for the same frequencies used in the air pure tone audiometry. Only patients with sensorineural hearing loss were included, defined as those with equal thresholds measured by air and bone audiometry.

Pure tone audiometry and SRT were also performed in free field. Patients were positioned in an acoustic cabin, this time without headphones [22]. They were instructed to press a button whenever they perceived a sound stimulus. Free-field evaluation allows the calculation of functional gain (FG), a procedure defined by Pascoe [23], and is used to evaluate the efficiency of HA interventions. It consists of computing the percentage change in free field by comparing aided and unaided thresholds, i.e., with and without HA in place.

We first performed the evaluation without HA in place and then with HA positioned in one ear only, while the other ear remained without HA. Functional gain (FG) = aided threshold minus the unaided threshold. Thresholds were obtained for each ear separately. Patients remained seated with one ear pointing to a speaker positioned in the horizontal plane of the ear. First, the tested ear had the HA in place, while the other ear was unaided. Then, HA was removed, and a new threshold was obtained, this time with both ears unaided. The same procedure was repeated with the other ear pointing to the speaker.

Between-group comparison (patients vs. control group) was assessed by the Mann–Whitney U test, while within-group differences (patients before HA use × patients after HA use) were inspected by the Wilcoxon test for two dependent samples.

2.3. fMRI Acquisition. There were two MRI sessions: right before HA fitting and after one year of HA use. Subjects were scanned in a 1.5 T scanner (Siemens, Magneton Vision, Erlangen, Germany) with a commercially available TX/RX head coil. fMRI acquisition used an echo-planar imaging (EPI) sequence, with the following parameters: 66 volumes, each one composed of 16 axial slices covering both hemispheres, TR = 4600 ms, TE = 60 ms, *flip angle* = 90°, FOV = 220 mm, matrix = 128 × 128, and slice thickness = 5 mm.

Whole brain anatomical T1-weighted images were also acquired using a 3D gradient-recalled echo (GRE) sequence, with the following parameters: TR = 9.7 ms, TE = 4.0 ms, matrix size = 256 × 256, *flip angle* = 12°, FOV = 256 mm, slice number = 154, and slice thickness = 1 mm.

2.4. Experimental Paradigm. fMRI auditory stimuli were delivered by MRI compatible headphones (Siemens, Erlangen, Germany) maintaining the same sound level in both ears and for both sessions: before and after HA fitting. The task consisted of listening to a story, presented in a block design, with five blocks of the story (27.5 seconds each) interrupted with five blocks of rest (27.5 seconds each) [24]. The same story was used in both sessions, recorded by a male voice, and delivered to both ears, using the same sound level in both sessions and for all patients (30 dB). Subjects were asked to report the story's content after each session, and story comprehension was rated using a 0–5 Likert scale (0—did not understand at all, 1—understood isolated words, 2—understood 25% of the story, 3—understood 50% of the story, 4—understood 75% of the story, and 5—understood the entire story). Prior to fMRI acquisition, subjects were carefully instructed not to move while in the scanner and to pay as much attention as possible to the story being told.

2.5. fMRI Analysis. fMRI data were processed using Brain-Voyager QX 1.86 (Brain Innovation, Maastricht, Netherlands) according to the same procedures described elsewhere [24, 25]. Preprocessing steps consisted of motion correction, high pass temporal filter at 0.01 Hz, spatial filtering (FWHM = 4 mm), and transformation into Talairach space. fMRI group differences were analyzed using a fixed-effect general linear model (GLM) with separate subject predictors. Clusters were selected using a threshold corrected for multiple comparisons (q[FDR] < 0.05) and with an extension of at least 50 mm^3. Group analysis included 2 orthogonal contrasts: (i) controls (CG) vs. patients before intervention (PB) and (ii) patients before intervention (PB) vs. patients after intervention (PA).

2.6. Correlation Analysis. A *Pearson* correlation analysis was used to assess whether individual fMRI β-values were correlated with individual changes in SRT with headphones, computed as a global difference between thresholds observed before and after intervention, according to [SRT (right ear before) + SRT (left ear before)] − [SRT (right ear after) + SRT (left ear after)]. Correlation was computed in specific regions of interest (ROI), involved in the auditory and Wernicke's area (BA22, BA41, and BA42), as well as in brain areas related to multimodal integration, such as the superior temporal sulcus (STS), the middle intraparietal sulcus (IT), and the insula.

2.7. Cortical Thickness (CT). In order to evaluate whether the use of the HA would also be associated with neuroanatomical changes, we used FreeSurfer image analysis suite for cortical reconstruction and volumetric segmentation, which is documented and freely available for download online (http://surfer.nmr.mgh.harvard.edu/). Processing was performed on a Mac-Pro OS X 10.8.2, 2 × 2.26 GHz Quad-Core Intel Xeon. Preprocessing steps included grey/white segmentation, segmentation of the pial surface, for final computation of cortical thickness (CT) maps [26]. Statistical significance was set at $p < 0.01$.

3. Results

3.1. Audiometric Evaluation. Figure 1(a) shows the pure tone averages (PTA) obtained with headphones for all groups. PTA with headphones in the control group (CG) revealed a threshold of 15.68 ± 8.34 dBHL for the right and 14.66 ± 8.47 dBHL for the left ear, which are within the range of normality for adults (0–25 dBHL). Supplementary Figure 1 shows the CG thresholds with headphones for all tested frequencies. Supplementary Table 2 shows individual CG PTA.

Before intervention, PTA with headphones in the patient group was 53.58 ± 12.94 dBHL for the right ear and 54.33 ± 12.10 dBHL for the left ear (Figure 1(a)). After one year of HA use, PTA changed to 53.03 ± 13.61 dBHL and 52.00 ± 11.77 dBHL, respectively, for the right and left ears, which were not significantly different from baseline (Figure 1(a)). We found statistically significant differences between controls and patients before intervention ($p < 0.001$, Figure 1(a)). All patients showed a tonal threshold superior to 25 dBHL for all frequencies tested, both before and after interventions (see Suppl. Figure 2 and Suppl. Table 3 for individual results).

Figure 1(b) shows Speech Reception Threshold (SRT) with headphones for all groups studied. The SRT measured with headphones in the CG is considered normal: 10.91 ± 7.01 dBHL and 11.36 ± 7.10 dBHL for the right ear and the left ear, respectively (Figure 1(b)). At baseline, patients showed SRT of 45.71 ± 14.92 and 46.43 ± 11.67 for the right and left ears, respectively (Figure 1(b)). These values reduced significantly after HA use and averaged 36.79 ± 15.14 for the right ear ($p < 0.001$) and 38.21 ± 11.03 ($p < 0.002$) for the left ear (Figure 1(b)). Although a significant improvement was observed, SRT with headphones was still significantly different between controls and patients after HA use, for both ears ($p < 0.0001$, Figure 1(b)). Supplementary Tables 2 and 4 show individual SRT with headphones for all groups studied.

Free-field PTA and SRT were evaluated in patients only (Figure 2). Before HA use, free-field PTA thresholds averaged 33.15 ± 8.48 dBHL (right ear) and 32.68 ± 10.29 dBHL (left ear). After HA use, free-field PTA improved significantly in both ears ($p < 0.001$), reaching 27.68 ± 5.64 dBHL (right ear) and 28.27 ± 7.40 dBHL (left ear). Supplementary Table 5 shows individual free-field PTA, and Supplementary Figure 3 shows free-field tonal audiometry for all frequencies.

Likewise, free-field SRT improved significantly after HA use for both ears ($p < 0.001$, Figure 2(b)). It changed from 24.93 ± 8.36 dBHL (right ear) and 25.71 ± 5.50 dBHL (left ear) to 17.86 ± 8.48 dBHL (right ear) and 18.21 ± 4.64 dBHL

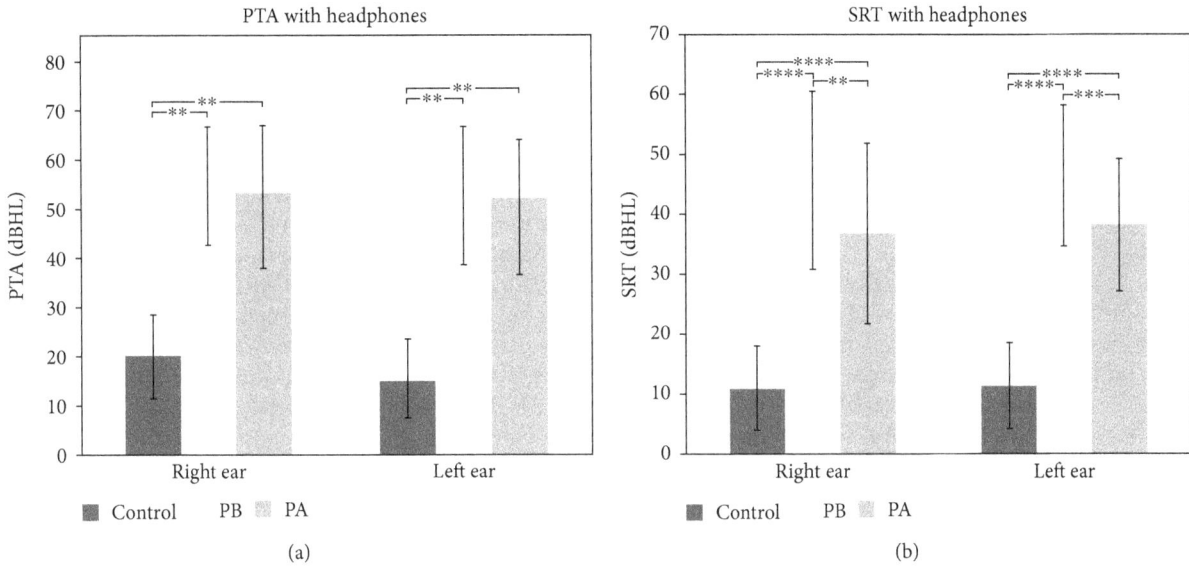

FIGURE 1: (a) PTA and (b) SRT with headphones of the control group, the patients before HA use (PB), and patients after HA use (PA). (a) Mean and standard deviations are shown for right and left ears. Results of PTA with headphones revealed statistical differences (**p < 0.001) in both ears between the CG and PB and PA. When comparing the PB with the PA, statistically significant difference was observed only for the left ear (*p < 0.04). (b) SRT results with headphones demonstrated statistically significant results between PB and PA for the right ear (**p < 0.001) and for the left ear (***p < 0.002). Moreover, statistical analysis indicated significant differences between the GC and PB and PA (*p < 0.0001, for both ears).

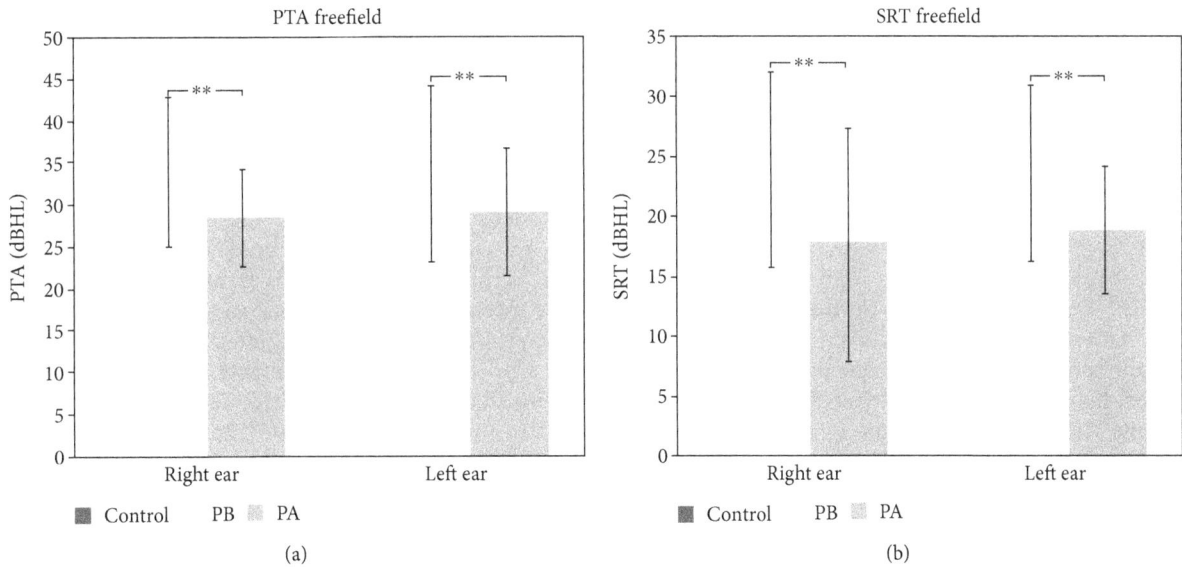

FIGURE 2: (a) PTA and (b) SRT in free field for the patients before (PB) and after (PA) HA use. Mean and standard deviation are shown for right and left ears before and after HA use. (a) PTA results in free field demonstrated statistically significant changes induced by HA use in both ears (**p < 0.001). (b) SRT evaluation in free field also showed a significant improvement in both ears (**p < 0.001).

(left ear) after HA use (Figure 2(b)). Supplementary Table 6 shows the individual free-field SRT results.

Both PTA and SRT functional gain (FG) improved significantly after HA use. PTA-FG improved significantly for both ears, from 33.15 ± 8.48 dB to 27.68 ± 5.64 dB (right ear, p = 0.001) and from 32.68 ± 10.29 dB to 28.27 ± 7.40 dB for the

left ear. SRT-FG also showed significant improvement from 23.93 ± 8.36 dB to 17.50 ± 9.15 dB (p = 0.001, right ear) and from 25.71 ± 5.49 dB to 18.21 ± 4.64 dB (p = 0.001, left ear).

3.2. fMRI. Two patients (#5 and #14) had to be excluded from further fMRI analysis due to excessive motion artifact (translation > 2 mm) in at least one of the two sessions, leaving 12 subjects in the final fMRI dataset.

The fMRI task was designed to engage auditory and language receptive fields [25, 27]. Indeed, in control subjects, it produced a robust activation in the auditory cortex for the contrast task (story) vs. baseline in the transverse temporal gyrus (BA41 and BA42) and language centers including Wernicke's area (BA22) (see Suppl. Figure 4 and Suppl. Table 7).

Figure 3 shows the fMRI results for the comparison between controls and patients before (PB) HA use. Statistical maps were much more diffuse in patients than in controls (Figure 3, Tables 1 and 2). Our results suggest that auditory deprivation is represented by decreased activity in the bilateral auditory cortex (BA41 and BA42) and Wernicke's area (Figure 3, Table 1). We also found increased activity in large portions of the frontal and occipital lobes, including bilateral visual areas (BA17, BA18, and BA19) and areas involved in multimodal integration, such as bilateral superior temporal sulcus (STS), middle intraparietal sulcus (IT, BA40), bilateral inferior frontal gyrus (IFG, BA44, BA45, and BA47), and the insula (BA13) (Figure 3, Table 2).

Figure 4 shows the fMRI results from the direct comparison between patients before (PB) vs. after (PA) HA use. Rehabilitation with HA leaded to increased activity of the left transverse temporal gyrus (BA40, BA41), Wernicke's area (left BA22), the left insula (BA13), and left superior frontal gyrus (BA8) (Figure 4, Table 3). We also found that intervention leads to reduced activity in left visual association areas (BA18, BA19), middle and superior frontal gyri (BA9, BA10, and BA46), and the thalamus (Figure 4, Table 4).

Figure 5 shows the correlation between individual changes in fMRI β-values and changes in SRT. We observed significant positive correlations in bilateral BA22 ($p < 0.006$, left; $p < 0.04$, right), left BA41 ($p < 0.04$), left BA42 ($p < 0.01$), left insula ($p < 0.05$), and left superior temporal gyrus ($p < 0.05$).

3.3. Cortical Thickness Analysis. Cortical thickness (CT) could not be estimated in two patients (#5 and #14) due excessive motion artifact in at least one of the sessions.

Figure 6 shows CT significant differences between controls and patients at baseline (PB). Before intervention, patients presented significant increased CT in bilateral prefrontal cortex (BA9 and BA10), precuneus/superior parietal gyrus (BA7), fusiform gyrus (BA37), and right posterior (BA39) and central portions (BA21) of the middle temporal gyrus (Figure 6, Table 5). We observed reduced CT bilaterally in portions of the visual cortex (BA17 and BA18), insula (BA13), supramarginal gyrus (BA40), left superior (BA41) and middle (BA21) temporal gyri, right parahippocampus (BA35), right posterior cingulate cortex (BA31), and the claustrum (Figure 6, Table 6).

When directly comparing patients before (PB) and after (PA) HA use, cortical thickness was increased in the left angular gyrus (BA39), located at the very caudal end of the superior temporal sulcus and in the right inferior parietal gyrus/superior temporal gyrus/posterior insula (BA13) (Figure 7, Table 7). We did not find areas of significant

reduced CT after interventions when compared to baseline values of the patients.

4. Discussion

In this study, we explored audiometric, anatomical, and functional brain changes following a one year of continuous HA use in postlingual deaf patients. We observed improved audiometric scores after intervention, particularly of speech recognition, together with fMRI signal increase in the primary auditory cortex, Wernicke's area, and visual areas. HA use also led to decreased fMRI activity in multimodal integration regions, such as the superior temporal sulcus (STS), the middle intraparietal sulcus (IT), and the insula. We observed significant positive correlations between changes in the speech recognition test and increased activity in the primary auditory cortex, Wernicke's area, left insula, and left STS. We also found increased cortical thickness after HA use in the left angular gyrus (BA39) and in the right posterior parietal/temporal junction, including the posterior insula.

Our measured pure tone averages (PTA) suggest that binaural HA fitting in individuals with postlingual sensorineural hearing loss steadies the deterioration of peripheral hearing, as already observed in previous reports [28]. In our study, patients also improved their SRT, both with headphones and in free field. It is well demonstrated that the rehabilitation with HA improves speech recognition, already at six to twelve weeks of HA use [29–31]. We also observed increased functional gain (FG), both for PTA and SRT measurements. Overall, our audiometric results suggest a significant benefit of HA use in speech recognition tasks, while the peripheral auditory system (cochlea, auditory nerve) may not evolve after HA use.

Compared to the control group, patients engaged much broader portions of the brain, including regions in the frontal, parietal, and occipital lobes (Tables 1 and 2). After HA use, activity was reduced in frontal and occipital regions and increased in the auditory cortex, Wernicke's area, and regions involved multimodal integration (Table 4).

Our observations are consistent with previous neuroimaging studies that reported increased activity in auditory-related cortices after CI [13–15]. Besides the auditory system, our results suggest increased activity in the primary and visual association occipital regions (Tables 3 and 4). Increased activity in visual areas has been reported in both fMRI and MEG, in patients with hearing loss [20]. Previous fMRI studies suggest that rehabilitation with CI increases the activity in the left middle occipitotemporal junction (BA37 and BA19) and in the posterior inferior temporal region (BA21 and BA37) [15]. Furthermore, the activity of visual cortex shortly after implantation seems to be related to the level of auditory recovery after cochlear implantation [19], and changes in functional connectivity across visual, temporal, and inferior frontal cortices have important consequences for subsequent CI outcome [32].

Such observations highlight the importance of multimodality as a fundamental aspect of human brain organization. Indeed, the old notion that sensory inputs are

(a)

(b)

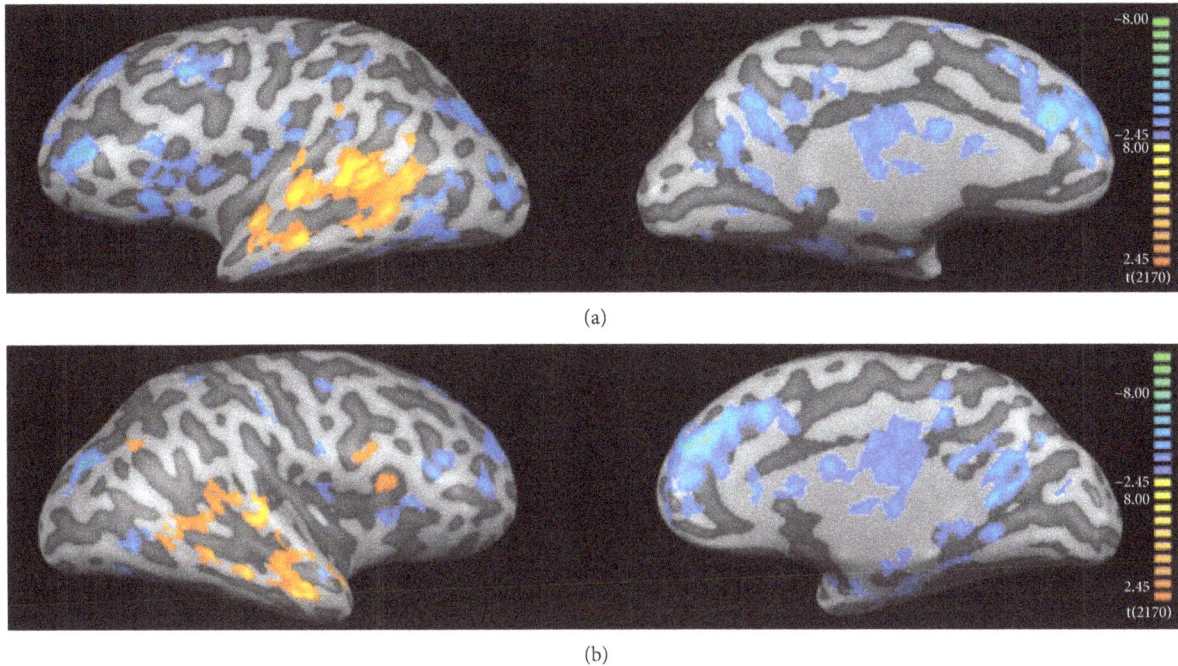

FIGURE 3: fMRI group analysis: controls versus patients before HA use. (a) Left and (b) right hemispheres, respectively. Color code indicates statistical significance. Warm colors (red-yellowish) show regions where activity was greater in controls than in PB, and cool colors (blue-greenish) show the opposite contrast (PB > CG). Clusters were selected with a q[FDR] < 0.05 and size of at least 50 mm^3.

TABLE 1: Brain regions with increased fMRI activity in controls (CG) when compared to patients before HA use (PB). The center of the cluster for each brain region is represented in Talairach coordinates (x, y, and z), followed by its respective standard deviations (in parentheses). Clusters were selected using a q[FDR] < 0.05 and a cluster size of at least 50 mm^3.

Brain region	Hem	Cluster size	Talairach coordinates			BA
			x	y	z	
Middle temporal gyrus	L	2403	−60 (5)	−33 (14)	0 (7)	21, 22, 37, 39
Middle temporal gyrus	R	855	59 (4)	−26 (15)	−3 (6)	21, 22, 37, 39
Transverse temporal gyrus	L	226	−53 (8)	−20 (4)	11 (1)	41, 42
Superior temporal gyrus	L	2893	−56 (6)	−18 (21)	3 (9)	22, 39, 41, 42
Superior temporal gyrus	R	1255	54 (6)	−12 (19)	0 (8)	22, 39, 41, 42
Inferior frontal gyrus	R	278	47 (2)	16 (4)	0 (14)	47
Inferior frontal gyrus	L	107	−51 (3)	15 (5)	0 (12)	47
Middle frontal gyrus	L	223	−2 (1)	−2 (4)	50 (2)	6

Hem = hemisphere; L = left; R = right; and BA = Brodmann area.

processed in specific and unimodal cortices is outdated [33]. For instance, studies in congenitally blind subjects have consistently found increased activity in the primary visual cortex during auditory stimulus processing [34, 35]. Moreover, several lines of evidence indicate that under certain circumstances and for specific visual tasks, hearing impairment leads to increased visual ability following congenital deafness [36]. In our study, we observed augmented fMRI activation of striate cortex (BA17) and extrastriate visual areas (BA18 and BA19), before rehabilitation. Increased recruitment of the visual system of hearing-impaired individuals in response to auditory stimuli has been reported in previous PET studies [37, 38]. Such findings have been interpreted as a result of the increased demand for visual cues during speech processing in individuals with hearing deficits [38]. Possibly as a

result of reduced demand, HA use was associated with reduced activity in the secondary and associative visual areas (BA18 and BA19).

Increased activity in frontal areas may reflect increased effort, inner speech with speech production, and/or increased audiovisual (AV) cooperation. In fact, after one year of HA use, we observed significant increased activity in bilateral auditory cortices. Besides, we have found increased activity in Wernicke's area (BA22) (Table 4) and reduced activity in visual areas, such as BA18 and BA19 (Table 3). Together, these results may show a different balance in AV interaction, with a reactivation of auditory speech areas and a more leftward lateralized network, i.e., a more physiological speech processing, less demanding after HA use. The recent study suggests that hearing loss impacts audiovisual speech

TABLE 2: Brain regions with increased fMRI activity in patients before HA use (PB) when compared to controls (CG). The center of the cluster for each brain region is represented in Talairach coordinates (x, y, and z), followed by its respective standard deviations (in parentheses). Clusters were selected using a q[FDR] < 0.05 and a cluster size of at least 50 mm^3.

Brain region	Hem	Cluster size	Talairach coordinates			BA
			x	y	z	
Cuneus	R	601	14 (5)	−78 (6)	11 (4)	17, 18
Lingual gyrus	R	872	20 (7)	−73 (11)	−2 (5)	17, 18, 19
Lingual gyrus	L	930	−19 (6)	−66 (11)	−3 (5)	17, 18, 19
Precuneus	R	355	12 (7)	−61 (8)	25 (5)	19
Precuneus	L	392	−13 (11)	−59 (8)	29 (7)	19
Fusiform gyrus	R	489	33 (7)	−60 (12)	−12 (3)	19, 37
Fusiform gyrus	L	770	−32 (9)	−62 (19)	−13 (3)	18, 19, 37
Middle occipital gyrus	L	565	−33 (8)	−80 (8)	3 (8)	18, 19
Superior temporal gyrus	L	178	−45 (5)	−43 (13)	19 (8)	13, 22, 41, 39
Superior temporal gyrus	R	152	43 (7)	−52 (5)	20 (3)	13, 22, 39
Inferior temporal gyrus	L	318	−53 (5)	−38 (27)	−10 (9)	19, 20
Middle temporal gyrus	L	374	−49 (10)	−45 (25)	2 (11)	19, 21
Parahippocampal gyrus	R	1131	24 (6)	−22 (14)	−14 (7)	28, 34, 35, 36, hippocampus, amygdala
Parahippocampal gyrus	L	1237	−25 (8)	−26 (12)	−12 (7)	27, 28, 34, 35, 36, hippocampus, amygdala
Cingulate gyrus	L	1206	−7 (5)	−2 (28)	34 (5)	23, 24, 31, 32
Cingulate gyrus	R	2492	7 (4)	−2 (22)	34 (5)	23, 24, 30, 31, 32
Anterior cingulate	L	482	−10 (5)	37 (3)	18 (5)	32
Anterior cingulate	R	935	8 (5)	35 (9)	15 (7)	24, 32, 33
Posterior cingulate	L	873	−6 (6)	−54 (6)	17 (5)	23, 29, 30, 31
Posterior cingulate	R	974	8 (7)	−54 (9)	15 (5)	23, 29, 30, 31
Insula	R	616	37 (4)	4 (18)	12 (6)	13
Insula	L	1213	−38 (5)	−5 (19)	12 (8)	13
Inferior frontal gyrus	L	796	−45 (8)	16 (6)	10 (13)	6, 9, 10, 44, 45, 46, 47
Middle frontal gyrus	L	2596	−6 (5)	39 (11)	28 (10)	6, 8, 9, 10
Middle frontal gyrus	R	2607	7 (4)	41 (10)	26 (11)	6, 8, 9, 10
Middle frontal gyrus	R	242	38 (7)	23 (20)	27 (12)	6, 9, 10, 46
Middle frontal gyrus	L	1416	−37 (8)	26 (20)	29 (14)	6, 8, 9, 10, 46
Superior frontal gyrus	R	882	11 (6)	53 (5)	29 (5)	8, 9, 10
Superior frontal gyrus	L	1932	−15 (10)	48 (13)	32 (10)	6, 8, 9, 10
Precentral gyrus	L	465	−44 (5)	2 (6)	32 (11)	4, 6, 9, 43
Precentral gyrus	R	497	45 (6)	−7 (7)	34 (9)	4, 6
Inferior parietal lobe	L	467	−44 (6)	−37 (7)	38 (7)	39, 40
Caudate	L	876	−14 (7)	−6 (16)	16 (6)	
Caudate	R	938	18 (6)	−11 (17)	17 (6)	
Thalamus	L	489	−7 (5)	−16 (8)	9 (5)	
Thalamus	R	1144	16 (6)	−17 (7)	10 (4)	

Hem = hemisphere; L = left; R = right; and BA = Brodmann area.

processing accompanied by changed activity in frontal brain areas, which are modulated by the level of hearing loss [39].

Clinical observations have demonstrated the impact of hearing impairment on higher cognitive processes [2], which can be at least partially recovered by auditory rehabilitation. For instance, it has been observed significant improvements of learning and speech in children after CI [15]. Interestingly, we observed significant correlations between individual fMRI signal changes in auditory (BA41 and BA41) and Wernicke's areas (BA22) and individual change in SRT. This finding

links, to our knowledge for the first time, clinical evidence of improved language abilities in patients with hearing loss after auditory rehabilitation with acoustic amplification.

Our results also suggest increased recruitment of brain areas involved in multimodal integration, after HA use, observed as increased fMRI activity in the superior temporal sulcus (STS), the middle intraparietal sulcus (IT, BA40), the inferior frontal gyrus (IFG, BA44, BA45, and BA47), and the insula (BA13). It is possible that HA use improved the quality of information provided by the auditory system to

(a)

(b)

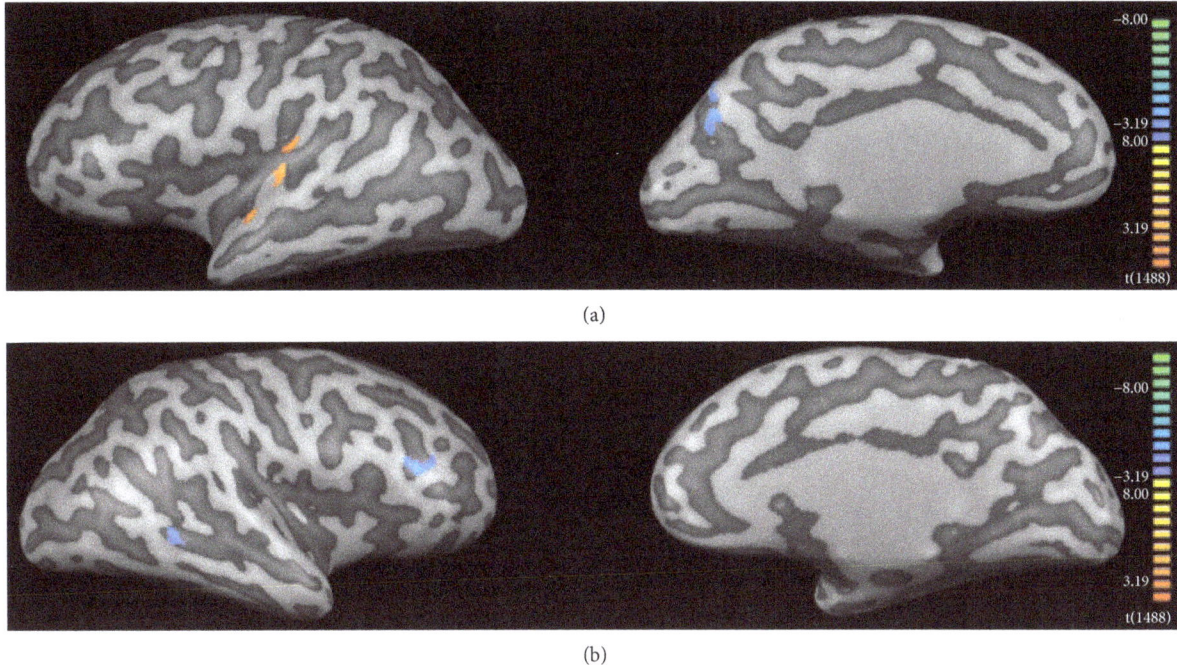

FIGURE 4: fMRI group analysis: patients before HA use (PB) versus patients after HA use (PA). (a) Left and (b) right hemispheres, respectively. Color code indicates statistical significance. Warm colors (red-yellowish) show regions where activity was greater in PA than in PB, and cool colors (blue-greenish) show the opposite contrast (PB > PA). Clusters were selected with a $q[\text{FDR}] < 0.05$ and size of at least $50\,\text{mm}^3$.

TABLE 3: Brain regions with increased fMRI activity in patients before HA use (PB) when compared to patients after HA use (PA). The center of the cluster for each brain region is represented in Talairach coordinates (x, y, and z), followed by its respective standard deviations (in parentheses). Clusters were selected using a $q[\text{FDR}] < 0.05$ and a cluster size of at least $50\,\text{mm}^3$.

Brain region	Hem	Cluster size	Talairach coordinates			BA
			x	y	z	
Cuneus	L	118	−12 (2)	−76 (2)	32 (1)	18, 19
Precuneus	L	156	−15 (2)	−73 (5)	33 (6)	19
Middle frontal gyrus	R	260	43 (3)	37 (5)	17 (2)	10, 46
Middle frontal gyrus	R	89	6 (2)	47 (1)	28 (2)	9
Superior frontal gyrus	R	70	6 (2)	49 (1)	30 (2)	9
Superior frontal gyrus	L	102	−4 (1)	55 (2)	25 (2)	9
Thalamus	R	325	12 (3)	−22 (3)	14 (2)	

Hem = hemisphere; L = left; R = right; and BA = Brodmann area.

TABLE 4: Brain regions with increased fMRI activity in patients after HA use (PA) when compared to patients before HA use (PB). The center of the cluster for each brain region is represented in Talairach coordinates (x, y, and z), followed by its respective standard deviations (in parentheses). Clusters were selected using a $q[\text{FDR}] < 0.05$ and a cluster size of at least $50\,\text{mm}^3$.

Brain region	Hem	Cluster size	Talairach coordinates			BA
			x	y	z	
Superior temporal gyrus	L	476	−51 (5)	−1 (10)	1 (4)	21, 22, 41
Transverse temporal gyrus	L	178	−42 (4)	−23 (2)	12 (1)	40, 41
Superior frontal gyrus	L	295	−6 (2)	40 (4)	46 (3)	8
Insula	L	109	−39 (4)	−23 (7)	12 (4)	13

Hem = hemisphere; L = left; R = right; and BA = Brodmann area.

speech integration centers, changing the balance between visual and auditory inputs. In fact, the process of multi-sensory integration is apparently based upon a weighed estimation of each sensorial input, which in turn depends on the reliability of the information contained in each modality [40]. In further supporting of this hypothesis is

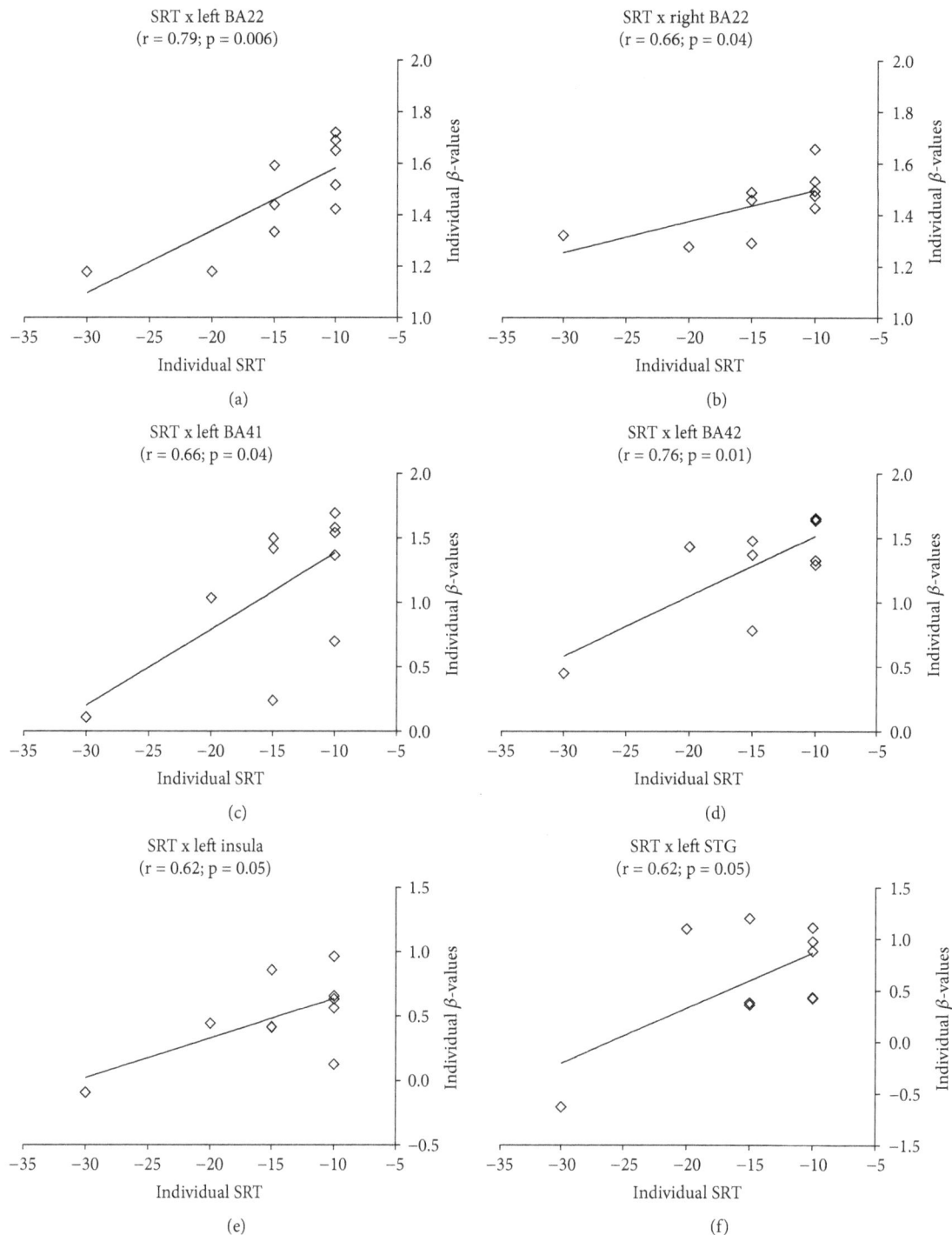

FIGURE 5: Pearson correlations between individual SRT changes and individual fMRI β-values changes. SRT with headphones changes were computed as a global difference between thresholds observed before and after intervention, according to [SRT (right ear before) + SRT (left ear before)] − [SRT (right ear after) + SRT (left ear after)]. Only regions that presented statistically significant correlation are shown. Significant correlations were found only after HA use in (a) left BA22, (b) right BA22, (c) left BA41, (d) left BA42, (e) left insula, and (f) left STG.

the significant positive correlation found between individual fMRI signal changes in the left insula and left STG with individual changes in SRT, such that the greater the SRT improvement, the greater was the fMRI signal change.

The aim of our study was not limited to investigate functional reorganization due to HA use, but it also explored

neuroanatomical changes. Before HA use, cortical thickness (CT) was reduced in the visual cortex (BA17 and BA18), primary auditory cortex (BA41), and multimodal cortex (BA13 and BA40) and increased CT was found in the associative somatosensory cortex (BA7), prefrontal cortex (BA9 and BA10), and middle temporal/fusiform gyrus (BA37). Only a

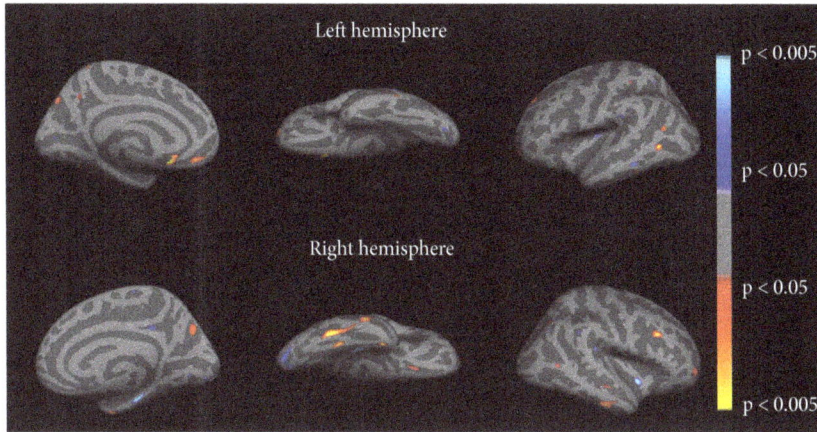

FIGURE 6: Cortical thickness changes of the patients before HA use (PB) when compared to the control group (CG). Color code indicates p values. Warm colors (red-yellowish) show regions where cortical thickness was greater in PB than in the controls, and cool colors (blue-greenish) show the opposite contrast (CG > PB).

TABLE 5: Regions of increased cortical thickness in patients at baseline (PB) when compared to controls (CG). Mean cortical thickness is expressed in mm. The numbers in parentheses correspond to standard deviations. Statistical significance was based at $p < 0.01$.

Brain region	Hem	Nvox	Talairach coordinates			BA	PB Mean (SD)	CG Mean (SD)	p value
			x	y	z				
Medial orbitofrontal gyrus	L	176	−9.0	37.8	−13.5	10	3.12 (0.36)	2.54 (0.35)	0.001
Middle frontal gyrus	L	111	−21.2	52.3	−9.7	10	2.83 (0.41)	2.45 (0.20)	0.010
Middle frontal gyrus	R	226	38.9	20.0	25.7	9	2.89 (0.22)	2.59 (0.21)	0.005
Superior parietal gyrus	L	209	−16.6	−70.1	37.3	7	2.35 (0.29)	2.00 (0.30)	0.010
Superior parietal gyrus	R	55	22.6	−53.5	57.5	7	2.28 (0.16)	2.01 (0.28)	0.010
Precuneus	L	58	−7.8	−52.7	37.5	7	2.96 (0.37)	2.50 (0.40)	0.010
Precuneus	R	279	18.8	−66.1	34.2	7	2.49 (0.29)	2.21 (0.16)	0.010
Fusiform gyrus	R	626	40.7	−48.7	−11.0	37	3.28 (0.16)	2.84 (0.25)	0.0002
Fusiform gyrus	L	127	−50.9	−58.3	3.3	37	3.08 (0.21)	2.59 (0.29)	0.0003
Middle temporal gyrus	R	281	54.5	−20.4	−18.6	21	3.34 (0.26)	2.95 (0.30)	0.005
Middle temporal gyrus	R	56	49.4	−59.1	7.4	39	3.11 (0.21)	2.73 (0.38)	0.010
Entorhinal gyrus	R	161	30.2	−3.5	−29.0	36	3.94 (0.50)	3.33 (0.31)	0.003

Hem = hemisphere; L = left; R = right; BA = Brodmann area; Nvox = number of voxels in the cluster; SD = standard deviation; PB = patients before HA use; CG = control group.

few studies have used MRI to investigate neuroanatomical changes due to auditory deprivation, and the results are not consistent. A seminal study used voxel-based morphometry (VBM) in prelingually deaf subjects and identified significant reduced volume only in the left posterior STG [41]. In a more recent study, VBM and CT analysis were applied to evaluate individuals with profound sensorineural hearing loss [42]. No brain structure in the patient group presented increased volume or CT, but the cortical thickness of the primary visual area (BA17) was significantly smaller in patients than in the control group [42]. In another study, CT was investigated in adolescents with prelingual deafness and significant CT differences were found in the right middle occipital gyrus, right precuneus, left gyrus rectus, and left posterior cingulate gyrus [43, 44].

After HA use, our results indicate increased CT at the very caudal end of the STS, including the left angular gyrus (BA39) and the inferior parietal gyrus/superior temporal gyrus/posterior insula (BA13). All of these regions are related to multimodality, and it is tempting to associate these anatomical changes to the functional ones detected by fMRI. Although there are evidence giving support to a possible link between functional and anatomical changes observed by MRI, this is still a matter of debate [45]. Indeed, in some brain areas, the observed increased fMRI activity was related to a reduced CT, as for instance BA17 before HA use. On the other hand, sensory integration areas, such as the left insula, showed increased CT and increased fMRI activity after HA use.

This study has a number of caveats and limitations worth mentioning. First, our sample size was limited to 12 patients in the final functional and anatomical datasets. Second, the absence of a control group (patients without intervention), where patients would be placed on a waiting list for follow-up intervention. However, the nature of this 1-year longitudinal study hinders such design. During audiologic assessments,

TABLE 6: Regions of reduced cortical thickness in patients at baseline (PB) when compared to controls (CG). Mean cortical thickness is expressed in mm. The numbers in parentheses correspond to standard deviations. Statistical significance was set at $p < 0.01$.

Brain region	Hem.	Nvox	Talairach coordinates			BA	PB Mean (SD)	CG Mean (SD)	p value
			x	y	z				
Insula	R	144	44.5	−35.3	19.9	13	2.54 (0.22)	2.87 (0.21)	0.003
Insula	L	166	−34.5	−14.9	13.5	13	2.93 (0.24)	3.35 (0.35)	0.005
Supramarginal gyrus	R	64	52.6	−39.3	30.6	40	2.66 (0.27)	3.09 (0.37)	0.007
Supramarginal gyrus	L	100	−55.8	−29.1	21.9	40	2.76 (0.34)	3.13 (0.29)	0.010
Superior temporal gyrus	L	55	−42.6	−28.7	5.0	41	2.71 (0.40)	3.34 (0.61)	0.010
Middle temporal gyrus	L	116	−58.4	−38.2	−9.3	21	2.92 (0.47)	3.61 (0.33)	0.001
Parahippocampal gyrus	R	336	23.8	−24.1	−19.0	35	3.06 (0.20)	3.43 (0.30)	0.004
Lateral occipital gyrus	R	462	21.5	−89.6	−2.2	17	2.13 (0.29)	2.55 (0.30)	0.004
Lingual gyrus	R	45	8.7	−69.9	3.9	18	2.15 (0.29)	2.55 (0.39)	0.010
Middle occipital gyrus	L	71	−23.1	−82.8	−6.5	18	2.19 (0.32)	2.69 (0.37)	0.004
Posterior cingulate	R	99	8.4	−34.9	33.0	31	3.00 (0.42)	3.67 (0.55)	0.006
Claustrum	R	187	35.5	−4.0	−4.6	—	3.40 (0.53)	4.16 (0.40)	0.001

Hem = hemisphere; L = left; R = right; BA = Brodmann area; Nvox = number of voxels in the cluster; SD = standard deviation; PB = patients before HA use; CG = control group.

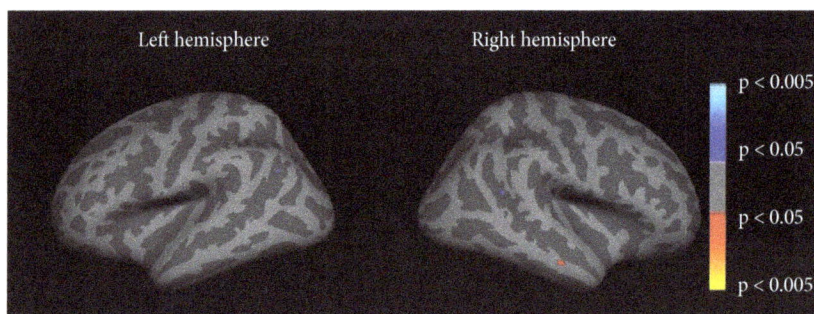

FIGURE 7: Cortical thickness changes of the patients before HA use (PB) when compared to patients after HA use (PA). Color code indicates p values. Warm colors (red-yellowish) show regions where cortical thickness was greater in PB than PA, and cool colors (blue-greenish) show the opposite contrast (PA > PB).

TABLE 7: Regions of increased cortical thickness in the patients after HA use (PA) when compared to patients before HA use (PB). Mean cortical thickness is expressed in mm. The numbers in parentheses correspond to standard deviations. Statistical significance was based at $p < 0.01$.

Brain region	Hem	Nvox	Talairach coordinates			BA	PB Mean (SD)	PA Mean (SD)	p value
			x	y	z				
Inferior parietal gyrus/superior temporal gyrus/posterior insula	R	36	44.7	−44.5	18.8	13	2.57 (0.28)	2.97 (0.29)	0.010
Angular gyrus	L	31	−38.6	−58.9	29.9	39	2.73 (0.37)	3.06 (0.29)	0.003

Hem = hemisphere; L = left; R = right; BA = Brodmann area; Nvox = number of voxels in the cluster; SD = standard deviation; PB = patients before HA use; PA = patients after HA use.

the nontested ear was not masked or plugged. Therefore, especially in case of mild HL, we might have observed an additive effect between the HA ear and the non-HA ear, and the observed audiometric changes may have been biased by the protocol we used. The same story was presented in both fMRI sessions (before and after HA use), and therefore, our fMRI results are susceptible to habituation. We used a fixed-effects model in the fMRI analysis, which limits our

conclusions to the population studied. We did not retest the control group after one year.

To our knowledge, this is the first study which is aimed at investigating audiometric and neuroimaging changes induced by HA use in patients with long-lasting auditory deprivation. Audiometric observations were complemented by neuroimaging investigation, both functional and anatomical cortical thicknesses, to assist in understanding the neurophysiological mechanisms behind hearing rehabilitation. Furthermore, the correlation found between individual fMRI and SRT further paves the perspective for the use of functional neuroimaging as a clinical tool in audiology.

Conflicts of Interest

The authors declare that there is no conflict of interest regarding the publication of this paper.

Acknowledgments

This work was supported by the São Paulo Research Foundation (FAPESP), Brazilian National Council for Scientific and Technological Development (CNPq), and CAPES, a foundation from the Ministry of Education, Brazil. Thanks are due to Sandra Moroti for MRI scanning, to Dr. Elson Rodrigues for helping with patient screening and for the diagnosis hearing loss type, and to the patients.

Supplementary Materials

Supplementary Figure 1: pure tone audiometry for each frequency tested with headphones in the control group. Supplementary Figure 2: pure tone audiometry for each frequency tested with headphones for the group of patients before (PB) and after (PA) HA use. Supplementary Figure 3: pure tone audiometry for each frequency tested in free field, for patients before (PB) and after (PA) HA use. Supplementary Figure 4: fMRI statistical maps of the control group. Supplementary Table 1: clinical and audiometric information of the patients. Supplementary Table 2: individual PTA and SRT with headphones for the control group (CG). Supplementary Table 3: individual PTA with headphones for patients before (PB) and after (PA) HA use. Supplementary Table 4: individual SRT with headphones of the group of patients before (PB) and after (PA) HA use. Supplementary Table 5: individual PTA in free field of the group of patients before (PB) and after (PA) HA use. Supplementary Table 6: individual SRT in free field for patients before (PB) and after (PA) HA use. Supplementary Table 7: statistically significant fMRI response in the control group. *(Supplementary Materials)*

References

[1] C. D. Mulrow, M. R. Tuley, and C. Aguilar, "Sustained benefits of hearing-aids," *Clinical Research*, vol. 39, pp. A593–A593, 1991.

[2] M. K. Pichora-Fuller and G. Singh, "Effects of age on auditory and cognitive processing: implications for hearing aid fitting and audiologic rehabilitation," *Trends in Amplification*, vol. 10, no. 1, pp. 29–59, 2006.

[3] A. Y. Choi, H. J. Shim, S. H. Lee, S. W. Yoon, and E. J. Joo, "Is cognitive function in adults with hearing impairment improved by the use of hearing aids?," *Clinical and Experimental Otorhinolaryngology*, vol. 4, no. 2, pp. 72–76, 2011.

[4] R. Rajan, D. R. F. Irvine, L. Z. Wise, and P. Heil, "Effect of unilateral partial cochlear lesions in adult cats on the representation of lesioned and unlesioned cochleas in primary auditory cortex," *The Journal of Comparative Neurology*, vol. 338, no. 1, pp. 17–49, 1993.

[5] M. K. Schwaber, P. E. Garraghty, and J. H. Kaas, "Neuroplasticity of the adult primate auditory cortex following cochlear hearing loss," *The American Journal of Otology*, vol. 14, no. 3, pp. 252–258, 1993.

[6] J. F. Willott, L. M. Aitkin, and S. L. McFadden, "Plasticity of auditory cortex associated with sensorineural hearing loss in adult C57BL/6J mice," *The Journal of Comparative Neurology*, vol. 329, no. 3, pp. 402–411, 1993.

[7] B. Ryals and E. Rubel, "Hair cell regeneration after acoustic trauma in adult *Coturnix* quail," *Science*, vol. 240, no. 4860, pp. 1774–1776, 1988.

[8] Y. Chung, K. E. Hancock, S. I. Nam, and B. Delgutte, "Coding of electric pulse trains presented through cochlear implants in the auditory midbrain of awake rabbit: comparison with anesthetized preparations," *The Journal of Neuroscience*, vol. 34, no. 1, pp. 218–231, 2014.

[9] J. B. Fallon, D. R. F. Irvine, and R. K. Shepherd, "Cochlear implant use following neonatal deafness influences the cochleotopic organization of the primary auditory cortex in cats," *Journal of Comparative Neurology*, vol. 512, no. 1, pp. 101–114, 2009.

[10] E. Amaro, S. C. R. Williams, S. S. Shergill et al., "Acoustic noise and functional magnetic resonance imaging: current strategies and future prospects," *Journal of Magnetic Resonance Imaging*, vol. 16, no. 5, pp. 497–510, 2002.

[11] D. Bilecen, E. Seifritz, E. W. Radu et al., "Cortical reorganization after acute unilateral hearing loss traced by fMRI," *Neurology*, vol. 54, no. 3, pp. 765–767, 2000.

[12] D. S. Lazard, H. J. Lee, E. Truy, and A. L. Giraud, "Bilateral reorganization of posterior temporal cortices in post-lingual deafness and its relation to cochlear implant outcome," *Human Brain Mapping*, vol. 34, no. 5, pp. 1208–1219, 2013.

[13] J. S. Lee, D. S. Lee, S. H. Oh et al., "PET evidence of neuroplasticity in adult auditory cortex of postlingual deafness," *The Journal of Nuclear Medicine*, vol. 44, no. 9, pp. 1435–1439, 2003.

[14] J. H. Hwang, C. W. Wu, J. H. Chen, and T. C. Liu, "Changes in activation of the auditory cortex following long-term amplification: an fMRI study," *Acta Oto-Laryngologica*, vol. 126, no. 12, pp. 1275–1280, 2006.

[15] E. Kang, D. S. Lee, H. Kang et al., "Neural changes associated with speech learning in deaf children following cochlear implantation," *NeuroImage*, vol. 22, no. 3, pp. 1173–1181, 2004.

[16] A. L. Giraud, C. J. Price, J. M. Graham, and R. S. J. Frackowiak, "Functional plasticity of language-related brain areas after cochlear implantation," *Brain*, vol. 124, no. 7, pp. 1307–1316, 2001.

[17] J. Rouger, S. Lagleyre, J. F. Démonet, B. Fraysse, O. Deguine, and P. Barone, "Evolution of crossmodal reorganization of the voice area in cochlear-implanted deaf patients," *Human Brain Mapping*, vol. 33, no. 8, pp. 1929–1940, 2012.

[18] G. A. Calvert, R. Campbell, and M. J. Brammer, "Evidence from functional magnetic resonance imaging of crossmodal

binding in the human heteromodal cortex," *Current Biology*, vol. 10, no. 11, pp. 649–657, 2000.

[19] K. Strelnikov, J. Rouger, J. F. Demonet et al., "Visual activity predicts auditory recovery from deafness after adult cochlear implantation," *Brain*, vol. 136, no. 12, pp. 3682–3695, 2013.

[20] Y. T. Zhang, Z. J. Geng, Q. Zhang, W. Li, and J. Zhang, "Auditory cortical responses evoked by pure tones in healthy and sensorineural hearing loss subjects: functional MRI and magnetoencephalography," *Chinese Medical Journal*, vol. 119, no. 18, pp. 1548–1554, 2006.

[21] H. Davis and S. R. Silverman, *Hearing and Deafness*, Holt, Rinehart & Winston of Canada Ltd, 1970.

[22] A. W. Bronkhorst and R. Plomp, "Binaural speech-intelligibility in noise for hearing-impaired listeners," *The Journal of the Acoustical Society of America*, vol. 86, no. 4, pp. 1374–1383, 1989.

[23] D. P. Pascoe, "Frequency responses of hearing aids and their effects on the speech perception of hearing-impaired subjects," *Annals of Otology, Rhinology & Laryngology*, vol. 84, no. 5, Supplement, pp. 5–40, 1975.

[24] D. Araujo, D. B. De Araujo, O. M. Pontes-Neto et al., "Language and motor *f*MRI activation in polymicrogyric cortex," *Epilepsia*, vol. 47, no. 3, pp. 589–592, 2006.

[25] C. A. Estombelo-Montesco, M. Sturzbecher Jr., A. K. D. Barros, and D. B. de Araujo, "Detection of auditory cortex activity by fMRI using a dependent component analysis," in *Advances in Experimental Medicine and Biology*, vol. 657, pp. 135–145, Springer, 2010.

[26] B. Fischl, M. I. Sereno, and A. M. Dale, "Cortical surface-based analysis: II: inflation, flattening, and a surface-based coordinate system," *NeuroImage*, vol. 9, no. 2, pp. 195–207, 1999.

[27] M. J. Sturzbecher, W. Tedeschi, B. C. T. Cabella, O. Baffa, U. P. C. Neves, and D. B. de Araujo, "Non-extensive entropy and the extraction of BOLD spatial information in event-related functional MRI," *Physics in Medicine & Biology*, vol. 54, no. 1, pp. 161–174, 2009.

[28] R. M. Hurley, "Onset of auditory deprivation," *Journal of the American Academy of Audiology*, vol. 10, no. 10, pp. 529–534, 1999.

[29] B. C. J. Moore, J. I. Alcántara, and J. Marriage, "Comparison of three procedures for initial fitting of compression hearing aids. I. Experienced users, fitted bilaterally," *British Journal of Audiology*, vol. 35, no. 6, pp. 339–353, 2001.

[30] G. H. Saunders and J. M. Kates, "Speech intelligibility enhancement using hearing-aid array processing," *The Journal of the Acoustical Society of America*, vol. 102, no. 3, pp. 1827–1837, 1997.

[31] T. Wittkop and V. Hohmann, "Strategy-selective noise reduction for binaural digital hearing aids," *Speech Communication*, vol. 39, no. 1-2, pp. 111–138, 2003.

[32] D. S. Lazard and A. L. Giraud, "Faster phonological processing and right occipito-temporal coupling in deaf adults signal poor cochlear implant outcome," *Nature Communications*, vol. 8, article 14872, 2017.

[33] A. Ghazanfar and C. Schroeder, "Is neocortex essentially multisensory?," *Trends in Cognitive Sciences*, vol. 10, no. 6, pp. 278–285, 2006.

[34] L. B. Merabet and A. Pascual-Leone, "Neural reorganization following sensory loss: the opportunity of change," *Nature Reviews Neuroscience*, vol. 11, no. 1, pp. 44–52, 2010.

[35] O. Collignon, G. Vandewalle, P. Voss et al., "Functional specialization for auditory–spatial processing in the occipital cortex of congenitally blind humans," *Proceedings of the National Academy of Sciences of the United States of America*, vol. 108, no. 11, pp. 4435–4440, 2011.

[36] D. Bavelier, M. W. G. Dye, and P. C. Hauser, "Do deaf individuals see better?," *Trends in Cognitive Sciences*, vol. 10, no. 11, pp. 512–518, 2006.

[37] A. L. Giraud, C. J. Price, J. M. Graham, E. Truy, and R. S. J. Frackowiak, "Cross-modal plasticity underpins language recovery after cochlear implantation," *Neuron*, vol. 30, no. 3, pp. 657–664, 2001.

[38] A. L. Giraud and E. Truy, "The contribution of visual areas to speech comprehension: a PET study in cochlear implants patients and normal-hearing subjects," *Neuropsychologia*, vol. 40, no. 9, pp. 1562–1569, 2002.

[39] S. Rosemann and C. M. Thiel, "Audio-visual speech processing in age-related hearing loss: stronger integration and increased frontal lobe recruitment," *NeuroImage*, vol. 175, pp. 425–437, 2018.

[40] N. W. Roach, J. Heron, and P. V. McGraw, "Resolving multisensory conflict: a strategy for balancing the costs and benefits of audio-visual integration," *Proceedings of the Royal Society B: Biological Sciences*, vol. 273, no. 1598, pp. 2159–2168, 2006.

[41] D. K. Shibata, "Differences in brain structure in deaf persons on MR imaging studied with voxel-based morphometry," *American Journal of Neuroradiology*, vol. 28, no. 2, pp. 243–249, 2007.

[42] J. Li, W. Li, J. Xian et al., "Cortical thickness analysis and optimized voxel-based morphometry in children and adolescents with prelingually profound sensorineural hearing loss," *Brain Research*, vol. 1430, pp. 35–42, 2012.

[43] W. Li, J. Li, J. Xian et al., "Alterations of grey matter asymmetries in adolescents with prelingual deafness: a combined VBM and cortical thickness analysis," *Restorative Neurology and Neuroscience*, vol. 31, no. 1, pp. 1–17, 2013.

[44] M. Yang, H. J. Chen, B. Liu et al., "Brain structural and functional alterations in patients with unilateral hearing loss," *Hearing Research*, vol. 316, pp. 37–43, 2014.

[45] M. P. Harms, L. Wang, J. G. Csernansky, and D. M. Barch, "Structure–function relationship of working memory activity with hippocampal and prefrontal cortex volumes," *Brain Structure and Function*, vol. 218, no. 1, pp. 173–186, 2013.

13

Contextual Fear Memory Formation and Destabilization Induce Hippocampal RyR2 Calcium Channel Upregulation

Jamileth More,[1] **María Mercedes Casas,**[1] **Gina Sánchez,**[2,3] **Cecilia Hidalgo** ⓘ**,**[1,3,4] **and Paola Haeger** ⓘ[5]

[1]*Biomedical Neuroscience Institute, Faculty of Medicine, Universidad de Chile, Santiago, Chile*
[2]*Pathophysiology Program, ICBM, Faculty of Medicine, Universidad de Chile, Santiago, Chile*
[3]*Center for Exercise, Metabolism and Cancer, Faculty of Medicine, Universidad de Chile, Santiago, Chile*
[4]*Department of Neurosciences and Physiology and Biophysics Program, ICBM, Faculty of Medicine, Universidad de Chile, Santiago, Chile*
[5]*Department of Biomedical Sciences, Faculty of Medicine, Universidad Católica del Norte, Coquimbo, Chile*

Correspondence should be addressed to Cecilia Hidalgo; chidalgo@med.uchile.cl and Paola Haeger; phaeger@ucn.cl

Academic Editor: Long-Jun Wu

Hippocampus-dependent spatial and aversive memory processes entail Ca^{2+} signals generated by ryanodine receptor (RyR) Ca^{2+} channels residing in the endoplasmic reticulum membrane. Rodents exposed to different spatial memory tasks exhibit significant hippocampal RyR upregulation. Contextual fear conditioning generates robust hippocampal memories through an associative learning process, but the effects of contextual fear memory acquisition, consolidation, or extinction on hippocampal RyR protein levels remain unreported. Accordingly, here we investigated if exposure of male rats to contextual fear protocols, or subsequent exposure to memory destabilization protocols, modified the hippocampal content of type-2 RyR (RyR2) channels, the predominant hippocampal RyR isoforms that hold key roles in synaptic plasticity and spatial memory processes. We found that contextual memory retention caused a transient increase in hippocampal RyR2 protein levels, determined 5 h after exposure to the conditioning protocol; this increase vanished 29 h after training. Context reexposure 24 h after training, for 3, 15, or 30 min without the aversive stimulus, decreased fear memory and increased RyR2 protein levels, determined 5 h after reexposure. We propose that both fear consolidation and extinction memories induce RyR2 protein upregulation in order to generate the intracellular Ca^{2+} signals required for these distinct memory processes.

1. Introduction

Fear conditioning, an associative learning process that produces robust memories, represents a form of Pavlovian conditioning that has received considerable attention over the last years [1, 2]. When exposed to fear conditioning protocols, animals acquire fear memory through the association between conditioned stimuli—a tone, a smell, or a context—with an unconditioned aversive stimulus, usually a foot shock. Evidence that the hippocampus forms part of the neuronal pathways involved in contextual fear conditioning came first from studies showing that lesions in the dorsal hippocampus prevent both the acquisition and the expression of context-dependent fear conditioning [3–5]. Recent optogenetic techniques support hippocampal involvement in context-dependent fear conditioning [6]. Other reports indicate that synaptic plasticity in the amygdala mediates the association between conditioned and unconditioned stimuli, whereas hippocampal synaptic plasticity mediates contextual coding [2, 7–9].

In agreement with the procedures developed by Pavlov many years ago [10], protocols to study memory destabilization entail special procedures, whereby animals previously exposed to fear conditioning protocols are reexposed subsequently to the conditioned stimulus in the absence of the unconditioned aversive stimulus. This procedure activates memory retrieval, a dynamic phenomenon that depending on the length of the reexposure session triggers two distinct processes, reconsolidation or extinction. Brief reexposition triggers a labile state that requires de novo protein synthesis to restabilize memory persistence in a process known as reconsolidation [11]. In contrast, prolonged, nonreinforced retrieval sessions induce memory extinction [12]. During the formation of extinction memory, a new learning process occurs, which interferes with the expression of the original memory [13–17]. In addition, it has been proposed that extinction does not destroy or erase the original association between conditioned and unconditioned stimuli, so that the expression of extinction memory represents the formation of a new memory that depends on the context [18]. Studies performed in rodents revealed that the dorsal hippocampus is involved in the acquisition, contextual encoding, and context-dependent retrieval of fear memory extinction [13]. Subsequent reports revealed that prefrontal modulation of amygdala activity mediates the context specificity of the extinction process and that the hippocampus has a fundamental role in contextual memory retrieval [19]. Furthermore, CA1 infusion with the $GABA_A$ agonist muscimol before the extinction session impaired extinction, showing that the hippocampal CA1 region plays an important role in the fear extinction process [20].

Neuronal Ca^{2+} signals play key roles in memory processes [21], including fear memory [22]. Activity-generated neuronal Ca^{2+} signals arise from Ca^{2+} influx mediated by N-methyl-D-aspartate receptors (NMDAR) and voltage-gated Ca^{2+} channels (VGCC). Calcium release from the endoplasmic reticulum (ER) mediated by inositol 1,4,5-tris-phosphate receptor (IP_3R) and ryanodine receptor (RyR) channels also contributes to generate Ca^{2+} signals in response to neuronal activation [23–25]. In a rodent brain, immunohistological techniques have revealed the heterogeneous expression pattern of both receptor types within neuronal cells [26, 27]. Mammals express three RyR isoforms; specific genes, identified and cloned, encode each isoform [28]. The brain expresses all three RyR isoforms; of these, the RyR2 isoform is the predominant isoform expressed in rat and chicken brain [29, 30]. As detailed below, the redox-sensitive RyR2 isoforms have key roles in hippocampal structural plasticity and spatial memory processes [31].

The generation of intracellular Ca^{2+} signals promotes RyR activity, giving rise to a cellular response known as Ca^{2+}-induced Ca^{2+} release (CICR). In neuronal cells, Ca^{2+} influx mediated by NMDAR and VGCC elicits RyR-mediated CICR, which operates as an amplification mechanism of postsynaptic Ca^{2+} entry signals [32]. The resulting amplification and propagation of the initial Ca^{2+} entry signals are presumably a necessary event for the induction of synaptic plasticity and for activity-induced gene expression in hippocampal neurons [32–37]. Hippocampal neurons possess in their soma, axons, dendrites, and dendritic spines the structural and molecular machinery that underlies CICR [33, 38, 39]. In effect, the ER forms an intricate continuous network in neuronal cells that is present in the soma and extends towards the axons, dendrites, and dendritic spines

[40, 41]. Treatment of primary hippocampal neurons with the RyR agonist caffeine or with brain-derived neurotrophic factor (BDNF) promotes RyR-dependent dendritic spine remodeling, leading to increased density and length of dendritic spines [38, 42, 43]. In addition, RyR2 downregulation abolishes BDNF-induced spine remodeling in primary hippocampal neurons [31]. These findings indicate that the RyR2 isoform plays a key role in hippocampal structural plasticity.

Calcium release mediated by RyR channels is becoming an important subject in the study of learning and memory under normal and pathological conditions. Several studies employing different paradigms or conditioning tasks have described that RyR-mediated Ca^{2+} release plays a central role in the acquisition and/or consolidation of memory processes [24, 25]. Training rats in the Morris water maze, a classical spatial memory task, increases hippocampal RyR2 protein levels and mRNA expression 12 and 24 h after training [44], suggesting RyR2 involvement in spatial memory processes. Rats trained in the Morris water maze also display significant RyR2 and RyR3 upregulation at the fifth day of training, and these changes persist until the memory consolidation phase (ninth day) [43]. In addition, successful long-term performance of a hippocampus-dependent spatial task (object location) increases the hippocampal protein levels of RyR2, RyR3, and IP_3R type-1 (IP_3R1) Ca^{2+} channels [45]. Other studies have shown that in a learning model, in which chickens were trained in a passive avoidance discrimination task, RyR channel inhibition with dantrolene (administered immediately after training) causes loss of memory retention [30]. In contrast, the RyR agonist 4-chloro-m-cresol (4-CMC) administered immediately after training chickens in a passive discrimination avoidance task results in high memory retention that persists for up to 24 h after training, an indication of enhanced memory consolidation [46]. In mice, RyR channel inhibition hampers memory retention in animals conditioned in inhibitory avoidance or radial arm-maze tasks [29, 47], while studies involving administration to mice of antisense oligodeoxynucleotides directed at each RyR isoform indicate that selective knockdown of RyR2 and RyR3, but not of RyR1, impairs memory retention in a passive avoidance test [29]. Highlighting the key role of the RyR2 isoform in memory processes, a recent study performed in rats showed that RyR2 downregulation by intrahippocampal injection of RyR2-directed antisense oligodeoxynucleotides causes conspicuous defects in a previously memorized spatial memory task [31]. To our knowledge, however, information is lacking regarding whether fear memory formation, consolidation, or extinction entail RyR channel function or expression.

In this work, we measured RyR2 protein content in the hippocampus isolated from rats exposed to context-dependent fear conditioning or to subsequent retrieval sessions aimed at destabilizing fear memory by triggering extinction memory. We found that both consolidation and destabilization of contextual fear conditioning resulted in significant increases of RyR2 protein content in the rat hippocampus.

2. Methods

2.1. Experimental Animals. Sprague-Dawley rats (males, 2.5-month average age) weighing 230–250 grams were used in this study. Animals housed in suitable cages (3 animals per cage) were maintained with a light/dark cycle of 12 h, at an average temperature of 22°C with food and water ad libitum. The animals were handled (habituation to the environment) 2 days before the initiation of conditioning protocols. All experimental protocols used in this work complied with the "Guiding Principles for Research Involving Animals and Human Beings" of the American Physiological Society and were approved by the Bioethics Committee on Animal Research, Faculty of Medicine, Universidad de Chile.

2.2. Context-Dependent Fear Conditioning. The animals were trained and tested in a conditioning chamber (Startle and Fear Conditioning System, PANLAB, Barcelona, Spain), equipped with stainless steel bars in the floor through which the animals received electrical stimulation. The "Freezing Software" program (PANLAB) was used to analyze the behavioral response known as freezing, defined as the complete absence of movement except breathing. The study engaged four different experimental groups: (1) control rats (C), which were exposed to the context but did not receive electrical stimulation; (2) rats exposed to the context unpaired with electrical stimulation (US); (3) trained rats (T5 and T29), which were exposed to the context paired with electrical stimulation, and (4) reexposed rats, which after exposure to the context paired with electrical stimulation, were reexposed 24 h later to the context without the aversive stimulus for 3 min (R3), 15 min (R15), or 30 min (R30).

Each group of rats underwent separately some of the following sessions (see Supplementary Figure 1 for a complete description of the experimental protocols employed). *Habituation session*: one day before exposure to the fear conditioning protocol, all animals were habituated to the conditioning chamber for a period of 3 min; the freezing behavior displayed in this habituation session was used to set up the equipment. After this initial exposure session without aversive electrical stimulus, all rats were returned to their respective cages. *Training sessions*: the animals were exposed 24 h after the habituation session to the conditioning chamber for 5 min. In this period, the animals of the control (C) group did not receive an aversive stimulus. The animals of the T5, T29, and the three R groups received two sets of paired electrical stimuli: the first stimulus (0.7 mA, for 2 s) was applied two min and the second stimulus (0.7 mA, for 2 s) four min after the rats entered the training chamber. The session concluded with a recovery time of 58 seconds; after this lapse, the animals were returned to their respective cages. The rats of the US group received only one unpaired electrical stimulus (0.7 mA, for 4 s) as soon as they entered the conditioning chamber and were removed immediately to their cages. *Reexposure sessions*: the animals were reexposed 24 h after the training session for 3 min (R3), 15 min (R15), or 30 min (R30) to the conditioning context, without the aversive stimulus. *Test sessions*: all test sessions

comprised exposure to the conditioning chamber without electric stimulus, as detailed below. In the test period, motor activity was measured continuously using the "Freezing Software" program. The freezing behavior of rats of the T5 and US groups was tested 5 h after training, while the rats of the T29 group were tested 29 h after training; in all cases, this last test session comprised 5 min of exposure to the context without the aversive stimulus. All the rats of the reexposed groups were tested 24 h after training, as detailed next. The freezing behavior of rats from the R3 group was measured during the 3 min period of reexposure and 5 h later. The freezing behavior of rats of the R15 and R30 groups was measured during the first 5 min of reexposure, during the entire duration of the respective reexposure session, and 5 h later in a test session that comprised 5 min of exposure to the context without the aversive stimulus. In all cases, the rats underwent euthanasia right after the last test session, and the hippocampus was removed for RyR2 protein determination.

2.3. Western Blot Analysis for RyR2 Protein Detection. The isolated hippocampus was homogenized with a glass/Teflon homogenizer in 200 μl of lysis solution (20 mM BAPTA; 10 mM MOPS-Tris, pH 7.5; leupeptin 100 μg/ml; and pepstatin 50 μg/ml). The resulting suspension was incubated on ice for 10 min, sonicated 3 times (20 s each time) and centrifuged at 3000 ×g for 25 min at 4°C. The supernatant was mixed with 1% NP40, shaken until dissolved (total extract), and aliquots were stored at −80°C. Protein concentration was measured with the sulfosalicylic acid Protein Assay Kit (Thermo Scientific, Rockford, IL, USA). For Western blot analysis, the above total extracts were denatured with 4x reducing buffer (34.8% glycerol, 1 M Tris base, 2 mM EDTA, 0.1 M dithiothreitol (DTT), 8% SDS, and 0.4% bromophenol blue). Electrophoresis was performed in 3.5–8% discontinuous gradient polyacrylamide gels, containing a 15% stacking layer to favor the separation of the different RyR isoforms without losing the β-actin band. Gels were immersed in Tris-Tricine buffer (6 mM Tricine, 1 mM EDTA, and 12.5 mM Bis-Tris propane, pH 8.0) and run for 4 h at 80 V. Next, protein bands were transferred (350 mA, 2.5 h) to PVDF membranes (Millipore Corp., Bedford, MA, USA) using the Transfer-Blot R Turbo System (Bio-Rad, Hercules, CA, USA) and Tris-Tricine transfer buffer with 10% methanol. PVDF membranes were incubated overnight at 4°C with blocking buffer containing 5% milk and were then incubated under constant stirring at room temperature for 2 h in 5% milk with specific antibodies against RyR2 (Anti-RyR2, Thermo, Waltham, CA, USA; 1 : 1000) or against β-actin used as loading control (Anti-β-actin, Sigma, San Luis, MI, USA; 1 : 12000). Membranes were washed next with 2% Tween in Tris-buffered saline (TBS, 3 washes, 10 min each) and were then incubated with conjugated secondary anti-mouse antibodies (Cell Signaling, Danvers, MA). The membranes were visualized with a chemiluminescence system (Amersham Biosciences, Piscataway, NJ, USA). Films were scanned and analyzed with the ImageJ software.

2.4. Immunofluorescence. Adult rats were perfused transcardially with 4% paraformaldehyde (Sigma, St. Louis, MI).

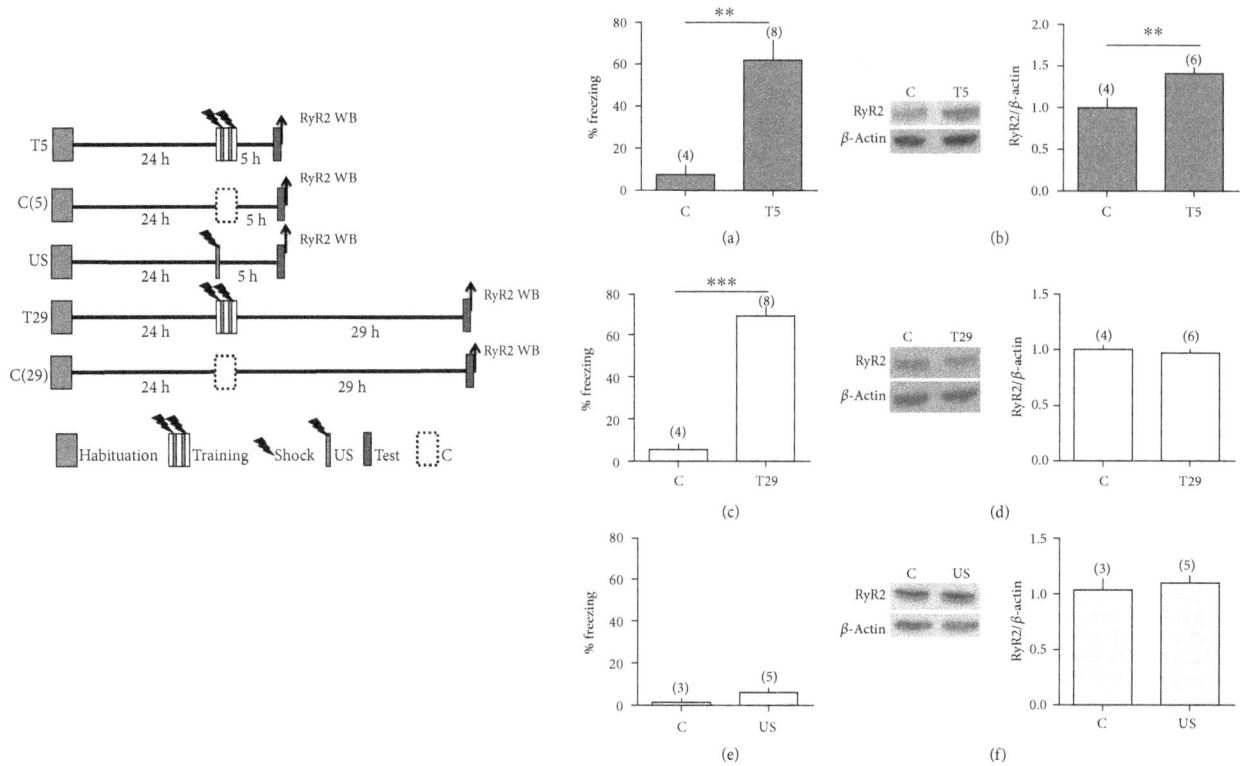

FIGURE 1: Context conditioned fear memory consolidation causes transient increases in RyR2 protein content. (a, c) Memory retention (% freezing) was measured 5 h (T5) or (c) 29 h (T29) after training or after context exposure without the aversive stimulus as control. (b, d) RyR2 protein content was analyzed 5 and 29 h after training, respectively. Representative blots and bar graphs illustrate RyR2 hippocampal content in each group of rats. (e, f) Memory retention and RyR2 hippocampal protein contents were measured (c) 5 h after exposure to the context or after unpaired stimulation (US). Values represent mean ± SE; the number of independent determinations is indicated in each graph. Statistical analysis was performed with unpaired Student's t-test; $^{**}p < 0.01$, $^{***}p < 0.001$.

The rats of the T5 fear-trained group, plus their respective untrained controls, were perfused 5 h after the 5 min training session. The rats of the reexposed R15 group were perfused 5 h after the 15 min reexposure session, while rats belonging to the T29 group were perfused right after the 5 min test session performed 29 h after the training session. As controls, naïve rats of the same age and weight were perfused as above. After perfusion, the brains were removed and placed in 4% paraformaldehyde for 2 h. The brains were incubated next for 72 h in a solution containing 30% sucrose, 0.001% sodium azide. Slices (30 μm) were cut with a microtome at −30°C. Free-floating sections were bathed in phosphate-based saline (PBS) buffer (mM: 137 NaCl, 2.7 KCl, 10 Na_2HPO_4, and 1.2 K_2HPO_4), containing 0.25% Triton X-100 (PBS-TX) plus 3% donkey serum, for 2 h at room temperature, and were incubated overnight at 4°C with PBS-TX containing RyR2 antibody (1 : 50, Thermo, Waltham, CA, USA). Sections were washed for 5 min in PBS and were incubated next for 2 h with Alexa Fluor 488 anti-mouse antibodies (1 : 300, Thermo, Waltham, CA, USA). Brain tissue slices, washed in PBS, were mounted on glass slides and covered with mounting medium. DAPI (Sigma, St. Louis, MI, USA) was employed for nuclear staining. Slices from −3.3 mm of the bregma [48] were chosen to analyze the expression of RyR2 in the CA1, CA3, and dentate gyrus (DG) hippocampal regions;

the dorsal third and lateral ventricles were taken as place references in the slices. A z-image stack of 1.5 μm sections was captured from the CA1, CA3, and DG regions using a confocal microscope (Nikon C2+). Fluorescence intensity was measured using the NIS-Elements software viewer 4.0 and ImageJ free viewer software.

2.5. Statistical Analysis. Results are expressed as mean ± SE. Statistical significance was evaluated with the GraphPad Prism 5 software. To test for statistical significance, unpaired or paired Student's t-test and one-way ANOVA followed by Tukey's multiple comparison post hoc test or repeated measures ANOVA were used, as detailed in the figure legends.

3. Results

3.1. Contextual Fear Conditioning Caused a Transient Increment of RyR2 Protein Content. Male rats exposed to the contextual fear conditioning protocol were tested 5 h or 29 h after the training session. In this test session, animals spent 5 min in the conditioning chamber in the absence of the aversive stimulus. Immediately after this test session, the rats underwent euthanasia and the hippocampus was isolated for Western blot (WB) analysis (Figure 1, left panel). The animals tested 5 h after training (T5) showed a significant (~7-fold) increase in freezing behavior compared to controls (Figure 1(a)), a clear-cut indication of fear memory retention.

The increased freezing behavior persisted in the group of animals tested 29 h after the training section (T29) (Figure 1(c)), indicating fear memory consolidation. Densitometry analysis of blots from hippocampal samples isolated 5 h after the training session (T5) revealed a significant increase (~1.5-fold) in RyR2 protein content compared to controls (Figure 1(b)), indicating that the RyR2 protein increase was due to contextual fear training and not to exposure to the context. This RyR2 increment was transient; 29 h after the training session, the hippocampal RyR2 protein levels in animals of the T29 group did not differ significantly from the levels displayed by the controls (Figure 1(d)). Additional analysis by immunohistochemistry of hippocampal sections isolated 5 h after the training session of the T5 group rats (see training scheme in Figure 1) showed that contextual fear (CF) training incremented RyR2 protein immunostaining (green) in the CA1 and CA3 hippocampal regions relative to their respective controls, as illustrated in Figure 2.

To assess if the RyR2 protein increase was due to an association between the electric shock and the context or occurred by an unspecific effect of the shock itself, we tested a separate group of animals, the US group. To this aim, rats from the US group received an electric shock (0.7 mA for 4 s) as soon as they entered the chamber and were removed immediately to their cages (Figure 1, left panel). As illustrated in Figure 1(e), this protocol did not generate associative learning in response to the context, as evidenced by the low freezing behavior exhibited by the US animals tested after 5 h, and did not result in increased RyR2 protein levels (Figure 1(f)). We interpret these combined findings as an indication that the RyR2 increase displayed by fear-trained animals 5 h after the training session stemmed from the associative learning induced by exposure to the contextual fear protocol.

3.2. Conditioned Fear Extinction Increases Hippocampal RyR2 Protein Levels.

To study whether an increase in hippocampal RyR2 protein content also occurred after exposure to retrieval sessions that promote memory destabilization, 24 h after the training session, the rats were reexposed for 3 min (R3), 15 min (R15), or 30 min (R30) to the conditioning context without the aversive stimulus. Control animals were reexposed for these same times (Figure 3, left panel). The freezing behavior of animals belonging to the R3 group was evaluated during the 3 min reexposure session; freezing in animals of the R15 and R30 groups was measured during the initial 5 min period and during the entire duration of the respective reexposure sessions. An additional 5 min test session was performed 5 h later for all animals. Immediately after this last test session, rats underwent euthanasia and the hippocampus was removed for RyR2 protein determination (Figure 3, left panel). Control animals presented under all situations low freezing behaviors during the respective reexposure sessions and the test sessions performed 5 h later (Figures 3(a), 3(c), and 3(e)). The animals reexposed for 3 min to the context without the aversive stimulus

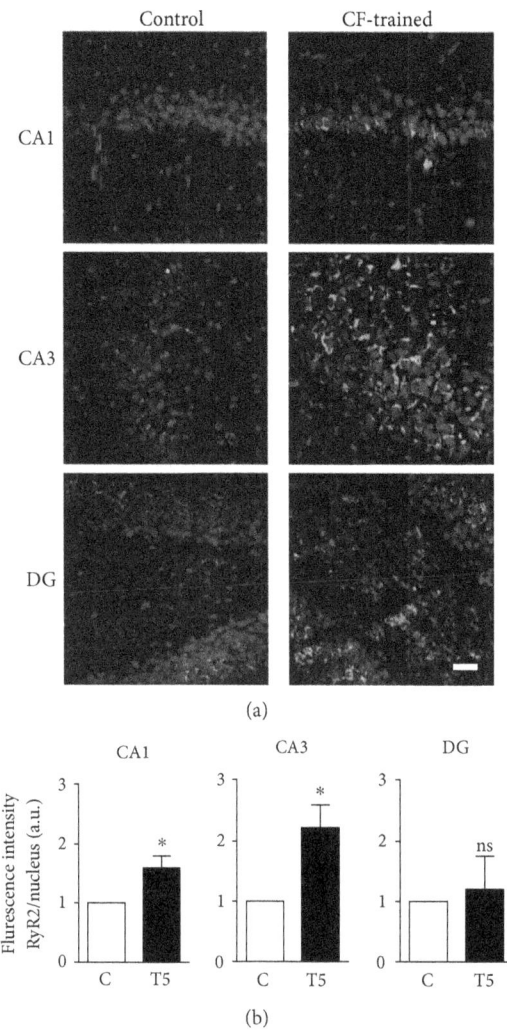

(a)

(b)

FIGURE 2: Contextual fear training promotes RyR2 upregulation in situ. (a) Representative confocal images of RyR2 immunofluorescence (green) and nuclear stain (blue) obtained from the CA1, CA3, and DG hippocampal regions. Samples were obtained 5 h after training animals (T5) in the contextual fear protocol or from controls similarly exposed to the context in the absence of the electric shock. Scale bar: 20 μm. (b) Normalized RyR2 immunofluorescence values. To calculate these values, RyR2 immunofluorescence in the entire image was divided in each case by the corresponding nuclear stain, and the control ratios were set as 1. Values represent mean ± SE; $N = 3$ for the T5 and the control groups. Statistical analysis was performed with paired one-tailed Student's t-test. $^*p < 0.05$; ns: not significant.

(R3) displayed in this period significant fear-associated memory retention, with prominent freezing behavior ($63.6 \pm 7.6\%$). Yet, when tested 5 h later, these animals displayed significantly lower freezing ($47.2 \pm 9.5\%$), as illustrated in Supplementary Figure 2B, and presented a significant increase (1.85 ± 0.23; $N = 6$) in RyR2 protein content (Figure 3(b)). In contrast, RyR2 protein content did not increase in the controls reexposed (24 h after the first exposure session) to the context for 3 min without a shock and tested 5 h later (Figure 3(b)).

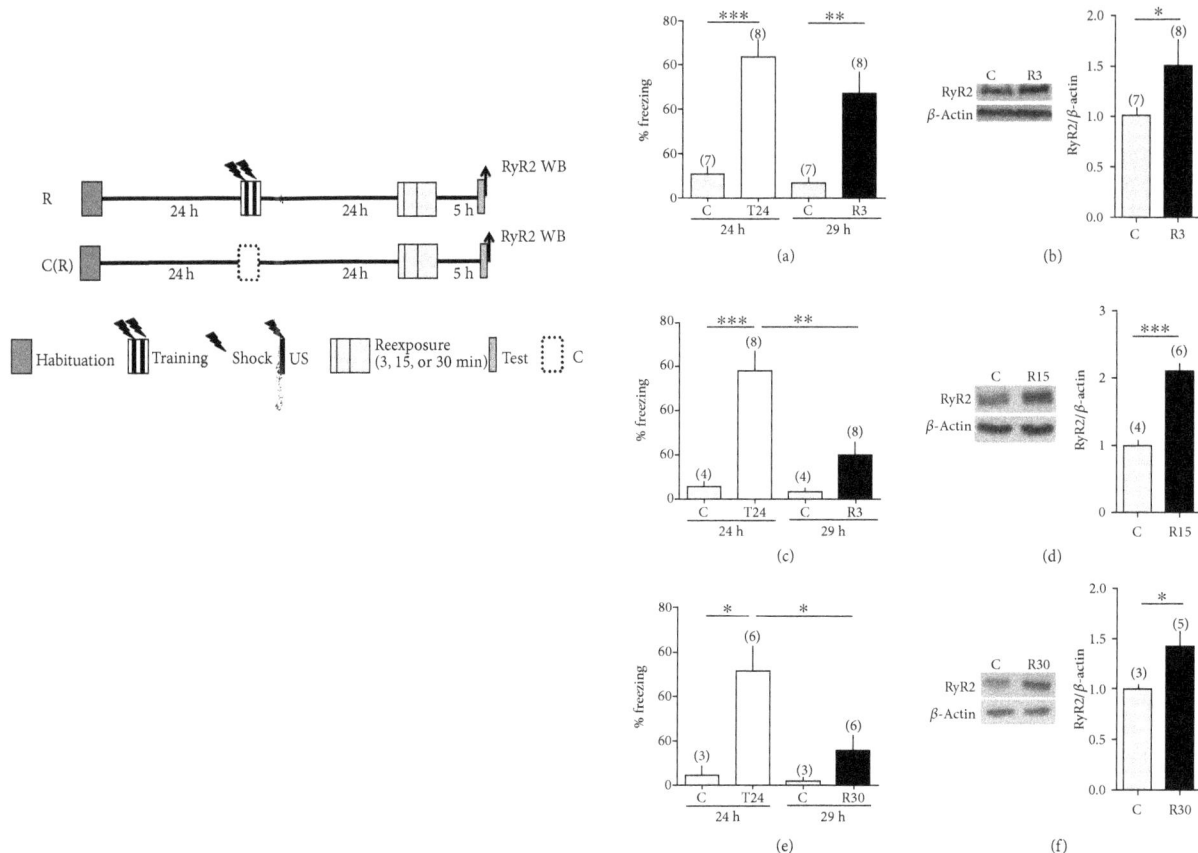

FIGURE 3: Context reexposure for 3, 15, or 30 min induces memory extinction and enhances RyR2 expression. (a, c, and e) Memory retention was evaluated 24 h after training (T24) or 5 h after reexposure to the context for 3 min (R3), 15 min (R15), or 30 min (R30). Control rats did not receive electrical stimulation during the training session and were evaluated 5 h after reexposure to the context for 3 min, 15 min, or 30 min. (b, d, and f) RyR2 expression was analyzed 5 h after performing the respective reexposure sessions (see scheme at left). Representative blots and quantification (bar graphs) showing hippocampal RyR2 protein content in each group of rats. Values represent mean ± SE. The number of independent determinations is indicated in each graph. Statistical analysis in (a, c, and e) was done with one-way ANOVA followed by Tukey's multiple comparison post hoc test; statistical analysis in (b, d, and f) was performed with Student's t-test. $^*p < 0.05$, $^{**}p < 0.01$, $^{***}p < 0.001$.

As an additional control, the RyR2 protein content was determined after the 3 min reexposure session (T24–3, Supplementary Figure 2A); no changes in RyR2 protein levels relative to the control were observed in these conditions. Accordingly, we conclude that the RyR2 protein content increase induced by the 3 min reexposure session did not happen immediately after the session but took place a few hours postreexposure. We propose (see "Discussion") that early extinction-dependent mechanisms mediate the RyR2 upregulation induced by this short reexposure session.

Animals reexposed to the context for 15 min (R15) exhibited a significant decrease in freezing behavior during the reexposure session, from $57.0 \pm 9.0\%$ during the first 5 min of reexposure to $35.0 \pm 6.7\%$ determined during the entire 15 min session (Supplementary Figure 2C). When tested 5 h later (Figure 3(c)), these same animals showed an even larger decrease in freezing ($19.9 \pm 6.3\%$), which was accompanied by a sizeable RyR2 protein increase (Figure 3(d)).

Likewise, the animals reexposed for 30 min (R30) displayed a significant decrease in freezing behavior during the

reexposure session, from $51.1 \pm 11.0\%$ freezing when measured during the first 5 min of reexposure to $21.0 \pm 4.0\%$ freezing when measured during the entire length of the reexposure session (Supplementary Figure 2D). When tested 5 h later, these rats displayed freezing behavior with values of $16.0 \pm 6.4\%$ (Figure 3(e)) and exhibited a significant increase in RyR2 protein content (Figure 3(f)).

Based on these combined results, we conclude that prolonging the retrieval session to 15 or 30 min without the aversive stimulus results in improved extinction of the previously acquired memory in comparison with reexposure for only 3 min (Supplementary Figures 2E and 2F). The extinction process was even more evident in animals tested 5 h after the reexposure sessions and was accompanied by significant RyR2 protein increases. The RyR2 increase peaked 15 min after reexposure to the context and did not increase further after the 30 min reexposure session (Figures 3(d) and 3(f)). In contrast, control rats reexposed to the context for 15 or 30 min without previous fear memory training did not present RyR2 upregulation (Figures 3(d) and 3(f)); we interpret

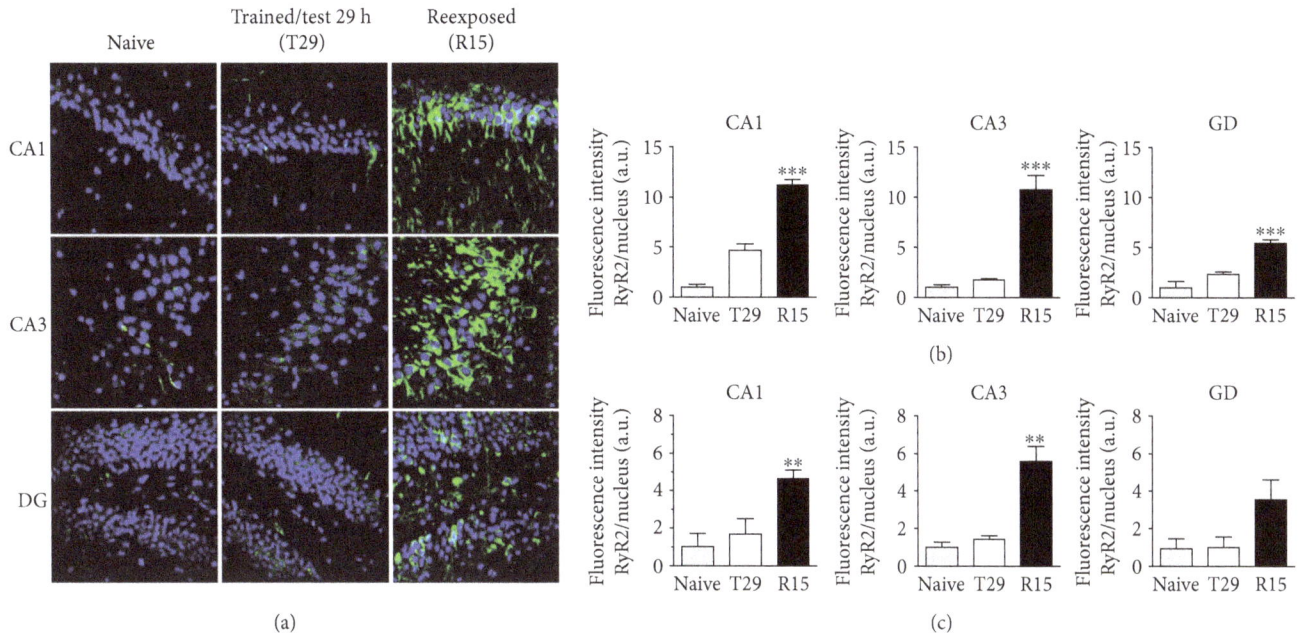

FIGURE 4: Memory extinction promotes RyR2 upregulation in situ. (a) Representative confocal images of RyR2 immunofluorescence (green) and Hoechst nucleus stain (blue) obtained from CA1, CA3, and DG region of the hippocampus. Samples were obtained 29 h after training (T29) or 5 h after the 15 min reexposure session (R15). Samples from naïve rats were used as control. Scale bar: 20 μm. (b) Bar graphs showing the quantification of RyR2 immunofluorescence pixels normalized by nuclear stain present in regions enriched in nuclei in CA1, CA3, and DG. (c) Bar graphs showing the quantification of RyR2 immunofluorescence pixels, normalized by the nuclear stain present in the entire images of CA1, CA3, and DG. Values represent mean ± SE; $N = 3$ for samples from the control and T29 groups; $N = 4$ for the R15 group. Statistical analysis was done with one-way ANOVA (CA1 $p = 0.0001$, CA3 $p = 0.0008$, and DG $p = 0.0009$) followed by Tukey's multiple comparison post hoc test; $^{**}p < 0.01$; $^{***}p < 0.001$ with respect to naïve and T29, respectively.

these findings as an indication that fear memory extinction caused this increase.

3.3. Conditioned Fear Extinction Increases RyR2 Immunofluorescence in the Hippocampal CA1, CA3, and DG Regions.

We used immunofluorescence assays of fixed brain samples to detect RyR2 protein levels in the different hippocampal regions. Samples from rats (R15) reexposed to the context for 15 min (24 h after training) and tested 5 h later were collected for RyR2 fluorescence immunodetection assays. Their immunofluorescence patterns were compared with those displayed by naïve rats or by rats (T29) trained in the contextual fear conditioning protocol, which exhibited robust memory in the test session performed 29 h later (Figure 1(c)) but presented no changes in hippocampal RyR2 protein content in immunoblots (Figure 1(d)).

The rats belonging to the R15 and T29 groups were perfused immediately after the last test sessions; in all cases, the aversive stimulus was applied only in the training sessions. Figure 4(a) illustrates RyR2 immunofluorescence staining (green) and nuclear staining (blue) in the hippocampal CA1, CA3, and DG regions. Although the naïve and T29 groups displayed some weak Ry2 protein staining, hippocampal RyR2 immunofluorescence was higher in sections from the R15 group.

The graph presented in Figure 4(b) illustrates the quantification of the immunofluorescence images acquired from regions enriched in nuclei; the graph presented in Figure 4(c) illustrates the quantification of the immunofluorescence

acquired from the complete images. All values represent the ratio between RyR2 immunofluorescence and nuclear stain. We conclude from these results that the 15 min reexposure session induced significant increments in RyR2 immunofluorescence in the CA1 and CA3 regions, which was particularly evident in regions enriched in nuclei (Figure 4(b)). The RyR2 immunofluorescence increase displayed by the DG region was less prominent when evaluated in nuclei-enriched regions (Figure 4(b)), but this increase did not reach statistical significance when evaluated in the entire image (Figure 4(c)).

Although a direct comparison between RyR2 immunoblot determinations (performed in whole hippocampus homogenates) and immunofluorescence images is not accurate, quantification of the whole immunofluorescence images (Figure 4(c)) yielded values closer to those presented in the immunoblots illustrated in Figure 3(d). In contrast, samples from rats tested 29 h after training, which did not undergo reexposure to the context (Supplementary Figure 1), displayed similar RyR2 immunofluorescence images as those exhibited by naïve rats (Figure 4(a); for details, see Supplementary Figure 3). Quantification of T29 RyR2 immunofluorescence images yielded values not significantly different from those displayed by the corresponding regions from naïve rats (Figures 4(b) and 4(c)). These results are in agreement with the immunoblot results (Figure 1(d)), which illustrate the lack of RyR2 protein increase displayed by the whole rat hippocampus isolated 29 h after contextual fear training.

4. Discussion

Based on the results shown in this work, we suggest that our model of context-conditioned fear memory, a task dependent on the hippocampus [9, 49], effectively promoted learning and memory acquisition, which became consolidated as indicated by the high percentage of freezing in animals evaluated 5, 24, or 29 h after training. Our novel results also show that a transient increase in RyR2 protein levels occurred during consolidation of fear-conditioned memory, since hippocampal RyR2 protein upregulation occurred 5 h posttraining but not 29 h after training. We suggest, accordingly, that the formation of long-term memory, or the early stages of the consolidation phase of fear-conditioned memory, requires transitory RyR2 upregulation in the whole hippocampus in order to generate the Ca^{2+} signals required for fear memory consolidation. Previous reports—showing increased RyR2 upregulation in animals exposed to different hippocampal-dependent memory protocols [31, 43–45]—support our proposal. These combined results place calcium release mediated by RyR2 channels and presumably RyR2 upregulation as well as important events in hippocampal-dependent memory processes.

Using different strategies and memory tasks, several authors have reported that protein synthesis is temporally required to elaborate long-term memory. Specifically, 1 h is the critical period for protein synthesis after contextual fear conditioning training [50]. Additionally, hippocampal inhibition of protein synthesis with anisomycin impairs memory formation when given either 15 min before training or 3 h posttraining in a one trial of inhibitory avoidance training task [51]. Furthermore, the expression of the immediate early genes (IEG) Zif268, c-Fos, and Arc peaks 90 min after the last training trial in the Morris water maze training [52] or in fear memory training [53]. In similarity to the current results, we described previously that the hippocampal RyR2 protein content increased 5 h after training rats in the Morris water maze [43]. Yet, the possibility of an even earlier RyR2 peak remains a subject of future studies, as does the analysis of a possible causal relationship between IEG and RyR2 expression in fear memory formation. A recent report described an important role of protein degradation in memory formation [54], but whether a decrease in RyR2 degradation underlies the transient RyR2 upregulation induced by fear memory training remains to be explored in future studies.

Moreover, when studying the process of conditioned fear extinction, we found that reexposure to the context for 3, 15, or 30 minutes without reinforcement of the electrical stimulus generated a decrease in the conditioned fear response and most likely promoted learning-associated fear memory extinction, as described in previous studies [14–16]. As all learning processes, extinction has three different phases: acquisition, consolidation, and retrieval [55]. In our experimental design, trained animals displayed decreased freezing with increasing times of reexposure to the context; freezing decreased more after reexposure for 15 or 30 min than after 3 min of reexposure, indicating increased formation of extinction memory with time. This freezing decrease was more evident at the test session performed 5 h after

reexposure, an indication of more effective extinction of fear-conditioned memory.

Both extinction of the learned response and original learning require acquisition of new information and protein synthesis, which promotes the consolidation of the new information [56]. The present results show that the 3, 15, and 30 min reexposure sessions resulted in marked extinction of fear memory and increased RyR2 protein levels in the whole hippocampus, determined by immunoblot assays. Moreover, reexposure for 15 min produced significant increments of RyR2 immunofluorescence in the CA1, CA3, and DG hippocampal regions, and these changes were especially evident in the regions enriched in nuclei. We suggest, therefore, that the hippocampal RyR2 protein increase forms part of the process of extinction memory generation related to contextual fear. In view of the current results showing the effects of the reexposure session on extinction memory generation, we evaluated the consequences of suppressing this session on RyR2 protein levels in different hippocampal regions. We found that the absence of the reexposure sessions generated high freezing behavior in the test session performed 29 h after training, indicating lack of extinction and significant retention of the original fear-associated memory. Nevertheless, the RyR2 upregulation induced by fear memory extinction did not occur in this case, a clear indication that the extinction process mediates the observed RyR2 protein increase.

Altogether, based on the present results, we suggest that RyR2 upregulation forms part of the processes underlying both fear-associated memory consolidation, which requires a transient increase in RyR2 protein content, and fear memory extinction, which implies the generation of new learning. Different spatial memory protocols induce RyR2 channel upregulation [43–45]. We now add to this list the formation as well as the destabilization of contextual fear memory. The molecular mechanisms underlying RyR2 upregulation in memory formation and extinction remain unreported. We propose that RyR2 upregulation would contribute, via RyR2-mediated CICR, to amplify the Ca^{2+} signals generated by NMDAR or L-type VGCC that are required for hippocampal-dependent fear extinction [57, 58]. The ensuing calcium-dependent signal transduction cascades may engage Scr kinase and CaMKII, both of which have been involved in fear extinction memory [57, 59]. Moreover, contextual fear memory extinction requires activity-dependent expression of BDNF [60], a neurotrophin that induces RyR2 upregulation, as does spatial memory consolidation [43]. Accordingly, RyR2 upregulation may form part of a common mechanism involved in BDNF-mediated memory formation and extinction. According to this view, RyR2 upregulation would ensure the proper amplification and propagation of the initial activity-generated Ca^{2+} signals elicited in postsynaptic neurons by ligand-dependent receptors or L-type VGCC that have been implicated in the learning process [55, 61–63].

A previous study reported that RyR type-3 (RyR3) knockout mice exhibited impairments of performance in contextual fear conditioning, passive avoidance, and Y-maze learning tests [64]. Furthermore, in mice, selective knockdown of RyR2 and RyR3, but not of RyR1, impairs memory retention in a passive avoidance test [29], while training rats in the Morris water maze causes significant RyR2 and RyR3 upregulation at the fifth day of training, and these changes persist until the memory consolidation phase (ninth day) [43]. Here, we present additional findings in wild-type rats showing that contextual fear memory acquisition or extinction upregulates the RyR2 isoform, which when downregulated causes striking spatial memory defects [31]. These combined results highlight the importance of the RyR2/RyR3 isoforms in hippocampal-dependent memory process.

To conclude, it is important to mention that extinction memory is a particularly interesting type of memory, which represents one of the most studied memory forms due to its relevance within the context of some psychiatric disorders such as panic disorders, anxiety, phobias, and posttraumatic stress disorder [65]. Additionally, the extinction memory process is also important for the attenuation of cue-induced drug craving and relapse behavior [66]. Hence, the participation of RyR2 channels as possible key pharmacological targets to these disorders is a relevant subject of future studies.

Conflicts of Interest

No competing financial interests exist.

Acknowledgments

The authors acknowledge the excellent technical support provided by Luis Montecinos and Alexander Riquelme, and the authors thank Dr. Erwin de la Fuente for his help in composing the figures. This work was supported by FONDECYT (Grant nos. 1140855, 1140545, and 1170053) and by BNI (P-09-015F).

Supplementary Materials

Complementary information regarding the additional results and protocols used to induce contextual fear memory acquisition and extinction. Supplementary Figure 1: the scheme illustrating the groups of rats exposed to each protocol and the times used to collect the hippocampus for RyR2 determinations. Supplementary Figure 2: results illustrating changes in freezing and RyR2 protein content under additional experimental conditions. Supplementary Figure 3: confocal images of RyR2 immunofluorescence and nuclear DAPI staining, collected in each hippocampal region isolated from different animals. (Supplementary Materials)

References

[1] M. S. Fanselow and A. M. Poulos, "The neuroscience of mammalian associative learning," *Annual Review of Psychology*, vol. 56, no. 1, pp. 207–234, 2005.

[2] B. F. Grewe, J. Grundemann, L. J. Kitch et al., "Neural ensemble dynamics underlying a long-term associative memory," *Nature*, vol. 543, no. 7647, pp. 670–675, 2017.

[3] R. G. Phillips and J. E. LeDoux, "Differential contribution of amygdala and hippocampus to cued and contextual fear conditioning," *Behavioral Neuroscience*, vol. 106, no. 2, pp. 274–285, 1992.

[4] N. R. W. Selden, B. J. Everitt, L. E. Jarrard, and T. W. Robbins, "Complementary roles for the amygdala and hippocampus in aversive conditioning to explicit and contextual cues," *Neuroscience*, vol. 42, no. 2, pp. 335–350, 1991.

[5] J. Kim and M. Fanselow, "Modality-specific retrograde amnesia of fear," *Science*, vol. 256, no. 5057, pp. 675–677, 1992.

[6] S. Ramirez, X. Liu, P. A. Lin et al., "Creating a false memory in the hippocampus," *Science*, vol. 341, no. 6144, pp. 387–391, 2013.

[7] C. Xu, S. Krabbe, J. Grundemann et al., "Distinct hippocampal pathways mediate dissociable roles of context in memory retrieval," *Cell*, vol. 167, no. 4, pp. 961–972.e16, 2016.

[8] T. Takeuchi, A. J. Duszkiewicz, and R. G. Morris, "The synaptic plasticity and memory hypothesis: encoding, storage and persistence," *Philosophical Transactions of the Royal Society of London. Series B, Biological Sciences*, vol. 369, no. 1633, article 20130288, 2014.

[9] S. Maren, "Neurobiology of Pavlovian fear conditioning," *Annual Review of Neuroscience*, vol. 24, no. 1, pp. 897–931, 2001.

[10] J. J. Kim and M. W. Jung, "Neural circuits and mechanisms involved in Pavlovian fear conditioning: a critical review," *Neuroscience and Biobehavioral Reviews*, vol. 30, no. 2, pp. 188–202, 2006.

[11] G. Valdivia, F. Simonetti, P. Cumsille et al., "Smoking habit in school age children, in Chile," *Revista Medica De Chile*, vol. 132, no. 2, pp. 171–182, 2004.

[12] M. Penkowa, A. Quintana, J. Carrasco, M. Giralt, A. Molinero, and J. Hidalgo, "Metallothionein prevents neurodegeneration and central nervous system cell death after treatment with gliotoxin 6-aminonicotinamide," *Journal of Neuroscience Research*, vol. 77, no. 1, pp. 35–53, 2004.

[13] K. A. Corcoran, T. J. Desmond, K. A. Frey, and S. Maren, "Hippocampal inactivation disrupts the acquisition and contextual encoding of fear extinction," *The Journal of Neuroscience: The Official Journal of the Society for Neuroscience*, vol. 25, no. 39, pp. 8978–8987, 2005.

[14] K. M. Myers and M. Davis, "Mechanisms of fear extinction," *Molecular Psychiatry*, vol. 12, no. 2, pp. 120–150, 2007.

[15] D. Eisenhardt and R. Menzel, "Extinction learning, reconsolidation and the internal reinforcement hypothesis," *Neurobiology of Learning and Memory*, vol. 87, no. 2, pp. 167–173, 2007.

[16] I. Izquierdo, M. Cammarota, M. R. M. Vianna, and L. R. M. Bevilaqua, "The inhibition of acquired fear," *Neurotoxicity Research*, vol. 6, no. 3, pp. 175–188, 2004.

[17] M. Cammarota, D. M. Barros, M. R. M. Vianna et al., "The transition from memory retrieval to extinction," *Anais da Academia Brasileira de Ciências*, vol. 76, no. 3, pp. 573–582, 2004.

[18] J. Ji and S. Maren, "Hippocampal involvement in contextual modulation of fear extinction," *Hippocampus*, vol. 17, no. 9, pp. 749–758, 2007.

[19] E. Knapska and S. Maren, "Reciprocal patterns of c-Fos expression in the medial prefrontal cortex and amygdala after

extinction and renewal of conditioned fear," *Learning & Memory*, vol. 16, no. 8, pp. 486–493, 2009.

[20] L. Xue, Z. D. Li, Z. X. Chen, X. G. Wang, Y. W. Shi, and H. Zhao, "Fear response failed to return in AAB extinction paradigm accompanied with increased NR2B and GluR1 per845 in hippocampal CA1," *Neuroscience*, vol. 260, pp. 1–11, 2014.

[21] A. M. Oliveira and H. Bading, "Calcium signaling in cognition and aging-dependent cognitive decline," *BioFactors*, vol. 37, no. 3, pp. 168–174, 2011.

[22] M. Davis, "Neural systems involved in fear and anxiety measured with fear-potentiated startle," *The American Psychologist*, vol. 61, no. 8, pp. 741–756, 2006.

[23] F. W. Johenning, A. K. Theis, U. Pannasch, M. Ruckl, S. Rudiger, and D. Schmitz, "Ryanodine receptor activation induces long-term plasticity of spine calcium dynamics," *PLoS Biology*, vol. 13, no. 6, article e1002181, 2015.

[24] K. D. Baker, T. M. Edwards, and N. S. Rickard, "The role of intracellular calcium stores in synaptic plasticity and memory consolidation," *Neuroscience and Biobehavioral Reviews*, vol. 37, no. 7, pp. 1211–1239, 2013.

[25] A. C. Paula-Lima, T. Adasme, and C. Hidalgo, "Contribution of Ca2+ release channels to hippocampal synaptic plasticity and spatial memory: potential redox modulation," *Antioxidants & Redox Signaling*, vol. 21, no. 6, pp. 892–914, 2014.

[26] G. Giannini and V. Sorrentino, "Molecular structure and tissue distribution of ryanodine receptors calcium channels," *Medicinal Research Reviews*, vol. 15, no. 4, pp. 313–323, 1995.

[27] G. Giannini, A. Conti, S. Mammarella, M. Scrobogna, and V. Sorrentino, "The ryanodine receptor/calcium channel genes are widely and differentially expressed in murine brain and peripheral tissues," *The Journal of Cell Biology*, vol. 128, no. 5, pp. 893–904, 1995.

[28] J. T. Lanner, D. K. Georgiou, A. D. Joshi, and S. L. Hamilton, "Ryanodine receptors: structure, expression, molecular details, and function in calcium release," *Cold Spring Harbor Perspectives in Biology*, vol. 2, no. 11, article a003996, 2010.

[29] N. Galeotti, A. Quattrone, E. Vivoli, M. Norcini, A. Bartolini, and C. Ghelardini, "Different involvement of type 1, 2, and 3 ryanodine receptors in memory processes," *Learning & Memory*, vol. 15, no. 5, pp. 315–323, 2008.

[30] T. M. Edwards and N. S. Rickard, "Pharmaco-behavioural evidence indicating a complex role for ryanodine receptor calcium release channels in memory processing for a passive avoidance task," *Neurobiology of Learning and Memory*, vol. 86, no. 1, pp. 1–8, 2006.

[31] J. Y. More, B. A. Bruna, P. E. Lobos et al., "Calcium release mediated by redox-sensitive RyR2 channels has a central role in hippocampal structural plasticity and spatial memory," *Antioxidants & Redox Signaling*, 2018.

[32] M. J. Berridge, "Neuronal calcium signaling," *Neuron*, vol. 21, no. 1, pp. 13–26, 1998.

[33] S. Bardo, M. G. Cavazzini, and N. Emptage, "The role of the endoplasmic reticulum Ca2+ store in the plasticity of central neurons," *Trends in Pharmacological Sciences*, vol. 27, no. 2, pp. 78–84, 2006.

[34] R. Bouchard, R. Pattarini, and J. D. Geiger, "Presence and functional significance of presynaptic ryanodine receptors," *Progress in Neurobiology*, vol. 69, no. 6, pp. 391–418, 2003.

[35] M. A. Carrasco, E. Jaimovich, U. Kemmerling, and C. Hidalgo, "Signal transduction and gene expression regulated by calcium release from internal stores in excitable cells," *Biological Research*, vol. 37, no. 4, pp. 701–712, 2004.

[36] M. Kubota, K. Narita, T. Murayama et al., "Type-3 ryanodine receptor involved in Ca2+-induced Ca2+ release and transmitter exocytosis at frog motor nerve terminals," *Cell Calcium*, vol. 38, no. 6, pp. 557–567, 2005.

[37] M. Shimuta, M. Yoshikawa, M. Fukaya, M. Watanabe, H. Takeshima, and T. Manabe, "Postsynaptic modulation of AMPA receptor-mediated synaptic responses and LTP by the type 3 ryanodine receptor," *Molecular and Cellular Neurosciences*, vol. 17, no. 5, pp. 921–930, 2001.

[38] E. Korkotian and M. Segal, "Fast confocal imaging of calcium released from stores in dendritic spines," *The European Journal of Neuroscience*, vol. 10, no. 6, pp. 2076–2084, 1998.

[39] H. Toresson and S. G. N. Grant, "Dynamic distribution of endoplasmic reticulum in hippocampal neuron dendritic spines," *European Journal of Neuroscience*, vol. 22, no. 7, pp. 1793–1798, 2005.

[40] O. A. Ramirez and A. Couve, "The endoplasmic reticulum and protein trafficking in dendrites and axons," *Trends in Cell Biology*, vol. 21, no. 4, pp. 219–227, 2011.

[41] A. Verkhratsky, "The endoplasmic reticulum and neuronal calcium signalling," *Cell Calcium*, vol. 32, no. 5-6, pp. 393–404, 2002.

[42] E. Korkotian and M. Segal, "Release of calcium from stores alters the morphology of dendritic spines in cultured hippocampal neurons," *Proceedings of the National Academy of Sciences of the United States of America*, vol. 96, no. 21, pp. 12068–12072, 1999.

[43] T. Adasme, P. Haeger, A. C. Paula-Lima et al., "Involvement of ryanodine receptors in neurotrophin-induced hippocampal synaptic plasticity and spatial memory formation," *Proceedings of the National Academy of Sciences of the United States of America*, vol. 108, no. 7, pp. 3029–3034, 2011.

[44] W. Zhao, N. Meiri, H. Xu et al., "Spatial learning induced changes in expression of the ryanodine type II receptor in the rat hippocampus," *The FASEB Journal*, vol. 14, no. 2, pp. 290–300, 2000.

[45] A. Arias-Cavieres, T. Adasme, G. Sanchez, P. Munoz, and C. Hidalgo, "Aging impairs hippocampal-dependent recognition memory and LTP and prevents the associated RyR up-regulation," *Frontiers in Aging Neuroscience*, vol. 9, p. 111, 2017.

[46] K. D. Baker, T. M. Edwards, and N. S. Rickard, "A ryanodine receptor agonist promotes the consolidation of long-term memory in young chicks," *Behavioural Brain Research*, vol. 206, no. 1, pp. 143–146, 2010.

[47] T. Ohnuki and Y. Nomura, "1-[[[5-(4-Nitrophenyl)-2-furanyl]methylene]imino]-2, 4-imidazolidinedione (dantrolene), an inhibitor of intracellular Ca2+ mobilization, impairs avoidance performance and spatial memory in mice," *Biological & Pharmaceutical Bulletin*, vol. 19, no. 8, pp. 1038–1040, 1996.

[48] G. Paxinos and C. Watson, *The Rat Brain in Stereotaxic Coordinates*, Academic Press, 1998.

[49] J. Radulovic and N. C. Tronson, "Molecular specificity of multiple hippocampal processes governing fear extinction," *Reviews in the Neurosciences*, vol. 21, no. 1, pp. 1–18, 2010.

[50] R. Bourtchouladze, T. Abel, N. Berman, R. Gordon, K. Lapidus, and E. R. Kandel, "Different training procedures recruit either one or two critical periods for contextual memory consolidation, each of which requires protein

synthesis and PKA," *Learning & Memory*, vol. 5, no. 4-5, pp. 365–374, 1998.

[51] P. Bekinschtein, M. Cammarota, L. M. Igaz, L. R. M. Bevilaqua, I. Izquierdo, and J. H. Medina, "Persistence of long-term memory storage requires a late protein synthesis- and BDNF-dependent phase in the hippocampus," *Neuron*, vol. 53, no. 2, pp. 261–277, 2007.

[52] D. N. Barry and S. Commins, "Temporal dynamics of immediate early gene expression during cellular consolidation of spatial memory," *Behavioural Brain Research*, vol. 327, pp. 44–53, 2017.

[53] M. E. Lonergan, G. M. Gafford, T. J. Jarome, and F. J. Helmstetter, "Time-dependent expression of Arc and zif268 after acquisition of fear conditioning," *Neural Plasticity*, vol. 2010, Article ID 139891, 12 pages, 2010.

[54] T. J. Jarome and F. J. Helmstetter, "Protein degradation and protein synthesis in long-term memory formation," *Frontiers in Molecular Neuroscience*, vol. 7, 2014.

[55] G. J. Quirk and D. Mueller, "Neural mechanisms of extinction learning and retrieval," *Neuropsychopharmacology*, vol. 33, no. 1, pp. 56–72, 2008.

[56] M. R. M. Vianna, G. Szapiro, J. L. McGaugh, J. H. Medina, and I. Izquierdo, "Retrieval of memory for fear-motivated training initiates extinction requiring protein synthesis in the rat hippocampus," *Proceedings of the National Academy of Sciences of the United States of America*, vol. 98, no. 21, pp. 12251–12254, 2001.

[57] J. de Carvalho Myskiw, C. R. G. Furini, F. Benetti, and I. Izquierdo, "Hippocampal molecular mechanisms involved in the enhancement of fear extinction caused by exposure to novelty," *Proceedings of the National Academy of Sciences of the United States of America*, vol. 111, no. 12, pp. 4572–4577, 2014.

[58] S. D. Schmidt, J. C. Myskiw, C. R. G. Furini, B. E. Schmidt, L. E. Cavalcante, and I. Izquierdo, "PACAP modulates the consolidation and extinction of the contextual fear conditioning through NMDA receptors," *Neurobiology of Learning and Memory*, vol. 118, pp. 120–124, 2015.

[59] B. Wang, R. C. Liang, Z. S. Liu et al., "Hippocampal Src kinase is required for novelty-induced enhancement of contextual fear extinction," *Biochemical and Biophysical Research Communications*, vol. 472, no. 4, pp. 656–661, 2016.

[60] K. Sakata, K. Martinowich, N. H. Woo et al., "Role of activity-dependent BDNF expression in hippocampal-prefrontal cortical regulation of behavioral perseverance," *Proceedings of the National Academy of Sciences of the United States of America*, vol. 110, no. 37, pp. 15103–15108, 2013.

[61] A. Suzuki, S. A. Josselyn, P. W. Frankland, S. Masushige, A. J. Silva, and S. Kida, "Memory reconsolidation and extinction have distinct temporal and biochemical signatures," *The Journal of Neuroscience*, vol. 24, no. 20, pp. 4787–4795, 2004.

[62] I. Izquierdo, L. R. M. Bevilaqua, J. I. Rossato, J. S. Bonini, J. H. Medina, and M. Cammarota, "Different molecular cascades in different sites of the brain control memory consolidation," *Trends in Neurosciences*, vol. 29, no. 9, pp. 496–505, 2006.

[63] J. L. C. Lee, A. L. Milton, and B. J. Everitt, "Reconsolidation and extinction of conditioned fear: inhibition and potentiation," *The Journal of Neuroscience*, vol. 26, no. 39, pp. 10051–10056, 2006.

[64] Y. Kouzu, T. Moriya, H. Takeshima, T. Yoshioka, and S. Shibata, "Mutant mice lacking ryanodine receptor type 3 exhibit deficits of contextual fear conditioning and activation of calcium/calmodulin-dependent protein kinase II in the hippocampus," *Brain Research. Molecular Brain Research*, vol. 76, no. 1, pp. 142–150, 2000.

[65] M. Wicking, F. Steiger, F. Nees et al., "Deficient fear extinction memory in posttraumatic stress disorder," *Neurobiology of Learning and Memory*, vol. 136, pp. 116–126, 2016.

[66] R. M. Cleva, J. T. Gass, J. J. Widholm, and M. F. Olive, "Glutamatergic targets for enhancing extinction learning in drug addiction," *Current Neuropharmacology*, vol. 8, no. 4, pp. 394–408, 2010.

14

Environmental Enrichment Induces Changes in Long-Term Memory for Social Transmission of Food Preference in Aged Mice through a Mechanism Associated with Epigenetic Processes

Simona Cintoli [1,2] Maria Cristina Cenni,[1] Bruno Pinto,[2,3] Silvia Morea,[2] Alessandro Sale,[1] Lamberto Maffei,[1,3] and Nicoletta Berardi [1,2]

[1]Neuroscience Institute, CNR, Via G. Moruzzi 1, 56124 Pisa, Italy
[2]Department of Neuroscience, Psychology, Drug Research and Child Health (NEUROFARBA), University of Florence, Florence, Italy
[3]Scuola Normale Superiore, Pisa, Italy

Correspondence should be addressed to Alessandro Sale; sale@in.cnr.it

Academic Editor: Claudio A. Mastronardi

Decline in declarative learning and memory performance is a typical feature of normal aging processes. Exposure of aged animals to an enriched environment (EE) counteracts this decline, an effect correlated with reduction of age-related changes in hippocampal dendritic branching, spine density, neurogenesis, gliogenesis, and neural plasticity, including its epigenetic underpinnings. Declarative memories depend on the medial temporal lobe system, including the hippocampus, for their formation, but, over days to weeks, they become increasingly dependent on other brain regions such as the neocortex and in particular the prefrontal cortex (PFC), a process known as system consolidation. Recently, it has been shown that early tagging of cortical networks is a crucial neurobiological process for remote memory formation and that this tagging involves epigenetic mechanisms in the recipient orbitofrontal (OFC) areas. Whether EE can enhance system consolidation in aged animals has not been tested; in particular, whether the early tagging mechanisms in OFC areas are deficient in aged animals and whether EE can ameliorate them is not known. This study aimed at testing whether EE could affect system consolidation in aged mice using the social transmission of food preference paradigm, which involves an ethologically based form of associative olfactory memory. We found that only EE mice successfully performed the remote memory recall task, showed neuronal activation in OFC, assessed with c-fos immunohistochemistry and early tagging of OFC, assessed with histone H3 acetylation, suggesting a defective system consolidation and early OFC tagging in aged mice which are ameliorated by EE.

1. Introduction

Aging of the brain is a complex biological process associated with decline in sensory, motor, and cognitive functions. In particular, a decline in declarative learning and memory performance is a typical feature of the normal aging process. Human and animal model data are in accordance to show that during aging, changes in neuronal morphology and density as well as changes in synaptic density, function, and plasticity are specific to each area of the brain [1–3]; brain areas crucial for declarative memory formation, such as hippocampus and other medial temporal lobe structures, show differential volume decline with age, associated with loss of synaptic density, changes in neuronal electrophysiological properties, deficits in synaptic plasticity [1, 3, 4], and changes in gene transcription [5, 6] and in epigenetic mechanisms, leading to reduction in plasticity factors necessary for the induction and local consolidation of synaptic efficacy changes [7, 8]. Aged rodents have contributed a crucial part of these data [1, 9, 10].

Environmental enrichment (EE) is an experimental protocol classically defined as "a combination of complex inanimate and social stimulation" [11] which provides animals with the opportunity to attain high levels of voluntary physical activity on running wheels and to enhance exploration, cognitive activity, and social interaction. EE causes brain changes at functional, anatomical, and molecular level, including changes in plasticity factors and mechanisms (see [9]), with clear benefits for learning and memory [12–15], particularly evident in aged animals [9, 12, 16]. Most of the studies have been conducted in aged rodents, but EE has been found to provide cognitive benefits also in other aged mammals (see [9]). Positive effects of EE on cognitive processes have been found in young, adult, and aged rodents both for hippocampal-dependent and hippocampal-independent learning and memory [9, 12–22]. For instance, EE improves spatial memory, (see [9, 23, 24]), object recognition memory [9, 24], social novelty [9, 24], and fear memory [25] in aged mice and in mouse models of neurodegeneration (see [26]). These beneficial effects in aged animals have been related to EE action on neurogenesis, neurotrophic factors (BDNF), IGF-I, synaptic plasticity, and neurotransmitter systems (see [9]). In particular, the improvement in declarative learning and memory performance in EE aged rodents has been correlated with EE attenuating the age-related changes in hippocampal dendritic branching, spine density, neurogenesis, gliogenesis, and neural plasticity, including its epigenetic underpinnings [9, 20–22, 26–31].

Declarative memories (memories for facts and events) are not acquired in their definitive form but undergo a gradual process of stabilization over time to allow long-term maintenance [32–34]. In animals, typical protocols to test declarative memory are those testing spatial memory, recognition memory, and in general associative memory. In the process of associative memory formation, consolidation, and maintenance, the hippocampus is believed to integrate, in the form of an anatomical index, information transmitted from distributed cortical networks that support the various features of a whole experience [34], rapidly merging these different features into a coherent memory trace. Consolidation of this new memory trace at the cortical level would then occur slowly via repeated and coordinated reactivation of hippocampal-cortical networks in order to progressively increase the strength and stability of corticocortical connections that represent the original experience. Therefore, these types of memories depend on the medial temporal lobe system, including the hippocampus, for their formation, but, over days to weeks, they become increasingly dependent on other brain regions such as the neocortex and in particular the prefrontal cortex (PFC) [20–23]. This process of time-dependent gradual reorganization of the brain regions supporting remote memory storage is known as systems-level memory consolidation or system consolidation [24–28]. Recently, it has been shown that early tagging of cortical networks is a necessary neurobiological process for remote associative olfactory memory formation using the social transmission of food preference (STFP) paradigm, an ethologically based form of associative olfactory memory [29–31], and that this tagging involves epigenetic mechanisms in the recipient orbitofrontal (OFC) areas [35, 36].

Whether EE can enhance system consolidation in aged animals has not been tested; in particular, whether the early tagging mechanisms in OFC areas demonstrated by Lesburgueres et al. [36] in young animals are deficient in aged animals and whether EE can ameliorate them is not known.

This study aimed at testing whether EE could affect system consolidation in STFP in aged mice. As already pointed out, aged mice are considered a good model of aging, with translation value [10]. For instance, deficits in the same types of memory appear in aged humans and mice, increases in oxidative stress parameters and neuroinflammation, which are typical alterations of the aged brain, are present in both aged humans and mice [9, 10], and, even if amyloid plaques are not found in aged mouse brain, recent work has shown that aged mice do show an increase in amyloid oligomers, which also characterize human aging [37]. Regarding the estimated correspondence between murine and human age, some comparative studies have estimated [38] that senescence begins in mice around eighteen months of age; the age of mice in the present paper (15-16 months) would then correspond, approximately, with the upper limit of human adulthood (65 years).

We have studied whether EE could affect system consolidation in STFP, a protocol particularly suitable to study recent and remote associative memory [39], in aged mice, using the same protocol used by Lesburgueres et al. [36] to demonstrate for the first time a role for histone acetylation in the early tagging of OFC in young animals. We found that only EE mice successfully performed the remote associative olfactory memory recall task and showed neuronal activation in OFC, assessed with c-fos immunohistochemistry. Early tagging of OFC, assessed with histone H3 acetylation [36], was found in EE but not in SC aged mice.

2. Materials and Methods

2.1. Animal Treatment. Male and female C57BL/6 mice of 14 months of age were used in this study. All the procedures were approved by the Italian Ministry of Health. Animals were housed in the animal house with a 12 h/12 h light/dark cycle and with food and water available ad libitum. At 14 months of age, animals were assigned to one of the following rearing conditions for 40 days: environmental enrichment (EE mice, $n = 32$) or standard condition (SC mice, $n = 40$). SC rearing condition consisted of $26 \times 18 \times 18$ cm cages housing 3 animals per cage. EE rearing condition was achieved using a large cage ($44 \times 62 \times 28$ cm) containing several food hoppers, one running wheel for voluntary physical exercise, and differently shaped objects (tunnels, toys, shelters, and stairs) that were repositioned twice a week and completely substituted with others once a week. The rearing conditions were maintained throughout the behavioral tests.

2.2. Social Transmission of Food Preference (STFP) Test. For the STFP test, mice, male and female, were transferred in same-sex littermate groups (2–5 animals per box) in Plexiglas cages. The test was performed during the light phase of the cycle. The STFP task is based on food neophobia in rodents. Mice show a preference for eating a food that is cued with an odor previously experienced in the breath of a conspecific, over a flavor cued with a novel scent [40, 41]. In this protocol, "observer" mice interact, during the learning phase, with a "demonstrator" mouse that has recently eaten a novel food. When observer mice are subsequently presented with a choice between the food eaten by the demonstrator and some other novel foods, they prefer the food eaten by the demonstrator, the familiar food. This phenomenon depends on the observer mice detecting olfactory cues in the breath of the demonstrator mouse during their interaction within the learning phase (sniff interaction). The subsequent food preference serves as a measure of memory for those olfactory cues. Before starting the test, one mouse from each cage was designated as the "demonstrator" and the others as the "observers." For the behavioral experiments we have used a total of 17 EE animals and 23 SC animals: in the EE group, 13 EE animals performed the behavioral tasks as observers and 4 EE mice served as demonstrator mice; in the SC group, 16 SC animals performed the task as observers and and 7 SC mice served as demonstrators.

The STFP task consisted of three distinct phases as described in the protocol of Wrenn et al. [41, 42]. To minimize neophobia during the experiments, mice were habituated to eat powdered rodent chow from 4 oz (113.40 g) glass food jar assemblies (Dyets Inc., Bethlehem, PA). Jars were approximately 7 cm in diameter and 5 cm in depth [41]. The jar assemblies have been selected in order to prevent mice from crawling and digging into the food and spilling the food from the jar.

Before the first phase, the experimenter prepared the food jar assemblies using flavored food and recorded the weights of the jars. Cocoa-flavored chow was obtained by mixing ground cocoa with plain powdered chow to give a 2% (w/w) cocoa mixture. Cumin-flavored chow was obtained by mixing cumin with plain powdered chow to give a 0.5% (w/w) cumin mixture [36].

In phase I, the demonstrators were exposed to cocoa-flavored food during a 1 h feeding session in a cage without water. At the end of phase I, the jar assemblies were removed and weighed: the demonstrator that did not eat at least 0.2 g of food was not used in the further steps of the experiment. In phase II, the learning phase, the demonstrators, immediately after the 1 h exposure to the flavored food, were placed into the cages containing their respective observers: mice were allowed to interact freely for 30 min. During phase II, the experimenter constantly watched the demonstrator from a distance of ≅50 cm and recorded the number of times that each "observer" sniffed the muzzle of the demonstrator. A sniff is defined as a close (<2 cm) orientation of the observer's nose toward the front or side of the demonstrator's muzzle [41]. The scoring of observer sniffs of the demonstrator's muzzle can provide critical data showing that the impairment in food preference is not due to changes in social behavior and insufficient social interaction. Phase III, the choice phase, started after a selected retention interval (1 h, 24 h, or 30 days). Each observer was placed in an individual cage with two jars in the opposite side of the cage for counterbalancing the position. One jar contained the familiar food (cocoa-flavored), consumed by the demonstrator

observer mice had interacted with, the other one the novel food (cumin-flavored). After 1 h of feeding period, the jars were removed from the cages and weighed; the amount of food eaten from each jar was recorded. The preference for the familiar food over the novel food was taken as an index of memory for the familiar food. For all three phases, the experimenter was blind to the rearing conditions of the mice.

To control for the effects of extra handling, novel food sniffing, and consumption and interaction with the demonstrator mouse on c-fos activation and histone H3 acetylation, we used pseudolearning (PL) mice; these animals experienced arena exploration, jar exploration, food consumption, and interaction with the demonstrator, but no learning was involved. Indeed, PL subjects (12 PL-EE and 12 PL-SC) did not detect any olfactory cue in the breath of the demonstrator mouse during the interaction period, since demonstrator mice (3 EE and 5 SC) did not eat any food before interaction. In this way, we can control for differences in c-fos expression or H3 acetylation simply due to extra handling, exposure to the arena, food, and demonstrator mouse, in the learning group and isolate the effect of learning on c-fos activation and H3 acetylation.

For c-fos-positive cell analysis, we used, at 24 h retention interval, EE ($n = 4$), SC ($n = 4$), PL-EE ($n = 4$), and PL-SC ($n = 4$); at 30-day retention interval, EE ($n = 4$), SC ($n = 4$), PL-EE ($n = 4$), and PL-SC ($n = 4$); for histone H3 acetylation analysis in the OFC, we used EE ($n = 4$), SC ($n = 4$), PL-EE ($n = 4$), and PL-SC ($n = 4$).

A possible confounding factor is the presence of an innate flavor preference for one of the flavors used in the experiment. Over the years, several different flavorants have been successfully used in the basic procedure of STFP [43]. The pairs of flavorant used in the present paper and their specific concentrations were based on literature data [36] and on pilot data indicating that by giving naïve mice a choice between the two flavors used in our experiment, mice ate the same amount of each flavored food in the absence of STFP training ($n = 5$, paired t-test cocoa-flavored versus cumin-flavored $p = 0.359$).

2.3. Immunohistochemistry. We used the procedure previously described in [44]. Mice were anaesthetized and perfused via intracardiac infusion with 0.1 M PBS and then 4% paraformaldehyde (PFA, dissolved in 0.1 M phosphate buffer, pH 7.4) 90 min after completion of phase III (choice phase) or 60 minutes after phase II (learning phase) for c-fos and histone H3 acetylation, respectively. Brains were removed, fixed overnight in PFA, and then transferred to 30% sucrose solution and stored at 4°C. Coronal sections were cut at 40 μm thickness on a freezing microtome (Sliding Leica microtome SM2010R, Leica Microsystems) and processed for immunohistochemistry.

For c-fos immunohistochemistry, after a blocking step in 10% NGS and 0.5% Triton X-100 in PBS, free-floating sections were incubated using anti-c-fos rabbit polyclonal antibody (1 : 3000 rabbit anti-c-fos polyclonal antibody, Calbiochem, USA) for 36 h at 4°C. Subsequently, sections were transferred in a solution containing 1% NGS,

0.1% Triton X-100, and 1 : 200 anti-rabbit biotinylated antibody (Vector Labs) in PBS. This was followed by incubation in ABC kit (Vector Labs) and final detection with DAB reaction kit (Vector Labs). Sections were finally mounted on gelatinized slides, dehydrated, and sealed with DPX mounting medium (VWR International, UK).

For acetyl-histone H3 immunohistochemistry, after a blocking step in 10% NGS and 0.05% Triton X-100 in PBS, sections were incubated in a solution containing 10% NGS, 0.05% Triton X-100, and anti-acetyl-histone H3 monoclonal rabbit antibodies (Lys14, 1 : 200 rabbit anti-acetyl-histone H3 monoclonal antibodies, Millipore, USA) overnight at 4°C. Subsequently, sections were transferred in a solution containing 3% NGS, 0.05% Triton X-100, and 1 : 400 Alexa Fluor 568 goat anti-rabbit IgG antibody (Life Technologies) in PBS (Ciccarelli et al., 2013). Sections were then mounted on gelatinized slides with VECTA-SHIELD (Vector Labs).

2.4. Quantitative Analysis of c-fos-Positive Cells. We used the procedure previously described in [44]. Counting of c-fos-positive cells in different brain areas was performed using a CCD camera (MBF Bioscience, Germany) mounted on a Zeiss Axioskop (Zeiss, Germany) microscope and the Stereo Investigator software (MBF Bioscience). Brain structures were anatomically defined according to a mouse brain atlas (Paxinos and Franklin, 1997), and the regions of interest selected for measurement of c-fos-positive nuclei in the orbitofrontal cortex (OFC) were (numbers indicate the distance in millimeters of the sections from bregma) medial orbital cortex (MO, +2.80 mm), ventral orbital cortex (VO, +2.80 mm), lateral orbital cortex (LO, +2.80 mm), and dorsolateral orbital cortex (DLO, +2.80 mm). The number of c-fos-positive cells was counted at 20x magnification, in 5–10 fields ($50 \times 50\,\mu m$ or $100 \times 100\,\mu m$) per section according to the size of brain structure and their density calculated (cells/mm^2), using at least 5 sections for each structure. The experimenter counting c-fos-positive cells was blind to the rearing condition and treatment of the animals.

2.5. Quantitative Analysis of Immunohistochemical Signal of Histone H3 Acetylation in the OFC. The imaging of brain areas was performed using a CCD camera (MBF Bioscience, Germany) mounted on a Zeiss Axioskop (Zeiss, Germany) microscope and QCapture software (QImaging, Canada). Brain structures were anatomically defined according to a mouse brain atlas (Paxinos and Franklin, 1997). Images were acquired at 20x magnification in one field of $200 \times 300\,\mu m$ per section, keeping constant both microscope settings and fluorescence-field intensity. The collected images were imported to the image analysis system MetaMorph (molecular devices), and for each animal, the relative signal intensity of AcH3-immunopositive cells was calculated using at least 5 sections for each structure. The relative signal intensity of AcH3-immunopositive cells was calculated as the ratio between the mean intensity of AcH3-immunopositive cells and the intensity of background signal measured in sample areas surrounding AcH3$^+$ cells. All image acquisition and analysis were carried out in blind.

2.6. Statistics. All results were expressed as mean ± SEM, and all statistical analyses were performed using statistical software package SigmaStat (SigmaStat, version 3.5). For STFP performance in phase III, a two-way analysis of variance (ANOVA) for repeated measures (RM) was performed for each retention interval (1 h, 24 h, or 30 days), considering both factor condition (EE or SC or PL-EE or PL-SC) and factor flavor (familiar or novel), with post hoc analysis Holm-Sidak method. The number of c-fos-positive cells in each OFC area was analyzed with a two-way ANOVA, factor condition and retention interval, with post hoc analysis Holm-Sidak method. The level of histone H3 acetylation in each OFC area was analyzed with a two-way ANOVA, factor condition, and area, with post hoc analysis Holm-Sidak method.

3. Results

3.1. Long-Term STFP Memory Deficit in Aged Mice Is Ameliorated by EE. Aged C57BL/6 mice, housed in EE or SC for 40 days, were subjected to the STFP task. During the learning phase (phase II), interactions between demonstrator and observer mice were scored to control for possible differences between EE and SC mice in the amount of interactions (a schematic diagram of the experimental protocol is reported in Figure 1).

Indeed, a difference in interaction with the demonstrator during the learning phase would affect performance in the choice phase: an observer mouse is expected not to show any preference for the cued food if it has not adequately interacted with the demonstrator during the learning phase. We found no difference in the amount of interactions between EE and SC mice (t-test, EE ($n = 13$) versus SC ($n = 16$), $p = 0.111$; data not shown).

Then, we evaluated olfactory memory abilities in the choice phase (phase III) of the STFP task: in this phase, observer mice, after a retention interval, were placed in individual cages allocating two jars: one jar contained a familiar food identical to that consumed by the demonstrator and the other containing a totally novel food. After 1 h spent in the choice phase, the jars were removed from the cage and weighed in order to assess the amount of food eaten from each jar. The choice phase was performed at three different intervals, that is, 1 h, 24 h (day 1), or 30 days (day 30) after the end of phase II.

At 1 h retention interval, we found a clear preference for the familiar food in both groups of animals which underwent associative learning of familiar food in the breath of the demonstrator, SC ($n = 8$) and EE ($n = 5$) (two-way RM ANOVA, post hoc analysis Holm-Sidak method, familiar food versus novel food, $p = 0.007$ for SC, $p < 0.001$ for EE; Figure 1); on the contrary, at retention intervals 24 h (day 1) and 30 days (day 30), we found a significant familiar food preference only for EE mice, while SC mice displayed no preference at either interval (two-way RM ANOVA post hoc analysis Holm-Sidak method, familiar food versus novel food at day 1, $p = 0.153$ for SC mice ($n = 4$), $p = 0.001$ for EE mice ($n = 4$); at day 30, $p = 0.095$ for SC mice ($n = 4$), $p = 0.021$ for EE mice ($n = 4$); Figure 2).

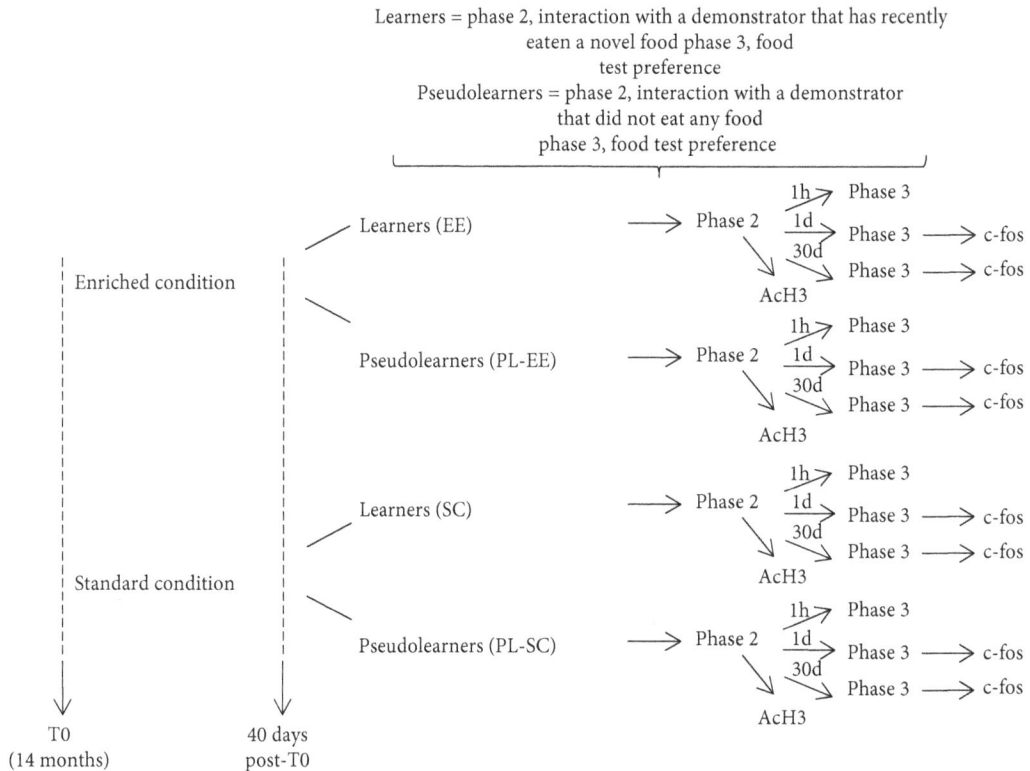

FIGURE 1: Schematic diagram of the experimental protocol.

As expected, no food preference was displayed by PL-SC and PL-EE mice, which did not undergo associative learning (two-way RM ANOVA, post hoc analysis Holm-Sidak method, novel versus familiar; $p > 0.05$ at both retention intervals; Figure 2).

The good performance of SC mice at 1 h retention interval rules out the possibility of olfactory deficits hampering the preference for the familiar food in aged SC mice. Thus, their failure in eating significantly more the familiar food at day 1 and day 30 indicates a long-term STFP memory deficit in aged SC mice, which is rescued by EE.

3.2. c-fos Expression in the OFC of Aged SC and EE Mice following a Retention Interval of 1 or 30 Days. After the end of the choice test at day 1 and day 30, when SC and EE mice significantly differed in their memory performance, mice were sacrificed and the expression of c-fos protein was assessed as an indicator of neuronal activity in the OFC, the final olfactory memory storage site. c-fos immunohistochemistry is currently used in developing adult and aging animals as a reliable, surrogate marker for neuronal activity, particularly when spatial distribution of neuronal activity and comparison of neural activation between different brain regions is of interest (see, e.g., [10, 44–50]). We separately counted c-fos-positive cells in 4 OFC subregions, medial orbital cortex (MO), ventral orbital cortex (VO), lateral orbital cortex (LO), and dorsolateral orbital cortex (DLO). No difference was present between the two control groups, PL-EE and PL-SC mice, in any OFC region at any retention interval (two-way ANOVA,

post hoc analysis Holm-Sidak method, PL-EE versus PL-SC, $p > 0.05$; Figure 3), suggesting that EE and SC condition per se does not affect c-fos expression in the areas of interest during the choice test.

At day 1, we found significant neuronal activation in OFC both for EE and SC mice: indeed, the number of c-fos-positive cells was higher in SC and EE mice with respect to their controls (PL-SC and PL-EE mice) in all OFC areas in EE mice and in LO and DLO in SC mice (two-way ANOVA, post hoc analysis Holm-Sidak method for condition, EE versus PL-EE ($p < 0.01$) for all areas; SC versus PL-SC ($p < 0.01$) for LO and DLO; SC versus PL-SC ($p > 0.05$) for MO and VO; Figure 3). No difference was present between EE and SC mice in any OFC regions (two-way ANOVA, post hoc analysis Holm-Sidak method for condition, EE versus SC ($p > 0.05$) for all areas; Figure 3).

At day 30 retention interval, we found significant neuronal activation only in EE mice: in particular, we found an increased number of c-fos-positive cells in all OFC areas of EE mice (two-way ANOVA, post hoc analysis Holm-Sidak method for condition, EE versus PL-EE ($p < 0.001$) in all areas; Figure 3). No increase in the number of c-fos-positive cells was present in any OFC area at day 30 in SC mice with respect to their controls (two-way ANOVA, post hoc analysis Holm-Sidak method for condition, SC versus PL-SC ($p > 0.05$) in all areas; Figure 2), indicating lack of neuronal activation. A comparison between EE and SC c-fos expression at day 30 showed a greater neuronal activation in EE with respect to SC mice in all OFC areas (two-way ANOVA, post hoc analysis Holm-Sidak method for housing

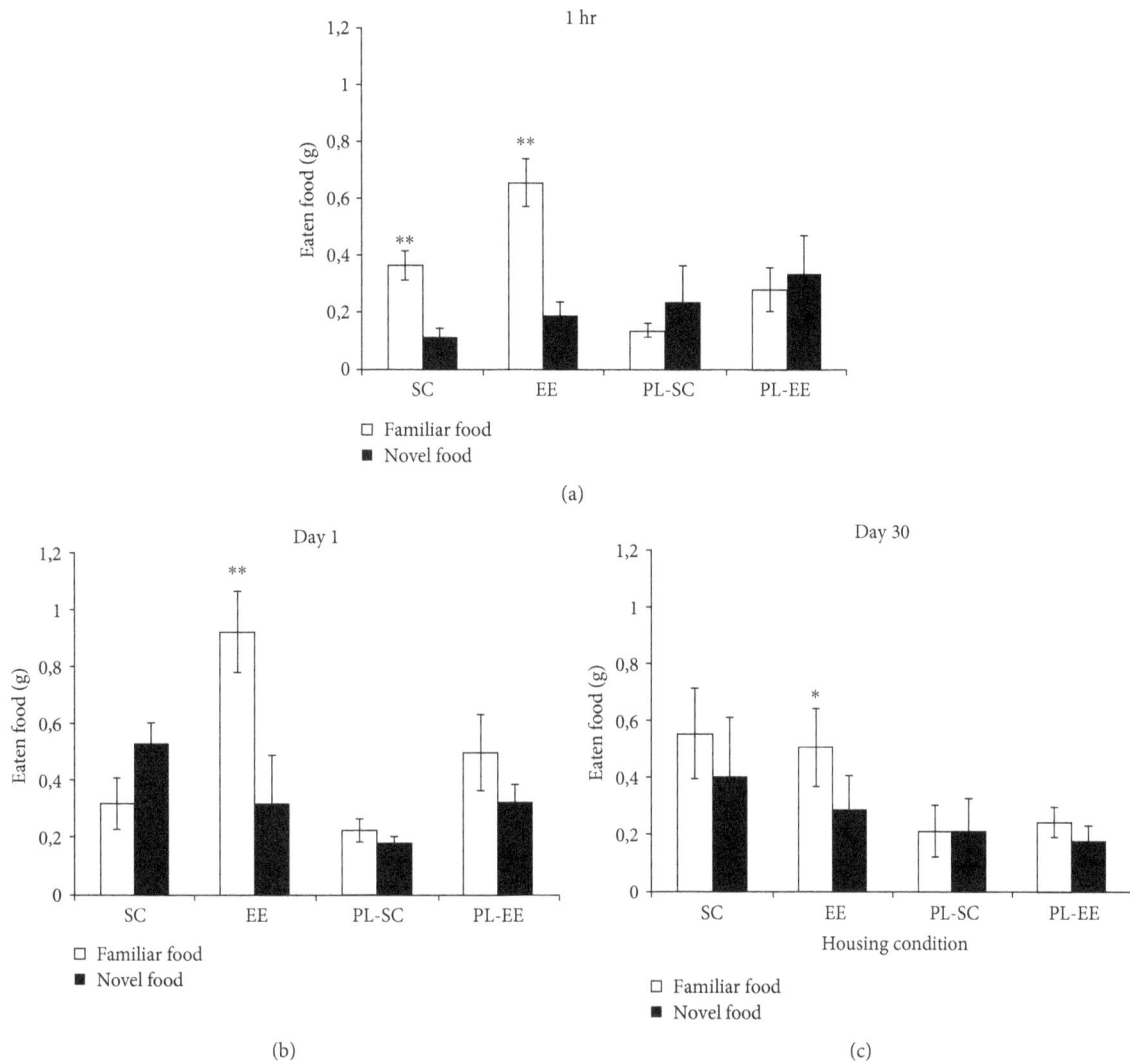

FIGURE 2: Performance of SC, EE, PL-SC, and PL-EE mice in the STFP. (a) 1-hour retention interval: there is a significant preference for the familiar food (open columns) with respect to the novel food (filled columns) for SC and EE groups, which underwent associative learning of familiar food in the breath of the demonstrator (two-way RM ANOVA post hoc analysis Holm-Sidak method, familiar food versus novel food for SC ($p = 0.007$) and EE ($p < 0.001$)). (b) 24-hour retention interval (day 1). There is a significant preference for the familiar food with respect to the novel food only for EE group (two-way RM ANOVA post hoc analysis Holm-Sidak method, familiar food versus novel food for EE ($p = 0.001$)). (c) 30-day retention interval (day 30): there is a significant preference for the familiar food with respect to the novel food only for EE group (two-way RM ANOVA post hoc analysis Holm-Sidak method, familiar food versus novel food for EE ($p = 0.021$)). There is no preference for the familiar food in pseudolearning mice, PL-SC and PL-EE, for any time interval (two-way RM ANOVA post hoc analysis Holm-Sidak method ($p > 0.05$) for all comparisons). $^{*}p < 0.05$; $^{**}p < 0.01$; error bars = SEM.

condition, EE versus SC, $p = 0.003$ for MO and $p < 0.001$ for VO, LO, and DLO; Figure 3).

In the comparison between c-fos activations at day 1 and day 30, we found a significantly higher number of c-fos-positive cells at day 30 with respect to day 1 in EE mice in all OFC areas but MO (two-way ANOVA, post hoc analysis Holm-Sidak method 30 versus 1 in EE, $p = 0.181$ in MO; $p < 0.001$ in VO; $p = 0.004$ in LO; $p = 0.035$ in DLO; Figure 3); on the contrary, no significantly higher activation of OFC areas was found at day 30 with respect to day 1 in SC mice; rather, we found a decrease in c-fos expression in LO for the SC group (two-way ANOVA, post hoc analysis Holm-Sidak method 30 versus 1 in SC, $p = 0.018$ in LO; $p > 0.05$ in MO, VO, and DLO; Figure 3).

Thus, preserved memory at day 30 in EE mice was associated with a significant activation of OFC and with increased OFC activation with respect to day 1 recall.

3.3. Increased Histone H3 Acetylation in the OFC of EE Aged Mice 1 h after the Learning Phase. Epigenetic changes are crucially involved in memory consolidation [35, 51]. Lesburgueres et al. [36] have shown that the setting of synaptic tags during system consolidation of STFP memory involves epigenetic mechanisms, in particular increased acetylation of histone H3 in the OFC shortly (1 h) after the learning phase; preventing the increase in H3 acetylation impaired remote memory, assessed 30 days later, while pharmacological maintenance of a higher level of acetylation resulted in

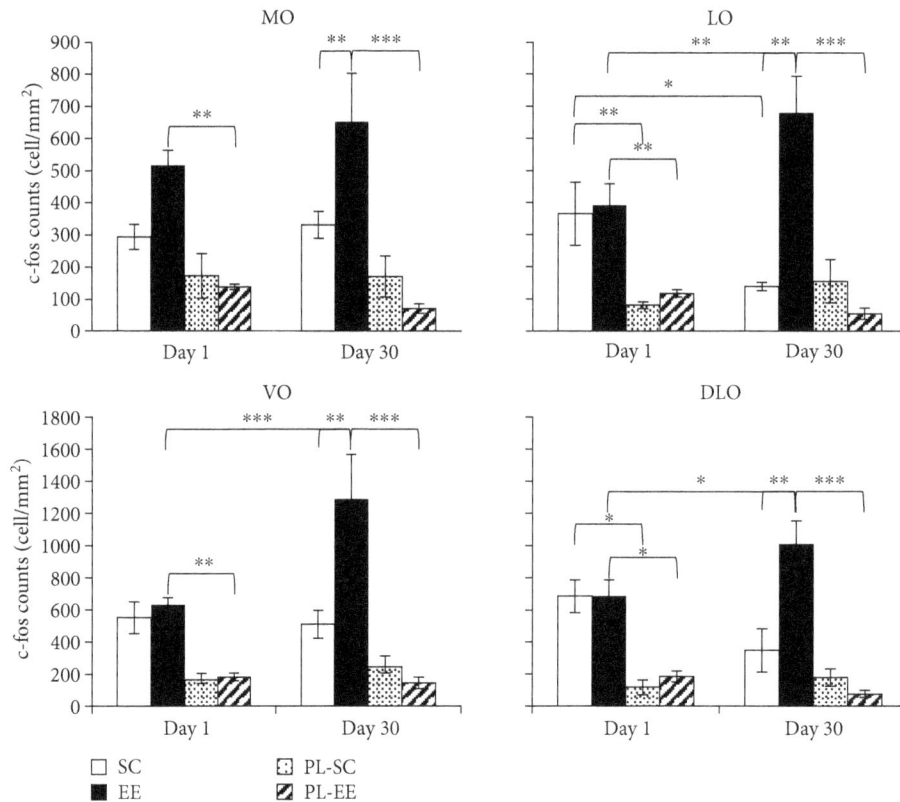

(a)

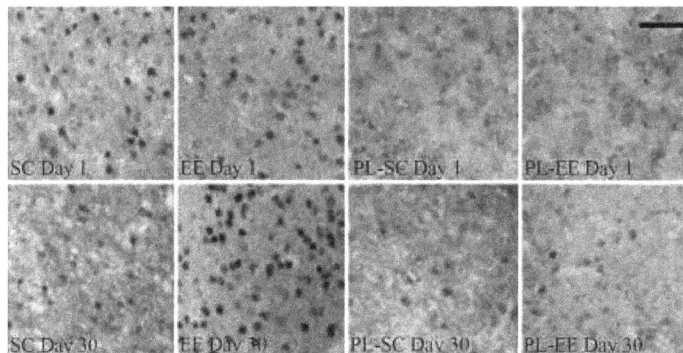

(b)

FIGURE 3: (a) c-fos expression in subregions of OFC for SC (open columns), EE (filled columns), PL-SC (dotted columns), and PL-EE (hatched columns) mice subjected to choice phase at day 1 and day 30. MO: two-way ANOVA, factor condition ($p < 0.001$), factor time ($p = 0.613$), condition × time ($p = 0.530$), post hoc analysis Holm-Sidak method. SC versus PL-SC and PL-SC versus PL-EE ($p > 0.05$) for all retention intervals. Statistical differences were found between EE versus PL-EE at day 1 ($p = 0.001$) and day 30 ($p < 0.001$); EE versus SC significant at day 30 ($p = 0.003$). LO: two-way ANOVA, factor condition ($p < 0.001$), factor time ($p = 0.688$), condition × time ($p = 0.004$), post hoc analysis Holm-Sidak method. PL-SC versus PL-EE ($p > 0.05$) for all retention intervals. Statistical differences were found between SC versus PL-SC at day 1 ($p = 0.004$); EE versus PL-EE at day 1 ($p = 0.001$) and day 30 ($p < 0.001$); EE versus SC significant at day 30 ($p < 0.001$). Statistical differences within group were found between day 1 and day 30 for SC group ($p = 0.018$) and for EE group ($p = 0.004$). VO: two-way ANOVA, factor condition ($p < 0.001$), factor time ($p = 0.054$), condition × time ($p = 0.015$), post hoc analysis Holm-Sidak method. SC versus PL-SC and PL-SC versus PL-EE ($p > 0.05$) for all retention intervals. Statistical differences were found between EE versus PL-EE at day 1 ($p = 0.001$) and day 30 ($p < 0.001$); EE versus SC significant at day 30 ($p < 0.001$). Statistical differences within EE group were found between day 1 and day 30 ($p < 0.001$). DLO: two-way ANOVA, factor condition ($p < 0.001$), factor time ($p = 0.913$), condition × time ($p = 0.059$), post hoc analysis Holm-Sidak method. PL-SC versus PL-EE ($p > 0.05$) for all retention intervals. Statistical differences were found between SC versus PL-SC at day 1 ($p = 0.003$); EE versus PL-EE at day 1 ($p = 0.002$) and day 30 ($p < 0.001$); EE versus SC significant at day 30 ($p < 0.001$). Statistical differences within EE group were found between day 1 and day 30 ($p = 0.035$). $^*p < 0.05$; $^{**}p < 0.01$; $^{***}p < 0.001$; error bars = SEM. (b) Representative panel of c-fos protein expression in DLO for SC, EE, PL-SC, and PL-EE mice, following recall at day 1 and day 30; scale bar: 50 μm.

AcH3 in OFC

(a)

(b)

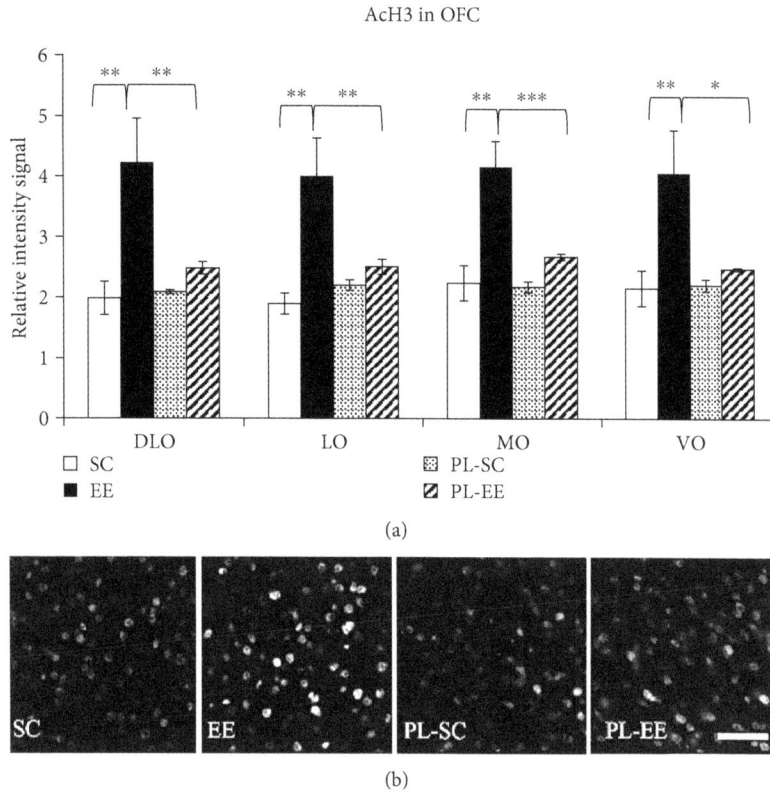

FIGURE 4: (a) H3 acetylation on L14 in subregions of OFC for SC (open columns), EE (filled columns), PL-SC (dotted columns), and PL-EE (hatched columns) mice 1 hour after the learning phase. PL-SC did not differ from PL-EE mice. Only EE animals showed significant differences with respect to their controls in OFC areas; (one-way ANOVA ($p < 0.01$), post hoc analysis Holm-Sidak method, SC versus PL-SC and PL-SC versus PL-EE ($p > 0.05$) for all subregions). MO: EE versus SC ($p < 0.001$), EE versus PL-EE ($p = 0.001$). LO: EE versus SC ($p < 0.001$), EE versus PL-EE ($p = 0.007$). VO: EE versus SC ($p = 0.004$), EE versus PL-EE ($p = 0.013$). DLO: EE versus SC ($p = 0.001$), EE versus PL-EE ($p = 0.008$). $^*p < 0.05$; $^{**}p < 0.01$; $^{***}p < 0.001$; error bars = SEM. (b) Representative panel of histone H3 acetylation in DLO for SC, EE, PL-SC, and PL-EE mice 1 h after learning; scale bar: 50 μm.

improved remote memory retrieval. Using Lesburgueres et al. protocol, we have assessed AcH3 levels in OFC 1 h after the learning phase.

We found that the signal intensity of histone H3 acetylation on lysine 14 was significantly increased with respect to control PL mice only in EE mice, and this was found in all subregions of OFC (one-way ANOVA, $p < 0.01$, post hoc analysis Holm-Sidak method, EE versus PL-EE, $p < 0.01$ for all subregions; Figure 4); no intensity difference was found between SC and PL-SC or between PL-EE and PL-SC mice (one-way ANOVA, $p < 0.01$, post hoc analysis Holm-Sidak method, SC versus PL-SC, $p > 0.05$ for all subregions; Figure 4). Intensity of H3 acetylation in EE mice was significantly higher than in SC mice in all OFC regions (one-way ANOVA, $p < 0.01$, post hoc analysis Holm-Sidak method, EE versus SC, $p < 0.01$ for all subregions; Figure 4).

Thus, the preserved remote memory recall in aged EE mice is associated with enhanced OFC histone acetylation early in the system consolidation process, which suggests a preserved early tagging of OFC.

4. Discussion

Brain aging is a complex physiological process characterized by a progressive deterioration of cognitive functions,

especially in the learning and memory domains. Major deficits are particularly evident at the level of declarative memory abilities requiring the precise recall of detailed information, a process initially mediated by the hippocampus and other medial temporal lobe structures [1, 4] and subsequently supported by the process of system consolidation. System consolidation consists in the functional and structural reorganization of cerebral regions prompted by the reactivation of hippocampal-cortical pathways and the strengthening of corticocortical connections, leading to formation of a cortical memory trace which supports remote memory recall [36, 52]. Many papers have investigated the effects of EE on local memory consolidation in the aged hippocampus, responsible for formation and early maintenance of hippocampus-dependent memory; for instance, EE ameliorates CA1 plasticity and cell excitability and reverses age-related epigenetic changes and other age-related negative processes (see, e.g., [20–22, 31, 53]). However, to our knowledge, the effects of EE on system consolidation, that is, on the recruitment of cortical activity to support remote memory, have not been investigated in aged animals. In particular, we found no study on the effects of EE on the early tagging in prefrontal cortex as a correlate of remote memory retrieval.

In this study, we showed that exposure to EE in aged mice modulates system consolidation and enhances performance in the STFP declarative memory task. STFP is a hippocampus-dependent task which exploits the natural tendency of rodents to prefer food sources based on a previous sampling of their odor in the breath of littermates. In this task, the behavioral performance can be efficiently measured in a single trial session and, given that the underlying memory traces are long-lasting, it allows researchers to perform a characterization of possible changes in the expression levels of potential transcription factors involved in memory acquisition and in the recall phases. Olfactory memories activated by STFP are eventually transferred to the OFC, via a system consolidation process which requires early tagging of cortical networks in this structure [36].

While early tagging of cortical networks has been previously investigated in adult rodents, no evidence for similar mechanisms has been provided, so far, in aged animals. We first report that, while aged SC animals displayed severe deficits in memory recall at both recent (1 day) and remote (30 days) time intervals, EE preserved cognitive performance in the STFP task at both intervals. The performance of aged EE mice thus resembles that of standard-reared young adult rats, performing well both recent and remote STFP memory recall [36].

Focusing on c-fos expression as a marker of neuronal activity, we analyzed the activation of the final recipient of SFTP memory, namely, OFC, during recent and remote recall. A marked environment-dependent effect was found in the OFC, with enriched mice displaying higher c-fos expression levels compared to SC animals at the 30-day interval, in agreement with the differences in recall abilities displayed by enriched versus SC animals in the SFTP declarative memory task at this time point. Importantly, the absence of OFC activation displayed by SC aged mice at the 30 days of retention interval was not dependent on general olfactory discrimination deficits, as demonstrated by the intact performance displayed by the same group at shorter intervals (1 h). Comparable amounts of OFC activation were instead found in SC and EE animals at the 1-day retention interval, when both groups displayed increased c-fos expression compared to their respective controls; however, this activation of OFC areas was paralleled by marked behavioral deficits evident at this time point. These results indicate that OFC activation recorded 24 h past the end of the acquisition phase is not sufficient for, or not correlated with, mouse mnemonic performance. This is in accordance with the late role for OFC in system consolidation and its dispensability for recent memory recall [36, 52, 54, 55].

Looking for possible epigenetic changes acting as an early tagging mechanism for memory formation in olfactory cortical networks, we found an increased H3 acetylation in all analyzed OFC areas of EE subjects compared to SC animals. H3 acetylation levels were found to be enhanced with respect to control animals in EE mice, but not in SC animals. These results suggest a deficit in the initial steps of cortical tagging of memory traces associated with brain aging in SC compared to EE animals and demonstrate that exposure to stimulating environmental conditions preserves remote recall of declarative memory abilities in aged mice by promoting

system consolidation through the activation of epigenetic regulatory processes crucial for coding and consolidation of cortical mnemonic traces. System consolidation is the process of time-dependent gradual reorganization of the brain regions supporting remote memory storage. Within this process, early tagging of cortical circuits is a necessary step for the formation of enduring associative memory [35, 36]. In particular, early tagging of OFC cortical networks is a prerequisite for the establishment of remote olfactory memory of the STFP. Synaptic tags may serve as an early and persistent signature of activity in the cortex that is necessary to ensure the progressive rewiring of cortical networks that support remote memory storage. The early increase in histone H3 acetylation following STFP learning phase is involved in the formation of the early synaptic tags in OFC supporting STFP remote memory retrieval: preventing the increase in H3 acetylation impaired remote memory, assessed 30 days later, while pharmacological maintenance of a higher level of acetylation resulted in improved remote memory retrieval probed 30 days later [36]. Our results show that in the absence of H3 acetylation following learning, as is the case of aged SC mice, there is a strong memory deficit. EE ameliorates memory performance in aged mice, allowing a good retrieval of memory 30 days after learning and this is associated with an increased H3 acetylation in OFC of EE mice. This suggests that EE preserves a good early tagging in aged mice and strengthens the hypothesis that early tagging is important for system consolidation.

It has been previously reported that an increased activity of histone acetyltransferase (HAT) enzymes during a hippocampus-dependent task can be accompanied by increased histone acetylation acting as a specific epigenetic tagging for memory consolidation [56]. It is well known that environment-induced beneficial effects on brain plasticity and memory abilities may involve HAT activation [9, 28]. The increased AcH3 found in our EE mice might suggest an involvement of HAT activation; however, further work would be necessary to elucidate the mechanisms underlying this increased acetylation.

At the 24 h retention interval, OFC activation in SC mice was enhanced with respect to their PL controls, reaching levels not significantly different from those displayed by EE mice; however, differently from EE mice, in SC mice, OFC activation at the 24 h of retention interval was not preceded by any early tagging process, suggesting that it is the lack of early tagging and not the lack of general recruitment of OFC areas that is responsible for the main deficits in remote associative memory formation displayed by SC aged mice. Indeed, the crucial and irreplaceable role of early tagging is that of topographically specifying, by means of epigenetic signature [35, 36], which sets of cortical neurons will participate to the hippocampal-cortical dialogue during the course of systems-level consolidation. In the absence of early tagging, that is, of the specification of the recipient circuits in OFC, the general activation of OFC would be unlikely to sustain the fine process of transferring specific information from the hippocampus to OFC to sustain formation of enduring associative memory.

EE is well known to affect synaptic function not only in young or adult but also in aged animals, where EE ameliorates many of the deficits in synaptic physiology, density, and plasticity induced by age (see [1, 9, 20, 22]). We cannot exclude that these effects of EE might have contributed to our results, for instance, via a better encoding/local consolidation process in the hippocampus, especially in the case of the better performance of EE animals at the 24 h interval, where early tagging in PFC is not supposed to play a key role; enhanced synaptic function and plasticity in EE animals might also have contributed to our results enhancing the efficacy of the hippocampal-cortical dialogue during formation of the cortical trace which supports remote memory.

In conclusion, our results show that exposure to stimulating environmental conditions can be used as a powerful paradigm to promote good system consolidation of associative memory in aged mice and suggest that system consolidation may be a crucial target for treatments aimed at ameliorating memory dysfunctions in elderly subjects.

Conflicts of Interest

The authors declare that they have no conflicts of interest.

Acknowledgments

This work was made possible by the generous funding of "Fondazione Pisa" to project "Train the Brain" and to project "Translational Assessment in Aging" (Bando Ricerca Scientifica in Neuroscienze 2007 and Bando Ricerca Scientifica e Tecnologica 2016, Fondazione Pisa).

References

[1] S. N. Burke and C. A. Barnes, "Neural plasticity in the ageing brain," *Nature Reviews Neuroscience*, vol. 7, no. 1, pp. 30–40, 2006.

[2] T. Hedden and J. D. E. Gabrieli, "Insights into the ageing mind: a view from cognitive neuroscience," *Nature Reviews Neuroscience*, vol. 5, no. 2, pp. 87–96, 2004.

[3] S. A. Small, S. A. Schobel, R. B. Buxton, M. P. Witter, and C. A. Barnes, "A pathophysiological framework of hippocampal dysfunction in ageing and disease," *Nature Reviews Neuroscience*, vol. 12, no. 10, pp. 585–601, 2011.

[4] C. A. Barnes, "Secrets of aging: what does a normally aging brain look like?," *F1000 Biology Reports*, vol. 3, p. 22, 2011.

[5] A. Fleischmann, O. Hvalby, V. Jensen et al., "Impaired long-term memory and NR2A-type NMDA receptor-dependent synaptic plasticity in mice lacking c-Fos in the CNS," *The Journal of Neuroscience*, vol. 23, no. 27, pp. 9116–9122, 2003.

[6] X. Zhou, C. Moon, F. Zheng et al., "N-methyl-D-aspartate-stimulated ERK1/2 signaling and the transcriptional upregulation of plasticity-related genes are developmentally regulated following in vitro neuronal maturation," *Journal*

of Neuroscience Research*, vol. 87, no. 12, pp. 2632–2644, 2009.

[7] J. Graff and L. H. Tsai, "Histone acetylation: molecular mnemonics on the chromatin," *Nature Reviews Neuroscience*, vol. 14, no. 2, pp. 97–111, 2013.

[8] S. K. Pirooznia and F. Elefant, "Targeting specific HATs for neurodegenerative disease treatment: translating basic biology to therapeutic possibilities," *Frontiers in Cellular Neuroscience*, vol. 7, p. 30, 2013.

[9] A. Sale, N. Berardi, and L. Maffei, "Environment and brain plasticity: towards an endogenous pharmacotherapy," *Physiological Reviews*, vol. 94, no. 1, pp. 189–234, 2014.

[10] M. Weber, T. Wu, J. E. Hanson et al., "Cognitive deficits, changes in synaptic function, and brain pathology in a mouse model of normal aging (1, 2, 3)," *eNeuro*, vol. 2, no. 5, 2015.

[11] M. R. Rosenzweig, E. L. Bennett, M. Hebert, and H. Morimoto, "Social grouping cannot account for cerebral effects of enriched environments," *Brain Research*, vol. 153, no. 3, pp. 563–576, 1978.

[12] J. Bennett, P. McRae, L. Levy, and K. Frick, "Long-term continuous, but not daily, environmental enrichment reduces spatial memory decline in aged male mice," *Neurobiology of Learning and Memory*, vol. 85, no. 2, pp. 139–152, 2006.

[13] S. N. Duffy, K. J. Craddock, T. Abel, and P. V. Nguyen, "Environmental enrichment modifies the PKA-dependence of hippocampal LTP and improves hippocampus-dependent memory," *Learning & Memory*, vol. 8, no. 1, pp. 26–34, 2001.

[14] H. van Praag, B. R. Christie, T. J. Sejnowski, and F. H. Gage, "Running enhances neurogenesis, learning, and long-term potentiation in mice," *Proceedings of the National Academy of Sciences of the United States of America*, vol. 96, no. 23, pp. 13427–13431, 1999.

[15] H. van Praag, G. Kempermann, and F. H. Gage, "Neural consequences of environmental enrichment," *Nature Reviews Neuroscience*, vol. 1, no. 3, pp. 191–198, 2000.

[16] K. M. Frick and S. M. Fernandez, "Enrichment enhances spatial memory and increases synaptophysin levels in aged female mice," *Neurobiology of Aging*, vol. 24, no. 4, pp. 615–626, 2003.

[17] G. Schoenbaum, M. R. Roesch, T. A. Stalnaker, and Y. K. Takahashi, "Orbitofrontal cortex and outcome expectancies: optimizing behavior and sensory perception," in *Neurobiology of Sensation and Reward*, J. A. Gottfried, Ed., CRC Press/Taylor & Francis, Boca Raton, FL, USA, 2011.

[18] Y. P. Tang, H. Wang, R. Feng, M. Kyin, and J. Z. Tsien, "Differential effects of enrichment on learning and memory function in NR2B transgenic mice," *Neuropharmacology*, vol. 41, no. 6, pp. 779–790, 2001.

[19] A. M. Birch and A. M. Kelly, "Lifelong environmental enrichment in the absence of exercise protects the brain from age-related cognitive decline," *Neuropharmacology*, 2018.

[20] L. E. B. Bettio, L. Rajendran, and J. Gil-Mohapel, "The effects of aging in the hippocampus and cognitive decline," *Neuroscience and Biobehavioral Reviews*, vol. 79, pp. 66–86, 2017.

[21] S. J. Morse, A. A. Butler, R. L. Davis, I. J. Soller, and F. D. Lubin, "Environmental enrichment reverses histone methylation changes in the aged hippocampus and restores age-related memory deficits," *Biology*, vol. 4, no. 2, pp. 298–313, 2015.

[22] A. Kumar, A. Rani, O. Tchigranova, W. H. Lee, and T. C. Foster, "Influence of late-life exposure to environmental enrichment or exercise on hippocampal function and CA1

senescent physiology," *Neurobiology of Aging*, vol. 33, no. 4, pp. 828.e1–828.e17, 2012.

[23] M. Hüttenrauch, G. Salinas, and O. Wirths, "Effects of long-term environmental enrichment on anxiety, memory, hippocampal plasticity and overall brain gene expression in C57BL6 mice," *Frontiers in Molecular Neuroscience*, vol. 9, 2016.

[24] C. Grinan-Ferre, D. Perez-Caceres, S. M. Gutierrez-Zetina et al., "Environmental enrichment improves behavior, cognition, and brain functional markers in young senescence-accelerated prone mice (SAMP8)," *Molecular Neurobiology*, vol. 53, no. 4, pp. 2435–2450, 2016.

[25] P. Obiang, E. Maubert, I. Bardou et al., "Enriched housing reverses age-associated impairment of cognitive functions and tPA-dependent maturation of BDNF," *Neurobiology of Learning and Memory*, vol. 96, no. 2, pp. 121–129, 2011.

[26] J. Nithianantharajah and A. J. Hannan, "Enriched environments, experience-dependent plasticity and disorders of the nervous system," *Nature Reviews Neuroscience*, vol. 7, no. 9, pp. 697–709, 2006.

[27] L. Baroncelli, C. Braschi, M. Spolidoro, T. Begenisic, A. Sale, and L. Maffei, "Nurturing brain plasticity: impact of environmental enrichment," *Cell Death and Differentiation*, vol. 17, no. 7, pp. 1092–1103, 2010.

[28] A. Fischer, F. Sananbenesi, X. Wang, M. Dobbin, and L. H. Tsai, "Recovery of learning and memory is associated with chromatin remodelling," *Nature*, vol. 447, no. 7141, pp. 178–182, 2007.

[29] B. Kolb, G. Gorny, A. H. V. Soderpalm, and T. E. Robinson, "Environmental complexity has different effects on the structure of neurons in the prefrontal cortex versus the parietal cortex or nucleus accumbens," *Synapse*, vol. 48, no. 3, pp. 149–153, 2003.

[30] F. Mora, G. Segovia, and A. del Arco, "Aging, plasticity and environmental enrichment: structural changes and neurotransmitter dynamics in several areas of the brain," *Brain Research Reviews*, vol. 55, no. 1, pp. 78–88, 2007.

[31] K. M. Frick, "Epigenetics, oestradiol and hippocampal memory consolidation," *Journal of Neuroendocrinology*, vol. 25, no. 11, pp. 1151–1162, 2013.

[32] Y. Dudai, "The neurobiology of consolidations, or, how stable is the engram?," *Annual Review of Psychology*, vol. 55, no. 1, pp. 51–86, 2004.

[33] S. H. Wang and R. G. M. Morris, "Hippocampal-neocortical interactions in memory formation, consolidation, and reconsolidation," *Annual Review of Psychology*, vol. 61, no. 1, pp. 49–79, 2010.

[34] L. R. Squire and P. J. Bayley, "The neuroscience of remote memory," *Current Opinion in Neurobiology*, vol. 17, no. 2, pp. 185–196, 2007.

[35] K. M. Lattal and M. A. Wood, "Epigenetics and persistent memory: implications for reconsolidation and silent extinction beyond the zero," *Nature Neuroscience*, vol. 16, no. 2, pp. 124–129, 2013.

[36] E. Lesburgueres, O. L. Gobbo, S. Alaux-Cantin, A. Hambucken, P. Trifilieff, and B. Bontempi, "Early tagging of cortical networks is required for the formation of enduring associative memory," *Science*, vol. 331, no. 6019, pp. 924–928, 2011.

[37] M. Mainardi, A. Di Garbo, M. Caleo, N. Berardi, A. Sale, and L. Maffei, "Environmental enrichment strengthens corticocortical interactions and reduces amyloid-β oligomers in aged mice," *Frontiers in Aging Neuroscience*, vol. 6, 2014.

[38] S. Dutta and P. Sengupta, "Men and mice: relating their ages," *Life Sciences*, vol. 152, pp. 244–248, 2016.

[39] B. Bessieres, O. Nicole, and B. Bontempi, "Assessing recent and remote associative olfactory memory in rats using the social transmission of food preference paradigm," *Nature Protocols*, vol. 12, no. 7, pp. 1415–1436, 2017.

[40] P. Valsecchi, M. Mainardi, A. Sgoifo, and A. Taticchi, "Maternal influences on food preferences in weanling mice Mus domesticus," *Behavioural Processes*, vol. 19, no. 1–3, pp. 155–166, 1989.

[41] C. C. Wrenn, A. P. Harris, M. C. Saavedra, and J. N. Crawley, "Social transmission of food preference in mice: methodology and application to galanin-overexpressing transgenic mice," *Behavioral Neuroscience*, vol. 117, no. 1, pp. 21–31, 2003.

[42] C. C. Wrenn, "Unit 8.5G Social transmission of food preference in mice," *Current Protocols in Neuroscience*, 2004.

[43] B. G. Galef and E. E. Whiskin, "Socially transmitted food preferences can be used to study long-term memory in rats," *Animal Learning & Behavior*, vol. 31, no. 2, pp. 160–164, 2003.

[44] J. Bonaccorsi, S. Cintoli, R. Mastrogiacomo et al., "System consolidation of spatial memories in mice: effects of enriched environment," *Neural Plasticity*, vol. 2013, Article ID 956312, 12 pages, 2013.

[45] J. P. Aggleton and M. W. Brown, "Contrasting hippocampal and perirhinalcortex function using immediate early gene imaging," *Quarterly Journal of Experimental Psychology*, vol. 58, no. 3-4b, pp. 218–233, 2005.

[46] R. Melani, G. Chelini, M. C. Cenni, and N. Berardi, "Enriched environment effects on remote object recognition memory," *Neuroscience*, vol. 352, pp. 296–305, 2017.

[47] A. S. Zannas, J. H. Kim, and A. E. West, "Regulation and function of MeCP2 Ser 421 phosphorylation in U50488-induced conditioned place aversion in mice," *Psychopharmacology*, vol. 234, no. 6, pp. 913–923, 2017.

[48] J. M. Stratford, J. A. Thompson, and T. E. Finger, "Immunocytochemical organization and sour taste activation in the rostral nucleus of the solitary tract of mice," *The Journal of Comparative Neurology*, vol. 525, no. 2, pp. 271–290, 2017.

[49] J. Y. Joo, K. Schaukowitch, L. Farbiak, G. Kilaru, and T. K. Kim, "Stimulus-specific combinatorial functionality of neuronal c-fos enhancers," *Nature Neuroscience*, vol. 19, no. 1, pp. 75–83, 2016.

[50] R. P. Haberman, M. T. Koh, and M. Gallagher, "Heightened cortical excitability in aged rodents with memory impairment," *Neurobiology of Aging*, vol. 54, pp. 144–151, 2017.

[51] M. Korte and D. Schmitz, "Cellular and system biology of memory: timing, molecules, and beyond," *Physiological Reviews*, vol. 96, no. 2, pp. 647–693, 2016.

[52] P. W. Frankland and B. Bontempi, "The organization of recent and remote memories," *Nature Reviews Neuroscience*, vol. 6, no. 2, pp. 119–130, 2005.

[53] S. Peleg, F. Sananbenesi, A. Zovoilis et al., "Altered histone acetylation is associated with age-dependent memory impairment in mice," *Science*, vol. 328, no. 5979, pp. 753–756, 2010.

[54] P. W. Frankland, B. Bontempi, L. E. Talton, L. Kaczmarek, and A. J. Silva, "The involvement of the anterior cingulate cortex in remote contextual fear memory," *Science*, vol. 304, no. 5672, pp. 881–883, 2004.

[55] P. W. Frankland, C. O'Brien, M. Ohno, A. Kirkwood, and A. J. Silva, "Alpha-CaMKII-dependent plasticity in the cortex is required for permanent memory," *Nature*, vol. 411, no. 6835, pp. 309–313, 2001.

[56] O. Bousiges, A. P. Vasconcelos, R. Neidl et al., "Spatial memory consolidation is associated with induction of several lysine-acetyltransferase (histone acetyltransferase) expression levels and H2B/H4 acetylation-dependent transcriptional events in the rat hippocampus," *Neuropsychopharmacology*, vol. 35, no. 13, pp. 2521–2537, 2010.

15

Testing rTMS-Induced Neuroplasticity: A Single Case Study of Focal Hand Dystonia

Sonia Betti,[1] **Andrea Spoto,**[1] **Umberto Castiello,**[1,2] **and Luisa Sartori** [ID][1,3]

[1]*Dipartimento di Psicologia Generale, Università di Padova, Padova, Italy*
[2]*Centro Beniamino Segre, Accademia Nazionale dei Lincei, Roma, Italy*
[3]*Centro di Neuroscienze Cognitive, Università di Padova, Padova, Italy*

Correspondence should be addressed to Luisa Sartori; luisa.sartori@unipd.it

Academic Editor: Toshiyuki Fujiwara

Focal hand dystonia in musicians is a neurological motor disorder in which aberrant plasticity is caused by excessive repetitive use. This work's purposes were to induce plasticity changes in a dystonic musician through five daily thirty-minute sessions of 1 Hz repetitive transcranial magnetic stimulation (rTMS) applied to the left M1 by using neuronavigated stimulation and to reliably measure the effect of these changes. To this aim, the relationship between neuroplasticity changes and motor recovery was investigated using fine-grained kinematic analysis. Our results suggest a statistically significant improvement in motor coordination both in a task resembling the dystonic-inducing symptoms and in a reach-to-grasp task. This single case study supports the safe and effective use of noninvasive brain stimulation in neurologic patients and highlights the importance of evaluating outcomes in measurable ways. This issue is a key aspect to focus on to classify the clinical expression of dystonia. These preliminary results promote the adoption of kinematic analysis as a valuable diagnostic tool.

1. Introduction

Dystonias are a group of disorders characterized by intermittent or sustained muscle contractions causing twisting and repetitive movements (for a review, see [1, 2]). The crucial catalyst behind dystonia is a multifactorial combination of excessive plasticity, intensive training, and failure of limiting plastic changes, as seen through noninvasive neurostimulation studies [3]. Once this abnormal plasticity process is brought under control, it could ultimately result in a clinical improvement [4].

Dystonia may be task-specific producing abnormal motor performance for only a specific task, such as in musician's dystonia (MD). MD affects isolated fingers that perform complex and repetitive motor tasks during actions associated with musical play, but can also lead to impaired adjacent finger flexion [2]. This overflow into adjacent muscles not specifically involved in the particular motor task is due to a loss of inhibition that manifests in the periphery with abnormally long muscle bursts [5]. In MD, abnormally prolonged muscle firing due to selective overtraining of an intended finger may prevent the ability to keep excitability within a useable range (i.e., homeostatic plasticity), a function which is specifically impaired in dystonia [6].

Although its underlying pathophysiology remains unclear, several studies in patients with MD have shown that repeated and prolonged hand use might result in abnormal activity in the cortical representation of the hand [7, 8]. In fact, important neural correlates of task-specific dystonia are the enlarged and partially overlapping fields revealed by brain imaging and transcranial magnetic stimulation (TMS) studies targeting the somatosensory and the motor cortices [8–14]. Whereas a typical homuncular organization reveals a distance of about 2.5 cm between the representations of the thumb and the little finger, these boundaries seem to be blurred for the dystonic fingers [10]. This lack of clearly defined somatosensory and motor cortical representations can lead to involuntary motor control [15]. The loss of control is particularly evident during fast passages, often leading to involuntary flexion or extension of one or more fingers [16]. In particular, stringed instrument players exhibit a use-dependent alteration in the cortical representational zones of the digits of the hand that engage in the dexterity-demanding task of fingering the strings [17]. While initial MD is only associated with impairment of highly practiced motor tasks, it can subsequently lead to severe deficits, eventually terminating a career for one percent of professional musicians [18].

Although prompt initiation of treatment could rescue some patients, dystonia is often misdiagnosed or neglected since the lack of objective diagnostic criteria and reliable biomarkers prohibits early diagnostic recognition [19]. So far, the extent of motor symptoms has mainly been estimated by means of visual inspection and rating procedures (e.g., [20]), without providing fine resolution (but see [21] for an example of kinematic analysis to assess a flautist performance). In addition, treatment responses are very patient-dependent. A precise quantification tool for objective and reliable diagnosis and for treatment evaluation is therefore needed to acquire highly precise data and to identify subtle differences in the symptomatology.

Given the sparse literature on this topic, there are no clinical practice guidelines on how to recover voluntary motor control. To date, the preferred treatment for dystonia is botulinum toxin injection, but it only transiently works in a minor fraction of patients and its application is limited by the spread of weakness to adjacent muscles, which causes further motor performance impairment [22].

Recently, motor training has been combined with neurostimulation methods in an attempt to normalize brain excitability and recover motor performance [23, 24]. Notably, since the effects of long-term treatment might differ from those of a single session [24], TMS is usually delivered in repeated daily sessions to prolong after effects. Therapeutic procedures with dystonic patients classically adopted daily sessions of low-frequency repetitive TMS (rTMS) over the primary motor cortex (M1; [5, 25–28]) or the premotor cortex (PM; [24, 29, 30]). Siebner and colleagues [25, 26] evaluated the effect of low-frequency (1 Hz) stimulation of M1 to increase inhibition in the motor areas of the cerebral cortex. Low-frequency rTMS set to 10% below the resting motor threshold of the target muscle restored intracortical inhibition. Treatment output on handwriting was quantified by means of a pressure-sensitive digitizing tablet.

Needless to say, the principle of the measurement must be based on the phenomenology of each patient. Motor assessment must be specifically related to the compromised movement (i.e., the particular exercise that most consistently induced the dystonic disorder), rather than to a more general skill (e.g., [21, 31]). As Pujol and colleagues (2000) convincingly demonstrated in an fMRI study, a tailored assessment of patients in the dystonia-inducing situation is necessary [8].

The aim of the present study was to test a multimethodological paradigm based on the combination of single-pulse transcranial magnetic stimulation (spTMS), low-frequency rTMS, and 3D motion analysis in a professional guitarist affected by MD. Single pulses of TMS were used to assess the excitability of synaptic connections within the motor cortex, providing indirect measures of changes produced by neural plasticity. In addition, TMS can also produce long-term changes in excitability if the TMS pulses are applied

repetitively [27]. In both cases, changes in excitability were monitored by computing the amplitude of the motor-evoked potential (MEP) in response to a standard TMS pulse. In particular, resting motor threshold MEPs reflect the degree of corticospinal system activation and potentially help in diagnosing motor symptoms and in monitoring treatment progress (i.e., whether interventions are safe and effective in slowing symptoms). Fine-grained 3D movement analysis has been adopted to specifically evaluate the treatment both in terms of improved motor coordination and cortical plasticity. The acquisition of MEPs induced by spTMS to the left M1 and recorded from the contralateral second dorsal interosseous (SDI) muscle before and after five daily sessions of rTMS protocol allowed to measure the variations on the resting motor threshold to obtain a physiological index of *neural plasticity*. Moreover, we considered two behavioral measures of *performance plasticity*: (i) a repetitive sequence of fingers' movement (task 1) and (ii) a reach-to-grasp action (task 2). Since guitar arpeggios involve a rapid succession of fine and isolated finger movements, the finger flexion task was conceived as a realistic attempt to execute the affected flexion pattern. As concerns the grip task, it was specifically chosen to investigate the distinct contribution of the two separate reaching and grasping components [32] on performed movements: the timing dissociation between these two components may in fact give useful hints to the underlying pathological state [33, 34]. Notably, problems to grasp and manipulate objects are frequent in movement disorders and a methodological approach providing highly standardized measures of natural movements is needed [35]. The outputs of both tasks were compared at local and general levels: across daily sessions and throughout the intervention, to provide a consistent measure of plasticity trend.

2. Method

2.1. Participants. A 55-year-old male right-handed classical guitarist (M.C.) diagnosed as suffering from MD in his right hand was recruited at the Neuroscience of Movement (NEMO) Laboratory at the Department of General Psychology, University of Padua. He specifically presented a painless and exaggerated involuntary flexion pattern in his right middle finger's metacarpophalangeal joint, which occurred exclusively in the task-specific context of playing the musical instrument (i.e., plucking the strings). The loss of synergistic muscle control was also evident as a cocontraction of adjacent muscles. The onset of the movement disorder had been three years before this study and had forced him to interrupt his career as a professional musician and especially as a concert performer. He reported no dystonic movement patterns in other activities. There was no evidence of any other neurologic disorder and he was not under medication. An additional guitarist served as control subject in this study. He was right-handed with comparable experience (40 years of practice) and age (50 years).

No adverse effects were reported during the experiment. Informed consent was obtained after they were fully informed, according to the Declaration of Helsinki, about

Daily experimental design

Prestimulation		Stimulation	Poststimulation	
Kinematic baseline (KB)	Neurophysiologic baseline (NB)	1 Hz rTMS (30 min)	Neurophysiologic test (NT)	Kinematic test (KT)
Task 1 Task 2	rMT		rMT	Task 1 Task 2

Time

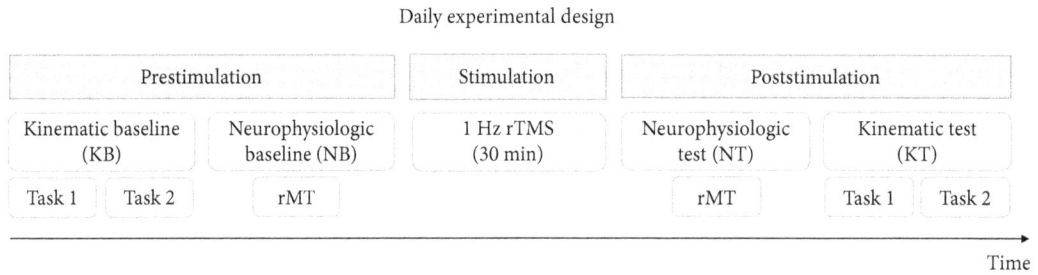

FIGURE 1: Daily experimental design for both MD patient and control participant. The graph represents the three daily phases of the experiment: behavioral and neurophysiological indexes were measured both before (prestimulation) and after (poststimulation) each stimulation session with low-frequency rTMS (1 Hz) on the left M1 (stimulation). The kinematic behavioral assessment (KB and KT) consisted of two tasks: finger abduction (task 1) and reach-to-grasp (task 2). In the neurophysiological assessment (NB and NT), the resting motor threshold was measured to assess corticospinal excitability variations. This protocol was repeated for five consecutive days.

the study's nature. The experimental protocol was approved by the University of Padua Ethics Review Board.

2.2. General Procedure. A daily protocol (Figure 1) entailing two evaluation sessions (prestimulation) of kinematic and resting motor threshold (rMT) baselines, followed by low-frequency rTMS (stimulation) and kinematic and rMT tests (poststimulation), was repeated for five consecutive days and was designed as follows:

(1) Prestimulation kinematic baseline (KB). A series of alternating finger flexion movements (i.e., the index, middle, and ring fingers, 15 movements per finger; task 1) with the palm upward and a sequence of 15 reach-to-grasp movements (task 2) were performed to test independent movements of the dystonic finger and motor coordination.

(2) Prestimulation neurophysiologic baseline (NB). TMS-induced motor-evoked potentials (MEPs) were recorded from the right second dorsal interosseous (SDI) muscle to measure the rMT, thus assessing corticospinal excitability before intervention.

(3) Stimulation. The participant underwent 30 minutes of rTMS (1 Hz) over the SDI muscle representation on the left primary motor cortex, delivered with intensity of 90% with respect to the rMT.

(4) Poststimulation neurophysiologic test (NT). The same procedure adopted during the prestimulation NB session was implemented for comparison purposes. We performed a trend analysis to evaluate changes in motor cortex plasticity.

(5) Poststimulation kinematic test (KT). The same procedure adopted during preintervention KB session was implemented for comparison purposes. We performed a day-by-day analysis and we compared the first and last day to evaluate both short- and long-term effects in motor coordination.

2.3. Kinematics Recording. A 3D optoelectronic SMART-D system (Bioengineering Technology and Systems, BTS) was

used to track the kinematics of the participants' right hand. During the KB and KT phases, the participants were seated in a height-adjustable chair in front of a table (900 mm × 900 mm) with the right hand placed on a designated position on the table surface so as to guarantee the consistency of the start position across participants. Three semispherical infrared-reflective markers (5 mm diameter) were attached to the right hand on the tip of the index, middle, and ring fingers, and one was attached to the radial aspect of the wrist. Six digital video cameras with a frequency of 140 Hz were placed in a semicircle around the table (at 1–1.2 m away) to detect the markers (see Figure 2(a)). Before the experimental sessions, cameras position, roll angle, focus, zoom, brightness, and threshold were adjusted to optimize markers' tracking. Static and dynamic calibrations were then performed. For the static calibration, a three-axis frame of reference at known distance was placed on the center of the table. For the dynamic calibration, a three-marker wand was moved in all directions throughout the workspace of interest for approximately one minute. The spatial resolution of the recording system was 0.3 mm over the field of view. The standard deviation (SD) of the reconstruction error was below 0.2 mm for all the axes (x, y, and z).

During each daily session of the KB and KT phases, the participants took part in two tasks:

(i) Task 1: A series of 45 randomly alternating finger flexion movements of the index, middle, and ring fingers (15 movements per finger) were performed to test independent movements of the dystonic and adjacent fingers. The participants' right wrists were placed over a wooden cylinder (7.5 mm diameter; 11 cm high) with the palm of the hand facing upwards.

(ii) Task 2: In the prehension task, a sequence of 15 reach-to-grasp movements was performed to test motor coordination. At the beginning of each trial, the hand was pronated with the palm resting on a starting platform (60 × 70 mm; 5 mm thick), which was shaped to allow for a comfortable and repeatable posture of all digits, that is, slightly flexed at the

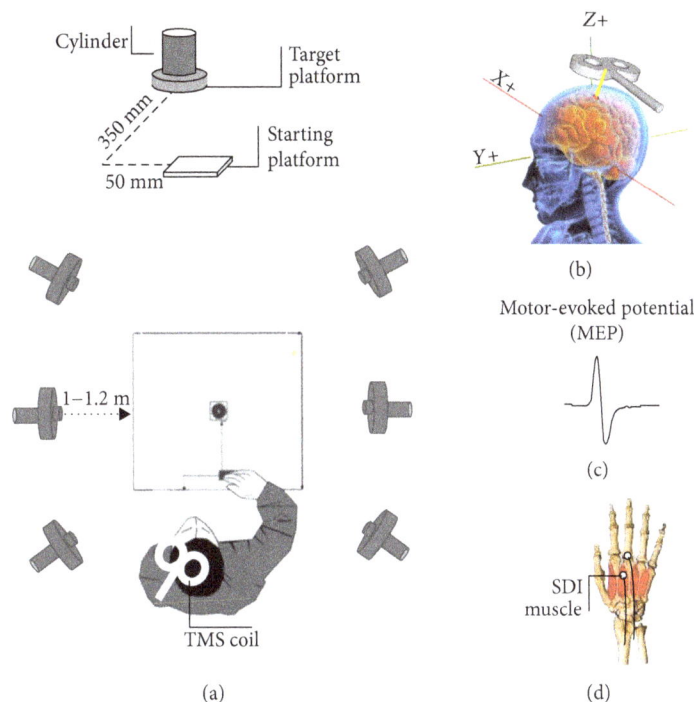

FIGURE 2: Experiment setup. A 3D optoelectronic SMART-D system was used to track the kinematics of the participant's right hand by means of six video cameras (a). TMS coil placement over the participant's left M1 hand area (b). Example of a TMS-evoked MEP (c). The targeted second dorsal interosseous (SDI) muscle (d).

metacarpal and proximal interphalangeal joints. Then, the participants were asked to reach and grasp the cylinder located frontally with a whole hand grasp (WHG). The starting platform was attached 90 mm away from the edge of the table surface 50 mm away from the midsection. The cylinder was placed on a target platform, located at a distance of 350 mm from the starting platform, for consistent replacing (Figure 2(a)). An affixed colored dot on the cylinder was signaling the required thumb's contact point in order to perform stable and consistent grasps across the experiment. An auditory signal (300 Hz; 200 ms) was adopted as the "go" signal.

2.4. Transcranial Magnetic Stimulation and Electromyographic Recording.
During both the MB and the MT phases, each participant was comfortably seated in an armchair with the right hand positioned on a pillow and the head kept stable by a neck pillow. The participant was asked to keep his muscles relaxed and to remain as still as possible during the delivery of the TMS pulses. While TMS pulses were delivered, he was asked to observe a white fixation cross on black background presented in the center of a monitor. TMS-induced MEPs were acquired from the participant's SDI muscle of the right hand (Figure 2(c)). EMG activity was recorded through pairs of surface Ag-AgCl surface electrodes (9 mm diameter) placed in a belly-tendon montage, with the active electrodes over the SDI muscle and the reference electrodes over the corresponding metacarpophalangeal joint (Figure 2(d)). The ground electrode was placed over the dorsal part of the right wrist. Electrodes were connected to an

isolable portable ExG input box linked to the main EMG amplifier for signal transmission via a twin fiber optic cable (Professional BrainAmp ExG MR, Munich, Germany). Single-pulse TMS was administered using a 70 mm figure-of-eight coil connected to a Magstim Bistim^2 stimulator (Magstim Co., Whitland, UK). Pulses were delivered to the hand region of the left M1. The coil was placed tangentially on the scalp, with the handle pointing laterally and caudally, so that the flow of induced electrical current in the brain travelled in a posterior-anterior direction [36, 37]. During the first session of the first day, the optimal cortical hotspot of the target muscle (OSP; i.e., the position at which larger and more stable MEPs are recorded from SDI with minimal stimulation intensity) was identified by delivering single TMS pulses at fixed intensity while moving the coil of 0.5 cm around the target area until the position was reached. To maintain an accurate and constant placement of the coil throughout the experimental sessions, it was kept over the OSP by a mechanical arm (Manfrotto, Italy) and its position and orientation were recorded and loaded into a neuronavigation system (SofTaxic Optic, EMS, Bologna, Italy; Figure 2(b)). Once the OSP was found, the individual resting motor threshold (rMT)—defined as the lowest stimulus intensity at which TMS is able to generate MEPs of at least 50 μV in relaxed muscles in 5 out of 10 consecutive pulses [38]—was determined. rMT was then measured every day before and after the rTMS protocol to test possible variations of corticospinal excitability. Repetitive TMS pulses were applied using a Magstim Rapid^2 stimulator (Magstim Co., Whitland, UK) with a figure-of-eight coil (70 mm outer diameter). Each rTMS session consisted of the application of off-line, low-frequency 1 Hz TMS for 30 min (1800 total pulses) at 90% of each participant's rMT. Both spTMS and rTMS were delivered on the side of the brain contralateral to the participant's dominant (and dystonia-affected) hand.

3. Data Analysis

3.1. Behavioral Measures. Following kinematic data collection, each trial was individually checked for correct marker identification and then run through a low-pass Butterworth filter with a 6 Hz cutoff. The SMART-D Tracker software package (Bioengineering Technology and Systems, BTS) was employed to reconstruct the 3D marker positions as a function of time. In task 1, the amplitude of maximum 3D distance between the dystonic fingertip and adjacent fingers (i.e., index and ring tips) was calculated as an index of abduction independence (AI). The amplitude of minimum distance between the dystonic finger and wrist was calculated as an index of abduction degree (AD) and compared to adjacent fingers' AD (see [21] for a similar approach). In task 2, we selected a set of standard measures universally reported in the literature for reach-to-grasp tasks, possibly enabling a productive comparison of results across participants (MD; control) and across experiments. We first computed movement onset (i.e., the first time point at which the wrist velocity crossed a 5 mm/sec threshold and remained above it for longer than 100 ms) and time of grip offset (i.e., the time at which the grip velocity dropped below a 5 mm/s threshold). Then, the following indexes were measured:

(i) Movement time (i.e., the time interval between onset and offset)

(ii) Maximum grip aperture (MGA, the maximum distance reached by the 3D coordinates of the thumb and index finger)

(iii) Time of maximum grip aperture (TMGA, the time at which the distance between the 3D coordinates of the thumb and index finger was maximum from movement onset)

(iv) Time of maximum grip velocity (TMGV, the time at which the tangential velocity of the 3D coordinates of the thumb and index finger was maximum from movement onset)

(v) Time of maximum wrist height (TMWH, the time at which the 3D coordinates of the wrist were maximum from movement onset)

(vi) Time of maximum wrist deceleration (TMWD, the time at which the deceleration of the 3D coordinates of the wrist was maximum from movement onset)

(vii) Delay grasping (DG, the time interval between the onset of the wrist movement and the onset of fingers' opening)

3.2. Neurophysiological Measures. Motor threshold at rest before (rMT pre) and after (rMT post) rTMS 1 Hz stimulation was evaluated in both MD and control participants.

3.3. Statistical Analyses. Behavioral data were analyzed using the R 3.3.9 statistical package [39]. More specifically, data were analyzed by means of an ad hoc function developed to implement the computation of the Young C test statistics [40]. This test, proposed by Young and Von Neumann, is used to evaluate the presence of a trend into a sequence of data collected on the same subject. It computes the probability that a sequence of data points follows a random, nonoriented distribution. If this probability is low, then the presence of some sort of either increasing or decreasing trend in the data can be argued. More specifically, the C test statistic is computed according to the following formula:

$$C = 1 - \frac{\sum_{i=1}^{N-1}(x_i - x_{i+1})^2}{2\sum_{i=1}^{N-1}(x_i - \bar{x})^2}, \tag{1}$$

where N is the number of observations; x_i and $\bar{x}$ are the average values of the observations. The value of C tends to increase as an inverse function of the ratio between the squared difference of each data point to its subsequent and the squared difference of each point to the mean. The smaller the ratio, the higher the C, the higher the probability that the data do follow some sort of oriented trend (Figure 3).

Given these premises, data analysis was carried out on the two different tasks. More specifically, with respect to task 1, a comparison between the trend of values obtained during the first and the last day of training was carried out separately for the data collected before (pre) and after (post) the administration of the rTMS protocol. Moreover, an analysis of the overall trend along all the five days of training was conducted. This analysis was carried out separately for the pre- and post-rTMS phases and for the variables measured in task 2. A pointwise difference (delta) between the values obtained at the pre- and post-rTMS phases has been computed in order to highlight the presence of any particular daily pattern. As concerns motor threshold at rest, the presence of a significant trend before (rMT pre) and after (rMT post) rTMS 1 Hz stimulation was evaluated by means of the test C in both MD and control participants.

4. Results

4.1. Behavioral Plasticity

4.1.1. Task 1: Finger Flexion Task. The main reference point of the analysis was the movement involving the middle finger. In the MD post phase, a significant increasing trend in the distance between the dystonia-affected finger and the index finger (AI) was observed on the first day of training ($C = .66$; $p < .01$). The evaluation of the overall trend showed that the measures collected throughout all the five days followed a significantly increasing trend ($C = .87$; $p < .01$). Reverse considerations can be referred to the pre-rTMS measures: a significantly increasing trend was not observed at the first day of training ($C = .20$; n.s.); however, the data collected the last day presented a significantly increasing trend ($C = .54$; $p < .05$); the overall trend was significantly increasing ($C = .81$; $p < .01$). Figure 4 shows the increasing

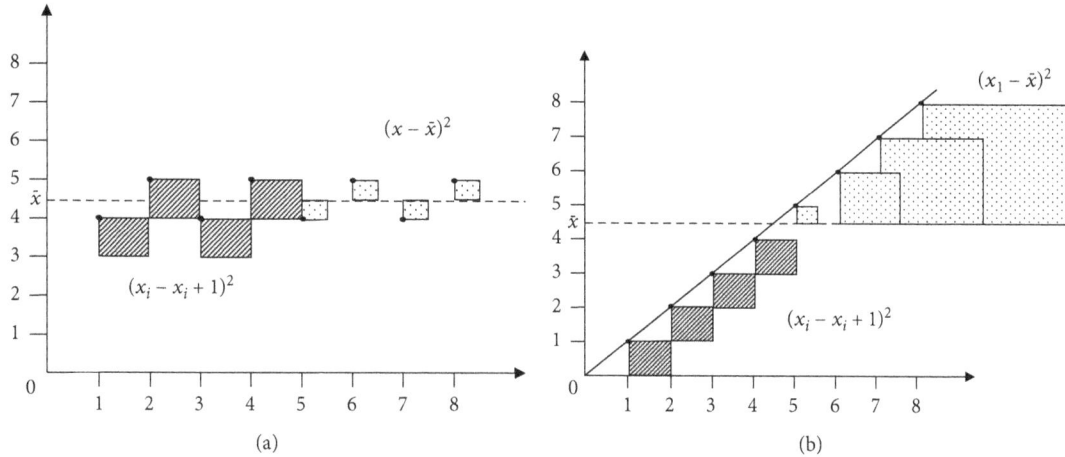

FIGURE 3: Graphical representation of the squared difference between (i) each data point and its subsequent value in the series (lined squares) and (ii) each data point and the average of the series (dotted squares) in the case of an oriented trend (a) and in the case of stationary data (b).

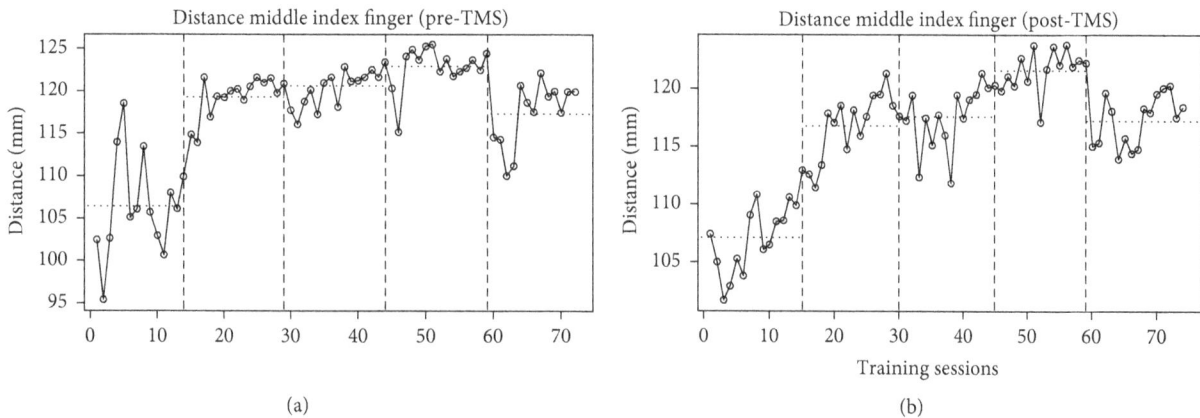

FIGURE 4: Graphical representation of the trend observed at the pre-rTMS (a) and post-rTMS (b) phases for the distance between the middle and index fingers when the former was flexed.

trend of this measure during the five days of training both at the pre-rTMS phase (a) and at the post-rTMS phase (b).

The same analysis conducted for the distance between the middle finger and the ring finger shows slightly different results. More specifically, while for the post measures the trend observed on the first day was significant (post: $C = .62$; $p < .01$), the measures collected in the pre phase did not show any trend (pre: $C = .33$; n.s.). Moreover, none of the trends were significant in the last days of training (day 5; post: $C = .40$; n.s.; pre: $C = .06$; n.s.). On the other hand, both the overall trends resulted significant (post: $C = .65$; $p < .01$; pre: $C = .64$; $p < .01$), showing an overall increase of the distance between the two fingers throughout the protocol. As concerns the control conditions (i.e., flexion of the adjacent fingers), no significantly increasing trend was observed in the distance between the index finger and the middle finger either at the first day of the training (pre: $C = .30$; n.s.; post: $C = .37$; n.s.) or at the last day (pre: $C = .32$; n.s.; post: $C = .33$; n.s.) when the index finger was flexed. Moreover, the overall analysis showed a significant trend in the pre-rTMS phase ($C = .57$; $p < .01$) while no effect was found in the post ($C = .37$; n.s.). The same results emerged from the analysis of the distance between the index finger

and the ring finger when the former was flexed. More precisely no significant trend was observed neither at the first day of the training phases (pre: $C = .28$; n.s.; post: $C = .01$; n.s.) or at the last day of training (pre: $C = .60$; n.s.; post: $C = .03$; n.s.). The overall analysis showed a significant trend in the pre-TMS phase ($C = .62$; $p < .01$) while no effect was found in the post ($C = .37$; n.s.). Finally, when the ring finger was flexed only, some of the overall trends were significantly increasing, namely, the distance between the ring finger and the index finger in the pre-rTMS phase ($C = .75$; $p < .01$) and the distance between the ring finger and the middle finger in both phases (pre: $C = .78$; $p < .01$; post: $C = .85$; $p < .01$). No significant overall trend was observed for the distance between the ring finger and the index finger during the post-rTMS phase ($C = .40$; n.s.). In terms of the middle finger abduction degree, a significant decreasing trend was observed the first day of training at the post-TMS phase ($C = .69$; $p < .01$). Moreover, both the overall trends were strong and significantly decreasing (pre: $C = .71$; $p < .01$; post: $C = .67$; $p < .01$). For the index finger AD, no significant trend was observed during the first day of training either at the pre- or post-TMS phases; similarly, no significant trend was observed the last day of the training. On the contrary, both the overall trends were significantly decreasing (pre: $C = .68$; $p < .01$; post: $C = .58$; $p < .01$). Finally, only the overall trends were significantly decreasing when considering the distance between the wrist and the ring finger (pre: $C = .82$; $p < .01$; post: $C = .84$; $p < .01$). When considering the control participant, data from day 1 were discarded due to a technical problem. Results showed no significant overall trend when the middle finger, the index finger, and the ring finger were moved. Such stable trends were observed in both the pre-TMS and post-TMS phases.

4.1.2. Task 2: Reach-to-Grasp Task. Several variables were considered during task 2. For such variables, the analysis was conducted by referring to the data collected throughout the five days of training before (pre) and after (post) the TMS stimulation. The results obtained from the selected kinematic variables in MD participant are reported as follows.

Movement time: A significantly decreasing trend was observed for the measures collected both pre-rTMS stimulation ($C = .73$; $p < .01$) and post-rTMS stimulation ($C = .62$; $p < .01$).

Maximum grip aperture: A significantly increasing trend was observed for the measures collected before the stimulation ($C = .64$; $p < .01$). No significant trend was observed for the measures collected after the rTMS ($C = .30$; n.s.).

Time of maximum grip aperture: Two clearly and significantly decreasing trends were observed for this variable. The first one involved the measures collected before the rTMS ($C = .79$; $p < .01$), while the second one involved the measures collected after the stimulation ($C = .62$; $p < .01$).

Time to maximum grip velocity: A clearly significant decreasing trend was observed for the data series collected before the TMS ($C = .72$; $p < .01$). The trend observed for the data series collected after the stimulation was significant, although more noisy ($C = .43$; $p < .01$).

Time of maximum wrist height: A significantly decreasing trend was observed at both the pre-rTMS ($C = .74$; $p < .01$) and the post-rTMS ($C = .69$; $p < .01$) phases.

Time of maximum wrist deceleration: With respect to this variable, a significant although very noisy decreasing trend was observed at both the pre-TMS measures ($C = .49$; $p < .01$) and the post-TMS ones ($C = .50$; $p < .01$).

Delay grasping: A significant decreasing trend was observed for this variable for the measures collected both pre-rTMS stimulation ($C = .57$; $p < .01$) and post-rTMS stimulation ($C = .57$; $p < .01$).

Figure 5 displays the trend of the pointwise delta computed for the main variables measured in task 2. It is noticeable the increase of the negative difference between the pre and the post measures during the first day of training, while an increase in the positive difference between the same values is observed during the second day of training. After these days, the difference tends to remain stable.

As concerns the control participant, no trend resulted statistically significant ($p_s > 0.05$). Figure 6 displays together the trends for the MD patient and the control participant. By the figure, it is clearly seen the difference of the two trends in the movement time variable. Similar results were observed for the remaining variables of task 2.

4.2. Neurophysiological Measures. No significant trend was observed in motor threshold at rest before (rMT pre) and after (rMT post) rTMS 1 Hz stimulation for either the MD ($C = .07$; n.s.; see Table 1) or the control ($C = .17$; n.s.; see Table 1) participant.

5. Conclusions

We set out to investigate neural plasticity in a professional guitarist affected by MD through a multimethodological paradigm. To this end, we combined spTMS, low-frequency rTMS, and 3D motion analysis. Results showed that although rTMS on M1 partially modulated resting motor threshold, a systematic normalization of various kinematic indexes during the 5-day treatment occurred for the MD participant. In particular, as concerns abduction independence, a significant increase in the distance between the dystonia-affected finger and the index and ring fingers was observed on the first day of training during the post-TMS session. The trend significantly increased throughout the five days, showing an overall increase of the distance between the fingers. These data were further confirmed by the distance between the affected finger and the wrist: a decreasing distance (abduction degree) was observed both on the first day of training during the post-TMS session and throughout the treatment's period. These results point to the presence of both a short-term and a long-term trend in the affected finger and not to a general effect of practice.

As regards the reach-to-grasp task, an increase in general motor coordination was hypothesized for the MD participant throughout the five days of training. No significant trend was instead expected for the control participant, since there was no room for improvement (ceiling effect). Results showed an increase in motor coordination only for the MD participant, as indexed by a significant decrease in the movement time. In terms of the reaching component, the time of maximum wrist height and the time of maximum wrist deceleration were anticipated, in line with previous studies demonstrating a significant anticipation when an object is approached more carefully (e.g., [41, 42]). For the grasping component, the amplitude of the maximum grip aperture revealed an increasing pattern of accuracy—as indexed by an appropriate finger scaling—throughout the 5-day training. The time of maximum grip aperture, the time of maximum grip velocity, and the delay grasping were anticipated as well as for the reaching parameters, indicating a temporal coupling between the reaching and the grasping components. These results are consistent with human literature suggesting that task constraints can modulate the proximal and distal components of a coordinated action. The failure to reduce variability as the target is being approached calls for coordination strategies amongst components, which might serve to partially dissipate errors [43].

An intriguing hypothesis points to a malfunctioning in the parietal-premotor pathway of dystonic patients [44]. Parietal-premotor connections are specialized for specific tasks, for example, reach-to-grasp movements, having separate pathways for each of the two components (i.e., reaching and grasping; [45]). Thus, a task-specific deficit

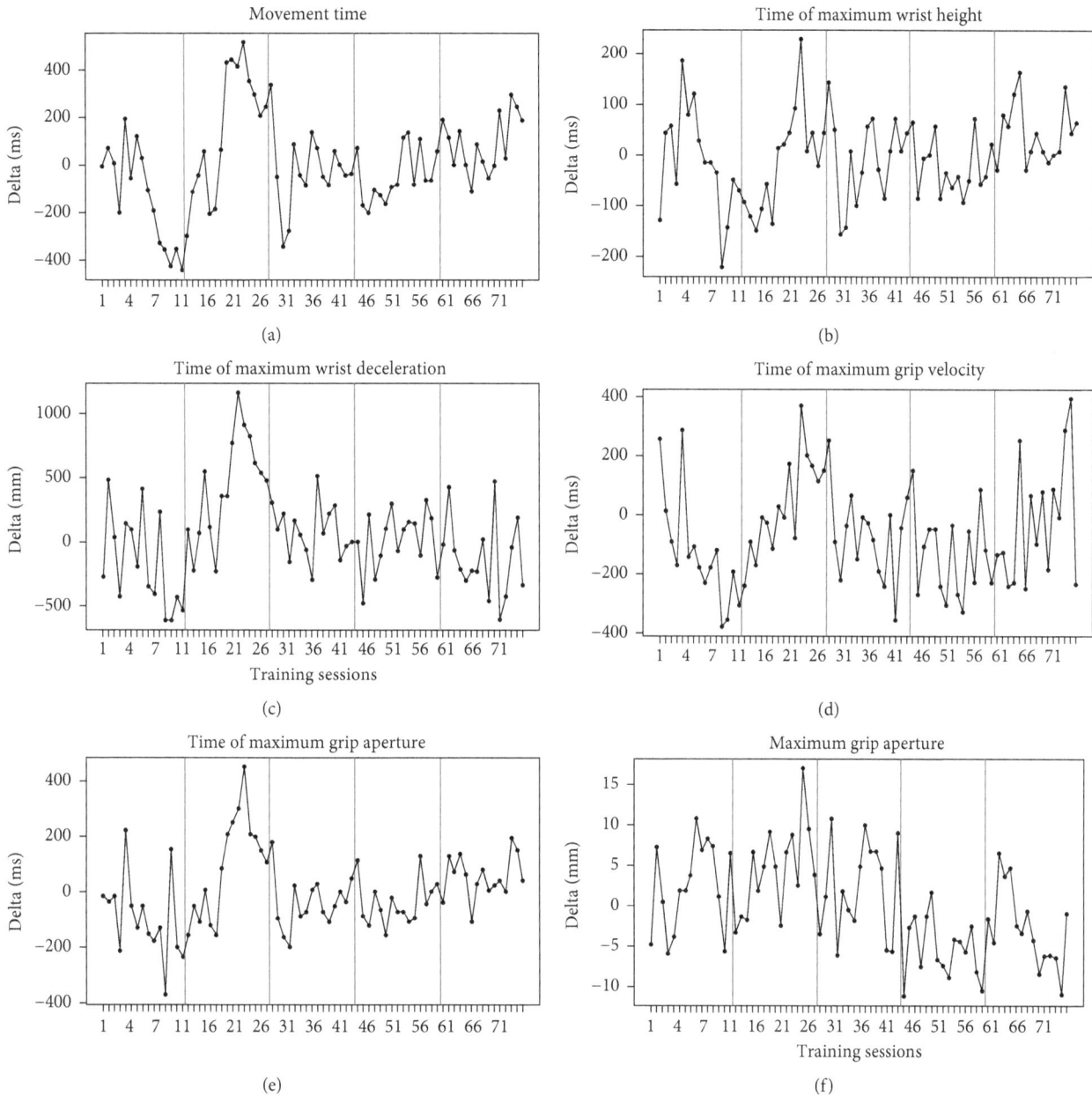

FIGURE 5: Pointwise delta between the measures, for the main variables of task 2, obtained at pre- and post-rTMS phases by the MD patient. Parameters referring to the reaching component are listed on (a), (b), and (c), whereas parameters for the grasping component are displayed on (d), (e), and (f).

could arise from the combination of excessive motor repetition of a particular task, together with disordered control of neural plasticity in the pathway where that specific task was learned [2]. Based on this hypothesis, we might suggest that future behavioral interventions should be based on restoring specific motor pathways through plasticity processes [22].

Notably, an initial positive outcome was observed during the post-TMS session of day 1, when all the parameters jointly showed a significant improvement. This effect, however, was neutralized and reversed during the post-TMS session of day 2, which was then followed by a stabilization phase for the remaining three days. The convergent

oscillation of all these parameters seems to indicate that rTMS inhibitory stimulation might be beneficial in the very short term, but it provides a stable advantage only in the course of a 5-day training. This result might suggest that it takes many days of intervention to rebalance motor activity.

Overall, these results suggest that kinematic assessments of abduction independence, abduction degree, and reaching and grasping components are useful parameters for objective quantification of MD before and after training. Moreover, the reach-to-grasp task might allow studying situations similar to those participants facing in their daily life motor activities. This points to the effectiveness of assessing kinematics in conjunction with individual clinical scores such as the Arm

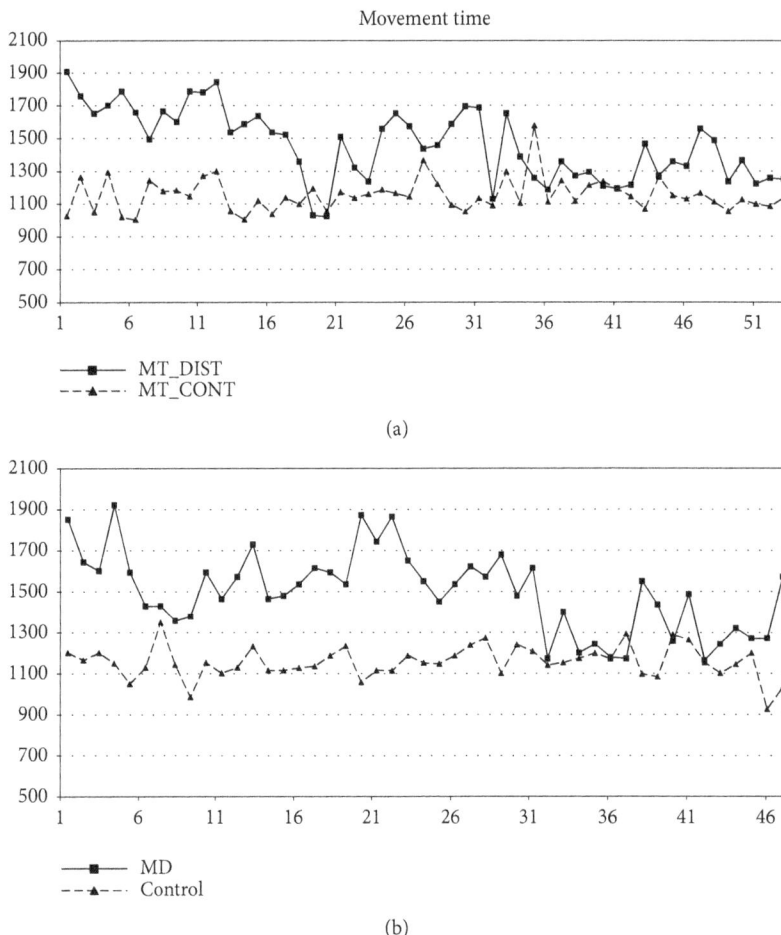

Figure 6: MD and control participant trends on the movement time (task 2).

Table 1: Resting motor threshold variations throughout the five-day protocol, before (rMT pre) and after (rMT post) the rTMS 1 Hz stimulation at the 90 percent of the rMT.

		Day 1	Day 2	Day 3	Day 4	Day 5
MD	rMT pre	43	43	43	44	44
	rMT post	46	44	46	46	46
Control	rMT pre	43	50	44	52	42
	rMT post	48	60	50	53	56

Dystonia Disability Scale (ADDS). Although they probe different aspects of motor impairment and might not correlate with each other [46], they should both be used to supplement the clinical diagnosis for monitoring the treatment and to assess the effectiveness of rehabilitation.

In neural terms, no trend was observed when considering rMT. This is a counterintuitive—though not rare—output. Veugen and colleagues [47] recently found that inhibition of the overactive dorsal premotor cortex partially recovered dystonic symptomatology despite having no influence on surround inhibition (i.e., the mechanism in the motor system which focuses neuronal activity to select the execution of the desired movement; [48]), as indexed by MEP sizes. In particular, stimulation improved writing performance in patients,

though there was no significant effect on rMT in either dystonic or control participants.

In this respect, the study described here highlights the importance of evaluating brain stimulation outcomes in a more systematic way, beyond classical measures of neural plasticity such as MEP size. The cause of MD is obscure, but a loss of inhibition in the central nervous system and a loss of the normal regulation of plasticity are classically reported [49–51]. Plasticity generally refers to the ability of the nervous system to change the effectiveness of transmission in neural circuits [3]. An increase of sensory and motor finger representations in musicians is usually described as an adaptive plastic change to conform to the new needs. However, when this change develops too far, brain plasticity might shift from a benefit to a maladaptive mechanism [52]. On the basis of this abnormal plasticity hypothesis, new treatment protocols have been designed aimed at the redifferentiation of the disturbed hand representations. Here, we propose a new procedure to investigate affected muscle activations in individuals with neurologic motor disorders after plastic changes induced by rTMS.

This line of intervention holds several advantages over pharmacologic therapy (e.g., injections of botulinum toxin into the intrinsic arm/hand muscles): It is safe and effective, as demonstrated by kinematic analysis, and there is no risk of impairing movement in adjacent fingers. Moreover, it can be applied to patients unresponsive to a variety of commonly used medical treatments. Noninvasive brain stimulation can transiently normalize corticospinal excitability to the affected muscles and can improve the degree of motor coordination over time. Objective quantifications of this treatment can be experimentally obtained with EMG and 3D movement analysis, paving the way for developing novel evaluation tools to optimize therapeutic strategies for motor disorders.

As the rehabilitation research in limb dystonia develops, it will be relevant to investigate comparative effectiveness of interventions to understand which approach holds the most promise.

The present results could support three future research aims:

(i) To develop an effective diagnostic tool based on neurophysiologic and behavioral measures for early identification of patients and for quantifying changes in symptoms

(ii) To investigate how dystonia affects the parietal-premotor pathway (reaching and grasping components)

(iii) To determine the best frequency and duration for interventions and after effects following rehabilitation.

A limit of the present study is the small sample adopted. However, according to Kimberley and colleagues [23, 53], studies in this field should utilize robust small n methodology such as single subject experimental design studies with repeated measures that allows for detailed analysis of within subject variability. Needless to say that definitive statements cannot yet be made regarding efficacy of this paradigm. Randomized controlled measurements are essential for future studies to compare different outcomes with similar frequency and duration.

Identifying the motor dynamics underlying this disorder will be helpful for moving forward both in diagnosis and in treatment, to optimize therapeutic outcomes. Since the available medical approaches are only moderately effective, preventing dystonia is just as much important.

We argue that an enhanced understanding of how neural plasticity can be assessed in FDH affected patients will provide helpful insights for designing more effective patient-tailored therapies based on noninvasive brain stimulation and for evaluating different treatment approaches.

Conflicts of Interest

The authors declare that there is no conflict of interest regarding the publication of this paper.

Acknowledgments

This work was supported by the Progetto Strategico, Università di Padova (N. 2010XPMFW4) to Umberto Castiello and by the SIR (Scientific Independence of Young Researchers) grant (N. RBSI141QKX) to Luisa Sartori. The authors would like to thank Dr. Paolo Fuschi for his precious advice.

References

[1] E. Altenmüller and H.-C. Jabusch, "Focal dystonia in musicians: phenomenology, pathophysiology and triggering factors," *European Journal of Neurology.*, vol. 17, pp. 31–36, 2010.

[2] S. Pirio Richardson, E. Altenmüller, K. Alter et al., "Research priorities in limb and task-specific dystonias," *Frontiers in Neurology*, vol. 8, p. 170, 2017.

[3] A. Quartarone, H. R. Siebner, and J. C. Rothwell, "Task-specific hand dystonia: can too much plasticity be bad for you?," *Trends in Neurosciences.*, vol. 29, no. 4, pp. 192–199, 2006.

[4] D. Ruge, S. Tisch, M. I. Hariz et al., "Deep brain stimulation effects in dystonia: time course of electrophysiological changes in early treatment," *Movement Disorders*, vol. 26, no. 10, pp. 1913–1921, 2011.

[5] A. Quartarone, S. Bagnato, V. Rizzo et al., "Abnormal associative plasticity of the human motor cortex in writer's cramp," *Brain*, vol. 126, no. 12, pp. 2586–2596, 2003.

[6] A. Quartarone, V. Rizzo, S. Bagnato et al., "Homeostatic-like plasticity of the primary motor hand area is impaired in focal hand dystonia," *Brain*, vol. 128, no. 8, pp. 1943–1950, 2005.

[7] A. Berardelli, J. C. Rothwell, M. Hallett, P. D. Thompson, M. Manfredi, and C. D. Marsden, "The pathophysiology of primary dystonia," *Brain*, vol. 121, no. 7, pp. 1195–1212, 1998.

[8] J. Pujol, J. Roset-Llobet, D. Rosinés-Cubells et al., "Brain cortical activation during guitar-induced hand dystonia studied by functional MRI," *NeuroImage*, vol. 12, no. 3, pp. 257–267, 2000.

[9] W. Bara-Jimenez, M. J. Catalan, M. Hallett, and C. Gerloff, "Abnormal somatosensory homunculus in dystonia of the hand," *Annals of Neurology*, vol. 44, no. 5, pp. 828–831, 1998.

[10] T. Elbert, V. Candia, E. Altenmüller et al., "Alteration of digital representations in somatosensory cortex in focal hand dystonia," *Neuroreport*, vol. 9, no. 16, pp. 3571–3575, 1998.

[11] M. L. Byrnes, G. W. Thickbroom, S. A. Wilson et al., "The corticomotor representation of upper limb muscles in writer's cramp and changes following botulinum toxin injection," *Brain*, vol. 121, no. 5, pp. 977–988, 1998.

[12] M. Sommer, D. Ruge, F. Tergau, W. Beuche, E. Altenmüller, and W. Paulus, "Intracortical excitability in the hand motor representation in hand dystonia and blepharospasm," *Movement Disorders*, vol. 17, no. 5, pp. 1017–1025, 2002.

[13] C. Pantev, A. Engelien, V. Candia, and T. Elbert, "Representational cortex in musicians," *Annals of the New York Academy of Sciences*, vol. 930, no. 1, pp. 300–314, 2001.

[14] A. Pascual-Leone, "The brain that plays music and is changed by it," *Annals of the New York Academy of Sciences*, vol. 930, no. 1, pp. 315–329, 2001.

[15] J. Konczak and G. Abbruzzese, "Focal dystonia in musicians: linking motor symptoms to somatosensory dysfunction," *Frontiers in Human Neuroscience*, vol. 7, p. 297, 2013.

[16] E. Altenmüller, "Focal dystonia: advances in brain imaging and understanding of fine motor control in musicians," *Hand Clinics*, vol. 19, no. 3, pp. 523–538, 2003.

[17] T. Elbert, C. Pantev, C. Wienbruch, B. Rockstroh, and E. Taub, "Increased cortical representation of the fingers of the left hand in string players," *Science*, vol. 270, no. 5234, pp. 305–307, 1995.

[18] E. Altenmüller, V. Baur, A. Hofmann, V. K. Lim, and H.-C. Jabusch, "Musician's cramp as manifestation of maladaptive brain plasticity: arguments from instrumental differences," *Annals of the New York Academy of Sciences*, vol. 1252, no. 1, pp. 259–265, 2012.

[19] S. J. Frucht, "Evaluating the musician with dystonia of the upper limb: a practical approach with video demonstration," *Journal of Clinical Movement Disorders*, vol. 2, no. 1, p. 16, 2015.

[20] N. N. Byl and A. McKenzie, "Treatment effectiveness for patients with a history of repetitive hand use and focal hand dystonia: a planned, prospective follow-up study," *Journal of Hand Therapy*, vol. 13, no. 4, pp. 289–301, 2000.

[21] H.-C. Jabusch and E. Altenmüller, "Three-dimensional movement analysis as a promising tool for treatment evaluation of musicians' dystonia," *Advances in Neurology*, vol. 94, pp. 239–245, 2004.

[22] F. Cogiamanian, S. Barbieri, and A. Priori, "Novel nonpharmacologic perspectives for the treatment of task-specific focal hand dystonia," *Journal of Hand Therapy*, vol. 22, no. 2, pp. 156–162, 2009.

[23] T. J. Kimberley, R. L. S. Schmidt, M. Chen, D. D. Dykstra, and C. M. Buetefisch, "Mixed effectiveness of rTMS and retraining in the treatment of focal hand dystonia," *Frontiers in Human Neuroscience*, vol. 9, p. 385, 2015.

[24] Y.-Z. Huang, C.-S. Lu, J. C. Rothwell et al., "Modulation of the disturbed motor network in dystonia by multisession suppression of premotor cortex," *PLoS One*, vol. 7, no. 10, article e47574, 2012.

[25] H. R. Siebner, J. M. Tormos, A. O. Ceballos-Baumann et al., "Low-frequency repetitive transcranial magnetic stimulation of the motor cortex in writer's cramp," *Neurology*, vol. 52, no. 3, pp. 529–537, 1999.

[26] H. R. Siebner, C. Auer, and B. Conrad, "Abnormal increase in the corticomotor output to the affected hand during repetitive transcranial magnetic stimulation of the primary motor cortex in patients with writer's cramp," *Neuroscience Letters*, vol. 262, no. 2, pp. 133–136, 1999.

[27] H. Siebner and J. Rothwell, "Transcranial magnetic stimulation: new insights into representational cortical plasticity," *Experimental Brain Research*, vol. 148, no. 1, pp. 1–16, 2003.

[28] H. R. Siebner, N. Lang, V. Rizzo et al., "Preconditioning of low-frequency repetitive transcranial magnetic stimulation with transcranial direct current stimulation: evidence for homeostatic plasticity in the human motor cortex," *The Journal of Neuroscience*, vol. 24, no. 13, pp. 3379–3385, 2004.

[29] M. Borich, S. Arora, and T. J. Kimberley, "Lasting effects of repeated rTMS application in focal hand dystonia," *Restorative Neurology and Neuroscience*, vol. 27, no. 1, pp. 55–65, 2009.

[30] N. Murase, J. C. Rothwell, R. Kaji et al., "Subthreshold low-frequency repetitive transcranial magnetic stimulation over the premotor cortex modulates writer's cramp," *Brain*, vol. 128, no. 1, pp. 104–115, 2005.

[31] A. S. Schneider, B. Baur, W. Fürholzer, I. Jasper, C. Marquardt, and J. Hermsdörfer, "Writing kinematics and pen forces in writer's cramp: effects of task and clinical subtype," *Clinical Neurophysiology*, vol. 121, no. 11, pp. 1898–1907, 2010.

[32] M. Jeannerod, "The timing of natural prehension movements," *Journal of Motor Behavior*, vol. 16, no. 3, pp. 235–254, 1984.

[33] D. A. Nowak and J. Hermsdörfer, "Coordination of grip and load forces during vertical point-to-point movements with a grasped object in Parkinson's disease," *Behavioral Neuroscience*, vol. 116, no. 5, pp. 837–850, 2002.

[34] D. A. Nowak and J. Hermsdörfer, "Grip force behavior during object manipulation in neurological disorders: toward an objective evaluation of manual performance deficits," *Movement Disorders*, vol. 20, no. 1, pp. 11–25, 2005.

[35] D. A. Nowak and J. Hermsdörfer, "Objective evaluation of manual performance deficits in neurological movement disorders," *Brain Research Reviews*, vol. 51, no. 1, pp. 108–124, 2006.

[36] J. P. Basil-Neto, L. G. Cohen, M. Panizza, J. Nilsson, B. J. Roth, and M. Hallett, "Optimal focal transcranial magnetic activation of the human motor cortex: effects of coil orientation, shape of the induced current pulse, and stimulus intensity," *Journal of Clinical Neurophysiology*, vol. 9, no. 1, pp. 132–136, 1992.

[37] K. R. Mills, S. J. Boniface, and M. Schubert, "Magnetic brain stimulation with a double coil: the importance of coil orientation," *Electroencephalography and Clinical Neurophysiology/ Evoked Potentials Section*, vol. 85, no. 1, pp. 17–21, 1992.

[38] P. M. Rossini, A. T. Barker, A. Berardelli et al., "Non-invasive electrical and magnetic stimulation of the brain, spinal cord and roots: basic principles and procedures for routine clinical application. Report of an IFCN committee," *Electroencephalography and Clinical Neurophysiology*, vol. 91, no. 2, pp. 79–92, 1994.

[39] R Core Team, R: A, *Language and Environment for Statistical Computing*, R Foundation for Statistical Computing, Vienna, Austria, 2014.

[40] L. C. Young, "On randomness in ordered sequences," *The Annals of Mathematical Statistics*, vol. 12, no. 3, pp. 293–300, 1941.

[41] C. Armbrüster and W. Spijkers, "Movement planning in prehension: do intended actions influence the initial reach and grasp movement?," *Motor Control*, vol. 10, no. 4, pp. 311–329, 2006.

[42] A. Schuboe, A. Maldonado, S. Stork, and M. Beetz, "Subsequent actions influence motor control parameters of a current grasping action," in *RO-MAN 2008 - The 17th IEEE International Symposium on Robot and Human Interactive Communication*, pp. 389–394, Munich, Germany, August 2008.

[43] A. M. Wing, A. Turton, and C. Fraser, "Grasp size and accuracy of approach in reaching," *Journal of Motor Behavior*, vol. 18, no. 3, pp. 245–260, 1986.

[44] C. Gallea, S. G. Horovitz, M. 'Ali Najee-Ullah, and M. Hallett, "Impairment of a parieto-premotor network specialized for handwriting in writer's cramp," *Human Brain Mapping*, vol. 37, no. 12, pp. 4363–4375, 2016.

[45] C. Cavina-Pratesi, S. Monaco, P. Fattori et al., "Functional magnetic resonance imaging reveals the neural substrates of arm transport and grip formation in reach-to-grasp actions in humans," *The Journal of Neuroscience*, vol. 30, no. 31, pp. 10306–10323, 2010.

[46] K. E. Zeuner, M. Peller, A. Knutzen et al., "How to assess motor impairment in writer's cramp," *Movement Disorders*, vol. 22, no. 8, pp. 1102–1109, 2007.

[47] L. C. Veugen, B. S. Hoffland, D. F. Stegeman, and B. P. van de Warrenburg, "Inhibition of the dorsal premotor cortex does not repair surround inhibition in writer's cramp patients," *Experimental Brain Research*, vol. 225, no. 1, pp. 85–92, 2013.

[48] S. Beck, S. P. Richardson, E. A. Shamim, N. Dang, M. Schubert, and M. Hallett, "Short intracortical and surround inhibition are selectively reduced during movement initiation in focal hand dystonia," *The Journal of Neuroscience*, vol. 28, no. 41, pp. 10363–10369, 2008.

[49] A. Quartarone and M. Hallett, "Emerging concepts in the physiological basis of dystonia," *Movement Disorders*, vol. 28, no. 7, pp. 958–967, 2013.

[50] P. T. Lin and M. Hallett, "The pathophysiology of focal hand dystonia," *Journal of Hand Therapy*, vol. 22, no. 2, pp. 109–114, 2009.

[51] M. Herrojo Ruiz, P. Senghaas, M. Grossbach et al., "Defective inhibition and inter-regional phase synchronization in pianists with musician's dystonia: an EEG study," *Human Brain Mapping*, vol. 30, no. 8, pp. 2689–2700, 2009.

[52] T. F. Münte, E. Altenmüller, and L. Jäncke, "The musician's brain as a model of neuroplasticity," *Nature Reviews Neuroscience*, vol. 3, no. 6, pp. 473–478, 2002.

[53] T. J. Kimberley and R. P. D. Fabio, "Visualizing the effects of rTMS in a patient sample: small N vs. group level analysis," *PLoS One*, vol. 5, no. 12, article e15155, 2010.

16

State-of-the-Art Techniques to Causally Link Neural Plasticity to Functional Recovery in Experimental Stroke Research

Anna-Sophia Wahl (ID) [1,2,3]

[1]*Brain Research Institute, University of Zurich, Winterthurerstr. 190, 8057 Zurich, Switzerland*
[2]*Department of Health Sciences and Technology, ETH Zurich, Winterthurerstr. 190, 8057 Zurich, Switzerland*
[3]*Central Institute of Mental Health, University of Heidelberg, J5, 68159 Mannheim, Germany*

Correspondence should be addressed to Anna-Sophia Wahl; wahl@hifo.uzh.ch

Academic Editor: Surjo R. Soekadar

Current experimental stroke research faces the same challenge as neuroscience: to transform correlative findings in causative ones. Research of recent years has shown the tremendous potential of the central nervous system to react to noxious stimuli such as a stroke: Increased plastic changes leading to reorganization in form of neuronal rewiring, neurogenesis, and synaptogenesis, accompanied by transcriptional and translational turnover in the affected cells, have been described both clinically and in experimental stroke research. However, only minor attempts have been made to connect distinct plastic remodeling processes as causative features for specific behavioral phenotypes. Here, we review current state-of the art techniques for the examination of cortical reorganization and for the manipulation of neuronal circuits as well as techniques which combine anatomical changes with molecular profiling. We provide the principles of the techniques together with studies in experimental stroke research which have already applied the described methodology. The tools discussed are useful to close the loop from our understanding of stroke pathology to the behavioral outcome and may allow discovering new targets for therapeutic approaches. The here presented methods open up new possibilities to assess the efficiency of rehabilitative strategies by understanding their external influence for intrinsic repair mechanisms on a neurobiological basis.

1. Introduction

Although huge efforts have been made in recent years, both by clinicians and basic researchers, we have still gained limited insights into a neurological disease such as stroke preventing us from developing specific cures and resulting in poor statistical numbers: Of 15 million people suffering from an ischemic brain attack every year, a third dies, a third remains permanently disabled, and a third recovers as the stroke itself has not been too devastating. On the clinical side, stroke units have been created, which combine experts in intensive care medicine, neurology, physiotherapy, and speech therapy, to accelerate and coordinate the diagnostic and therapeutical processes aiming at improving recovery rates for patients. According to the neurologists' saying "time is brain," even mobile units have been established to bring the hospital to the patient [1]. These efforts aim at increasing the number of patients

being eligible for the only currently approved acute treatment—thrombolysis or thrombectomy—within a very early time window of 4.5 h after stroke [2, 3].

On the side of basic research, we study the neurobiology of stroke, but seem to be stuck in a "black box" situation: We have accumulated data showing the tremendous capacities of the brain to reorganize by synaptogenesis and even neurogenesis and by neuronal circuit rewiring and new circuit formation. We find cortical map shifts and hyperactive brain regions after stroke; we detect genetic and proteomic turnover within a distinct spatiotemporal profile and sequence of events [4]. However, only minor attempts have been made to transform pure correlative data into causative ones, which would enable a causal connection of plastic remodeling processes in the brain with distinct behavioral outcomes. Not only would this allow us to form a new understanding of the functional brain status after stroke, but also it opens up possibilities to develop and test the efficiency of new therapeutic approaches. Today's basic stroke research is part of neuroscience that faces the challenges to first describe the broad morphological features, then study fine cellular and molecular events, find genes which are active in a specific neuron or cell type, and link it to the behavioral phenotype. But as the philosopher of science Karl Popper might have argued: Before we can provide answers, we need the power to ask new questions.

In recent years, new technology has been designed which is starting to fill the gap between correlative and causative research.

The aim of this review is to first discuss current state-of-the-art technology of experimental stroke research which enables a deeper understanding of neuronal reorganization and circuit formation. In the second part, techniques for distinct neuronal circuit manipulation are introduced which help to reveal causal relationships between anatomy and behavior. Finally, new approaches combining cytology with molecular profiles are provided which elucidate the underlying molecular mechanisms of neuronal rewiring and repair. The principles of the techniques are explained together with exemplary studies in experimental stroke research which have already applied the described methodology. The here discussed tools may not only enhance our understanding of stroke pathology but also help to identify crucial anchor points for new therapeutic interventions.

2. State-of-the-Art Techniques to Study Neuronal Reorganization and Circuit Formation after Experimental Stroke

2.1. Approaches to Examine Brain-Wide Remodeling. A classical approach to study reorganizational processes across the whole brain is functional resonance imaging (fMRI), allowing the monitoring of neuronal rewiring processes on a macroanatomical level within the same animal. However, although significant contributions to the understanding of the interplay between altered functional status and structural connectivity have been made in stroke models [5, 6] using this technique, the spatial and temporal resolution level remains low.

In contrast, intrinsic optical imaging sticks out by a high spatial resolution enabling the visualization of small domains within larger brain areas demonstrating the functional organization and the spatial relationships among those smaller domains, for example, in the barrel or visual cortex [7]. Intrinsic optical imaging uses the effect that more active brain tissue reflects less light than does less active tissue. Thus, the most active areas appear as the darkest ones. Optical imaging has been used to show disrupted functional connectivity in rodent mouse models of stroke [8, 9].

Another technique to study in particular sensory map shifts is millisecond-timescale voltage-sensitive dye (VSD) imaging which unlike functional fMRI and intrinsic optical signal imaging measures electrical activity with relatively high spatial and temporal resolution [10]. VSD imaging has recently been applied to measure spontaneous activity over large regions of the mouse cortex to reveal fast, complex,

localized, and bilaterally synchronized patterns of depolarization [10]. In a study by Gosh et al. [11], VSD imaging was used to show the expansion of the forelimb sensory map towards parts of the hindlimb cortex after a large thoracic spinal cord injury, indicating incorporation of axotomized hindlimb neurons into sensory circuits of the forelimb. In another study by Brown et al. [12], the function of the sensorimotor cortex was visualized with VSD imaging. The mouse forelimb sensory cortex was targeted by stroke leading to a new sensory representation in the territory previously occupied by the forelimb motor cortex. VSD imaging revealed slower kinetics in remapped sensory circuits accompanied by high levels of dendritic spines as visualized with two-photon microscopy.

While VSD imaging was the first demonstration of wide-field optical imaging of neural activity [13], the necessity to apply VSDs prior to imaging, their very fast response time, and their very small signal ratios made them difficult to use. However, recent developments of exogenous and in particular genetically encoded fluorescent indicators of neuronal activity such as GCaMP and YC-Nano have revolutionized the targeted expression of fluorescence with much higher signal levels. And even transgenetic lines exist [14]. Furthermore, recent work has shown that the dynamics of flavoprotein fluorescence can be optically mapped in wild-type CNS tissue as an indicator of oxidative metabolism [15, 16], which might be also a useful tool in experimental stroke research. As wide-field neuroimaging methods are also relatively easily combined with optogenetics to modify brain activity in the behaving animal, studies have been conducted using camera-based "mesoscopic" optical recording of neuronal activity examining a large part of the cortical surface. These mesoscopic optical recordings became possible by extensive chronic window implantations [17] and improved high-speed sensitive camera technology. Vanni et al. [18] measured cortical functional connectivity using wide-field imaging in lightly anesthetized GCaMP3 mice and correlated calcium signals recoded in the primary sensory cortex to the other sensorimotor areas bilaterally. The coactivation of areas was interpreted as an indication that areas might be functionally connected. However, a final proof for a functional connection, shutting-off correlated areas, was missing in this study. Balbi et al. [19] used the same approach in awake GCaMP6 mice studying mososcopic functional connectivity longitudinally in a microinfarct model.

That wide-field calcium imaging might be also a powerful tool to study brain-wide cortical reorganization on a high-resolution level over time in animals monitoring their rehabilitative courses or recording rehabilitative training after stroke was demonstrated by Murphy et al. [20]. His lab presented a home cage system, where mice could initiate mesoscopic functional imaging by themselves over days being unsupervised.

2.2. Methods to Understand Regional Reorganization. Intracortical microstimulation (ICMS) and surface stimulation with electrode arrays have been used for many years to map cortical regions, to study cortical reorganization, and to find first hints if projections in the motor cortex are functionally relevant. This technique applies electrical stimulation of cortical sites to induce, for example, stimulus-evoked movement responses, which can be detected visually, by EMG responses or by the usage of accelerometers. Several studies have used this technique to either examine cortical map shifts in sensorimotor areas after spontaneous recovery or different therapeutical applications [21–24] or used the stimulation itself as a method to increase plastic processes [25]. However, ICMS has its disadvantages such as the inability to selectively target neuronal subtypes as well as the indiscriminate activation of axons of passage. Furthermore, due to electrode penetration, intracortical electric stimulation remains an invasive procedure causing tissue damage [26]. ICMS is also limited to perform cortical representation of body function at a distinct time point after stroke constraining longitudinal experiments within the same animal.

A new noninvasive strategy to study the reorganization of the motor cortex after stroke in the same animal over time is light-based motor mapping: This technique makes usage of the possibility to stimulate neurons by light, either by uncaging neurotransmitters [27, 28] or by directly activating light-sensitive channels, such as channelrhodopsin-2 (ChR-2). Ayling et al. [26] used transgenic channelrhodopsin-2 mice which express ChR-2 in layer 5B pyramidal neurons of the motor cortex. Thus, light-based stimulation directly targets corticofugal cells, enabling the analysis of their contribution to motor cortex topography. Light-based motor mapping has the advantage of sampling stimulus-evoked movements at hundreds of cortical locations in mere minutes objectively and in a reproducible manner [29]. It is faster and less invasive than electrode-based mapping and can be combined with intrinsic signal imaging in animals with cranial window preparations [30]. In addition, it enables repeated mapping of the motor cortex over a timescale of minutes to months, opening up possibilities to examine the dynamics of movement representations at distinct conditions such as learning over time, pharmacological intervention or reorganization before, during, and after cortical damage. In a first study by Harrison et al. [29] light-based motor mapping revealed a functional subdivision of the forelimb motor cortex based on the direction of movements evoked by brief light pulses (10 ms), while prolonged stimulation (100–500 ms) resulted in complex movements of the forelimb to specific positions in space. In a follow-up study [30], light-based mapping was for the first time used to perform a longitudinal experiment studying the reorganization of the sensorimotor cortex after a focal sensory stroke. The sensory stroke caused the establishment of a new sensory map in prior parts of the forelimb motor cortex, which preserved its center position but became more dispersed.

2.3. Studying Poststroke Neuronal Circuit Formation and Network Activity. However, although all described mapping approaches are powerful tools, they can only provide information about map shifts and representation of general movement dynamics. They stay far beyond cellular resolution and do not allow studying local neuronal circuitry or single neuron contribution to neuronal networks. In particular after stroke, it is not clear how activity in single neurons changes

in relation to cortical map shifts. The analysis of single neurons in relation to the neuronal circuit in which they are embedded may elucidate whether stroke-induced plasticity is a result of the capacity of surviving neurons to process multiple functional streams. In vivo two-photon calcium imaging is a potent method which not only allows studying activity of a single neuron or ensembles of neurons in a network but also enables cell type and neuronal subtype-specific analysis. Only a few in vivo two-photon calcium imaging studies focusing on neuronal reorganization and circuit rewiring after stroke have been conducted so far. In an acute in vivo calcium imaging experiment during the induction of a transient global ischemia model in mice, Murphy et al. [31] saw a widespread loss of mouse somatosensory cortex apical dendritic structure during the phase of ischemic depolarization. This was accompanied by increased intracellular calcium levels which coincidently occurred with the loss of dendritic structure. In a second study [32], in vivo two-photon calcium imaging was used to examine how response properties of individual neurons and glial cells in reorganized forelimb and hindlimb functional somatosensory maps modified during the recovery period from ischemic damage in the sensory cortex. However, all studies have been conducted in animals under anesthesia which itself influences neuronal activity. An experiment which examines single neuron activity in the behaving animal before stroke and during the recovery phase after insult is lacking so far.

Two-photon calcium imaging enables recordings of individual neuronal activity within a neuronal network and allows subtype-specific functional analysis of brain tissue. However, neuronal activity with cellular resolution level can only be examined in small (<1 millimeter) fields of view. Collective dynamics across different brain regions are inaccessible. Recent advances in two-photon microscopy allow the simultaneous imaging of neuronal networks with cellular resolution level in the active animal in multiple areas, which are even not directly connected [33–35]. This technological progress also provides new promises for experimental stroke research.

3. State-of-the-Art Techniques for Manipulating Neuronal Circuits

In a 1979 Scientific American article, Nobel laureate Francis Crick stated that the major challenge facing neuroscience was the need to control one type of cell in the brain while leaving others unaltered. In a lecture from 1999, he further confined: "One of the next requirements is to be able to turn the firing of one or more types of neuron on and off in the alert animal in a rapid manner. The ideal signal would be light, probably at an infrared wavelength to allow the light to penetrate far enough. This seems rather farfetched but it is conceivable that molecular biologists could engineer a particular cell type to be sensitive to light in this way" [36].

Manipulation of neuronal circuits or single neurons has two prerequisites: Manipulation has to be quick and very specific. Over the years, a very diverse set of tools has been developed to manipulate whole brain regions as well as the activity of individual cells and subtypes in the alert behaving animal.

3.1. Manipulating with Specific Spatial Control. The first constraint for specific manipulation implies a high spatial control allowing the selective modulation of a whole brain area, a distinct anatomical sub region (e.g., layer 5 pyramidal cells in the sensorimotor cortex) or a particular cell type (e.g., a parvalbumin-positive interneuron).

For inhibiting neuronal activity in whole brain regions, agents such as the GABA agonist muscimol have been used [37, 38] resulting in a loss of motor function, indicating a causal relationship between anatomy and behavior. Other approaches block synapse remodeling through protein synthesis inhibitors such as anisomycin, for example, inducing the disruption of synapses and motor maps in a rat forelimb stroke model [39]. However, for a better spatial control to target distinct circuits and individual cell types, researchers have either created transgenic mouse lines or locally injected viruses with cell-type specific promotors [40]. These promotors induce gene expression directly—as in the case of transgenic mice—or indirectly via, for example, Tet- (tetracycline-controlled transcriptional activation-) on/off or Cre-flox systems.

The Tet system uses at least two viral vectors plus an antibiotic drug which in a sequential way activate each other to induce the transcription and translation of the gene of interest: A tissue-specific promoter initiates the expression of a transcription factor, either the tetracycline transactivator (tTA) or the reverse tetracycline transactivator (rtTA). The tTA or rtTA then becomes the key player for the transcription of a tetracycline response element (TRE) promotor, which in dependence of the presence of tetracycline or doxycycline drives the expression of the gene of interest. Expression of the gene of interest is fully reversible as administration or removal of tetracycline or doxycycline will turn its expression on or off. In a study by Kinoshita et al. [41] a Tet-on system was used to selectively express the synaptotoxin tetanus toxin in propriospinal (PN) neurons innervated by the motor cortex. The researchers could show that upon doxycycline administration in the drinking water reaching performance of monkeys significantly declined due to temporal blockade of the motor cortex–PN–motor neuron pathway. The same Tet-on system was used by Wahl et al. [42] in a rat stroke model to selectively shut off rewired corticospinal fibers originating in the contralesional pre- and motor cortex and targeting the stroke-denervated hemispinal cord: When doxycycline was administered to the rats in the drinking water after the rehabilitative treatment for impaired skilled motor function, the recovered grasping skills of the impaired paw decreased again over time. The effect was reversible, when doxycycline was removed from the drinking water. This study showed for the first time the specific and reversible inactivating of newly out-sprouting corticospinal fibers after stroke. In another study by Ishida et al. [43] ipsilesional corticorubral fibers were shut off after forced rehabilitation in a rat stroke model revealing the functional importance of the red nucleus for the recovery of impaired motor function.

Similar to the Tet system, the Cre-flox system also requires two transgenes: A tissue-specific promotor regulates the expression of Cre recombinase, a bacteriophage enzyme which recombines DNA at specific recognition sequences called loxP sites. Cre recombinase then excises DNA within two loxP sites ("floxed"). As in most cases, floxed-stop constructs are knocked in by homologous recombination to a gene of interest [40]; the stop signal is excised in the presence of Cre and the transgene expression can be initiated. Cre-mediated expression only occurs in cells expressing Cre, which are also those cells in which the tissue-specific promotor is active, indicating the high cell-type specificity of this technique.

3.2. Manipulating with High Spatial and Temporal Control

3.2.1. DREADDs. As the second prerequisite for specific neuronal manipulation in addition to a high degree of spatial resolution, temporal resolution and directional modulation of signaling are required for remotely controlling neuronal firing. Temporal resolution implies the precise control when a receptor or pathway is active or inactive and for how long it should be in a specific active status. Temporal resolution can vary from milliseconds (see "opsins" described below) to hours (e.g., designer receptors exclusively activated by designer drugs, DREADDs). Important are also "onset" kinetics (the time between the experimental manipulation and the modulation of the receptor or signaling pathway) and "offset" kinetics (the time between the initiation of the signaling modulation and the termination of the modulation [40]). Directional regulation describes the effect of the tool on neuronal activity (either activating or inhibiting), while bidirectional control would be the optimal case: Turning on and off the same cell population would elucidate the full spectrum of function that a cell provides within a particular network for perception or execution of a distinct behavior.

For manipulation of neuronal networks for minutes to hours, designer G protein-coupled receptors have been developed. G protein-coupled receptor pathways are involved in a multitude of cellular functions. Unlike opsins, which are functionally silent without excitation in vivo as they are not directly activated by endogenous compounds, G protein-coupled receptors (GCPRs) are constantly modulated by endogenous ligands in vivo or reveal ligand-independent activity [44, 45]. In vitro and in vivo pharmacological studies have described GPCRs as the most important class of druggable targets in the human genome [46], through which 50% of prescribed therapeutics act [47]. These facts made the development of highly selective orthologous ligand-receptor pairs, which would enable a high spatiotemporal control over GPCR signaling pathways in vivo challenging [48]. In recent years, mutations to more than a dozen native GPCRs have opened the field for the development of selectively activated designer receptors. Most of these receptors are divided in two classes: the first-generation RASSLs (receptors activated solely by synthetic ligands) and the second-generation DREADDs (designer receptors exclusively activated by designer drugs), which were evolved through directed molecular evolution in yeast [40]. RASSLs were first engineered on the basis of serotonin receptors [49], histamine receptors [50], and melanocortin-4 receptors [51]. However, the first generation of orthologous ligand-GPCR pairs revealed potential shortcomings: Although the receptors were activated solely by the synthetic ligands, the ligands themselves did not solely activate the designer receptors (as reviewed by Rogan and Roth [40]). Thus, for the development of second-generation DREADDs, Armbruster et al. took a designer ligand, clozapine n-oxide (CNO), which was known to be inert at endogenous targets and highly bioavailable and blood-brain barrier-permeant in both humans and mice [52, 53]. As CNO had a modified structure of clozapine, which is known to be a weak partial agonist at muscarinic receptors, [54] mutations were induced in the five members of the muscarinic cholinergic receptor family and tested upon their selective responsiveness to the CNO application. Introducing two mutations transformed the hM3 receptor into a designer receptor which was insensitive to its native ligands, but highly sensitive to the designer ligand CNO. In smooth muscles cells the G_q-coupled hM3 DREADD receptor stimulated a cascade of inositol phosphate hydrolysis, calcium release and ERK1/2 activation, while the hM4Di DREADD receptor, derived from the G_i-coupled human muscarinic M4 receptor, inhibited forskolin-induced cAMP formation and activation of GIRK causing hyperpolarization and inhibition of neuronal firing [54].

Since the first development of DREADD receptors, reports of their usage in vivo are now appearing: The pharmacokinetic properties of the DREADD ligands and the particular route of administration (oral administration, subcutaneous, intraperitoneal, or even local stereotaxic infusion) determine how quickly neurons response to experimental manipulation by ligand application. Responses typically emerge 5 to 15 min after systematic application, for example, of CNO and usually last for 2 h—but this time period can be further enlarged upon dose-dependent increase of CNO [55]. When Ferguson et al. [56] used virus-mediated expression of the hM4Di receptor in the direct and indirect pathway neurons of the striatum, they found altered behavioral plasticity associated with repeated drug treatment. In particular, decreasing striatopallidal neuronal activity facilitated behavioral sensitization to drug treatment. Expression of the hM4Di receptor in rewired corticospinal projecting neurons was recently used to shut off regained grasping function in rats which had gained nearly full recovery of impaired skilled forelimb function due to a large stroke after the sequential application of a growth-promoting therapy and intense rehabilitative training [42].

3.2.2. Optogenetics. Although manipulation of GPCR signaling pathways by DREADD receptor induction and activation is highly efficient and shows a very specific spatial resolution (depending on the constructs or transgenic mouse lines used), the temporal resolution remains limited to an activation within minutes—due to the slower nature of GPCR signaling—and the necessary ligand delivery to the location of neuronal manipulation. In contrast, high-temporal (milliseconds) and cellular precision within intact mammalian neural tissue for fast, specific excitation or inhibition even within a freely moving animal can only be achieved with optogenetics [57].

Early approaches to use light to stimulate neuron activity included the selective photostimulation of neurons in *Drosophila* by coexpression of the drosophila photoreceptor genes encoding arrestin-2, rhodopsin, and the alpha subunit of the cognate heterotrimeric G protein which enabled the sensitization of neurons to light [58]. In a second approach, action potentials in hippocampal neurons were induced in a reliable and temporarily precise manner by uncaging a caged capsaicin derivate by light [59]. However, depolarization occurred within 5 s after a 1 s light pulse, lasting for 2–3 s and did not attenuate with multiple light pulses. Other approaches such as UV light-isomerizable chemicals linked to genetically encoded channels [60, 61] had also shown limitations due to reduced speed, targeting, tissue penetration, or applicability because of their multicomponent nature [57]. In 2003, Nagel et al. [62] cloned channelrhodopsin-2 (ChR2), a cation channel from the green alga *Chlamydomonas reinhardtii* which depicted similarities to the vertebrate rhodopsin which opens in response to blue light allowing potassium ions to enter the cell. Two years later, the first optogenetic experiment in neuroscience was conducted by expressing ChR2 using a lentiviral vector in cultured rat hippocampal neurons [63]. Illumination of these cultures with shorter wavelength blue light (450–490 nm) initiated large and rapid depolarization, while light with longer wavelengths (490–510 nm) induced smaller currents. Light stimulation of neurons was selective to those neurons expressing ChR2. Since then, neuroscientists rapidly adapted the possibilities of this new technology to in vivo experiments. In addition, the palette of available light-sensitive channels and ion pumps for neuronal inhibition and activation, for fast- and slow-acting opsins, and for opsins activated at distinct wavelengths has been extensively augmented in recent years [64–68].

However, although the numerous advantages of optogenetics are evident—such as the highest specificity, the ultrafast millisecond time scale dissection, and basically no adverse effects due to the light (unless the light source is not too strong or applied too long)—optogenetics stays an invasive procedure for many in vivo experiments: As the light source has to be brought close to the neuronal tissue, targeting deep brain areas or diffuse neuronal populations remains challenging. New development of step function or bistable opsins and opsins such as Jaws—an inhibitory opsin, which is activated by light of infrared wavelength [66]—opens up new possibilities for noninvasive manipulation in-vivo.

Only very few studies have applied optogenetics in experimental stroke research so far: Optogenetics was mainly used in the context of light-based motor mapping as described above [30]. Other studies used optogenetics as a therapeutic approach to increase neuronal activity aiming at enhancing functional recovery: In a first study by Cheng et al. [69], optogenetic stimulation of the ipsilateral primary motor cortex in ChR2 transgenic mice promoted functional recovery and the induction of growth-promoting genes after stroke induction in the striatum and somatosensory cortex. Shah et al. [70]

could furthermore show that selectively stimulating neurons in the lateral cerebellar nucleus (LCN), a deep cerebellar nucleus that sends major excitatory output to multiple motor and sensory areas in the forebrain, results in persistent recovery on the rotating beam after stroke in a transgenic mouse line (Thy1-ChR2-YFP-channelrhodopsin fused to yellow fluorescent protein under the Thy1 pan-neuronal promoter). Tennant et al. [71] revealed that optogenetic stimulation of thalamocortical axons could facilitate recovery. In another study [72], optogenetic stimulation of the intact corticospinal tract was sufficient to promote functional recovery after a large photothrombotic stroke in rats. Optogenetics were also used to drive the excitatory outputs of the grafted neural stem cells and increase forelimb use on the stroke-affected side and motor activity in a rat stroke model [73]. Reducing the inhibitory striatal output by optogenetics enhanced neurogenesis in the subventribular zone and behavioral recovery in mice after middle cerebral artery occlusion [74–76].

That optogenetics can also be used to demonstrate a causal relationship between a rewiring neuronal circuit and recovery of a specific (sensorimotor) behavior was demonstrated by Wahl et al. [72]: The authors used the inhibitory light-sensitive proton pump ArchT to reveal the functional relevance and regionalized organization of rewired corticospinal circuitry for the recovery of distinct grasping features.

New advanced technology in microscopy allows the precise optogenetic stimulation of individual neurons [77] and even dendritic spines and nerve cell somata [78, 79] using holographic photostimulation. In addition, the development of parallel illumination methods [80] which combine the preservation of the spatial targeting capability of beam-scanning systems and the rapid stimulation of multiple neurons now enable the simultaneous excitation of neurons in selected target regions.

3.2.3. Magnetogenetics. Although optogenetics have revolutionized the field of neuroscience, the examination of deeper, subcortical brain regions remains a challenge, as the light has to be somehow delivered to the tissue often requiring invasive implantation of fiber optics causing collateral damage of the surrounding brain tissue. A new emerging method which overcomes the spatial limitations is magnetogenetics: It relies on a principle known as thermal relaxation [81], implying that an alternating magnetic field is able to heat up small magnetic nanoparticles. As key elements the specific frequency of the magnetic field, the size and composition of the nanoparticles are required. Huang et al. [82] activated a heat-sensitive TRPV1 channel expressed in human embryonic kidney (HEK) cells by induction of thermal relaxation of manganese oxide nanoparticles, which enhanced the temperature at the plasma membrane and initiated the calcium influx through the heat-sensitive ion channels. Chen et al. [83] used this technique to stimulate a defined neuronal population activity in the ventral tegmental area in behaving mice demonstrating the potential of magnetogenetics for deep brain stimulation.

However, although individual neuron and specific neuronal circuit manipulation with high spatial and temporal control is possible as discussed above, there still is a need for good behavioral readouts: In particular, in experimental stroke research studying, for example, motor impairment and recovery, it is crucial to quantitatively understand true recovery versus compensation of impaired function [84]: While analyzing video recordings of motor behavior using scores is not only time consuming but also often very subjective, even the analysis of movement trajectories might not provide the full picture [72]: When manipulating with high precision control on a cellular and even subcellular level on the neurobiological side, there is a need for precise analysis of the behavioral phenotype. The dramatic development of Computer Vision algorithms and artificial intelligence may allow further steps beyond for a detailed analysis of kinematics including the sequence of postures, shape and trajectories, which is missed by the human eye.

4. State-of-the-Art Techniques to Combine Anatomy and Molecular Biology

So far, we have discussed how stroke reorganization can be examined on the macrolevel of map shifts or by studying single neurons in neuronal circuits using 2-photon calcium imaging approaches. We have reviewed how individual neurons and whole neuronal populations can be manipulated with high spatiotemporal resolution disclosing new possibilities of causally linking individual neuronal activity with a distinct behavioral phenotype. However, an understanding of the underlying molecular crosstalk which induces anatomical and behavioral changes is still lacking. Classically, tracing techniques (e.g., dextran tracers) have been applied to visualize cells involved in structural reorganization after stroke [22, 23]. Li et al. [85] found a way to exclusively study molecular changes in newly out-sprouting neurons ("the sprouting transcriptome") in the peri-infarct cortex by injecting two different fluorescent conjugates of the tracer cholera toxin B (CTB) into forelimb sensorimotor cortex at different times points: One CTB tracer was injected at the time of stroke, the second differently labeled one either 7 or 21 days afterwards. Neurons which expressed only the second tracer were those which missed an axonal projection to the injection site at the time of the injection of the first tracer and thus represented neurons which established a new projection pattern after stroke. Both neuron types (single- and double-labeled ones) were laser captured to identify the distinct transcriptional profile of an out-sprouting neuron in the peri-infarct cortex.

In addition, new constructs have been recently developed for molecular profiling of projecting neurons and thus bridging the gap between anatomical modifications and underlying molecular mechanisms. Using, for example, bacterial artificial chromosome (BAC) transgenic mice which express EGFP-tagged ribosomal protein L10a in defined cell populations allowed purification of polysomal mRNAs from genetically defined cell populations in the brain [86, 87]. In another study by Ekstrand et al. [88], ribosomes were tagged with a camelid nanobody raised against GFP enabling the selective capture of translating mRNAs in projecting neurons.

5. Conclusion

Here, we have reviewed current and new promising state-of-the-art techniques for studying reorganization after stroke, for the identification and manipulation of distinct neuronal populations and approaches which allow examining molecular profiles of neurons being part of the cortical reorganization process. While for decades studies in basic stroke research have only described and reported correlative findings, these techniques open up tremendous possibilities to analyze plastic processes and identify and target key players for the development of new therapies in stroke.

Conflicts of Interest

The author excludes any competing interest.

Funding

This work was supported by the Swiss National Science Foundation Grant no. 31003A-149315-1.

References

[1] S. Walter, P. Kostopoulos, A. Haass et al., "Diagnosis and treatment of patients with stroke in a mobile stroke unit versus in hospital: a randomised controlled trial," *The Lancet Neurology*, vol. 11, no. 5, pp. 397–404, 2012.

[2] O. A. Berkhemer, P. S. Fransen, D. Beumer et al., "A randomized trial of intraarterial treatment for acute ischemic stroke," *The New England Journal of Medicine*, vol. 372, no. 1, pp. 11–20, 2015.

[3] W. Hacke, M. Kaste, E. Bluhmki et al., "Thrombolysis with alteplase 3 to 4.5 hours after acute ischemic stroke," *The New England Journal of Medicine*, vol. 359, no. 13, pp. 1317–1329, 2008.

[4] S. T. Carmichael, I. Archibeque, L. Luke, T. Nolan, J. Momiy, and S. Li, "Growth-associated gene expression after stroke: evidence for a growth-promoting region in peri-infarct cortex," *Experimental Neurology*, vol. 193, no. 2, pp. 291–311, 2005.

[5] M. P. van Meer, K. van der Marel, W. M. Otte, J. W. Berkelbach van der Sprenkel, and R. M. Dijkhuizen, "Correspondence between altered functional and structural connectivity in the contralesional sensorimotor cortex after unilateral stroke in rats: a combined resting-state functional MRI and manganese-enhanced MRI study," *Journal of Cerebral Blood Flow & Metabolism*, vol. 30, no. 10, pp. 1707–1711, 2010.

[6] M. P. A. van Meer, W. M. Otte, K. van der Marel et al., "Extent of bilateral neuronal network reorganization and functional recovery in relation to stroke severity," *The Journal of Neuroscience*, vol. 32, no. 13, pp. 4495–4507, 2012.

[7] R. D. Frostig and C. H. Chen-Bee, "Visualizing adult cortical plasticity using intrinsic signal optical imaging," in *In Vivo Optical Imaging of Brain Function*, R. D. Frostig, Ed., CRC Press, Boca Raton, FL, USA, 2009.

[8] A. Q. Bauer, A. W. Kraft, P. W. Wright, A. Z. Snyder, J. M. Lee, and J. P. Culver, "Optical imaging of disrupted functional connectivity following ischemic stroke in mice," *NeuroImage*, vol. 99, pp. 388–401, 2014.

[9] J. Hakon, M. J. Quattromani, C. Sjölund et al., "Multisensory stimulation improves functional recovery and resting-state functional connectivity in the mouse brain after stroke," *NeuroImage: Clinical*, vol. 17, pp. 717–730, 2018.

[10] M. H. Mohajerani, A. W. Chan, M. Mohsenvand et al., "Spontaneous cortical activity alternates between motifs defined by regional axonal projections," *Nature Neuroscience*, vol. 16, no. 10, pp. 1426–1435, 2013.

[11] A. Ghosh, F. Haiss, E. Sydekum et al., "Rewiring of hindlimb corticospinal neurons after spinal cord injury," *Nature Neuroscience*, vol. 13, no. 1, pp. 97–104, 2010.

[12] C. E. Brown, K. Aminoltejari, H. Erb, I. R. Winship, and T. H. Murphy, "*In vivo* voltage-sensitive dye imaging in adult mice reveals that somatosensory maps lost to stroke are replaced over weeks by new structural and functional circuits with prolonged modes of activation within both the peri-infarct zone and distant sites," *The Journal of Neuroscience*, vol. 29, no. 6, pp. 1719–1734, 2009.

[13] Y. Ma, M. A. Shaik, S. H. Kim et al., "Wide-field optical mapping of neural activity and brain haemodynamics: considerations and novel approaches," *Philosophical Transactions of the Royal Society of London Series B, Biological Sciences*, vol. 371, no. 1705, p. 20150360, 2016.

[14] K. Horikawa, "Recent progress in the development of genetically encoded Ca^{2+} indicators," *The Journal of Medical Investigation*, vol. 62, no. 1.2, pp. 24–28, 2015.

[15] M. Kozberg and E. Hillman, "Chapter 10 - neurovascular coupling and energy metabolism in the developing brain," *Progress in Brain Research*, vol. 225, pp. 213–242, 2016.

[16] M. G. Kozberg, Y. Ma, M. A. Shaik, S. H. Kim, and E. M. C. Hillman, "Rapid postnatal expansion of neural networks occurs in an environment of altered neurovascular and neurometabolic coupling," *The Journal of Neuroscience*, vol. 36, no. 25, pp. 6704–6717, 2016.

[17] G. Silasi, D. Xiao, M. P. Vanni, A. C. N. Chen, and T. H. Murphy, "Intact skull chronic windows for mesoscopic wide-field imaging in awake mice," *Journal of Neuroscience Methods*, vol. 267, pp. 141–149, 2016.

[18] M. P. Vanni and T. H. Murphy, "Mesoscale transcranial spontaneous activity mapping in GCaMP3 transgenic mice reveals extensive reciprocal connections between areas of somatomotor cortex," *The Journal of Neuroscience*, vol. 34, no. 48, pp. 15931–15946, 2014.

[19] M. Balbi, M. P. Vanni, M. J. Vega et al., "Longitudinal monitoring of mesoscopic cortical activity in a mouse model of microinfarcts reveals dissociations with behavioral and motor function," *Journal of Cerebral Blood Flow & Metabolism*, 2018.

[20] T. H. Murphy, J. D. Boyd, F. Bolaños et al., "High-throughput automated home-cage mesoscopic functional imaging of mouse cortex," *Nature Communications*, vol. 7, article 11611, 2016.

[21] A. J. Emerick, E. J. Neafsey, M. E. Schwab, and G. L. Kartje, "Functional reorganization of the motor cortex in adult rats after cortical lesion and treatment with monoclonal antibody IN-1," *The Journal of Neuroscience*, vol. 23, no. 12, pp. 4826–4830, 2003.

[22] N. T. Lindau, B. J. Bänninger, M. Gullo et al., "Rewiring of the corticospinal tract in the adult rat after unilateral stroke and anti-Nogo-A therapy," *Brain*, vol. 137, no. 3, pp. 739–756, 2014.

[23] M. L. Starkey, C. Bleul, B. Zörner et al., "Back seat driving: hindlimb corticospinal neurons assume forelimb control following ischaemic stroke," *Brain*, vol. 135, no. 11, pp. 3265–3281, 2012.

[24] K. A. Tennant, D. A. L. Adkins, N. A. Donlan et al., "The organization of the forelimb representation of the C57BL/6 mouse motor cortex as defined by intracortical microstimulation and cytoarchitecture," *Cerebral Cortex*, vol. 21, no. 4, pp. 865–876, 2011.

[25] M. Brus-Ramer, J. B. Carmel, S. Chakrabarty, and J. H. Martin, "Electrical stimulation of spared corticospinal axons augments connections with ipsilateral spinal motor circuits after injury," *The Journal of Neuroscience*, vol. 27, no. 50, pp. 13793–13801, 2007.

[26] O. G. S. Ayling, T. C. Harrison, J. D. Boyd, A. Goroshkov, and T. H. Murphy, "Automated light-based mapping of motor cortex by photoactivation of channelrhodopsin-2 transgenic mice," *Nature Methods*, vol. 6, no. 3, pp. 219–224, 2009.

[27] G. M. G. Shepherd, T. A. Pologruto, and K. Svoboda, "Circuit analysis of experience-dependent plasticity in the developing rat barrel cortex," *Neuron*, vol. 38, no. 2, pp. 277–289, 2003.

[28] L. Luo, E. M. Callaway, and K. Svoboda, "Genetic dissection of neural circuits," *Neuron*, vol. 57, no. 5, pp. 634–660, 2008.

[29] T. C. Harrison, O. G. S. Ayling, and T. H. Murphy, "Distinct cortical circuit mechanisms for complex forelimb movement and motor map topography," *Neuron*, vol. 74, no. 2, pp. 397–409, 2012.

[30] T. C. Harrison, G. Silasi, J. D. Boyd, and T. H. Murphy, "Displacement of sensory maps and disorganization of motor cortex after targeted stroke in mice," *Stroke*, vol. 44, no. 8, pp. 2300–2306, 2013.

[31] T. H. Murphy, P. Li, K. Betts, and R. Liu, "Two-photon imaging of stroke onset *in vivo* reveals that NMDA-receptor independent ischemic depolarization is the major cause of rapid reversible damage to dendrites and spines," *The Journal of Neuroscience*, vol. 28, no. 7, pp. 1756–1772, 2008.

[32] I. R. Winship and T. H. Murphy, "*In vivo* calcium imaging reveals functional rewiring of single somatosensory neurons after stroke," *The Journal of Neuroscience*, vol. 28, no. 26, pp. 6592–6606, 2008.

[33] N. J. Sofroniew, D. Flickinger, J. King, and K. Svoboda, "A large field of view two-photon mesoscope with subcellular resolution for in vivo imaging," *eLife*, vol. 5, 2016.

[34] J. Lecoq, J. Savall, D. Vučinić et al., "Visualizing mammalian brain area interactions by dual-axis two-photon calcium imaging," *Nature Neuroscience*, vol. 17, no. 12, pp. 1825–1829, 2014.

[35] J. L. Chen, F. F. Voigt, M. Javadzadeh, R. Krueppel, and F. Helmchen, "Long-range population dynamics of anatomically defined neocortical networks," *eLife*, vol. 5, 2016.

[36] F. Crick, "The impact of molecular biology on neuroscience," *Philosophical Transactions of the Royal Society of London Series B, Biological Sciences*, vol. 354, no. 1392, pp. 2021–2025, 1999.

[37] J. B. Carmel, H. Kimura, and J. H. Martin, "Electrical stimulation of motor cortex in the uninjured hemisphere after chronic unilateral injury promotes recovery of skilled locomotion through ipsilateral control," *The Journal of Neuroscience*, vol. 34, no. 2, pp. 462–466, 2014.

[38] B. K. Mansoori, L. Jean-Charles, B. Touvykine, A. Liu, S. Quessy, and N. Dancause, "Acute inactivation of the contralesional hemisphere for longer durations improves recovery after cortical injury," *Experimental Neurology*, vol. 254, pp. 18–28, 2014.

[39] S. Y. Kim, J. E. Hsu, L. C. Husbands, J. A. Kleim, and T. A. Jones, "Coordinated plasticity of synapses and astrocytes underlies practice-driven functional vicariation in peri-infarct motor cortex," *The Journal of Neuroscience*, vol. 38, no. 1, pp. 93–107, 2018.

[40] S. C. Rogan and B. L. Roth, "Remote control of neuronal signaling," *Pharmacological Reviews*, vol. 63, no. 2, pp. 291–315, 2011.

[41] M. Kinoshita, R. Matsui, S. Kato et al., "Genetic dissection of the circuit for hand dexterity in primates," *Nature*, vol. 487, no. 7406, pp. 235–238, 2012.

[42] A. S. Wahl, W. Omlor, J. C. Rubio et al., "Neuronal repair. Asynchronous therapy restores motor control by rewiring of the rat corticospinal tract after stroke," *Science*, vol. 344, no. 6189, pp. 1250–1255, 2014.

[43] A. Ishida, K. Isa, T. Umeda et al., "Causal link between the cortico-rubral pathway and functional recovery through forced impaired limb use in rats with stroke," *The Journal of Neuroscience*, vol. 36, no. 2, pp. 455–467, 2016.

[44] R. Seifert and K. Wenzel-Seifert, "Constitutive activity of G-protein-coupled receptors: cause of disease and common property of wild-type receptors," *Naunyn-Schmiedeberg's Archives of Pharmacology*, vol. 366, no. 5, pp. 381–416, 2002.

[45] M. J. Smit, H. F. Vischer, R. A. Bakker et al., "Pharmacogenomic and structural analysis of constitutive G protein-coupled receptor activity," *Annual Review of Pharmacology and Toxicology*, vol. 47, no. 1, pp. 53–87, 2007.

[46] P. M. Giguere, W. K. Kroeze, and B. L. Roth, "Tuning up the right signal: chemical and genetic approaches to study GPCR functions," *Current Opinion in Cell Biology*, vol. 27, pp. 51–55, 2014.

[47] J. P. Overington, B. Al-Lazikani, and A. L. Hopkins, "How many drug targets are there?," *Nature Reviews Drug Discovery*, vol. 5, no. 12, pp. 993–996, 2006.

[48] B. R. Conklin, E. C. Hsiao, S. Claeysen et al., "Engineering GPCR signaling pathways with RASSLs," *Nature Methods*, vol. 5, no. 8, pp. 673–8, 2008.

[49] K. Kristiansen, W. K. Kroeze, D. L. Willins et al., "A highly conserved aspartic acid (Asp-155) anchors the terminal amine moiety of tryptamines and is involved in membrane targeting of the 5-HT$_{2A}$ serotonin receptor but does not participate in activation via a "salt-bridge disruption" mechanism," *The Journal of Pharmacology and Experimental Therapeutics*, vol. 293, no. 3, pp. 735–746, 2000.

[50] M. Bruysters, A. Jongejan, A. Akdemir, R. A. Bakker, and R. Leurs, "A G$_{q/11}$-coupled mutant histamine H$_1$ receptor F435A activated solely by synthetic ligands (RASSL)," *Journal of Biological Chemistry*, vol. 280, no. 41, pp. 34741–34746, 2005.

[51] S. Srinivasan, C. Vaisse, and B. R. Conklin, "Engineering the melanocortin-4 receptor to control G$_s$ signaling *in vivo*," *Annals of the New York Academy of Sciences*, vol. 994, no. 1, pp. 225–232, 2003.

[52] W. H. Chang, S. K. Lin, H. Y. Lane et al., "Reversible metabolism of clozapine and clozapine N-oxide in schizophrenic patients," *Progress in Neuro-Psychopharmacology & Biological Psychiatry*, vol. 22, no. 5, pp. 723–739, 1998.

[53] D. M. Weiner, H. Y. Meltzer, I. Veinbergs et al., "The role of M1 muscarinic receptor agonism of *N*-desmethylclozapine in the unique clinical effects of clozapine," *Psychopharmacology*, vol. 177, no. 1-2, pp. 207–216, 2004.

[54] B. N. Armbruster, X. Li, M. H. Pausch, S. Herlitze, and B. L. Roth, "Evolving the lock to fit the key to create a family of G protein-coupled receptors potently activated by an inert ligand," *Proceedings of the National Academy of Sciences of the United States of America*, vol. 104, no. 12, pp. 5163–5168, 2007.

[55] J. M. Guettier, D. Gautam, M. Scarselli et al., "A chemical-genetic approach to study G protein regulation of *β* cell function in vivo," *Proceedings of the National Academy of Sciences of the United States of America*, vol. 106, no. 45, pp. 19197–19202, 2009.

[56] S. M. Ferguson, D. Eskenazi, M. Ishikawa et al., "Transient neuronal inhibition reveals opposing roles of indirect and direct pathways in sensitization," *Nature Neuroscience*, vol. 14, no. 1, pp. 22–24, 2011.

[57] L. Fenno, O. Yizhar, and K. Deisseroth, "The development and application of optogenetics," *Annual Review of Neuroscience*, vol. 34, no. 1, pp. 389–412, 2011.

[58] B. V. Zemelman, G. A. Lee, M. Ng, and G. Miesenböck, "Selective photostimulation of genetically chARGed neurons," *Neuron*, vol. 33, no. 1, pp. 15–22, 2002.

[59] B. V. Zemelman, N. Nesnas, G. A. Lee, and G. Miesenbock, "Photochemical gating of heterologous ion channels: remote control over genetically designated populations of neurons," *Proceedings of the National Academy of Sciences of the United States of America*, vol. 100, no. 3, pp. 1352–1357, 2003.

[60] S. Szobota, P. Gorostiza, F. del Bene et al., "Remote control of neuronal activity with a light-gated glutamate receptor," *Neuron*, vol. 54, no. 4, pp. 535–545, 2007.

[61] P. Gorostiza and E. Y. Isacoff, "Optical switches for remote and noninvasive control of cell signaling," *Science*, vol. 322, no. 5900, pp. 395–399, 2008.

[62] G. Nagel, T. Szellas, W. Huhn et al., "Channelrhodopsin-2, a directly light-gated cation-selective membrane channel," *Proceedings of the National Academy of Sciences of the United States of America*, vol. 100, no. 24, pp. 13940–13945, 2003.

[63] E. S. Boyden, F. Zhang, E. Bamberg, G. Nagel, and K. Deisseroth, "Millisecond-timescale, genetically targeted optical control of neural activity," *Nature Neuroscience*, vol. 8, no. 9, pp. 1263–1268, 2005.

[64] O. Yizhar, L. Fenno, F. Zhang, P. Hegemann, and K. Deisseroth, "Microbial opsins: a family of single-component tools for optical control of neural activity," *Cold Spring Harbor Protocols*, vol. 2011, no. 3, article top102, 2011.

[65] D. Schmidt, P. W. Tillberg, F. Chen, and E. S. Boyden, "A fully genetically encoded protein architecture for optical control of peptide ligand concentration," *Nature Communications*, vol. 5, p. 3019, 2014.

[66] A. S. Chuong, M. L. Miri, V. Busskamp et al., "Noninvasive optical inhibition with a red-shifted microbial rhodopsin," *Nature Neuroscience*, vol. 17, no. 8, pp. 1123–1129, 2014.

[67] N. C. Klapoetke, Y. Murata, S. S. Kim et al., "Independent optical excitation of distinct neural populations," *Nature Methods*, vol. 11, no. 3, pp. 338–346, 2014.

[68] C. K. Kim, A. Adhikari, and K. Deisseroth, "Integration of optogenetics with complementary methodologies in systems neuroscience," *Nature Reviews Neuroscience*, vol. 18, no. 4, pp. 222–235, 2017.

[69] M. Y. Cheng, E. H. Wang, W. J. Woodson et al., "Optogenetic neuronal stimulation promotes functional recovery after stroke," *Proceedings of the National Academy of Sciences of the United States of America*, vol. 111, no. 35, pp. 12913–12918, 2014.

[70] A. M. Shah, S. Ishizaka, M. Y. Cheng et al., "Optogenetic neuronal stimulation of the lateral cerebellar nucleus promotes persistent functional recovery after stroke," *Scientific Reports*, vol. 7, article 46612, 2017.

[71] K. A. Tennant, S. L. Taylor, E. R. White, and C. E. Brown, "Optogenetic rewiring of thalamocortical circuits to restore function in the stroke injured brain," *Nature Communications*, vol. 8, article 15879, 2017.

[72] A. S. Wahl, U. Büchler, A. Brändli et al., "Optogenetically stimulating intact rat corticospinal tract post-stroke restores motor control through regionalized functional circuit formation," *Nature Communications*, vol. 8, no. 1, p. 1187, 2017.

[73] M. M. Daadi, J. Q. Klausner, B. Bajar et al., "Optogenetic stimulation of neural grafts enhances neurotransmission and downregulates the inflammatory response in experimental stroke model," *Cell Transplantation*, vol. 25, no. 7, pp. 1371–1380, 2016.

[74] L. Jiang, W. Li, M. Mamtilahun et al., "Optogenetic inhibition of striatal GABAergic neuronal activity improves outcomes after ischemic brain injury," *Stroke*, vol. 48, no. 12, pp. 3375–3383, 2017.

[75] Y. Lu, L. Jiang, W. Li et al., "Optogenetic inhibition of striatal neuronal activity improves the survival of transplanted neural stem cells and neurological outcomes after ischemic stroke in mice," *Stem Cells International*, vol. 2017, Article ID 4364302, 11 pages, 2017.

[76] M. Song, S. P. Yu, O. Mohamad et al., "Optogenetic stimulation of glutamatergic neuronal activity in the striatum enhances neurogenesis in the subventricular zone of normal and stroke mice," *Neurobiology of Disease*, vol. 98, pp. 9–24, 2017.

[77] O. A. Shemesh, D. Tanese, V. Zampini et al., "Temporally precise single-cell-resolution optogenetics," *Nature Neuroscience*, vol. 20, no. 12, pp. 1796–1806, 2017.

[78] A. M. Packer, D. S. Peterka, J. J. Hirtz, R. Prakash, K. Deisseroth, and R. Yuste, "Two-photon optogenetics of dendritic spines and neural circuits," *Nature Methods*, vol. 9, no. 12, pp. 1202–1205, 2012.

[79] A. M. Packer, L. E. Russell, H. W. P. Dalgleish, and M. Häusser, "Simultaneous all-optical manipulation and recording of neural circuit activity with cellular resolution *in vivo*," *Nature Methods*, vol. 12, no. 2, pp. 140–146, 2015.

[80] V. Emiliani, A. E. Cohen, K. Deisseroth, and M. Hausser, "All-optical interrogation of neural circuits," *The Journal of Neuroscience*, vol. 35, no. 41, pp. 13917–13926, 2015.

[81] S. Nimpf and D. A. Keays, "Is magnetogenetics the new optogenetics?," *The EMBO Journal*, vol. 36, no. 12, pp. 1643–1646, 2017.

[82] H. Huang, S. Delikanli, H. Zeng, D. M. Ferkey, and A. Pralle, "Remote control of ion channels and neurons through magnetic-field heating of nanoparticles," *Nature Nanotechnology*, vol. 5, no. 8, pp. 602–606, 2010.

[83] R. Chen, G. Romero, M. G. Christiansen, A. Mohr, and P. Anikeeva, "Wireless magnetothermal deep brain stimulation," *Science*, vol. 347, no. 6229, pp. 1477–1480, 2015.

[84] T. A. Jones, "Motor compensation and its effects on neural reorganization after stroke," *Nature Reviews Neuroscience*, vol. 18, no. 5, pp. 267–280, 2017.

[85] S. Li, J. J. Overman, D. Katsman et al., "An age-related sprouting transcriptome provides molecular control of axonal sprouting after stroke," *Nature Neuroscience*, vol. 13, no. 12, pp. 1496–1504, 2010.

[86] J. P. Doyle, J. D. Dougherty, M. Heiman et al., "Application of a translational profiling approach for the comparative analysis of CNS cell types," *Cell*, vol. 135, no. 4, pp. 749–762, 2008.

[87] M. Heiman, A. Schaefer, S. Gong et al., "A translational profiling approach for the molecular characterization of CNS cell types," *Cell*, vol. 135, no. 4, pp. 738–748, 2008.

[88] M. I. Ekstrand, A. R. Nectow, Z. A. Knight, K. N. Latcha, L. E. Pomeranz, and J. M. Friedman, "Molecular profiling of neurons based on connectivity," *Cell*, vol. 157, no. 5, pp. 1230–1242, 2014.

17

Functional Brain Connectivity during Multiple Motor Imagery Tasks in Spinal Cord Injury

Alkinoos Athanasiou [ID],[1,2] Nikos Terzopoulos,[1] Niki Pandria [ID],[1] Ioannis Xygonakis,[1] Nicolas Foroglou,[2] Konstantinos Polyzoidis,[2] and Panagiotis D. Bamidis [ID][1]

[1]Biomedical Electronics Robotics & Devices (BERD) Group, Lab of Medical Physics, School of Medicine, Faculty of Health Sciences, Aristotle University of Thessaloniki (AUTH), 54124 Thessaloniki, Greece
[2]1st Department of Neurosurgery, "AHEPA" University General Hospital, Aristotle University of Thessaloniki (AUTH), 54636 Thessaloniki, Greece

Correspondence should be addressed to Alkinoos Athanasiou; athalkinoos@auth.gr

Academic Editor: Thierry Pozzo

Reciprocal communication of the central and peripheral nervous systems is compromised during spinal cord injury due to neurotrauma of ascending and descending pathways. Changes in brain organization after spinal cord injury have been associated with differences in prognosis. Changes in functional connectivity may also serve as injury biomarkers. Most studies on functional connectivity have focused on chronic complete injury or resting-state condition. In our study, ten right-handed patients with incomplete spinal cord injury and ten age- and gender-matched healthy controls performed multiple visual motor imagery tasks of upper extremities and walking under high-resolution electroencephalography recording. Directed transfer function was used to study connectivity at the cortical source space between sensorimotor nodes. Chronic disruption of reciprocal communication in incomplete injury could result in permanent significant decrease of connectivity in a subset of the sensorimotor network, regardless of positive or negative neurological outcome. Cingulate motor areas consistently contributed the larger outflow (right) and received the higher inflow (left) among all nodes, across all motor imagery categories, in both groups. Injured subjects had higher outflow from left cingulate than healthy subjects and higher inflow in right cingulate than healthy subjects. Alpha networks were less dense, showing less integration and more segregation than beta networks. Spinal cord injury patients showed signs of increased local processing as adaptive mechanism. This trial is registered with NCT02443558.

1. Introduction

Reciprocal communication of the central and peripheral nervous systems is compromised during spinal cord injury (SCI), a condition that often causes permanent disability due to massive neurotrauma of ascending and descending pathways [1, 2]. While changes in brain activity and brain organization may seem trivial, when compared to the underlying injury of the pathways, they have nevertheless been consistently associated with SCI [3–5]. Such changes have also been observed at the early stages after the injury and have been associated with differences regarding the prognosis of SCI patients' recovery [4–6]. Demonstrated structural changes of the brain include atrophy of afferent neural pathways, microstructural changes of efferent axons, and disorder of white matter integrity in multiple nodes of the sensorimotor cortex that involve the primary motor and somatosensory areas [7] and also diffuse neuronal degeneration [8].

Functional connectivity (FC) after SCI has been studied by means of electroencephalography (EEG) [9–15] and functional magnetic resonance imaging (fMRI) [6, 16–21]. Poor recovery after SCI has been associated with decreased FC strengths between midline sensorimotor network nodes during resting state, while the opposite pattern has been associated with good recovery [6]. Supplementary and cingulate motor areas have been shown to play important roles during the sensorimotor neurophysiological process [9, 11], while unique interactions and temporal dynamics have been identified in the functional networks of SCI patients [12, 14]. Connectivity changes have been hypothesized to be able to serve as injury biomarkers [22] while novel methods have been developed and have been proposed in order to study the brain's connectome following SCI in hopes of providing more reliable evidence of these changes [23].

Most studies on functional connectivity after SCI have focused on patients with chronic complete injury, including the majority of EEG studies. Only a couple of studies employing fMRI as a modality to detect brain activity have assessed patients with incomplete injury but those have only studied connectivity during resting-state condition so far [6, 16–18]. Moreover, the pioneer EEG studies on functional cortical connectivity of SCI patients during motor imagery have employed a robust but rather limited study design [9]. In this design, the motor imagery task involved an attempt to move the paralyzed right foot and was performed simultaneously with one motor execution task (lip protrusion), while the functional networks were subsequently analyzed using a variety of tools. So far, to the authors' best knowledge, no study has been performed employing multiple motor imagery tasks, especially of the upper extremities, aiming to analyze differences in the formed networks. Moreover, incomplete injury at the chronic phases remains understudied compared to chronic complete injury with regard to functional connectivity networks. Despite the clinical and social impact of SCI, so far published studies have been unable to form a complete model regarding the effect of the injury on brain networks, although effort has been made into modeling-specific aspects, like resting-state connectivity and chronic injury [3, 22]. It can be hypothesized—and there are also indications—that even incomplete spinal cord injury may show measurable effects on the functional sensorimotor network [24] that could be important for modeling the condition in relation to prognosis [3, 6, 16].

Motor imagery, apart from its importance to the study of brain activity after neurotrauma, has shown great potential in motor skill learning and in rehabilitation of upper and lower limb paralysis [25, 26]. It has been established that motor imagery produces patterns of brain activation and brain connectivity similar to those of motor execution [27, 28], while the visual motor imagery class also activates a distinct task-dependent neural system [29, 30]. Motor imagery has been used as a modality to induce plasticity and recovery in a range of conditions [31], including complete cervical spinal cord injury [32] and stroke [33]. Moreover, motor imagery has been also used as a control modality for brain-computer interface implementations of exoskeletons for complete [34] and incomplete spinal cord injury [35]. Functional recovery has been induced even in the case of complete injuries using such an approach [34]. Such results demonstrate the importance of motor imagery functional networks studies to accurately model the plastic changes that occur after SCI.

In our previous work, we have presented our study with a cohort of SCI patients and healthy control subjects that exercised motor imagery to achieve control of anthropomorphic robotic arms in various movement tasks. We have accounted

for development [36], pilot experiments, and brain network analysis [37, 38], and we have presented a detailed user perception and performance assessment study, based on neurological and psychometric evaluation [39]. In the current paper, we present an elaborate analysis of the functional connectivity networks formed on the sensorimotor cortex during visual motor imagery of multiple motor tasks performed by subjects with SCI and healthy controls. In Materials and Methods, we briefly present the experimental setup and detail our signal processing computational workflow, network analysis, and statistical comparisons. In Results, we detail important findings with regard to the effect of injury, motor imagery category, brainwave rhythm, and timing of imagery. In Discussion, we attempt to interpret our results in the context of already published studies in the field, and we note the limitations of this approach.

2. Materials and Methods

2.1. Experimental Setup

2.1.1. Recruitment and Subject Assessment. The experimental setup has been previously described in detail, including subject assessment [39] and procedures [36, 37], so we will hereby provide only a brief overview. Our experimental protocol was approved by the institutional ethical committee [40], and all subjects signed an informed consent form. We recruited 8 male and 2 female patients with SCI (age: mean 46.0, SD 17.64, range 28–74 years) and ten gender- and age-matched healthy controls. All participants were right-handed and reported no prior experience in mental imagery (Table 1).

For both groups, we collected demographics and medical history; also, a specialist physician performed neurological examination using the International Standards for Neurological Classification of Spinal Cord Injury, to document classification in American Spinal Injury Association Impairment Scale (AIS) and the Neurological Level of Injury (NLI). Subject assessment also included subjective reporting of imagery capacity, using Vividness of Visual Imagery Questionnaire (VVIQ) [41] with eyes open (Table 1). Within the SCI group, 60% of the patients were grouped into positive outcome based on the neurological assessment (4 AIS D, 2 AIS E), and 40% of the patients were grouped into negative outcome (1 AIS A, 2 AIS B, and 1 AIS C).

2.1.2. Experimental Procedure. The experiment took place inside a magnetic shielded room for EEG recording, specially designed for presentation capability and audiovisual monitoring of the participants. The subjects sat at a 1 m distance across a 21″ computer monitor. They wore an active electrode cap (Brain Products, Germany) and were connected to a 128-channel EEG (Nihon-Kohden, Japan) according to the high-resolution EEG 10–5 international electrode system [42]. Recordings were taken at a sampling rate of 1000 Hz and an impedance threshold of 10 kohm [36]. Initially, we recorded resting-state activity, 1.5 min with open eyes and 1.5 min with closed eyes.

TABLE 1: Demographic data and reported imagery capacity of subject groups (SCI and healthy).

(a)

SCI group	Age	Gender	Cause	AIS	NLI	VVIQ
CSI-02-001	28	f	MVA	C	C4	54
CSI-02-002	52	m	MVA	D	C4	69
CSI-02-003	42	m	MVA	D	C8	68
CSI-02-004	70	m	Fall	D	C5	76
CSI-02-005	60	m	Fall	E	C6	70
CSI-02-006	28	m	MVA	D	C5	56
CSI-02-007	30	m	MVA	E	C5	67
CSI-03-001	47	m	Fall	A	T7	72
CSI-03-002	29	f	MVA	B	T4	60
CSI-03-003	74	m	Other	B	T4	65
Mean (SD)	46.00 (17.64)					65.70 (7.04)

(b)

Healthy group	Age	Gender	VVIQ
CSI-04-001	27	f	77
CSI-04-007	51	m	75
CSI-04-003	43	m	56
CSI-04-006	71	m	70
CSI-04-009	63	m	70
CSI-04-004	28	m	46
CSI-04-005	31	m	58
CSI-04-008	47	m	80
CSI-04-002	27	f	75
CSI-04-010	74	m	63
Mean (SD)	46.20 (18.27)		67.00 (10.09)

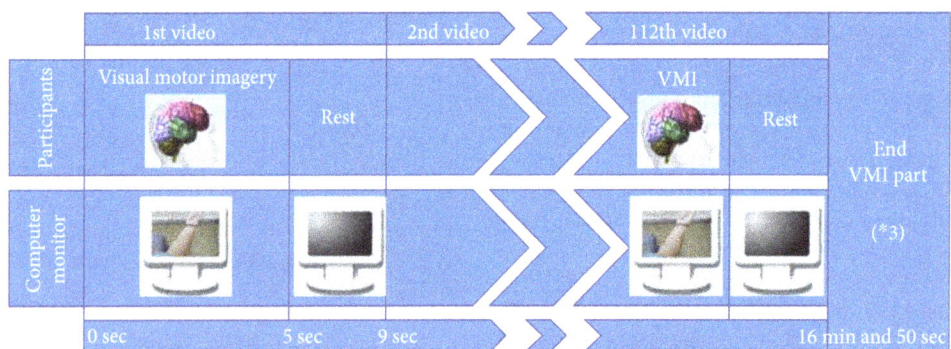

FIGURE 1: Flow diagram of the experimental procedure of one part of the visual motor imagery presentation. Each presented video lasted 5 seconds and was followed by 4 seconds of black resting screen. The videos were presented 9 times each, in a random order. The presentation was divided into three parts, lasting approximately 17 minutes each, with an intermission between them.

In the main experimental part, the subjects watched videos of 32 different arm motor tasks, a walking task video, and an oddball video. The videos were presented in random order. All arm motor task videos were presented from the perspective of the participant watching his or her own arms and were gender-matched. The walking task video presented a pair of gender-matched legs walking, while seeing them from the perspective of watching one's own legs. The oddball video showed a wildlife documentary. The videos lasted 5 sec, each followed by a black screen with duration of 4 sec. A trigger channel was recorded at the onset of each visual cue (the start of each video) through an optic diode. The presentation was separated in three parts of about 17 min each, with 5 min of rest between them (Figure 1). At conclusion, each task had been presented 9 times in total. The subjects were asked to perform visual motor imagery (VMI), while watching a motor task, without actually moving their limbs (regardless of neurological status or group) and were instructed to rest while watching the black screen. They already knew that the videos would be presented at random but not of the presence of an oddball video (video showing wildlife). Moreover, the subjects' arms, torso, and legs were covered with a black curtain during the whole procedure in order to facilitate mental registration of the presented arms and legs into their perceived body schema [43].

The 32 upper extremity motor tasks consisted of 8 independent movements (degrees of freedom) * 2 directions of movement * 2 extremities, comprising the full range of motion of the human arms and were classified into categories for further analysis [39]. In short, the 8 categories of motor tasks were "Hands," "Left," "Right," "Proximal," "Distal," "Rotational," "Linear," and "Walking."

The "Hands" category included all 32 tasks of both upper extremities. The "Left" and "Right" categories included 16 motor tasks each of the respective upper extremity (left or right). The "Proximal" category included 16 motor tasks of the shoulder and elbow joints of both extremities, while the "Distal" category included the remaining 16 motor tasks of wrist joints and fingers. Further, the "Rotational" category included those 8 motor tasks that result in rotational motion, and the "Linear" category included those 24 motor tasks of both extremities that resulted in linear motion (Table 2). Finally, the "Walking" category was also defined as a separate category of motor imagery, consisting only of the walking motor imagery task, for a total of 8 categories. Table 2 lists in summary all presented motor tasks of one upper extremity (16 tasks), for each showing the degree of freedom, direction of movement, classification by proximity, and resulted motion.

2.2. Signal Analysis

2.2.1. Signal Preprocessing.
Signal analysis was performed on a subset of the 10–5 international electrode system that is overlying the cortical sensorimotor areas [44] that were later defined as regions of interest (ROIs) for this study (Figure 2). This subset included 64 electrodes: AFF5h, AFF3h, AFF1h, AFz, AFF2h, AFF4h, AFF6h, F5, F3, F1, Fz, F2, F4, F6, FFT7h, FFC3h, FFC1h, FFC2h, FFC4h, FFT8h, FT7, FC5, FC3, FC1, FC2, FC4, FC6, FT8, FTT7h, FCC5h, FCC3h, FCC1h, FCC4h, FCC6h, FTT8h, C5, C3, C1, Cz, C2, C4, C6, CCP3h, CCP1h, CCP2h, CCP4h, CP5, CP3, CP1, CPz, CP2, CP4, CP6, CPP3h, CPP1h, CPP2h, CPP4h, P3, P1, Pz, P2, P4, PPO1h, and PPO2h. As scalp electrodes capture mixed activity from unknown cortical and subcortical brain sources, recording brain activity related to motor tasks only from the sensors overlying the sensorimotor area presents some risk for loss of information but also presents certain advantages. This approach has been used in EEG source imaging studies regarding motor tasks with good results [45–48], as the signal of interest is less attenuated and signal to noise ratio is higher than in distant sensors, while contaminated channels closer to muscular artifact generators are excluded.

TABLE 2: Presented motor tasks for one upper extremity (left or right): 16 motor tasks were presented (8 independent movements (degrees of freedom) * 2 directions of movement) and were then classified by proximity (proximal or distal tasks) and resulting motion (linear or rotational). For both upper extremities, the subjects watched and performed visual imagery of 32 motor tasks in total.

Independent movement	Direction	Proximal/ distal	Linear/ rotational
Shoulder	Arm down	Proximal	Linear
Shoulder	Arm up	Proximal	Linear
Shoulder	Arm left	Proximal	Linear
Shoulder	Arm right	Proximal	Linear
Elbow	Forearm down	Proximal	Linear
Elbow	Forearm up	Proximal	Linear
Forearm	External rotation	Proximal	Rotational
Forearm	Internal rotation	Proximal	Rotational
Wrist	Hand down	Distal	Linear
Wrist	Hand up	Distal	Linear
Wrist	External rotation	Distal	Rotational
Wrist	Internal rotation	Distal	Rotational
Thumb	Open	Distal	Linear
Thumb	Close	Distal	Linear
Fingers	Open	Distal	Linear
Fingers	Close	Distal	Linear

All signal preprocessing was performed using a custom script on the FieldTrip toolbox for MATLAB [49]. Raw data from those selected channels was band-pass filtered at 0.5–30 Hz using a zero-phase FIR filter and subsequently downsampled at 100 Hz. We visually examined continuous EEG signal time series of each subject to detect bad electrodes that showed large drifts from their mean value and then removed these electrodes. Epochs were then initially extracted from −2000 msec to +5000 msec centered on the trigger (visual cue). Subsequently, independent component analysis was performed on the concatenated continuous data (of each session) using the second-order blind identification method [50]. Independent components corresponding to eye blinks and muscle artifacts were identified and removed from the epoched data. Bad electrodes were then interpolated using spherical splines interpolation [51]. Finally, the epoched data were split into two time intervals (Figure 3), which will be referred to as "early" (early onset imagery from −1000 msec to +2000 msec around the trigger) and "late" (late continuous imagery from +2000 msec to +5000 msec after the trigger). While shorter time windows have also been used in similar analyses [52], differences in the behavior of alpha and beta rhythms between the window around the imagery onset and later windows have been identified with regard to networks [53], relative power [54], and

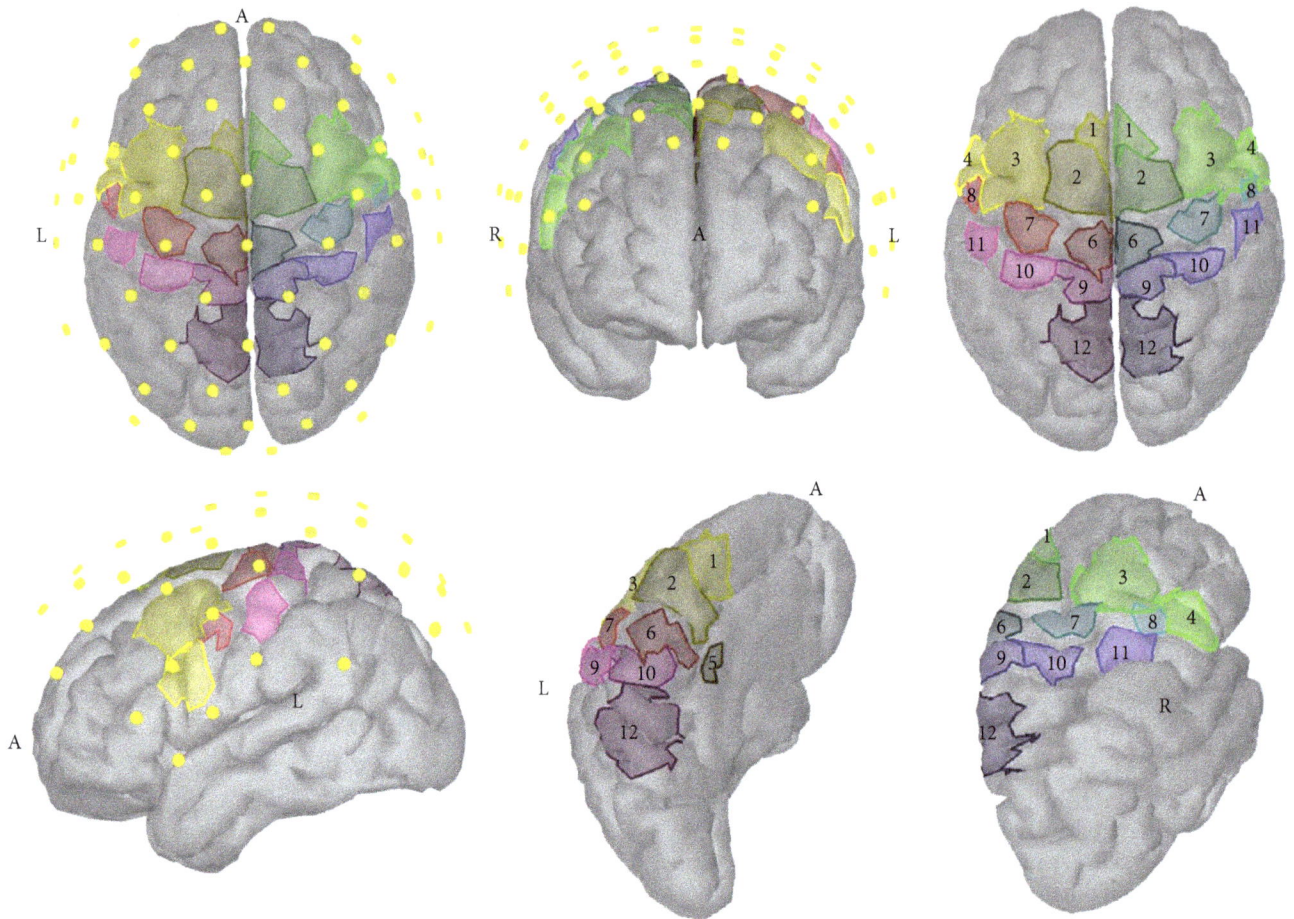

FIGURE 2: Regions of interest (ROIs) of the sensorimotor cortex and the overlying subset of electrodes that was used for signal analysis in our study. 1: presupplementary motor area (pSMA); 2: supplementary motor area (SMA); 3: dorsal premotor area (PMd); 4: ventral premotor area (PMv); 5: cingulate motor area (CMA); 6: primary foot motor area (M1F); 7: primary hand motor area (M1H); 8: primary lip motor area (M1L); 9: primary foot somatosensory area (S1F); 10: primary hand somatosensory area (S1H); 11: secondary somatosensory area (S2); 12: somatosensory association area (SAC).

event-related desynchronization [55]. The data from one subject (from the healthy group) was exempted from further analysis, as this preprocessing methodology did not result in sufficiently clean epoched data.

2.2.2. Current Cortical Density. The solution of the forward problem, the lead field matrix that best describes the conduction from the current cortical density (CCD) source model (Table 3) to scalp potentials, is based on the following equation:

$$m = Ld + b, \qquad (1)$$

where m refers to the M simultaneous electrode voltage recordings, d refers to the N current dipoles in the current cortical density model, b is the noise vector, and L is the abovementioned lead field matrix [56]. We used the solution applied in eConnectome toolbox for MATLAB [57, 58] of the forward problem which is a high-resolution lead field matrix relating 2054 scalp triangles to 7850 cortical dipoles. The lead field matrix is derived using a three-layer block element modifier model based on the Colin27 Montreal Neurological Institute brain [59]. The dipoles were constrained to the gray

matter with orientations perpendicular to the local cortical surface, under the assumption that the primary source of measured EEG signal is local groups of pyramidal neurons of the cortex firing synchronously and is arranged perpendicular to its surface [60]. In our case, a subset of the lead field matrix was used for the 64 selected EEG electrodes.

Weighted minimum norm estimate was used to solve the ill-posed inverse problem (Table 3) by minimizing the source space energy based on the fact that the power of the source dipoles is limited by the cortex physiology [61]. Minimum norm estimate aims at minimizing the following equation:

$$J(d) = \|m - Ld\|^2 + \lambda \|d\|^2, \qquad (2)$$

where m refers to the actual recordings from the scalp, d is the simultaneous current dipoles to be calculated, L is the lead field matrix, λ is the regularization parameter, and $|d|^2$ is the regularization term which in our case refers to the energy of the solution's dipoles. The first term in the above equation represents the error between the actual and predicted electrode recordings. The second term is the penalization term, which aims at enforcing the abovementioned

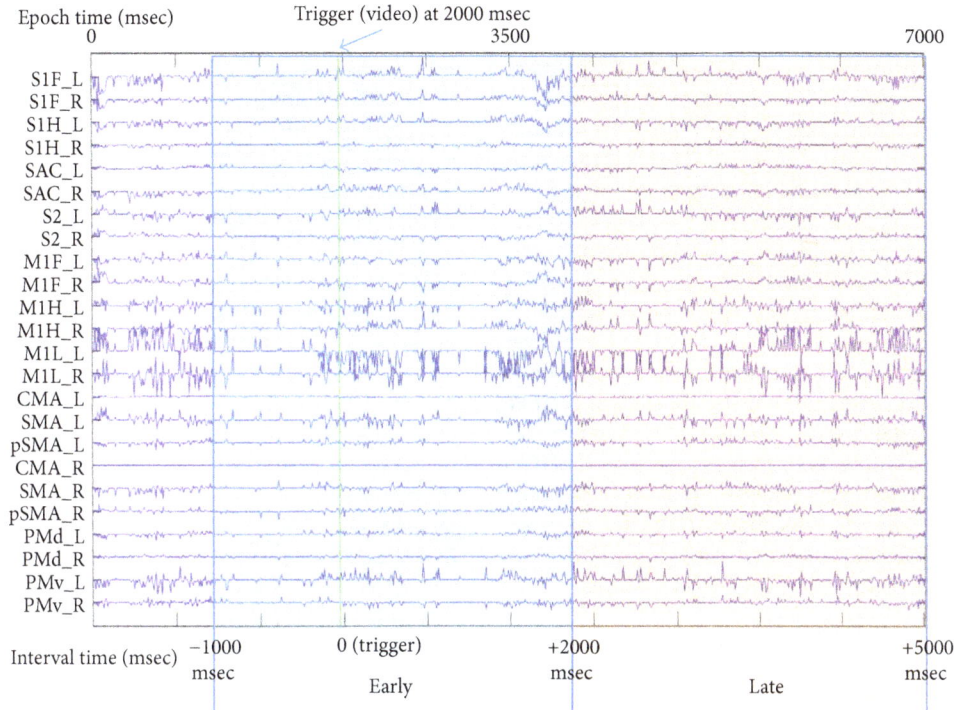

FIGURE 3: Activation time series of all regions of interest (ROIs) of the sensorimotor cortex during a random epoch and definition of time intervals around the trigger (onset of the video presenting the motor imagery task).

TABLE 3: Summary presentation and description of the most important models and connectivity metrics or measures that were used in the methodological section of this study.

Metric or model name	Acronym		Description
Current cortical density	CCD	Forward problem solution	A model that aims to explain the correspondence of cortical source activity to scalp electrical potentials, taking account of skull and scalp conductivity.
Weighted minimum norm estimate	wMNE	Inverse problem solution	An estimation of how signals captured at the scalp correspond to source activations, with their power limited by the cortical physiology.
Directed transfer function	DTF	Granger causality measure	A metric of effective network connectivity (functional connectivity that incorporates causal relations instead of statistical inference alone) that produces directed networks with weighted edges.
Characteristic path length	CPL	Network integration	A representative measure of shortest distances between network nodes that are connected to each other.
Clustering coefficient	CC	Network segregation	A measure of the tendency of network nodes to become organized into functionally separated clusters.
Density	D	Network density	A measure of existing connections against the theoretical maximum number of possible connections if the network was fully connected.
Small-worldness	SW	Overall network effectiveness	A model of network behavior, where short paths and increased forming of functional clusters lead to optimization and resilience of information transfer.
Out-strength and in-strength	OS and IS		The total nodal sum of weights from outgoing and incoming connections, respectively.

energy restriction. Lastly, λ, which balances the effect of the penalization term, was calculated using the L-curve method [62]. The solution of minimum norm estimate was derived using Tikhonov regularization in the regularization toolbox [63]. 24 custom-defined ROIs were created at the surface of the cortex model, in order to proceed to connectivity analysis, as illustrated in Figure 2. The ROI time series signal

(Figure 3) was calculated by averaging the amplitude from all included cortical current dipoles.

2.2.3. Functional Connectivity. In total, 24 ROIs were defined on the cortical source model, consisting of the following areas bilaterally: presupplementary motor area (pSMA), supplementary motor area (SMA), dorsal premotor area (PMd), ventral premotor area (PMv), cingulate motor area (CMA), primary foot motor area (M1F), primary hand motor area (M1H), primary lip motor area (M1L), primary foot somatosensory area (S1F), primary hand somatosensory area (S1H), secondary somatosensory area (S2), and somatosensory association area (SAC) (Figure 2). Their average activation time series were computed for every time interval.

Directed transfer function (DTF) [64] was used (Table 3) in order to calculate functional cortical connectivity of the sensorimotor network consisting of the 24 ROIs as nodes [44], computing causal relations among the nodal activation time series. The produced connectivity matrices were thresholded, using the surrogate data method with testing of significance of connections, instead of using absolute or relative thresholding [65–67]. During computation of DTF, a number of 1000 surrogate permutations and a significance level of 0.05 were set, resulting in partially connected matrices with only the most significant causal connections. DTF is a measure based on Granger causality [68] that uses the multivariate autoregressive model described by the following function:

$$X(t) = \sum_{j=1}^{p} A(j)X(t-j) + E(t), \qquad (3)$$

where p is the model order, $X(t)$ contains the ROIs values at time t, $E(t)$ is the residual noise vector, and A is a coefficient $k \times k$-sized matrix [44]. Using the above equation, the A matrices are computed by means of the minimalization of the residual noise E.

The order of the multivariate autoregressive model [69] was chosen to be 8 after considering the following criterions [70]: (a) tests that demonstrated an optimal order of 10 for a sampling rate of 128 Hz for modeling EEG spectra [71, 72]; (b) the model order should be smaller than $\tau \times \text{Fs}$, where τ is the expected lag between two brain processes and Fs the sampling rate; (c) better to err on the side of selecting a larger model order, (d) using the same model order for all DTF computations.

Equation (3) is described in the frequency domain as

$$\begin{aligned} E(f) &= A(f)X(f), \\ X(f) &= A^{-1}(f)E(f) = H(f)E(f), \end{aligned} \qquad (4)$$

where $H(f)$ is a transfer matrix of the system, and it contains information about the relationships between signals. It is nonsymmetric, so it allows for finding causal dependencies. DTF is then computed by the equation:

$$\text{DTF}_{j \to i}^2(f) = \frac{\|H_{ij}(f)\|^2}{\sum_{m=1}^{k} \|H_{im}(f)\|^2}. \qquad (5)$$

DTF describes casual influence of channel j on channel i at frequency f. For our analysis, DTF was computed for the networks formed at the frequency bands of alpha rhythm at 8–12 Hz ("alpha networks") and beta rhythm at 13–30 Hz ("beta networks"), as those are considered the brainwaves most relevant to the sensorimotor processes [73].

2.2.4. Network Analysis. Network analysis in terms of descriptors of the weighted directed graphs ("network properties") was performed with the brain connectivity toolbox for MATLAB [74] for the *alpha* and *beta* networks formed during *early* and *late* time intervals. Out-strength (OS), in-strength (IS), and clustering coefficient were computed for each of the 24 nodes of the network during each task of imagery. Characteristic path length (CPL), mean clustering coefficient (CC), and density (D) were also computed at the level of graphs of each task of imagery. Topology of small-worldness (SW) was then derived from these network properties for each task of imagery [44]. To facilitate further analysis, all properties were averaged for the 8 imagery categories mentioned in Experimental Procedure. A summary of the interpretation of these network properties is also presented in Table 3.

CPL, a measure of integration, calculates the sum of the shortest distances among connected graph nodes, divided by the number of nodes [75, 76]. It is described by (6), where Li is the average distance between node i and the other node, and d_{ij} is the shortest path between nodes i and j. The distance matrix was computed using the logarithmic conversion of weights by the Floyd-Warshall algorithm [77], as implemented in the BCT [78].

$$\text{CPL} = \frac{1}{n} \sum_{i \in N} Li = \frac{1}{n} \sum_{i \in N} \frac{\sum_{j \in N, j \neq i} d_{ij}}{n-1}. \qquad (6)$$

Global CC, a measure of segregation, estimates the tendency of the graph nodes to organize into clusters [79, 80]. It is described by (7), where Ci is the clustering value for a node i, k_i is the node's degree, and t_i is the number of neighboring nodes that connect to each other in triangles around node i.

$$\text{CC} = \frac{1}{n} \sum_{i \in N} Ci = \frac{1}{n} \sum_{i \in N} \frac{2t_i}{k_i(k_i - 1)}. \qquad (7)$$

D is the ratio of a network's actual connections to the maximum possible connections. In our example, the graphs were only partially connected, and the connection weights were ignored, since all connections were considered significant as computed by DTF with testing for statistical significance ($p = 0.05$) by surrogate data. It is therefore described by (8), where E is the ensemble of the network's connections, and V is the ensemble of the network's nodes.

$$D = \frac{|E|}{|V|(|V|-1)}. \qquad (8)$$

SW is defined as the combination of short paths and high clustering in a network, when compared to random networks with comparable paths constructed by the same number of nodes and connections. This property has commanded attention as an important brain network characteristic that models the brain's effective communication patterns [81–83]. It is described by (9), and in our study, the comparison of CPL and CC was made against 10,000 random networks. These random networks were directed graphs, with the same number of nodes and edges as the original, and they were generated using the brain connectivity toolbox [84]. CPL and CC were computed for each random network and compared against the original, in a process that was iterated 10,000 times to produce a range of SW values. The range of values was then averaged to produce a single robust value of the SW property for each original network.

$$SW = \frac{CC/CC_{rand}}{CPL/CPL_{rand}}. \qquad (9)$$

The strength of node strength is the sum of the weights of connections to or from that node. The IS, therefore, is the sum of incoming connection weights, and the OS is the sum of outgoing connection weights [74]. They are described by (10) and (11), respectively, where C_{ij} is the weighted directed N^*M connectivity matrix, with a direction of $i \rightarrow j$, N is the number of columns, and M is the number of rows.

$$IS = \sum_{j=1}^{N} C_{ij}, \qquad (10)$$

$$OS = \sum_{i=1}^{M} C_{ij}. \qquad (11)$$

2.3. Statistical Analysis. Adjacency matrices computed by directed transfer function were compared between healthy and patient groups using the network-based statistic toolbox for MATLAB [85]. We performed the statistical analysis using the false discovery rate on the general linear model with t-test [86], a significance level of 0.05 and 50,000 permutations. Using a between-group design, we compared alpha and beta networks of healthy subjects to alpha and beta networks of SCI subjects for each imagery category, elaborating the comparisons for the effect of early and late intervals. We also compared alpha to beta networks of each category and time interval using a within-group design. Differences in networks were visualized using the BrainNet Viewer for MATLAB [87].

Statistical analysis of age, imagery capacity, and computed network properties was performed in IBM SPSS Statistics (version 23), and we set a significance level of 0.05 for all statistical tests. All variables were explored for normality assumption (healthy and SCI groups as grouping factor) using visual inspection of histograms, normal Q-Q plots and box-plots, skewness and kurtosis [88–90], and normality tests (Shapiro-Wilk test and Kolmogorov-Smirnov test) [91, 92]. Depending on normality assumption, different analyses were performed (paired t-tests or Wilcoxon signed-rank tests). Normality assumption was met for the variable age and for the VVIQ score for both groups. Independent sample t-tests were performed to reveal significant age and VVIQ differences between the two groups. As the groups did not differ either for age distributions (healthy-skewness: 0.407 (SE = 0.687), kurtosis: −1.418 (SE = 1.334); SCI-skewness: 0.651 (SE = 0.687), kurtosis: −0.752 (SE = 1.334)) or for their reported imagery capacity (VVIQ: $t = -1.094$, df = 8, and $p = 0.306$), the rest of the statistical analysis was planned accordingly.

We planned within-group comparisons of brain network properties using as grouping factor the rhythm (alpha, beta). Differences of variables between the two rhythms were calculated for the categories of visual motor imagery tasks, separately at early and late time intervals. Subsequently, we calculated within-group comparisons of brain network properties using as grouping factor the time interval (early, late). Between-group comparisons were performed using the calculated differences of variables at the two time intervals with either independent samples t-tests or Mann–Whitney U tests.

Nodal strengths, both incoming and outgoing, were averaged across different motor imagery tasks, rhythms, and time intervals, and total nodal strengths were calculated. They were tested for normality assumption for both groups and analyzed within groups using descriptive statistics and between groups (SCI, healthy) using Mann–Whitney U test. Targeted differences between nodes CMA_L and CMA_R were tested for statistical significance using either Pearson or Spearman correlation coefficient depending on normality assumption.

3. Results

3.1. Functional Connectivity. Visualizations of connectivity maps for the two groups (SCI, healthy) were made using the eConnectome toolbox for alpha and beta networks during both time intervals averaged across the motor imagery categories (Figure 4). The highest information transfer in all examined networks came from the bilateral cingulate motor areas including their reciprocal communication. In both groups, the maximum incoming nodal strength was observed in right CMA (Table 4), whereas the maximum outgoing nodal strength was found in left CMA (Table 5). Between-group comparisons revealed significant differences in total nodal strengths, both incoming and outgoing.

More precisely, significant differences in incoming strengths were found bilaterally in CMA, SMA, S1H, PMd, and PMv as well as in the left S1F. Healthy participants showed higher incoming strengths in all aforementioned nodes apart from the left CMA (Figure 5) compared to the SCI participants (Table 4).

Outgoing strengths were found to be significantly different between groups in all nodes (Table 5) apart from the right S1F. In more detail, SCI group showed considerably higher outgoing strengths in the S1F and SAC in the left hemisphere, in S1H and CMA in the right hemisphere as well as in S2, PMd and PMv bilaterally. In the remaining nodes, healthy participants were found to have increased outgoing strengths compared to SCI participants.

When calculating differences of group averages (healthy group-SCI group) of in-strength (IS) and out-strength (OS) of cingulate motor areas (CMAs) during all motor imagery categories, a possible trend was revealed. OS of CMA_R was consistently higher in the healthy group, while OS of CMA_L was consistently higher in the SCI group. The opposite held true for IS of those nodes (Figure 6). Between-group differences in CMA_R were negatively correlated to those in CMA_L in targeted imagery categories (early alpha walking ($r = -0.867$, $p = 0.002$), late alpha walking ($r = -0.250$ $p = 0.517$), early beta walking ($r = -0.502$, $p = 0.169$), and late beta walking ($r = -0.827$, $p = 0.006$)).

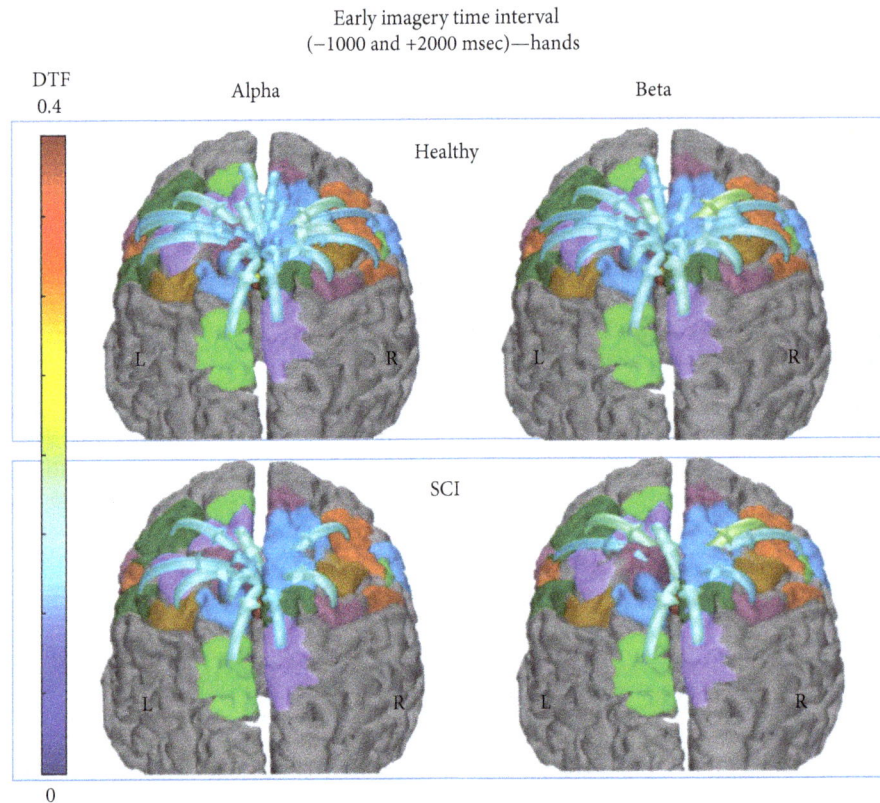

FIGURE 4: Average information transfer (calculated by directed transfer function) of healthy and SCI groups calculated for alpha (left) and beta (right) rhythm networks during the early imagery time interval, for the hands motor imagery category. Connections between the bilateral cingulate motor areas (CMA_R ← → CMA_L) presented the highest information transfer. Only connections with at least 25% of max information transfer among all statistically significant connections are displayed.

TABLE 4: Descriptive statistics of nodal incoming strengths with statistically significant differences between healthy and SCI participants and between-group comparison results.

Nodes	Median		Mean ranks		IQR: [Q_1, Q_2]		Healthy versus SCI
	Healthy	SCI	Healthy	SCI	Healthy	SCI	
SIF L	**0.235**	0.230	37.72	27.28	[0.231, 0.253]	[0.226, 0.238]	$U = 345.0$, $p = 0.025$
SIH L	**0.263**	0.246	44.13	20.88	[0.258, 0.270]	[0.239, 0.256]	$U = 140.0$, $p < 0.001$
SIH R	**0.256**	0.233	40.94	24.06	[0.243, 0.265]	[0.229, 0.248]	$U = 242.0$, $p < 0.001$
CMA L	0.410	**0.438**	18.84	46.16	[0.402, 0.419]	[0.431, 0.445]	$U = 75.0$, $p < 0.001$
CMA R	**0.486**	0.473	38.38	26.63	[0.475, 0.509]	[0.458, 0.489]	$U = 324.0$, $p = 0.012$
SMA L	**0.236**	0.217	41.34	23.66	[0.230, 0.243]	[0.213, 0.229]	$U = 229.0$, $p < 0.001$
SMA R	**0.305**	0.289	39.50	25.50	[0.296, 0.314]	[0.281, 0.297]	$U = 288.0$, $p = 0.003$
PMd L	**0.309**	0.272	46.84	18.16	[0.296, 0.320]	[0.260, 0.278]	$U = 53.0$, $p < 0.001$
PMd R	**0.299**	0.284	37.78	27.22	[0.290, 0.304]	[0.274, 0.299]	$U = 343.0$, $p = 0.023$
PMv L	**0.252**	0.232	40.53	24.47	[0.236, 0.259]	[0.220, 0.243]	$U = 255.0$, $p = 0.001$
PMv R	**0.262**	0.247	41.81	23.19	[0.254, 0.267]	[0.240, 0.255]	$U = 214.0$, $p < 0.001$

3.2. Network-Based Statistics between Groups and within Groups. Important differences of connectivity were found only in between groups (SCI against healthy), where a subset of connections had significantly higher FC in the healthy group than in the SCI group in the hands motor imagery category (Figure 7). This subset included connections with lower FC in the SCI group of M1H_R to bilateral primary foot motor areas (M1F), primary foot and hand sensory areas (S1H, S1F), the somatosensory association areas (SAC), and the secondary sensory areas (S2). This finding persisted in both alpha and beta networks when testing with *t*-test.

TABLE 5: Descriptive statistics of nodal outgoing strengths with statistically significant differences between healthy and SCI participants and between-group comparison results.

Nodes	Median		Mean ranks		IQR: $[Q_1, Q_2]$		Healthy versus SCI
	Healthy	SCI	Healthy	SCI	Healthy	SCI	
S1F L	0.073	**0.084**	21.34	43.66	[0.080, 0.095]	[0.080, 0.095]	$U = 155.000, p < 0.001$
S1F R	0.131	0.133	31.81	33.19	[0.123, 0.146]	[0.123, 0.146]	$U = 490.000, p = 0.768$
S1H L	**0.090**	0.084	38.38	26.63	[0.084, 0.100]	[0.077, 0.091]	$U = 324.000, p = 0.012$
S1H R	0.091	**0.166**	16.50	48.50	[0.086, 0.096]	[0.153, 0.181]	$U = 0.000, p < 0.001$
SAC L	0.071	**0.087**	18.28	46.72	[0.069, 0.074]	[0.084, 0.092]	$U = 57.000, p < 0.001$
SAC R	**0.025**	0.015	47.41	17.59	[0.023, 0.027]	[0.014, 0.016]	$U = 35.000, p < 0.001$
S2 L	0.010	**0.022**	17.41	47.59	[0.009, 0.012]	[0.020, 0.024]	$U = 29.000, p < 0.001$
S2 R	0.128	**0.148**	20.91	44.09	[0.124, 0.138]	[0.139, 0.159]	$U = 141.000, p < 0.001$
M1F L	**0.078**	0.073	38.13	26.88	[0.072, 0.088]	[0.069, 0.076]	$U = 332.000, p = 0.016$
M1F R	**0.294**	0.236	47.69	17.31	[0.286, 0.324]	[0.230, 0.263]	$U = 26.000, p < 0.001$
M1H L	**0.311**	0.170	47.59	17.41	[0.283, 0.339]	[0.163, 0.181]	$U = 29.000, p < 0.001$
M1H R	**0.061**	0.059	38.34	26.66	[0.059, 0.066]	[0.058, 0.061]	$U = 325.000, p = 0.012$
M1L L	**0.003**	0.003	26.25	38.75	[0.003, 0.003]	[0.003, 0.004]	$U = 312.000, p = 0.007$
M1L R	**0.011**	0.010	42.78	22.22	[0.010, 0.013]	[0.009, 0.010]	$U = 183.000, p < 0.001$
CMA L	**2.927**	2.519	47.28	17.72	[2.805, 3.008]	[2.404, 2.581]	$U = 39.000, p < 0.001$
CMA R	0.879	**1.156**	18.41	46.59	[0.784, 0.973]	[1.082, 1.261]	$U = 61.000, p < 0.001$
SMA L	**0.350**	0.276	46.25	18.75	[0.326, 0.375]	[0.267, 0.295]	$U = 72.000, p < 0.001$
SMA R	**0.206**	0.187	41.72	23.28	[0.191, 0.226]	[0.176, 0.194]	$U = 217.000, p < 0.001$
pSMA L	**0.044**	0.031	46.50	18.50	[0.040, 0.048]	[0.030, 0.035]	$U = 64.000, p < 0.001$
pSMA R	0.026	**0.031**	19.28	45.72	[0.024, 0.027]	[0.030, 0.033]	$U = 89.000, p < 0.001$
PMd L	0.149	**0.187**	21.13	43.88	[0.141, 0.167]	[0.179, 0.201]	$U = 148.000, p < 0.001$
PMd R	0.484	**0.577**	18.25	46.75	[0.448, 0.521]	[0.559, 0.606]	$U = 56.000, p < 0.001$
PMv L	0.014	**0.024**	16.50	48.50	[0.013, 0.014]	[0.022, 0.025]	$U = 0.000, p < 0.001$
PMv R	0.016	**0.032**	17.91	47.09	[0.014, 0.018]	[0.028, 0.035]	$U = 45.000, p < 0.001$

When we further tested the networks of our participants by grouping the SCI subjects by outcome (positive and negative), no differences were found between the networks of the two groups. During all permutations, the p value of the false discovery rate did not approach statistical significance ($p > 0.05$). Also, testing for other imagery categories did not reveal significant differences, with the exception of the walking category. Comparing the networks of healthy and patients during the walking imagery category, significantly greater S2_L-PMv_R connectivity was found in the SCI group.

Furthermore, when testing for main effect of within time interval and brainwave rhythm within the healthy and patient groups, no further statistical significant differences of the connectivity weights of the network were observed.

3.3. Analysis of Network Properties

3.3.1. Within-Group Comparisons of Graph Properties between Alpha and Beta Showed Less Segregation, Less Integration, Greater Density, and Less Effectiveness of Beta Networks. When exploring within-group differences of graph properties using as grouping factor the rhythm (alpha, beta),

beta networks showed *less segregation, less integration,* and *less overall effectiveness* compared to alpha networks. CPL, CC, and SW showed significantly lower values in beta compared to alpha networks, *in both early and late time intervals.* These findings were observed during nearly all imagery categories in both SCI and healthy group.

On the opposite, beta networks showed *greater density* compared to alpha networks. *D* was significantly greater in beta networks in both early and late time intervals of all imagery categories in both SCI and healthy group (Figure 8). Aggregated statistical test results and p values for abovementioned findings can be found in supplementary material (available here). Specific exemptions are detailed below, as differences of graph properties in beta network compared to alpha did not reach statistical significance only in walking category, in the following cases: (a) in SCI group, CPL during the late interval, (b) in SCI group, CC and SW during the early interval, and (c) in healthy group, CC during the late interval.

3.3.2. Within-Group Comparisons of Graph Properties between Early and Late Time Intervals Showed (1) Less SCI Network Integration during Late Walking Imagery, (2)

(a)

(b)

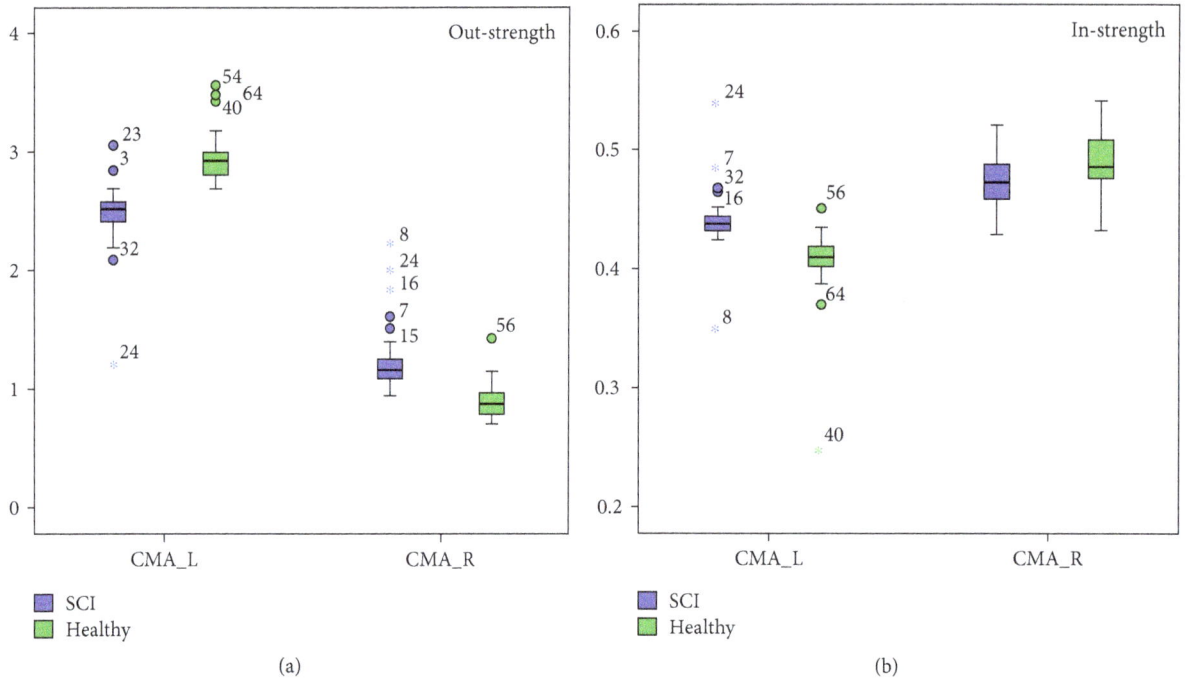

FIGURE 5: Nodal strengths (a: out-strength, b: in-strength) of bilateral cingulate motor areas for both subject groups. Left cingulate motor area (CMA_L) showed the highest out-strength and right cingulate motor area (CMA_R) showed the highest in-strength in the network. SCI subjects presented significantly higher CMA_R out-strength and CMA_L in-strength than healthy subjects. " ∗ " represent extreme values and "o" represent outliers.

Greater SCI Network Segregation and Stable Effectiveness for Distal Tasks during Late Imagery, and (3) Less Healthy Network Segregation and Effectiveness for Distal Tasks during Late Imagery. When exploring within-group differences of graph properties using as grouping factor the time interval (early, late), few significant differences were observed.

Regarding network integration, significant difference of CPL values was shown only SCI group's alpha networks during the *walking* task ($t = 2.743$, df $= 9$, and $p = 0.023$). More precisely, SCI subjects were characterized by lower path lengths at the second stage of the task (late) (early alpha walking CPL: 7.809; late alpha walking CPL: 7.032). Changes in the CPL in the beta rhythm comparing the two time intervals were not observed. Also, no significant difference was found for healthy subjects.

Regarding network segregation, significantly higher CC values in the SCI group were observed in the alpha band of *distal* imagery category ($t = -2.574$, df $= 9$, and $p = 0.030$; early alpha distal CC: 0.0076; late alpha distal CC: 0.0082). Considerable differences in mean CC at the beta band were not found. In healthy participants, considerably lower CC value was found only in alpha band of the *left* category ($t = 2.435$, df $= 8$, and $p = 0.041$; early alpha left CC: 0.0094; late alpha left CC: 0.0086).

Regarding network density, healthy group showed significantly higher D values at the late stage of *linear* imagery tasks in alpha rhythm ($t = -2.543$, df $= 8$, and $p = 0.035$; early alpha linear D: 0.3595; late alpha linear D: 0.3713), whereas density was considerably less at the late stage of *proximal* tasks in beta rhythm ($t = 3.038$, df $= 8$, and $p = 0.016$; early beta proximal

D: 0.5904; late beta proximal D: 0.5784). SCI group showed greater density when comparing the two time intervals of *right* imagery category in alpha band ($t = -2.962$, df $= 9$, and $p = 0.016$; early alpha right D: 0.3663; late alpha right D: 0.3801), but no alterations were found in beta networks.

Regarding overall network effectiveness, significant results of SW were found for healthy subjects at *distal* imagery tasks in both alpha and beta rhythms (alpha: $t = 2.201$, df $= 8$, and $p = 0.059$; beta: $t = 3.044$, df $= 8$, and $p = 0.016$). In more detail, significantly lower values of SW were observed in distal imagery tasks between the two time intervals (early alpha distal SW: 1.553; late alpha distal SW: 1.406; early beta distal SW: 1.159; late beta distal SW: 1.137). For the SCI group, considerable differences were not observed.

3.3.3. Between-Group Comparisons of Graph Properties Showed Not Only Similar Network Integration and Density But Also Greater Segregation and Effectiveness of Alpha Band Networks in Some Imagery Categories for the Patients. When exploring between-group differences of graph properties, few significant differences were observed. Comparisons of CPL and D did not reveal any considerable difference across any imagery category (supplementary material), showing similar network integration and network density of the networks of healthy and patient subjects.

Regarding network segregation, significant changes in CC were observed at the *left* imagery tasks ($t = 2.672$, df $= 17$, and $p = 0.016$), at the *rotational* imagery tasks ($t = 2.104$, df $= 17$, and $p = 0.051$), and at *distal* imagery tasks ($U = 20.00$, $p = 0.041$), all appearing in alpha band. In more detail, SCI subjects seem to show greater CC of alpha networks in the

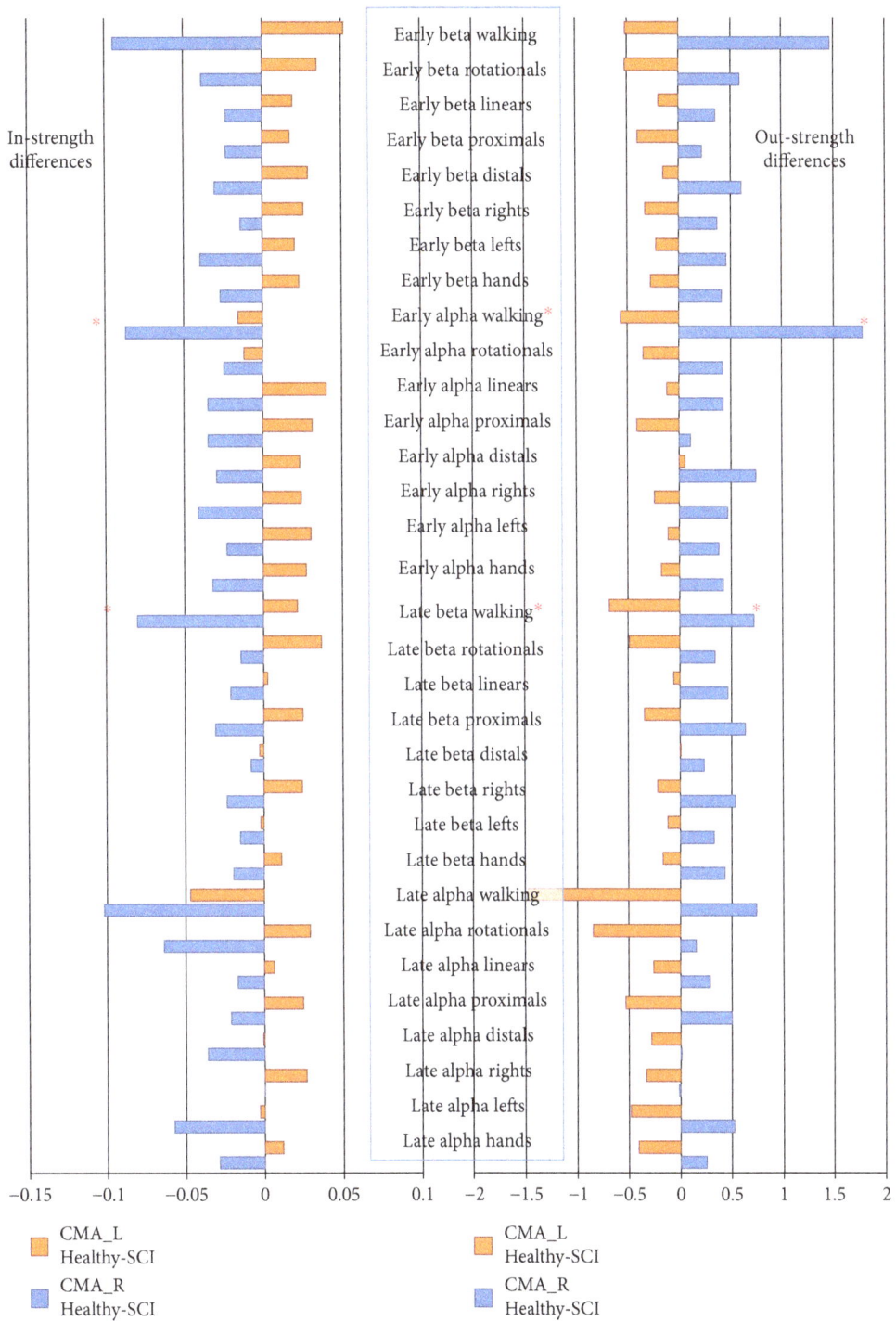

FIGURE 6: Differences of group averages (healthy-SCI) of in-strength (IS) and out-strength (OS) of cingulate motor areas (CMAs) during all motor imagery categories. A trend was revealed, in which OS of CMA_R was consistently higher in the healthy than the SCI group. OS of CMA_L was consistently lower in the healthy than the SCI group. The opposite held true for IS of those nodes. This trend reached statistical significance only for early alpha walking ($p = 0.002$) and late beta walking ($p = 0.006$) tasks.

late part of the aforementioned imagery tasks (alpha left dif (mean)—SCI: 0.00019, healthy: −0.00084; alpha distal dif (median)—SCI: 0.00049, healthy: −0.00075; alpha rotational dif (mean)—SCI: 0.00061, healthy: −0.0010). Significant differences were not found between groups in the beta networks of all tasks.

Regarding overall network effectiveness, the SCI group seems to have only a significant change in mean SW of alpha network while performing VMI on *distal* imagery tasks compared to healthy ($t = 2.365$, df $= 17$, and $p = 0.030$). More precisely, SCI group seems to show greater SW of alpha networks in the late part of the distal tasks (alpha distal dif (mean)—SCI:

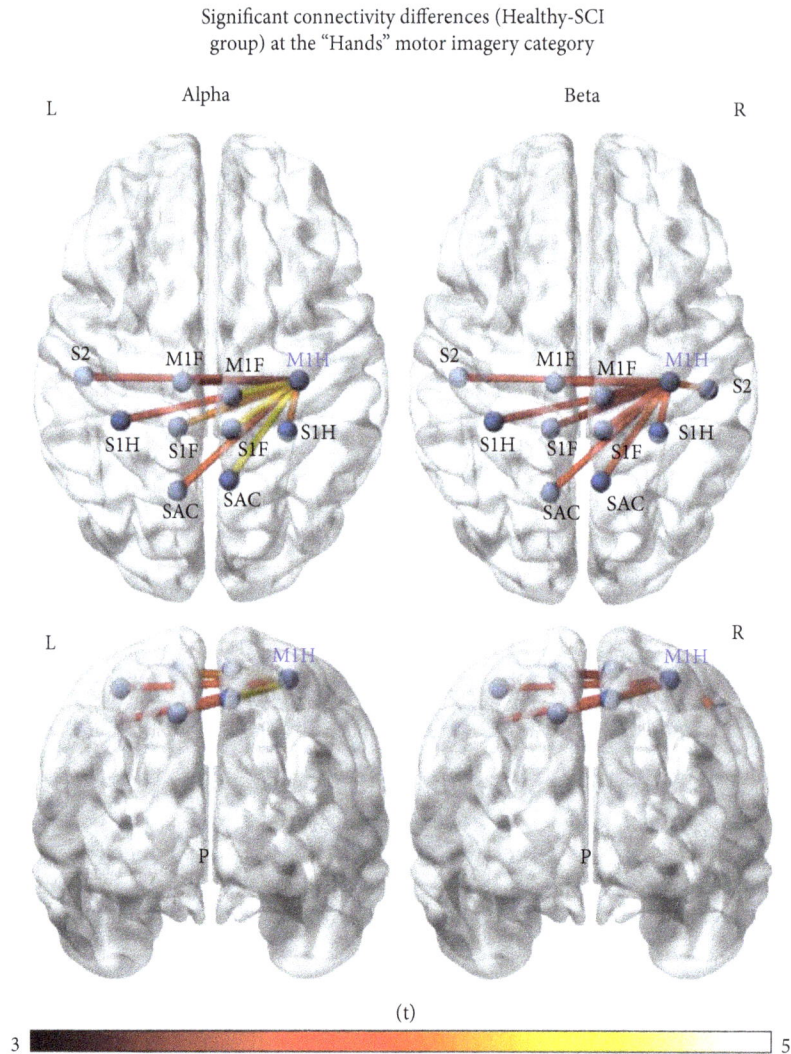

FIGURE 7: From the comparison of the networks of healthy and SCI subjects, a subset of network connections emerged as significantly stronger in the healthy group than in the SCI group for both the alpha and beta networks of "hands" motor imagery category, as calculated by network-based statistics—false discovery rate methodology.

0.0253, healthy: −0.1467). Other between-group differences were not observed (supplementary material).

4. Discussion

4.1. Functional Connectivity. A subset of the sensorimotor network during hands motor imagery was shown to have significantly lower functional connectivity power in the SCI group compared to the healthy group, a finding from analyses of the general linear model. This subset included connections of the M1H_R cortical area (theoretically the nondominant hand primary motor area for right-handed subjects) with other motor and sensory cortical areas. This subset also excluded the "assistive" motor nodes (CMA/SMA/pSMA/PMv/PMd). Interestingly, among these excluded nodes were also the ones that were shown to have consistently higher OS and IS, for all imagery categories, as we will discuss later on. The subset of connected nodes to M1H_R included bilateral primary foot motor areas (M1F),

primary foot and hand sensory areas (S1H, S1F), the somatosensory association areas (SAC) located in superior parietal cortex (SPC), and the secondary sensory areas (S2). Small differences between alpha and beta rhythm networks can be observed, whereas most of those connections' lower FC reached statistical significance for either rhythm. These cortical areas can be identified as the point of origin of the pyramidal tract and the point of conclusion of the major somatosensory tracts. This finding could suggest that chronic disruption of reciprocal communication between the brain and spinal cord, even in noncomplete injuries, could result in permanent significant decrease of connectivity between a subset of the functional sensorimotor network at the cortical level. This effect was observed regardless of positive or negative neurological outcome since grouping SCI subjects by outcome did not reveal any differences regarding this finding. While the lack of difference between those two clinically and functionally different subgroups of patients could be affected by a lack of statistical power when comparing small samples,

Network density (*D*) of "Hands" motor imagery category
all *p* values < 0.001

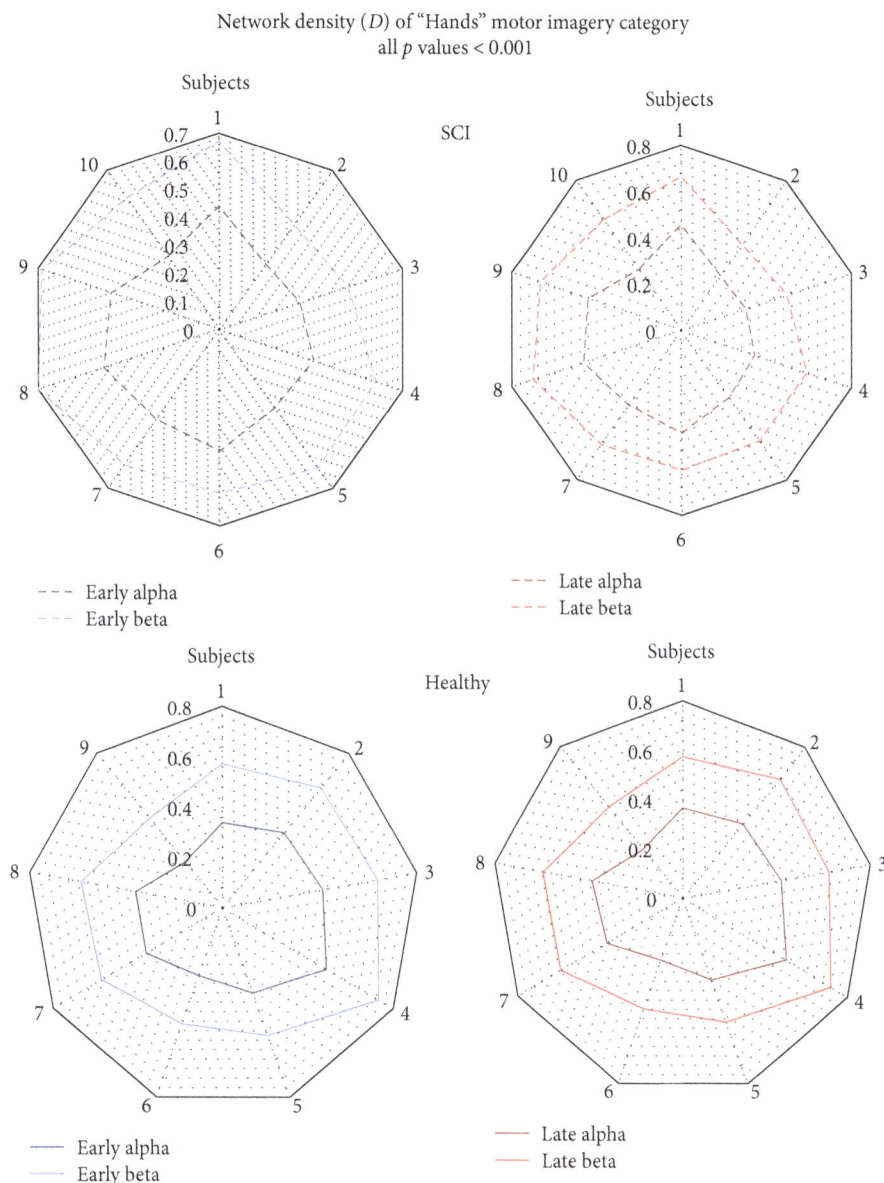

FIGURE 8: Network density was significantly higher in beta than alpha networks (all *p* values < 0.001) of the "hands" motor imagery category during both early and late time intervals for all subjects of both the SCI and the healthy group (all *p* values < 0.001). This finding was also consistent across every other motor imagery categories in both groups (all *p* values < 0.001).

a possible explanation could also be explored along the lines of mental imagery capacity. Motor execution and motor imagery do present differences in the level of neural networks that are affected by the subjects' quality and intensity of imagination [93]. In our study, the patients did not report differences in vividness of visual imagery to that of the healthy participants, as measured by the VVIQ questionnaire at the time of the experimental procedure. A degree of "though extinction process" has been reported in chronic paralysis [94], but since this is not the case in our investigation, it is possible that the lack of difference in the networks of patients with positive and negative outcomes could be due to the unaffected mental capacity of the participants.

Further significant differences between the healthy and patient groups were found with regard to nodal strengths. Almost all nodes had significantly different out-strength between the two groups. An interesting pattern can be identified. Primary motor areas, supplementary motor areas, left presupplementary motor area, and left cingulate motor area show significantly higher out-strength in the healthy group. On the contrary, premotor areas, right presupplementary motor area, and right cingulate motor area show significantly higher out-strength in the SCI group. Incoming connection strengths to primary somatosensory areas, premotor areas, supplementary motor areas, and right cingulate motor area are higher for healthy participants, while in-strength of left cingulate motor area is higher for SCI participants. Despite the differences in strengths of those nodes, similar patterns of connectivity were found for both groups [12, 13]. The significantly reduced nodal strengths could reflect the disconnection itself and the reduced input and output of the sensorimotor pathways in spinal cord injury. Nonetheless, the higher in-strengths of left cingulate motor area and out-strengths of premotor areas and right pSMA and CMA in SCI group could indicate an attempt of the sensorimotor network to compensate for the impaired function [10, 11, 95].

CMA areas have been previously identified as important information hubs for sensorimotor networks, especially those of beta rhythm [9, 11]. In our study, this attribute is confirmed, since bilateral CMA areas consistently received the greater inflow and contributed the greater outflow in terms of connection strengths for all categories of motor imagery. Moreover, their reciprocal communication constituted the most powerful connections of every examined network. On the other hand, an important role has been identified for the SMAs [11–13] that have been shown to present notable outflow during motor imagery tasks and form clusters with the CMAs. Their role was asserted in our work previously too [44, 96], but it is not so apparent in our current study, where the SMAs were not among the top contributors in either outflow or inflow. Although not easily explained, the meaning of this finding can be explored along possible factors: (a) the random-oddball (unexpected imagery task) paradigm of presentation, (b) the MVAR model order set, and (c) the definitions of the midline network nodes themselves. The degree that each factor possibly contributed to this finding is an issue for further investigation. An example of SMAs and primary motor areas not presenting the greatest strength during hands motor imagery has also been recently reported in a study [97] where the authors used transcranial direct current stimulation to affect the connectivity of a broader definition of sensorimotor ROIs.

With regard to differentiating different upper limb motor imagery tasks, our results did not produce significant differences in terms of spatial patterns specific to certain tasks. Moreover, network-based differences between healthy and patients, although significant for the all-inclusive upper limb imagery category, did not reach statistical significance for specific categories, suggesting possibly a lack of statistical power for these categorical differences. This is not unexpected, since connectivity features, in general, have so far shown only moderate success in classification of motor imagery tasks [98, 99]. It should be also noted that some effort has been made in analyzing effective networks of compound motor imagery tasks [100]. Differentiating anatomical levels and consecutive classification should perhaps be better explored along the lines of time-varying connectivity [95, 101–103] instead of spatial pattern analysis.

Walking motor imagery, while it also did not reveal specific connectivity patterns, produced the most promising results in terms of classification, in accordance to previous studies suggesting that maximally different conditions should be explored [98]. Walking motor imagery category was the only one where the negative correlation

between-group differences of the two cingulate motor area strengths reach statistical significance in half of the studied cases, those of early alpha rhythm walking networks ($p = 0.002$) and of late beta walking networks ($p = 0.006$). Moreover, the comparison of networks of healthy and patient subjects produced at least one significantly stronger connection, between the right ventral premotor area and the left secondary somatosensory area, although it is unclear whether this can be attributed to plasticity or merely to SCI-induced disconnection sequelae. To the best of the authors' knowledge, this is the first electroencephalographic study of functional cortical connectivity after incomplete spinal cord injury, and it is also the first functional cortical connectivity study examining multiple motor imagery tasks in those patients regardless of recording modality.

4.2. Analysis of Network Properties. Analysis of within-group effect of rhythm produced the most consistent results. According to the revealed pattern, alpha networks present lower integration (as measured by CPL), higher segregation (as measured by CC), while being less dense and more "effective" (as measured by SW) than beta networks. These findings are present across all motor imagery categories and they closely match findings from our previous study on the role of alpha and beta rhythms in sensorimotor networks [44, 104]. Our previous work suggested a pattern where alpha rhythm engaged local information processing using greater wiring costs [105], and that beta rhythm assumes a coordinative role during the sensorimotor process [106]. These findings were then observed on different ROI models and during simpler but far more repetitive motor imagery and motor execution tasks. They are also now replicated on a wider definition of the model of ROIs and during multiple, more complex, random motor imagery tasks. More importantly, these findings have now also been confirmed on networks of SCI patients with incomplete injury, allowing us to attempt to model the behavior of other between-group and within-group findings based on this pattern of alpha and beta organization.

Between the two groups, the fact that CPL and D were not significantly different, neither in alpha nor in beta networks, allows us to make direct comparisons of their sensorimotor network organization since they reach the same level of wiring costs and node integration. Moreover, the few between-group differences were observed mostly in alpha rhythm, which could be interpreted as differences only in local processing in the sensorimotor network of SCI patients. Increased functional segregation (CC in left, rotational and distal categories) and increased "effectiveness" of the network (SW in distal) were found for certain categories of motor imagery. More importantly, they were observed for *distal* arm imagery tasks, those that correspond to spinal cord levels below the level of injury, as the majority of the SCI subjects included in our study suffered from mid to low cervical SCI (C4–C8). As those differences were also observed during the late time interval, they can possibly be interpreted as an effect for delayed adaptation (compensation) of the sensorimotor network at the cortical level. This could possibly fall in line with reported increased network fault tolerance [10] and an increase of local efficiency and communication between closest cortical areas [15] during paralyzed foot motor imagery that has been reported in chronic complete SCI subjects.

Regarding the walking imagery category in our study, walking networks were the only where alpha and beta rhythm differences did not reach statistical significance in certain cases. Indeed, this previously reported increase of local efficiency and close communication in complete SCI appears to also be possible in incomplete injuries as well. The walking beta networks did not show less segregation and effectiveness than the walking alpha networks of incomplete SCI subjects during the early imagery part and also did not show less integration during the late imagery part, as was the case with the upper limb imagery categories. These findings suggest the presence of a phenomenon that has been attributed to adaptive plasticity and compensation when it regards patients with complete injuries [10, 15]. Within-group effect of time interval for upper limb motor imagery categories was far more sporadic, showing greater network segregation and less network integration of the alpha rhythm network in the patient group during the late imagery in some categories. What could interestingly fall into place with the rest of the interpretation is that healthy subjects display a drop of overall network effectiveness (as depicted by SW) in both alpha and beta networks during the late imagery part. In the SCI group, such a difference was not observed, an observation that could possibly be attributed to the same delayed compensatory effect induced by the injury. Since indeed the rest of the observed effects are not consistent, our reported findings cannot be obligatory attributed to neuroplasticity effects. Therefore, it is evident that more investigation in the direction of modeling the effect of spinal cord injury on the effective connectivity of the brain during different time points and injury severity conditions is needed before drawing accurate conclusions.

4.3. Limitations and Future Work. Among limitations of our study, one investigating functional connectivity should remain wary when the analysis reveals significant differences between the groups, as those differences are usually very small and not always clear if functionally or clinically meaningful. As such, it remains difficult to identify compelling advantages of graph theory-based analysis of brain activity over other approaches to provide additional important insight into the effects of SCI on brain activity. Functional connectivity at the source level also suffers from certain disadvantages including localization error, smoothing effect, and a degree of uncertainty of the connectivity between spatially close nodes [107]. There are several factors contributing to source localization errors, induced most importantly by the forward model but also by the inverse. The resolution of the source reconstruction is determined by the source space, with 4.69 mm of average source spacing and 22.04 mm^2 average surface area per source. Nonetheless, resolution of the source space is considered sufficient for the purpose of the study, and the same model has been previously used by similar studies [9–15]. The 3-layer block

element modifier forward model introduces errors through the use of a general template anatomy, modeling of skull conductivity as isotropic, not modeling cerebrospinal fluid and conductivity ratios. Moreover, it is known that EEG boasts great temporal but suffers from low spatial resolution and has been traditionally considered able to detect rapid brain dynamics in a trade-off with source estimation and low signal to noise ratio due to volume conduction effect [108, 109]. EEG in general greatly suffers from anisotropic conductivity of skull leading to signals blurring and to low EEG spatial resolution. In accordance, the localization error of deeper sources is considered greater than swallower ones. An interesting approach to address these problems would be the investigation of time-adaptive connectivity with a focus on temporal alterations of important connections rather than spatial [64], while using individual subject anatomy, an approach that we aim to explore in our future work.

5. Conclusions

We observed that chronic disruption of reciprocal communication between the brain and spinal cord, even in the context of incomplete injuries, could result in permanent significant decrease of connectivity between a subset of the functional sensorimotor network at the cortical level. This effect was observed regardless of positive or negative neurological outcome since grouping SCI subjects by outcome did not reveal any further difference. Cingulate motor areas were identified as important information hubs in different categories of motor imagery as they consistently showed the highest in-strengths (CMA_L) and out-strengths (CMA_R) in both groups of participants. While SCI subjects also followed the same pattern, they had higher outflow from left CMA and higher inflow to right CMA than healthy subjects. For both groups, alpha networks were less dense while having both longer average paths and more clustering than beta networks in almost all imagery categories. SCI patients showed signs of increased local processing in the late part of imagery, possibly an adaptive compensatory mechanism of injury-induced neuroplasticity.

Consent

All experiments were conducted with the subjects' understanding and written informed consent.

Conflicts of Interest

The authors declare that there is no conflict of interest regarding the publication of this article.

Acknowledgments

Early phases of the study were supported in part by a Mario Boni grant from the Cervical Spine Research Society-

European Section, awarded to CSI: Brainwave Project. This study was supported by 2018 "Brihaye" EANS Research Fund Grant from the European Association of Neurosurgical Societies. This work was supported by European Union's Horizon 2020 research and innovation programme under grant agreement No 681120 of the SmokeFreeBrain project (http://smokefreebrain.eu).

Supplementary Materials

Statistical analysis: methodology and results for CPL, CC. D, SW, and correlations. Figure 1: SCI group shows increase in mean global clustering coefficient compared to healthy group in late time interval of the alpha networks, during "left," "distal," and "rotational" motor imagery categories. Figure 2: SCI group shows increased small-worldness (SW) compared to healthy group in the late time interval of alpha networks for "distal" imagery category. Figure 3: between-group differences in CMA_L were negatively correlated to those in CMA_R in early alpha walking and late beta walking. Table 1: descriptive statistics of total nodal out-strengths and in-strengths of the networks of the SCI subjects. Table 2: descriptive statistics of total nodal out-strengths and in-strengths of the networks of the healthy subjects. *(Supplementary Materials)*

References

[1] K. D. Anderson, M. E. Acuff, B. G. Arp et al., "United States (US) multi-center study to assess the validity and reliability of the spinal cord independence measure (SCIM III)," *Spinal Cord*, vol. 49, no. 8, pp. 880–885, 2011.

[2] R. Nardone, Y. Höller, F. Brigo et al., "Descending motor pathways and cortical physiology after spinal cord injury assessed by transcranial magnetic stimulation: a systematic review," *Brain Research*, vol. 1619, pp. 139–154, 2015.

[3] A. Athanasiou, M. A. Klados, N. Pandria et al., "A systematic review of investigations into functional brain connectivity following spinal cord injury," *Frontiers in Human Neuroscience*, vol. 11, p. 517, 2017.

[4] R. Nardone, Y. Höller, F. Brigo et al., "Functional brain reorganization after spinal cord injury: systematic review of animal and human studies," *Brain Research*, vol. 1504, pp. 58–73, 2013.

[5] P. Freund, N. Weiskopf, J. Ashburner et al., "MRI investigation of the sensorimotor cortex and the corticospinal tract after acute spinal cord injury: a prospective longitudinal study," *The Lancet Neurology*, vol. 12, no. 9, pp. 873–881, 2013.

[6] J. Hou, Z. Xiang, R. Yan et al., "Motor recovery at 6 months after admission is related to structural and functional reorganization of the spine and brain in patients with spinal cord injury," *Human Brain Mapping*, vol. 37, no. 6, pp. 2195–2209, 2016.

[7] W. Zheng, Q. Chen, X. Chen et al., "Brain white matter impairment in patients with spinal cord injury," *Neural Plasticity*, vol. 2017, Article ID 4671607, 8 pages, 2017.

[8] T. Ilvesmäki, E. Koskinen, A. Brander, T. Luoto, J. Öhman, and H. Eskola, "Spinal cord injury induces widespread chronic changes in cerebral white matter," *Human Brain Mapping*, vol. 38, no. 7, pp. 3637–3647, 2017.

[9] L. Astolfi, H. Bakardjian, F. Cincotti et al., "Estimate of causality between independent cortical spatial patterns during movement volition in spinal cord injured patients," *Brain Topography*, vol. 19, no. 3, pp. 107–123, 2007.

[10] F. D. V. Fallani, L. Astolfi, F. Cincotti et al., "Cortical functional connectivity networks in normal and spinal cord injured patients: evaluation by graph analysis," *Human Brain Mapping*, vol. 28, no. 12, pp. 1334–1346, 2007.

[11] F. De Vico Fallani, L. Astolfi, F. Cincotti et al., "Extracting information from cortical connectivity patterns estimated from high resolution EEG recordings: a theoretical graph approach," *Brain Topography*, vol. 19, no. 3, pp. 125–136, 2007.

[12] D. Mattia, F. Cincotti, L. Astolfi et al., "Motor cortical responsiveness to attempted movements in tetraplegia: evidence from neuroelectrical imaging," *Clinical Neurophysiology*, vol. 120, no. 1, pp. 181–189, 2009.

[13] R. Sinatra, F. de Vico Fallani, L. Astolfi et al., "Cluster structure of functional networks estimated from high-resolution EEG data," *International Journal of Bifurcation and Chaos*, vol. 19, no. 2, pp. 665–676, 2009.

[14] L. Astolfi, F. Cincotti, D. Mattia et al., "Time-varying cortical connectivity estimation from noninvasive, high-resolution EEG recordings," *Journal of Psychophysiology*, vol. 24, no. 2, pp. 83–90, 2010.

[15] F. De Vico Fallani, F. A. Rodrigues, L. da Fontoura Costa et al., "Multiple pathways analysis of brain functional networks from EEG signals: an application to real data," *Brain Topography*, vol. 23, no. 4, pp. 344–354, 2011.

[16] J.-M. Hou, T.-S. Sun, Z.-M. Xiang et al., "Alterations of resting-state regional and network-level neural function after acute spinal cord injury," *Neuroscience*, vol. 277, pp. 446–454, 2014.

[17] Y.-S. Min, J. W. Park, S. U. Jin et al., "Alteration of resting-state brain sensorimotor connectivity following spinal cord injury: a resting-state functional magnetic resonance imaging study," *Journal of Neurotrauma*, vol. 32, no. 18, pp. 1422–1427, 2015.

[18] Y.-S. Min, Y. Chang, J. W. Park et al., "Change of brain functional connectivity in patients with spinal cord injury: graph theory based approach," *Annals of Rehabilitation Medicine*, vol. 39, no. 3, pp. 374–383, 2015.

[19] A. Oni-Orisan, M. Kaushal, W. Li et al., "Alterations in cortical sensorimotor connectivity following complete cervical spinal cord injury: a prospective resting-state fMRI study," *PLoS One*, vol. 11, no. 3, article e0150351, 2016.

[20] M. Kaushal, A. Oni-Orisan, G. Chen et al., "Evaluation of whole-brain resting-state functional connectivity in spinal cord injury: a large-scale network analysis using network-based statistic," *Journal of Neurotrauma*, vol. 34, no. 6, pp. 1278–1282, 2017.

[21] M. Kaushal, A. Oni-Orisan, G. Chen et al., "Large-scale network analysis of whole-brain resting-state functional connectivity in spinal cord injury: a comparative study," *Brain Connectivity*, vol. 7, no. 7, pp. 413–423, 2017.

[22] A. H. Hawasli, J. Rutlin, J. L. Roland et al., "Spinal cord injury disrupts resting-state networks in the human brain," *Journal of Neurotrauma*, vol. 35, no. 6, pp. 864–873, 2018.

[23] H. Luo, W. Dou, Y. Pan et al., "Joint analysis of multi-level functional brain networks," in *2016 9th International Congress on Image and Signal Processing, BioMedical Engineering and Informatics (CISP-BMEI)*, pp. 1521–1526, Datong, China, 2016.

[24] Y. Pan, W. Dou, Y. Wang et al., "Non-concomitant cortical structural and functional alterations in sensorimotor areas following incomplete spinal cord injury," *Neural Regeneration Research*, vol. 12, no. 12, pp. 2059–2066, 2017.

[25] S. Hétu, M. Grégoire, A. Saimpont et al., "The neural network of motor imagery: an ALE meta-analysis," *Neuroscience & Biobehavioral Reviews*, vol. 37, no. 5, pp. 930–949, 2013.

[26] M. Lotze and U. Halsband, "Motor imagery," *Journal of Physiology-Paris*, vol. 99, no. 4–6, pp. 386–395, 2006.

[27] S. Kraeutner, A. Gionfriddo, T. Bardouille, and S. Boe, "Motor imagery-based brain activity parallels that of motor execution: evidence from magnetic source imaging of cortical oscillations," *Brain Research*, vol. 1588, pp. 81–91, 2014.

[28] L. Xu, H. Zhang, M. Hui et al., "Motor execution and motor imagery: a comparison of functional connectivity patterns based on graph theory," *Neuroscience*, vol. 261, pp. 184–194, 2014.

[29] A. Guillot, C. Collet, V. A. Nguyen, F. Malouin, C. Richards, and J. Doyon, "Brain activity during visual versus kinesthetic imagery: an fMRI study," *Human Brain Mapping*, vol. 30, no. 7, pp. 2157–2172, 2009.

[30] N. Mizuguchi, M. Nakamura, and K. Kanosue, "Task-dependent engagements of the primary visual cortex during kinesthetic and visual motor imagery," *Neuroscience Letters*, vol. 636, pp. 108–112, 2017.

[31] J. Harris and A. Hebert, "Utilization of motor imagery in upper limb rehabilitation: a systematic scoping review," *Clinical Rehabilitation*, vol. 29, no. 11, pp. 1092–1107, 2015.

[32] L. Bunketorp Käll, R. J. Cooper, J. Wangdell, J. Fridén, and M. Björnsdotter, "Adaptive motor cortex plasticity following grip reconstruction in individuals with tetraplegia," *Restorative Neurology and Neuroscience*, vol. 36, no. 1, pp. 73–82, 2018.

[33] S. W. Tung, C. Guan, K. K. Ang et al., "Motor imagery BCI for upper limb stroke rehabilitation: an evaluation of the EEG recordings using coherence analysis," in *2013 35th Annual International Conference of the IEEE Engineering in Medicine and Biology Society (EMBC)*, pp. 261–264, Osaka, Japan, 2013.

[34] A. R. C. Donati, S. Shokur, E. Morya et al., "Long-term training with a brain-machine interface-based gait protocol induces partial neurological recovery in paraplegic patients," *Scientific Reports*, vol. 6, no. 1, article 30383, 2016.

[35] V. Rajasekaran, E. López-Larraz, F. Trincado-Alonso et al., "Volition-adaptive control for gait training using wearable exoskeleton: preliminary tests with incomplete spinal cord injury individuals," *Journal of NeuroEngineering and Rehabilitation*, vol. 15, no. 1, p. 4, 2018.

[36] A. Athanasiou, I. Xygonakis, N. Pandria et al., "Towards rehabilitation robotics: off-the-shelf BCI control of anthropomorphic robotic arms," *BioMed Research International*, vol. 2017, Article ID 5708937, 17 pages, 2017.

[37] G. Arfaras, A. Athanasiou, P. Niki et al., "Visual versus kinesthetic motor imagery for BCI control of robotic arms (Mercury 2.0)," in *2017 IEEE 30th International Symposium on Computer-Based Medical Systems (CBMS)*, pp. 440–445, Thessaloniki, Greece, 2017.

[38] A. Athanasiou, G. Arfaras, I. Xygonakis et al., "Commercial BCI control and functional brain networks in spinal cord injury: a proof-of-concept," in *2017 IEEE 30th International Symposium on Computer-Based Medical Systems (CBMS)*, pp. 262–267, Thessaloniki, Greece, 2017.

[39] A. Athanasiou, G. Arfaras, N. Pandria et al., "Wireless brain-robot interface: user perception and performance assessment of spinal cord injury patients," *Wireless Communications and Mobile Computing*, vol. 2017, Article ID 2986423, 16 pages, 2017.

[40] "Brainwave control of a wearable robotic arm for rehabilitation and neurophysiological study in cervical spine injury (CSI:Brainwave)," https://clinicaltrials.gov/ct2/show/NCT02443558.

[41] D. F. Marks, "New directions in mental imagery research," *Journal of Mental Imagery*, vol. 19, no. 3-4, pp. 153–167, 1995.

[42] R. Oostenveld and P. Praamstra, "The five percent electrode system for high-resolution EEG and ERP measurements," *Clinical Neurophysiology*, vol. 112, no. 4, pp. 713–719, 2001.

[43] O. Christ and M. Reiner, "Perspectives and possible applications of the rubber hand and virtual hand illusion in non-invasive rehabilitation: technological improvements and their consequences," *Neuroscience & Biobehavioral Reviews*, vol. 44, pp. 33–44, 2014.

[44] A. Athanasiou, M. A. Klados, C. Styliadis, N. Foroglou, K. Polyzoidis, and P. D. Bamidis, "Investigating the role of alpha and beta rhythms in functional motor networks," *Neuroscience*, 2016, In press.

[45] L. Qin, L. Ding, and B. He, "Motor imagery classification by means of source analysis for brain–computer interface applications," *Journal of Neural Engineering*, vol. 1, no. 3, pp. 135–141, 2004.

[46] B. Kamousi, A. N. Amini, and B. He, "Classification of motor imagery by means of cortical current density estimation and Von Neumann entropy," *Journal of Neural Engineering*, vol. 4, no. 2, pp. 17–25, 2007.

[47] B. Kamousi, Z. Liu, and B. He, "Classification of motor imagery tasks for brain-computer interface applications by means of two equivalent dipoles analysis," *IEEE Transactions on Neural Systems and Rehabilitation Engineering*, vol. 13, no. 2, pp. 166–171, 2005.

[48] B. J. Edelman, B. Baxter, and B. He, "EEG source imaging enhances the decoding of complex right-hand motor imagery tasks," *IEEE Transactions on Biomedical Engineering*, vol. 63, no. 1, pp. 4–14, 2016.

[49] R. Oostenveld, P. Fries, E. Maris, and J.-M. Schoffelen, "FieldTrip: open source software for advanced analysis of MEG, EEG, and invasive electrophysiological data," *Computational Intelligence and Neuroscience*, vol. 2011, Article ID 156869, 9 pages, 2011.

[50] A. Belouchrani and A. Cichocki, "Robust whitening procedure in blind source separation context," *Electronics Letters*, vol. 36, no. 24, p. 2050, 2000.

[51] F. Perrin, J. Pernier, O. Bertrand, and J. F. Echallier, "Spherical splines for scalp potential and current density mapping," *Electroencephalography and Clinical Neurophysiology*, vol. 72, no. 2, pp. 184–187, 1989.

[52] M. Hamedi, S.-H. Salleh, and A. M. Noor, "Electroencephalographic motor imagery brain connectivity analysis for BCI: a

review," *Neural Computation*, vol. 28, no. 6, pp. 999–1041, 2016.

[53] J. Ginter Jr., K. J. Blinowska, M. Kamiński, P. J. Durka, G. Pfurtscheller, and C. Neuper, "Propagation of EEG activity in the beta and gamma band during movement imagery in humans," *Methods of Information in Medicine*, vol. 44, no. 1, pp. 106–113, 2005.

[54] P. Avanzini, M. Fabbri-Destro, R. Dalla Volta, E. Daprati, G. Rizzolatti, and G. Cantalupo, "The dynamics of sensorimotor cortical oscillations during the observation of hand movements: an EEG study," *PLoS One*, vol. 7, no. 5, article e37534, 2012.

[55] K. Sakihara and M. Inagaki, "Mu rhythm desynchronization by tongue thrust observation," *Frontiers in Human Neuroscience*, vol. 9, p. 501, 2015.

[56] R. Grech, T. Cassar, J. Muscat et al., "Review on solving the inverse problem in EEG source analysis," *Journal of NeuroEngineering and Rehabilitation*, vol. 5, no. 1, p. 25, 2008.

[57] B. He, Y. Dai, L. Astolfi, F. Babiloni, H. Yuan, and L. Yang, "*eConnectome*: a MATLAB toolbox for mapping and imaging of brain functional connectivity," *Journal of Neuroscience Methods*, vol. 195, no. 2, pp. 261–269, 2011.

[58] F. Babiloni, F. Cincotti, C. Babiloni et al., "Estimation of the cortical functional connectivity with the multimodal integration of high-resolution EEG and fMRI data by directed transfer function," *NeuroImage*, vol. 24, no. 1, pp. 118–131, 2005.

[59] A. C. Evans, D. L. Collins, S. R. Mills, E. D. Brown, R. L. Kelly, and T. M. Peters, "3D statistical neuroanatomical models from 305 MRI volumes," in *1993 IEEE Conference Record Nuclear Science Symposium and Medical Imaging Conference*, pp. 1813–1817, San Francisco, CA, USA, 1993.

[60] G. Buzsáki, C. A. Anastassiou, and C. Koch, "The origin of extracellular fields and currents—EEG, ECoG, LFP and spikes," *Nature Reviews Neuroscience*, vol. 13, no. 6, pp. 407–420, 2012.

[61] H. Becker, L. Albera, P. Comon, R. Gribonval, F. Wendling, and I. Merlet, "Brain-source imaging: from sparse to tensor models," *IEEE Signal Processing Magazine*, vol. 32, no. 6, pp. 100–112, 2015.

[62] P. C. Hansen, T. K. Jensen, and G. Rodriguez, "An adaptive pruning algorithm for the discrete L-curve criterion," *Journal of Computational and Applied Mathematics*, vol. 198, no. 2, pp. 483–492, 2007.

[63] P. C. Hansen, "Regularization tools version 4.0 for Matlab 7.3," *Numerical Algorithms*, vol. 46, no. 2, pp. 189–194, 2007.

[64] C. Wilke, L. Ding, and B. He, "Estimation of time-varying connectivity patterns through the use of an adaptive directed transfer function," *IEEE Transactions on Biomedical Engineering*, vol. 55, no. 11, pp. 2557–2564, 2008.

[65] D. Kugiumtzis, "On the reliability of the surrogate data test for nonlinearity in the analysis of noisy time series," *International Journal of Bifurcation and Chaos*, vol. 11, no. 7, pp. 1881–1896, 2001.

[66] D. Kugiumtzis, "Surrogate data test on time series," in *Modelling and Forecasting Financial Data*, pp. 267–282, Springer, Boston, MA, USA, 2002.

[67] M. Kamiński, M. Ding, W. A. Truccolo, and S. L. Bressler, "Evaluating causal relations in neural systems: granger causality, directed transfer function and statistical assessment

of significance," *Biological Cybernetics*, vol. 85, no. 2, pp. 145–157, 2001.

[68] C. W. J. Granger, "Investigating causal relations by econometric models and cross-spectral methods," *Econometrica*, vol. 37, no. 3, p. 424, 1969.

[69] T. Schneider and A. Neumaier, "Algorithm 808: ARfit—a matlab package for the estimation of parameters and eigenmodes of multivariate autoregressive models," *ACM Transactions on Mathematical Software*, vol. 27, no. 1, pp. 58–65, 2001.

[70] A. Delorme, T. Mullen, C. Kothe et al., "EEGLAB, SIFT, NFT, BCILAB, and ERICA: new tools for advanced EEG processing," *Computational Intelligence and Neuroscience*, vol. 2011, Article ID 130714, 12 pages, 2011.

[71] B. H. Jansen, J. R. Bourne, and J. W. Ward, "Spectral decomposition of EEG intervals using Walsh and Fourier transforms," *IEEE Transactions on Biomedical Engineering*, vol. 28, no. 12, pp. 836–838, 1981.

[72] G. Florian and G. Pfurtscheller, "Dynamic spectral analysis of event-related EEG data," *Electroencephalography and Clinical Neurophysiology*, vol. 95, no. 5, pp. 393–396, 1995.

[73] M. Sabate, C. Llanos, E. Enriquez, B. Gonzalez, and M. Rodriguez, "Fast modulation of alpha activity during visual processing and motor control," *Neuroscience*, vol. 189, pp. 236–249, 2011.

[74] M. Rubinov and O. Sporns, "Complex network measures of brain connectivity: uses and interpretations," *NeuroImage*, vol. 52, no. 3, pp. 1059–1069, 2010.

[75] O. Sporns, "Graph theory methods for the analysis of neural connectivity patterns," in *Neuroscience Databases: a Practical Guide*, R. Kötter, Ed., pp. 171–185, Springer, Boston, MA, USA, 2003.

[76] O. Sporns and R. Kötter, "Motifs in brain networks," *PLoS Biology*, vol. 2, no. 11, article e369, 2004.

[77] R. W. Floyd, "Algorithm 97: shortest path," *Communications of the ACM*, vol. 5, no. 6, p. 345, 1962.

[78] J. Goni, M. P. van den Heuvel, A. Avena-Koenigsberger et al., "Resting-brain functional connectivity predicted by analytic measures of network communication," *Proceedings of the National Academy of Sciences*, vol. 111, no. 2, pp. 833–838, 2014.

[79] J.-P. Onnela, J. Saramäki, J. Kertész, and K. Kaski, "Intensity and coherence of motifs in weighted complex networks," *Physical Review E*, vol. 71, no. 6, article 065103, 2005.

[80] G. Fagiolo, "Clustering in complex directed networks," *Physical Review E*, vol. 76, no. 2, article 026107, 2007.

[81] D. J. Watts and S. H. Strogatz, "Collective dynamics of 'small-world' networks," *Nature*, vol. 393, no. 6684, pp. 440–442, 1998.

[82] S. Achard, R. Salvador, B. Whitcher, J. Suckling, and E. Bullmore, "A resilient, low-frequency, small-world human brain functional network with highly connected association cortical hubs," *The Journal of Neuroscience*, vol. 26, no. 1, pp. 63–72, 2006.

[83] M. D. Humphries and K. Gurney, "Network 'small-world-ness': a quantitative method for determining canonical network equivalence," *PLoS One*, vol. 3, no. 4, article e0002051, 2008.

[84] O. Sporns, C. J. Honey, and R. Kötter, "Identification and classification of hubs in brain networks," *PLoS One*, vol. 2, no. 10, article e1049, 2007.

[85] A. Zalesky, A. Fornito, and E. T. Bullmore, "Network-based statistic: identifying differences in brain networks," *Neuro-Image*, vol. 53, no. 4, pp. 1197–1207, 2010.

[86] Y. Benjamini and Y. Hochberg, "Controlling the false discovery rate: a practical and powerful approach to multiple testing," *Journal of the Royal Statistical Society: Series B (Methodological)*, vol. 57, no. 1, pp. 289–300, 1995.

[87] M. Xia, J. Wang, and Y. He, "BrainNet Viewer: a network visualization tool for human brain connectomics," *PLoS One*, vol. 8, no. 7, article e68910, 2013.

[88] D. Cramer, *Fundamental Statistics for Social Research: Step-By-Step Calculations and Computer Techniques Using SPSS for Windows*, Routledge, New York, NY, USA, 1998.

[89] D. Cramer and D. Howitt, *The SAGE Dictionary of Statistics*, SAGE Publications Ltd, London, UK, 2004.

[90] D. P. Doane and L. E. Seward, "Measuring skewness : a forgotten statistic?," *Journal of Statistics Education*, vol. 19, no. 2, 2011.

[91] N. M. Razali, Y. B. Wah, and M. Sciences, "Power comparisons of Shapiro-Wilk, Kolmogorov-Smirnov, Lilliefors and Anderson-Darling tests," *Journal of Statistical Modeling and Analytics*, vol. 2, no. 1, pp. 21–33, 2011.

[92] S. S. Shapiro and M. B. Wilk, "An analysis of variance test for normality (complete samples)," *Biometrika*, vol. 52, no. 3-4, pp. 591–611, 1965.

[93] N. Kordjazi, A. Koravand, and H. Sveistrup, "Enhancing the representational similarity between execution and imagination of movement using network-based brain computer interfacing," *bioRxiv*, 2017, In press.

[94] N. Birbaumer and P. Sauseng, "Brain–computer interface in neurorehabilitation," in *Brain-Computer Interfaces*, pp. 155–169, Springer, Berlin, Heidelberg, 2009.

[95] F. De Vico Fallani, V. Latora, L. Astolfi et al., "Persistent patterns of interconnection in time-varying cortical networks estimated from high-resolution EEG recordings in humans during a simple motor act," *Journal of Physics A: Mathematical and Theoretical*, vol. 41, no. 22, article 224014, 2008.

[96] A. Athanasiou, C. Lithari, K. Kalogianni, M. A. Klados, and P. D. Bamidis, "Source detection and functional connectivity of the sensorimotor cortex during actual and imaginary limb movement: a preliminary study on the implementation of econnectome in motor imagery protocols," *Advances in Human-Computer Interaction*, vol. 2012, Article ID 127627, 10 pages, 2012.

[97] B. S. Baxter, B. J. Edelman, A. Sohrabpour, and B. He, "Anodal transcranial direct current stimulation increases bilateral directed brain connectivity during motor-imagery based brain-computer interface control," *Frontiers in Neuroscience*, vol. 11, p. 691, 2017.

[98] M. Grosse-wentrup, "Understanding brain connectivity patterns during motor imagery for brain-computer interfacing," in *Advances in Neural Information Processing Systems 21 (NIPS 2008)*, D. Koller, D. Schuurmans, Y. Bengio, and L. Bottou, Eds., pp. 561–568, Curran Associates, Inc., Red Hook, NY, USA, 2009.

[99] Y. K. Kim, E. Park, A. Lee, C.-H. Im, and Y.-H. Kim, "Changes in network connectivity during motor imagery and execution," *PLoS One*, vol. 13, no. 1, article e0190715, 2018.

[100] W. Yi, S. Qiu, K. Wang et al., "Evaluation of EEG oscillatory patterns and cognitive process during simple and compound limb motor imagery," *PLoS One*, vol. 9, no. 12, article e114853, 2014.

[101] M. Hamedi, S.-H. Salleh, S. B. Samdin, and A. M. Noor, "Motor imagery brain functional connectivity analysis via coherence," in *2015 IEEE International Conference on Signal and Image Processing Applications (ICSIPA)*, pp. 269–273, Kuala Lumpur, Malaysia, 2015.

[102] S. B. Samdin, C.-M. Ting, S.-H. Salleh, M. Hamedi, and A. B. M. Noor, "Estimating dynamic cortical connectivity from motor imagery EEG using KALMAN smoother & EM algorithm," in *2014 IEEE Workshop on Statistical Signal Processing (SSP)*, pp. 181–184, Gold Coast, VIC, Australia, 2014.

[103] B. K. Kang, J. S. Kim, S. Ryun, and C. K. Chung, "Prediction of movement intention using connectivity within motor-related network: an electrocorticography study," *PLoS One*, vol. 13, no. 1, article e0191480, 2018.

[104] A. Athanasiou, N. Foroglou, K. Polyzoidis, and P. D. Bamidis, "Graph analysis of sensorimotor cortex functional networks – comparison of alpha vs beta rhythm in motor imagery and execution," in *SAN/NIHC 2014 Meeting*, pp. 64-65, Utrecht, Netherlands, 2014.

[105] R. B. Willemse, J. C. de Munck, J. P. A. Verbunt et al., "Topographical organization of mu and beta band activity associated with hand and foot movements in patients with perirolandic lesions," *The Open Neuroimaging Journal*, vol. 4, pp. 93–99, 2010.

[106] F. De Vico Fallani, F. Pichiorri, G. Morone et al., "Multiscale topological properties of functional brain networks during motor imagery after stroke," *NeuroImage*, vol. 83, pp. 438–449, 2013.

[107] A. M. Bastos and J.-M. Schoffelen, "A tutorial review of functional connectivity analysis methods and their interpretational pitfalls," *Frontiers in Systems Neuroscience*, vol. 9, p. 175, 2016.

[108] B. He, Ed., *Modeling and Imaging of Bioelectrical Activity*, Springer, Boston, MA, USA, 2005.

[109] P. L. Nunez and R. Srinivasan, *Electric Fields of the Brain: the Neurophysics of EEG*, Oxford University Press, New York, NY, USA, 2006.

Permissions

All chapters in this book were first published in NP, by Hindawi Publishing Corporation; hereby published with permission under the Creative Commons Attribution License or equivalent. Every chapter published in this book has been scrutinized by our experts. Their significance has been extensively debated. The topics covered herein carry significant findings which will fuel the growth of the discipline. They may even be implemented as practical applications or may be referred to as a beginning point for another development.

The contributors of this book come from diverse backgrounds, making this book a truly international effort. This book will bring forth new frontiers with its revolutionizing research information and detailed analysis of the nascent developments around the world.

We would like to thank all the contributing authors for lending their expertise to make the book truly unique. They have played a crucial role in the development of this book. Without their invaluable contributions this book wouldn't have been possible. They have made vital efforts to compile up to date information on the varied aspects of this subject to make this book a valuable addition to the collection of many professionals and students.

This book was conceptualized with the vision of imparting up-to-date information and advanced data in this field. To ensure the same, a matchless editorial board was set up. Every individual on the board went through rigorous rounds of assessment to prove their worth. After which they invested a large part of their time researching and compiling the most relevant data for our readers.

The editorial board has been involved in producing this book since its inception. They have spent rigorous hours researching and exploring the diverse topics which have resulted in the successful publishing of this book. They have passed on their knowledge of decades through this book. To expedite this challenging task, the publisher supported the team at every step. A small team of assistant editors was also appointed to further simplify the editing procedure and attain best results for the readers.

Apart from the editorial board, the designing team has also invested a significant amount of their time in understanding the subject and creating the most relevant covers. They scrutinized every image to scout for the most suitable representation of the subject and create an appropriate cover for the book.

The publishing team has been an ardent support to the editorial, designing and production team. Their endless efforts to recruit the best for this project, has resulted in the accomplishment of this book. They are a veteran in the field of academics and their pool of knowledge is as vast as their experience in printing. Their expertise and guidance has proved useful at every step. Their uncompromising quality standards have made this book an exceptional effort. Their encouragement from time to time has been an inspiration for everyone.

The publisher and the editorial board hope that this book will prove to be a valuable piece of knowledge for researchers, students, practitioners and scholars across the globe.

List of Contributors

Olga Borodovitsyna, Neal Joshi and Daniel Chandler
Department of Cell Biology and Neuroscience, Rowan University School of Osteopathic Medicine, Stratford, NJ 08084, USA

Yun Qin, Bo Sun, Hui He, Rui Peng, Tao Zhang, Jianfu Li, Cheng Luo and Dezhong Yao
The Clinical Hospital of Chengdu Brain Science Institute, MOE Key Lab for Neuroinformation, High-Field Magnetic Resonance Brain Imaging Key Laboratory of Sichuan Province, University of Electronic Science and Technology of China, Chengdu 610054, China

Yanan Li and Chengyan Sun
Sichuan Rehabilitation Hospital, Chengdu, China

Andrea Guerra
Neuromed Institute IRCCS, Pozzilli, Italy

Giulia Paparella and Donato Colella
Department of Human Neurosciences, Sapienza University of Rome, Rome, Italy

Matteo Bologna, Antonio Suppa and Alfredo Berardelli
Neuromed Institute IRCCS, Pozzilli, Italy
Department of Human Neurosciences, Sapienza University of Rome, Rome, Italy

Vincenzo Di Lazzaro
Unit of Neurology, Neurophysiology, Neurobiology, Department of Medicine, University Campus Bio-Medico, Rome, Italy

Peter Brown
Nuffield Department of Clinical Neurosciences, John Radcliffe Hospital, University of Oxford, Oxford, UK
Medical Research Council Brain Network Dynamics Unit, Department of Pharmacology, University of Oxford, Mansfield Road, Oxford, UK

Carla Sanjurjo-Soriano and Vasiliki Kalatzis
Inserm U1051, Institute for Neurosciences of Montpellier, Montpellier, France
University of Montpellier, Montpellier, France

Enrico Sangiovanni, Paola Brivio, Mario Dell'Agli and Francesca Calabrese
Department of Pharmacological and Biomolecular Sciences, Università degli Studi di Milano, Milan, Italy

Sook-Lei Liew, Kaori L. Ito, Panthea Heydari, Mona Sobhani, Hanna Damasio, Carolee J. Winstein and Lisa Aziz-Zadeh
University of Southern California, Los Angeles, CA, USA

Kathleen A. Garrison
Yale University, New Haven, CT, USA

Julie Werner
California State University, Dominguez Hills, Carson, CA, USA
Children's Hospital Los Angeles, Los Angeles, CA, USA

E. Traverse, F. Lebon and A. Martin
INSERM UMR1093-CAPS, UFR des Sciences du Sport, Université Bourgogne Franche-Comté, 21000 Dijon, France

Jong Whi Kim, Dae Young Yoo and Hyo Young Jung
Department of Anatomy and Cell Biology, College of Veterinary Medicine, Research Institute for Veterinary Science, Seoul National University, Seoul 08826, Republic of Korea

Sung Min Nam
Department of Anatomy and Cell Biology, College of Veterinary Medicine, Research Institute for Veterinary Science, Seoul National University, Seoul 08826, Republic of Korea
Department of Anatomy, College of Veterinary Medicine, Konkuk University, Seoul 05030, Republic of Korea

Il Yong Kim
KMPC (Korea Mouse Phenotyping Center), Seoul National University, Seoul 08826, Republic of Korea

In Koo Hwang, Je Kyung Seong and Yeo Sung Yoon
Department of Anatomy and Cell Biology, College of Veterinary Medicine, Research Institute for Veterinary Science, Seoul National University, Seoul 08826, Republic of Korea
KMPC (Korea Mouse Phenotyping Center), Seoul National University, Seoul 08826, Republic of Korea

Bei Li, Yang Guo, Guang Yang, Yanmei Feng and Shankai Yin
Department of Otolaryngology Head and Neck Surgery, Shanghai Jiao Tong University Affiliated Sixth People's Hospital, No. 600, Yishan Road, Xuhui District, Shanghai 200233, China

Giovanni Buccino
Department of Medical and Surgical Sciences, University of Magna Graecia, Catanzaro, Italy

Anna Molinaro, Elisa Fazzi and Jessica Galli
Unit of Child Neurology and Psychiatry, ASST Spedali Civili, Brescia, Italy
Department of Clinical and Experimental Sciences, University of Brescia, Brescia, Italy

Claudia Ambrosi and Roberto Gasparotti
Department of Diagnostic Imaging, Neuroradiology Unit, University of Brescia, Brescia, Italy

Daniele Arisi
Department of Paediatrics, Ospedale di Cremona, Cremona, Italy

Lorella Mascaro
Department of Diagnostic Imaging, Medical Physics Unit, ASST Spedali Civili, Brescia, Italy

Chiara Pinardi
Neuroscience Unit, Department of Medicine and Surgery, University of Parma, Parma, Italy

Andrea Rossi
Unit of Child Neurology and Psychiatry, ASST Spedali Civili, Brescia, Italy

Jingyuan Ren and Jing Luo
School of Psychology, Capital Normal University, Beijing, China

Jun Zhan
School of Psychology, Capital Normal University, Beijing, China
School of Marxism, Fujian Agriculture and Forestry University, Fuzhou, China

Pei Sun
Department of Psychology, Tsinghua University, Beijing, China

Jin Fan
Department of Psychology, The City University of New York, New York City, NY, USA

Chang Liu
School of Psychology, Nanjing Normal University, Nanjing, China

M. R. Pereira-Jorge and M. Sturzbecher
Department of Neuroscience and Behavior, University of São Paulo, Ribeirao Preto, SP, Brazil

K. C. Andrade, F. X. Palhano-Fontes and D. B. Araujo
Brain Institute/Onofre Lopes University Hospital, Federal University of Rio Grande do Norte (UFRN), Natal, RN, Brazil

P. R. B. Diniz
Department of Internal Medicine, Federal University of Pernambuco, Recife, PE, Brazil

A. C. Santos
Department of Neuroscience and Behavior, University of São Paulo, Ribeirao Preto, SP, Brazil
Department of Internal Medicine, University of São Paulo, Ribeirao Preto, SP, Brazil

Jamileth More and María Mercedes Casas
Biomedical Neuroscience Institute, Faculty of Medicine, Universidad de Chile, Santiago, Chile

Gina Sánchez
Pathophysiology Program, ICBM, Faculty of Medicine, Universidad de Chile, Santiago, Chile
Center for Exercise, Metabolism and Cancer, Faculty of Medicine, Universidad de Chile, Santiago, Chile

Cecilia Hidalgo
Biomedical Neuroscience Institute, Faculty of Medicine, Universidad de Chile, Santiago, Chile
Center for Exercise, Metabolism and Cancer, Faculty of Medicine, Universidad de Chile, Santiago, Chile
Department of Neurosciences and Physiology and Biophysics Program, ICBM, Faculty of Medicine, Universidad de Chile, Santiago, Chile

Paola Haeger
Department of Biomedical Sciences, Faculty of Medicine, Universidad Católica del Norte, Coquimbo, Chile

Maria Cristina Cenni and Alessandro Sale
Neuroscience Institute, CNR, Via G. Moruzzi 1, 56124 Pisa, Italy

Silvia Morea
Department of Neuroscience, Psychology, Drug Research and Child Health (NEUROFARBA), University of Florence, Florence, Italy

Simona Cintoli and Nicoletta Berardi
Neuroscience Institute, CNR, Via G. Moruzzi 1, 56124 Pisa, Italy
Department of Neuroscience, Psychology, Drug Research and Child Health (NEUROFARBA), University of Florence, Florence, Italy

Bruno Pinto
Department of Neuroscience, Psychology, Drug Research and Child Health (NEUROFARBA), University of Florence, Florence, Italy
Scuola Normale Superiore, Pisa, Italy

Lamberto Maffei
Neuroscience Institute, CNR, Via G. Moruzzi 1, 56124 Pisa, Italy
Scuola Normale Superiore, Pisa, Italy

Sonia Betti and Andrea Spoto
Dipartimento di Psicologia Generale, Università di Padova, Padova, Italy

Umberto Castiello
Dipartimento di Psicologia Generale, Università di Padova, Padova, Italy
Centro Beniamino Segre, Accademia Nazionale dei Lincei, Roma, Italy

Luisa Sartori
Dipartimento di Psicologia Generale, Università di Padova, Padova, Italy
Centro di Neuroscienze Cognitive, Università di Padova, Padova, Italy

Anna-Sophia Wahl
Brain Research Institute, University of Zurich, Winterthurerstr. 190, 8057 Zurich, Switzerland
Department of Health Sciences and Technology, ETH Zurich, Winterthurerstr. 190, 8057 Zurich, Switzerland
Central Institute of Mental Health, University of Heidelberg, J5, 68159 Mannheim, Germany

Nikos Terzopoulos, Niki Pandria, Ioannis Xygonakis and Panagiotis D. Bamidis
Biomedical Electronics Robotics & Devices (BERD) Group, Lab of Medical Physics, School of Medicine, Faculty of Health Sciences, Aristotle University of Thessaloniki (AUTH), 54124 Thessaloniki, Greece

Nicolas Foroglou and Konstantinos Polyzoidis
1st Department of Neurosurgery, "AHEPA" University General Hospital, Aristotle University of Thessaloniki (AUTH), 54636 Thessaloniki, Greece

Alkinoos Athanasiou
Biomedical Electronics Robotics & Devices (BERD) Group, Lab of Medical Physics, School of Medicine, Faculty of Health Sciences, Aristotle University of Thessaloniki (AUTH), 54124 Thessaloniki, Greece
1st Department of Neurosurgery, "AHEPA" University General Hospital, Aristotle University of Thessaloniki (AUTH), 54636 Thessaloniki, Greece

Index